THE CANADIAN GUIDE TO

CLINICAL
PREVENTIVE
HEALTH CARE

The Canadian Task Force on the Periodic Health Examination

The technical reports including a full reference for chapters 38, 44, 57, 63, 72 and 73 are sold by Canada Communication Group — Publishing, Ottawa, Canada, K1A 0S9.

Canadian Cataloguing in Publication Data

Canadian Task Force on the Periodic Health Examination

The Canadian Guide to Clinical Preventive Health Care

Issued also in French under title: *Guide canadien de médecine clinique préventive*
ISBN 0-660-15732-2
Cat. no. H21-117/1994E

1. Medecine, Preventive — Canada — Handbooks, manuals, etc.
2. Periodic health examination — Canada — Handbooks, manuals, etc.
3. Preventive health services — Canada — Handbooks, manuals, etc.
I. Canada, Health Canada.
II. Title.

RA449.C32 1994   614.44′0971   C94-980322-7

TELEPHONE/TÉLÉPHONE	PO Box/C.P. 8650
(613) 731-9331	Ottawa ON K1G 0G8
FAX/TÉLÉCOPIEUR	1867 Alta Vista
(613) 731-1779	Ottawa ON K1G 3Y6

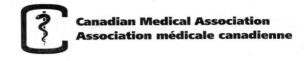

Canadian Medical Association
Association médicale canadienne

September 1994

Dear Reader:

On behalf of the Canadian Medical Association I welcome the publication of the *Canadian Guide to Clinical Preventive Health Care*. This book represents the synthesis of many years of effort by the Canadian Task Force on the Periodic Health Examination, a world pioneer in the field of preventive medicine. The Canadian Medical Association Journal has published the recommendations of the Task Force since 1979, a partnership of which the CMA is very proud.

The CMA strongly supports the development of materials to enhance the practice of preventive care by physicians and other clinicians. The importance of prevention in medical practice has already been articulated by the CMA, most recently in its 1994 policy paper "Strengthening the Foundation: the Role of the Physician in Primary Health Care in Canada". While it is not the role of the CMA to endorse the specific recommendations in the Task Force report, we recognize the excellent process that the Task Force has developed in reviewing emerging evidence, and feel that the *Canadian Guide* will be a valuable resource to the physician in practice.

We congratulate the Task Force and Health Canada on the publication of this book, and look forward to further productive association in the enhancement of prevention as a component of high-quality health care.

Yours truly,

Bruno J. L'Heureux, MD
President

Table of Contents

Prenatal and Perinatal Preventive Care

Pediatric Preventive Care

Metabolic/Nutritional Disorders

Circulatory Disorders

Other Infectious Diseases

Neoplasms

Conditions Affecting Primarily the Elderly

Appendices

Note: ‡ = Original review by U.S. Preventive Services Task Force
             † = Original review by another agency or association

Introduction

This book is designed to serve as a practical guide to clinicians, health professionals, professional associations and health care planners in determining the inclusion or exclusion, content and frequency of a wide variety of preventive health interventions.

The Canadian Task Force on the Periodic Health Examination was established in September, 1976 by the Conference of Deputy Ministers of Health of the ten Canadian provinces. Its stated mandate was "to determine how the periodic health examination might enhance or protect the health of Canadians and to recommend a plan for a lifetime program of periodic health assessments for all persons living in Canada".

The original Task Force was chaired by Dr. Walter O. Spitzer. Its membership included epidemiologists, health care researchers and clinicians, both primary caregivers and specialists.

The Task Force spent the first two years of its existence developing a methodology for weighing the scientific evidence for and against the effectiveness of an intervention in the prevention of a disease or disorder. The methodology that evolved from this process included a bi-directional system for grading the strength of any recommendation for or against the inclusion of a particular maneuver in the periodic health examination. The Task Force recognized then, as it does now, that in clinical practice, caregivers dealing with individual patients, must make binary decisions ("do it" or "don't do it"). It also recognizes, however, that for many preventive interventions, the scientific evidence does not lend itself to such simple two-dimensional alternatives. What may be an advisable preventive intervention for one individual or population group may be totally inappropriate for another. The particular characteristic that distinguishes the Task Force methodology from traditional approaches to decision-making on prevention issues is that evidence takes precedence over consensus. What at first seemed like an inordinate amount of time spent developing a rigorous evidence-based methodology turned out (with the wisdom of hindsight) to have been time very well spent. Several years later, the Canadian Task Force methodology was adopted with minimal modification by the U.S. Preventive Services Task Force. It has now been applied successfully by the two task forces to evaluate the preventability of over 200 conditions adversely affecting health, and has achieved international recognition as a basis for developing guidelines for clinical practice and public health policy.

Specific criteria have guided the selection of particular conditions for assessment by the Task Force. These have included the current burden of suffering (prevalence, morbidity and mortality) and the effectiveness and acceptability of the preventive maneuver.

The first Task Force report, published in 1979, reviewed the scientific evidence for preventability of 78 conditions and arrived at an important central recommendation, namely that the undefined "annual check-up" should be abandoned. In its stead, the Task Force recommended a series of age-specific "health protection packages" that could be implemented in the course of medical visits for other purposes.

Since 1979, the Canadian Task Force has published 9 updates, evaluating the preventability of 19 conditions not considered previously and revising 28 earlier reports in the light of new evidence. For many years the Canadian Task Force and its American counterpart, the U.S. Preventive Services Task Force have worked together in a close, constructive collaboration. The strength of this association has grown with the passing years. Each group has built on the virtues of the other, often adopting reviews and recommendations of the other body with little or no change when both were essentially in agreement, as was usually the case. Most meetings of either Task Force have been attended by representatives of the other. Further tangible evidence of the strength of this binational collaboration was the publication of the book, "Preventing Disease: Beyond the Rhetoric" (Springer-Verlag, New York, 1990), containing extensive scientific reviews on the preventability of over 40 conditions and detailed discussions of issues such as scientific admissibility of evidence, technology assessment, integration of preventive services in primary care and the role of counselling in prevention. Most contributors were members of the Canadian or U.S. Task Force, and some chapters were co-authored by members of the two bodies. The book was edited jointly by the Chairpersons of the Canadian and U.S. Task Forces.

The Canadian Guide to Clinical Preventive Health Care has also benefitted from the strength of the Canadian-U.S. collaboration. Both task forces have updated their analyses of the scientific evidence and recommendations concerning most conditions reviewed previously and have added reviews of additional conditions. Again, each group has borrowed freely from the work of the other to avoid unnecessary duplication of effort. Through a similar process, the U.S. Task Force is currently updating its 1989 Guide to Clinical Preventive Services.

Readers will be struck by the remarkably small number of conditions for which high quality (Type I) scientific evidence for effective prevention is available, and for which it can be stated that "there is *good* evidence that the condition be included in the context of the periodic health examinations" (an A Recommendation).

By the same token, clinicians may be frustrated by the large number of C Recommendations ("poor or insufficient evidence to exclude or include") – leaving the decision to be made on other grounds. In some instances, we have indicated the type of other considerations that may help decide whether a particular preventive maneuver should be performed. But the Task Force methodology by its very nature, does not permit us to go beyond what is supported by solid scientific evidence.

What some may consider an unduly conservative position on C Recommendations should, however, carry significant benefits for the future of preventive health care. Every equivocal recommendation automatically generates an agenda for future research, designed to establish or refute a positive benefit : harm ratio of a particular preventive intervention. Also, a C Recommendation can serve as a caution to those who have to decide which preventive measures justify public funding.

The largest number of A Recommendations apply to preventive maneuvers performed at the beginning of the life cycle, such as newborn screening for inherited metabolic disorders and congenital hypothyroidism and childhood immunizations. Generally speaking, the later in life a preventive maneuver is applied, the less dramatic its benefits are likely to be. Finally, many preventive interventions that have the potential to improve the health of the nation's citizens undoubtedly lie outside the context of the clinician-patient encounter – the prevention of poverty, of violence and of pollution are striking examples.

Although cost-effectiveness analysis has not been a major focus of Task Force evaluations, the issue is inescapable in an era of acute concern over the need to control health care expenditures. Sooner or later, everyone involved in health care will have to face difficult choices between unrelated interventions. The mere demonstration that a particular intervention may offer *some* excess of benefit over harm may be insufficient justification for population-wide implementation, especially if the costs are high and the benefits modest. Unlike several preventive maneuvers applied in the early years of life, many preventive interventions aimed at adults represent add-on costs to the health care budget rather than the savings that some would have us believe. This is not to suggest that monetary costs should be the principal or the sole criterion for adoption or rejection of an effective preventive measure. Nevertheless, these are inescapable and serious considerations. When preventive maneuvers are costly, especially if applied widely, we will have to ask how great is the margin of good over harm?

We also underline the need for honest comprehensiveness in accounting for *all* varieties of benefit and harm associated with any preventive maneuver. Benefits may include improved quality or length of life, anxiety relieved or money saved. Possible adverse effects that must be taken into account include cost, "labelling" associated with false positive tests and the attendant anxiety generated, and, for some interventions the added anxiety induced by earlier diagnosis when such diagnosis does not lead to a better outcome. These issues are especially important when screening to identify conditions in the pre-symptomatic stage.

The mathematical terms used to express benefit or harm must not be misleading. A 30% reduction in mortality may sound very worthwhile, but in fact may be neither statistically nor clinically significant if the incidence and/or mortality of the condition is low to begin with. Caregivers, planners and the public must be told the odds in terms that are not misleading so that sensible, rational decisions can be made both for individuals and for society.

Task Force members have repeatedly had to confront the question of whether early detection of disease leads to a better outcome or merely advances the onset of anxiety and prolongs its duration for the patient and family. Examples abound: Is earlier diagnosis of Alzheimer's disease a provable benefit? Does detection of diabetes in the pre-symptomatic phase improve health prospects for the patient? Where various cancers are concerned, is it plausible (as we naturally *wish* to believe) that early detection regularly improves the probability of a successful response to treatment. It has been said, for instance, that more men die *with* prostate cancer than die *of* it. At this time of writing, we are still unsure whether the new and more sensitive detection methods for prostate cancer will lead to more good than harm. The history of preventive health care is replete with examples of interventions whose proponents failed to look before they leaped. These instances are important items on our agendas for future research.

In weighing the balance of good versus harm for any preventive intervention we must also look beyond the impact of the intervention on the target condition alone. The issue of preventing coronary artery disease is a case in point. Lowering of serum cholesterol may reduce the incidence and mortality of coronary heart disease. But if, as some studies have suggested, the intervention fails to reduce mortality from all causes, can it be recommended unhesitatingly as the road to better health. Every one of us must grow old, wither and die. We may be edging toward a time when society may have to choose the diseases from which they prefer to die. Prevention is not without its ethical dilemmas. Like it or not, choices may have to be made, on both monetary and ethical grounds, between preventive interventions for unrelated conditions. It is more than hypothetical to suggest that Canadians and others might soon have to decide whether they prefer to put their limited resources into smoking cessation or extensive mammography programs; into universal immunization against various infections or education programs on AIDS prevention or prevention of child maltreatment. Such comparisons and decisions can be counted on to generate a good deal of emotion. But if the comprehensive benefits and disadvantages of every program are weighed in the balance, the priorities should become much clearer and the decisions more acceptable. This is where the evidence-based approach of the Canadian and U.S. Task Forces serves society best. By giving scientific evidence precedence over consensus, reason supersedes emotion when wise decisions have to be made.

Richard B. Goldbloom, O.C., M.D., F.R.C.P.C.,
Editor and Chairman, The Canadian Task Force
on the Periodic Health Examination

Canadian Task Force on the Periodic Health Examination Membership

Richard B. Goldbloom, O.C., M.D.,
  F.R.C.P.C., *Chairman*
Professor, Department of Pediatrics
Dalhousie University
Halifax, N.S.

Renaldo N. Battista, M.D., Sc.D.,
  F.R.C.P.C., *Vice-Chairman*
Director
Division of Clinical Epidemiology
Montreal General Hospital
McGill University
Montreal, Quebec

Geoffrey Anderson, M.D., Ph.D.
Senior Scientist
Institute for Clinical Evaluative Sciences
Associate Professor
Department of Health Administration,
University of Toronto
Toronto, Ontario

Marie-Dominique Beaulieu, M.D.,
  F.C.F.P., M.Sc.
Associate Professor
Department of Family Medicine
University of Montreal
Montreal, Quebec

R. Wayne Elford, M.D., C.C.F.P., F.C.F.P.
Professor, Director of Research and
  Faculty Development
Department of Family Medicine
University of Calgary
Calgary, Alberta

John W. Feightner, M.D., M.Sc., F.C.F.P.
Professor
Department of Family Medicine
McMaster University
Hamilton, Ontario

William Feldman, M.D., F.R.C.P.C.
Professor of Pediatrics and of Preventive
  Medicine and Biostatistics
University of Toronto
Toronto, Ontario

Alexander G. Logan, M.D., F.R.C.P.C.
Professor of Medicine
Department of Medicine
University of Toronto
Toronto, Ontario

Brenda J. Morrison, Ph.D.
Professor
Department of Health Care and
  Epidemiology
University of British Columbia
Vancouver, B.C.

David R. (Dan) Offord, M.D., F.R.C.P.C.
Professor
Department of Psychiatry
McMaster University
Hamilton, Ontario

Christopher Patterson, M.D., F.R.C.P.C.
Professor and Head
Division of Geriatric Medicine
Department of Medicine
McMaster University
Hamilton, Ontario

Walter O. Spitzer, M.D., M.P.H.
Professor
Department of Epidemiology and
  Biostatistics
McGill University
Montreal, Quebec

Elaine E. L. Wang, M.D., C.M., F.R.C.P.C.
Associate Professor
Department of Pediatrics and of
  Preventive Medicine and Biostatistics
Faculty of Medicine
University of Toronto
Toronto, Ontario

Liaison to Health Canada

Wm. Phillip Mickelson, M.D., M.A.
Medical Consultant, Health Standards
Preventive Health Services Division
Health Programs and Services Branch
Health Canada
Ottawa, Ontario

Task Force Staff

Jennifer L. Dingle, M.B.A.
Coordinator

Patricia Randel, M.Sc.
Research Associate

Acknowledgements

Funding for the Canadian Task Force on the Periodic Health Examination has been provided by the Health Programs and Services Branch (HPSB), Health Canada.[1] In HPSB, the Preventive Health Services Division, Health Services Directorate, and the National Health Research and Development Program (Research grants 6605-2702-57X and 6603-1375-57X) have been primarily responsible for supporting the work of the Task Force. Additional funding for specific chapters has been provided by the Mental Health Division, Health Services Directorate, under the Government of Canada's Brighter Futures, and Family Violence, Initiatives, and by the Family and Child Health Unit, Health Promotion Directorate, under the Brighter Futures Initiative. We thank the Izaak Walton Killam Children's Hospital, Halifax, Nova Scotia, for generously providing office space.

Dr. Wm. Phillip Mickelson of Health Canada has served with great dedication as liaison between the Task Force and Health Canada since 1986. The Task Force also acknowledges with deep gratitude the contributions of its research staff Jennifer Dingle, Patricia Randel, and Heather Davis, and of former research associate Brenda Beagan. The Task Force also thanks Lise Talbot-Bélair and her associates at Translation Services, Public Works and Government Services Canada for their adept handling of the French translation of the Guide.

Finally, the Task Force would like to thank members and staff of the U.S. Preventive Services Task Force for their interest, support and collaboration.

---

[1] Formerly Health and Welfare Canada (until June 1993)

Preventive Guidelines: Their Role in Clinical Prevention and Health Promotion

Prepared by Sylvie Stachenko, MD, MSc, FCFP[1]

Over the past fifteen years, the Canadian Task Force on the Periodic Health Examination has had a seminal impact on the practice of clinical preventive medicine in Canada and around the world. The Task Force has provided health professionals and health care planners with leadership and guidance on the value of preventive interventions in the practice setting.

A key finding of the Task Force was that a periodic health examination (PHE) targeted at preventing, detecting, and controlling specific conditions or risk factors for different age-, sex- and high-risk groups was likely to be more effective than a routine annual physical examination.[1] As a result of the work of the Task Force, health practitioners now have access to a comprehensive package of preventive interventions for use over the life-cycle of individuals.

This guide may be regarded as an atlas of preventive interventions. It also contributes to the systematic evaluation of preventive medicine by analyzing a number of issues including the quality of scientific data on prevention, and the efficacy, effectiveness and efficiency of preventive procedures. The rigorous scientific evaluation upon which the Task Force recommendations are based has enhanced the credibility of preventive medicine.[2]

Clinical Prevention and Health Promotion

In Canada, the leading causes of death among adults younger than 65 years of age – cardiovascular disease, some common types of cancer, and unintentional injuries – are largely preventable.[3] A number of primary and secondary preventive interventions in the clinical setting have been shown to reduce morbidity and mortality. The integration of prevention into clinical practice is recognized as an efficient, or cost effective way of providing comprehensive care and meeting current health care concerns.

In its broadest sense, clinical prevention can be defined as a clinician/patient interaction that promotes health and prevents illness or injuries. Clinical prevention includes an array of procedures ranging from counselling, screening, and immunization to chemoprophylaxis in asymptomatic individuals.

---

[1] Director, Preventive Health Services, Health Canada, Ottawa, Ontario

The Periodic Health Examination incorporates primary and secondary preventive measures. Primary prevention addresses factors that lead to the onset of a disease (e.g., cigarette smoking). Secondary prevention aims at detecting latent conditions and either reducing or halting their progression (e.g., detecting and treating hypertension).

Primary prevention poses a challenge for the busy physician. This type of intervention requires an efficient and personalized patient education effort.[4] Persuading patients to quit smoking and to achieve and maintain a healthy weight requires more than merely providing information. To encourage behaviour change, the physician must assume the role of change agent.[5] It is clear that to help patients with lifestyle change, clinicians will need to expand their skills in counselling and communication. The patient must also become actively involved in his or her own health.[6]

A number of the preventive procedures recommended by the Canadian Task Force focus on counselling for behaviour-related risk factors. Clinicians' efforts to counsel patients in areas such as dietary habits, alcohol consumption, physical activity, and tobacco use may have a significant impact on cardiovascular disease and other chronic diseases.

Two out of three Canadians have one or more of the major risk factors for cardiovascular disease.[7] An appreciable proportion of Canadian adults have concomitant risk factors.[8] The clustering of risk factors is clinically significant because of their synergistic effect on risk. This suggests the need for health professionals to assess overall risk rather than focussing on single risk factors.

Clearly, there is no single strategy for improving the delivery of preventive services; multiple approaches are necessary.[9] Strategies directed towards health professionals are complemented by patient-centred approaches. Effective counselling requires an appreciation of the full spectrum of the public's perceptions, their health concerns and the factors influencing their lifestyles. Data from the two national health promotion surveys (1985, 1990) have contributed to our understanding of how people view health and how they respond to the prevention message.[10,11] These survey findings indicate that behaviour change is mainly influenced by knowledge of the risk factors, role models, support from family and friends, and advice from health professionals.

In recent years, the public's tremendous interest in health promotion and disease prevention has helped highlight the role of prevention in clinical settings. The benefit of incorporating prevention into clinical practice has become more apparent with the decline in the incidence of a number of diseases. Age-adjusted mortality from stroke has decreased by 50% in the last 20 years,[12] a trend that may be attributed, in part, to the early detection and treatment of hypertension. Cervical cancer mortality has also fallen by 50% since Papanicolau testing of women has become widespread.<13>

In Canada, the primary care setting offers an excellent opportunity for implementing prevention. Over 50 percent of physicians are either general practitioners or family physicians. They can play a pivotal role in prevention. Physicians are also perceived by the general public as a reliable and credible source of health information. They have the opportunity to take advantage of the "teachable" moment when patients are concerned about their health. They have contact with a large percentage of the population each year. It is estimated that 80 percent of Canadian adults see a physician at least once a year.<14> Among those who see a doctor, the average number of visits per year is about four.<14>

A number of studies have shown that the provision of preventive services by physicians is far from optimal.<15,16> This has been attributed to a variety of factors including time constraints, practice organization issues, patient non-compliance, a lack of counselling skills, and gaps in knowledge about which interventions to provide. Contradictory recommendations and a lack of consensus contribute to clinicians' confusion and skepticism concerning the value of prevention.

Implementation of preventive activities in clinical practice continues to be a challenge. To address this issue, Health Canada established a National Coalition of Health Professional Organizations in 1989. The purpose was to develop a strategy to enhance the preventive practices of health professionals. Two national workshops were held. The first focused on strengthening the provision of preventive services by Canadian physicians. The second addressed the need for collaboration among all health professionals. This process led to the development of a framework or "blueprint for action" for strengthening the delivery of preventive services in Canada.<17> It is a milestone for professional associations and one that will have a major impact on the development of preventive policies in this country.

In practice, preventive interventions of health professionals do not take place in a vacuum. Clinical prevention must be seen in the broader context of public health and healthy public policy. Preventive interventions occur in combination with health promotion efforts implemented through a variety of channels including the media, the workplace, and schools. A comprehensive approach to prevention involves the coordination of these individual efforts with those of the community. The one-to-one doctor/patient relationship serves to reinforce large-scale public education and community wide health promotion efforts. It is well recognized that it is the interplay among multiple reinforcing approaches and the collaboration of numerous partners in both the public and private sectors that ultimately lead to a change in individuals' behaviour.

Practice Guidelines and Quality of Care

Practice guidelines have been defined as "systematically developed statements to assist practitioner and patient decisions about appropriate health care for specific clinical circumstances."[18] They are becoming an integral part of the clinical decision-making process. There is growing interest in using guidelines as a means of reducing inappropriate care, assessing geographic variations in practice patterns, and using health care resources more effectively. With the current attention being given to quality of care, practice guidelines should play an increasingly prominent role in medical care policy.

Over the years, professional, scientific, and voluntary organizations, as well as government health agencies and licensing authorities, have attempted to resolve clinical uncertainty by issuing guidelines on effective interventions. In Canada, forty organizations are involved in developing practice guidelines.[19] The guidelines issued by the Canadian Task Force on the Periodic Health Examination are the most comprehensive recommendations available on preventive care.

The process developed by the Task Force to evaluate effectiveness may be as important a contribution to clinical policy making as the recommendations themselves. The techniques developed and used by the Task Force to review evidence and develop recommendations are applicable far beyond the sphere of prevention. They are particularly relevant at this time when increasing attention is being paid to evaluating the effectiveness of clinical diagnostic and therapeutic interventions.

In 1991 the Canadian Medical Association spearheaded the creation of a National Partnership for Quality in Health to coordinate the development and implementation of practice guidelines in Canada.[20] This partnership includes the following: the Association of Canadian Medical Colleges, the College of Family Physicians of Canada, the Federation of Medical Licensing Authorities of Canada, the Royal College of Physicians and Surgeons of Canada, the Canadian Council on Health Facilities Accreditation, and the Canadian Medical Association.

The existence of guidelines is no guarantee they will be used. The dissemination and diffusion of guidelines is a critical task and requires innovative approaches and concerted effort on the part of professional associations and health care professionals. Continuing education is one avenue for the dissemination of guidelines. Local physician leaders, educational outreach programs, and computerized reminder systems may complement more traditional methods such as lectures and written materials.

Public education programs should also support the process of guideline dissemination. In this context, rapidly expanding information technology, such as interactive video or computerized information systems with telephone voice output, presents opportunities for innovative patient education. The media may also be allies in the communication of some relevant aspects of guidelines to the public. All of these technologies should be evaluated.

The implementation of multiple strategies for promoting the use of practice guidelines requires marshalling the efforts of governments, administrators, and health professionals at national, provincial and local levels. It is up to physicians and other health professionals to adopt approaches for the implementation of guidelines in clinical practice and to support research efforts in this direction.

The compilation of preventive guidelines in this book is a significant step toward making health promotion and disease prevention a reality.

Selected References

1. Canadian Task Force on the Periodic Health Examination: The periodic health examination. *Can Med Assoc J* 1979; 121: 1193-1254

2. Woolf SH, Battista RN, Anderson GM, *et al*: Assessing the clinical effectiveness of preventive maneuvers: analytic principles and systematic methods in reviewing evidence and developing clinical practice recommendations. *J Clin Epidemiol* 1990; 43(9): 891-905

3. Working Group on Policy Development: *Positioning CINDI to Meet the Challenges: A WHO Policy Framework for Noncommunicable Disease Prevention.* December 1992

4. American College of Physicians, Medical Practice Committee: Periodic health examination: a guide for designing individualized preventive health care in the asymptomatic patient. *Ann Intern Med* 1981; 95: 729-732

5. Kamerow DB, Woolf SH, Mickalide AD: *Preventive Medicine.* AAFP Home Study Self Assessment, 1989

6. Charles C and Demaio S: *Lay Participation in Health Care Decision Making: A Conceptual Framework.* McMaster University Centre for Health Economics and Policy Analysis. Working Paper # 92-16, June 1992

7. MacDonald S, Joffres MR, Stachenko SJ, *et al*: Multiple cardiovascular disease risk factors in Canadian adults. *Can Med Assoc J* 1992; 146: 2021-2029

8. Stachenko SJ, Reeder BA, Lindsay E, *et al*: Smoking prevalence and associated risk factors in Canadian adults. *Can Med Assoc J* 1992; 146: 1989-1996

9. Lomas J: *Teaching Old (and not so old) Docs New Tricks: Effective Ways to Implement Research Findings.* McMaster University Centre for Health Economics and Policy Analysis. Working Paper 93-4, April 1993

10. Department of National Health and Welfare, Rootman I, Warren R, Stephens T, Peters L (ed): *Canada's Health Promotion Survey 1985: Technical Report*. Minister of Supply and Services, Ottawa, 1988 [Cat no. H39-119/1988]

11. Department of National Health and Welfare, Stephens T, Graham DF (ed): *Canada's Health Promotion Survey 1990: Technical Report*. Minister of Supply and Services, Ottawa, 1993 [Cat no. H39-263/2-1990]

12. Heart and Stroke Foundation of Canada: *Cardiovascular Disease In Canada*. Heart and Stroke Foundation of Canada. February 1993

13. National Cancer Institute of Canada: *Canadian Cancer Statistics 1993*. Toronto, 1993

14. Statistics Canada: *1991 General Social Survey on Health*.

15. Battista RN, Tannenbaum TN, Rosenberg E, *et al*: *Survey of physician practices regarding early detection and treatment of hyperlipidemia*. Research report submitted to Merck Frosst Canada. Personal communication from Battista RN, Division of Clinical Epidemiology of the Montreal General Hospital, 1989

16. Reeder BA, Horlick L, Laxdal A: *A Saskatchewan Survey of Current Management of Hyperlipidemia*. Personal Communication from Reeder B, University of Saskatchewan, Saskatoon, 1989

17. Stachenko S (ed): *Enhancing Prevention in the Practice of Health Professionals: Strategies for Today and Tomorrow*. Health and Welfare Canada, Ottawa, 1992

18. National Academy of Sciences, Institute of Medicine: Clinical Practice Guidelines: Directions for a New Program. Natl Acad Pr, Washington, 1990

19. Supply and Services Canada: *An Inventory of Quality Initiatives in Canada: Towards a Quality and Effectiveness*. Health and Welfare Canada, Ottawa, 1993 [Cat no. H39-274/1993E]

20. Quality of Care Program: *Proceedings of the Workshop on Clinical Practice Guidelines*. Ottawa, Ontario, November 15-17, 1992

Methodology

Adapted from the report of the Canadian Task Force on the Periodic Health Examination (Principal authors: Steven H. Woolf, MD, MPH[1]; Renaldo N. Battista, MD, ScD, FRCPC[2]; Geoffrey M. Anderson, MD, PhD[3]; Alexander G. Logan, MD, FRCPC[4]; and Elaine E.L. Wang, MD, MSc, CM, FRCPC[5])[1]
by Jennifer L. Dingle, MBA[6]

The Canadian Task Force on the Periodic Health Examination uses a standardized methodology for evaluating the effectiveness of preventive health care interventions and for developing clinical practice guidelines based on the evidence from published medical research. This chapter reviews the process used by the Task Force to develop guidelines and introduces concepts of clinical epidemiology and statistics involved in the reviews that follow.

The periodic health examination includes a group of activities designed either to determine a person's risk of developing disease at a later date or to identify early, asymptomatic disease. It encompasses both primary and secondary prevention activities. The aim of *primary prevention* is to prevent the occurrence of disease through immunization or by reducing exposure to risk factors or modifying behaviours; the aim of *secondary prevention* is to identify asymptomatic individuals with early stage disease when such early identification promises a significantly better response to treatment than in those who first present with symptoms.

With its inception in 1976, the Canadian Task Force on the Periodic Health Examination adopted a plan to use explicit analytic criteria to guide its evaluation of effectiveness.[2] The rules were refined in collaboration with the U.S. Preventive Services Task Force in the 1980s,[3-6] but the basic premise of forming recommendations of graded strength based on the quality of published medical evidence remains unaltered. The greatest weight has been placed on the

[1] Assistant Clinical Professor, Department of Family Practice, Medical College of Virginia, Richmond, Virginia and Science Advisor, U.S. Preventive Services Task Force, Washington, D.C.
[2] Director, Division of Clinical Epidemiology, Montreal General Hospital, McGill University, Montreal, Quebec
[3] Senior Scientist, Institute for Clinical Evaluative Sciences, Associate Professor, Department of Health Administration, University of Toronto, Toronto, Ontario
[4] Professor of Medicine, Department of Medicine, University of Toronto, Toronto, Ontario
[5] Associate Professor, Department of Pediatrics and of Preventive Medicine and Biostatistics, Faculty of Medicine, University of Toronto, Toronto, Ontario
[6] Coordinator, Canadian Task Force on the Periodic Health Examination, Department of Pediatrics, Dalhousie University, Halifax, Nova Scotia

features of study design and analysis that tend to eliminate or minimize biased results. Table 1 provides a summary of grades of evidence and the classification of recommendations. The Task Force strives to provide a bridge between research findings and clinical preventive practice. When research does not provide clear guidance, this lack of evidence is articulated. A major objective is to help physicians choose tests, counselling strategies or other preventive interventions of proven utility and avoid those that lack demonstrated value. For example, the performance of a routine electrocardiogram in an asymptomatic individual may work to the patient's disadvantage by consuming time that could be devoted to considerably more effective interventions for preventing heart disease, such as counselling regarding smoking, dietary fat intake or exercise. Of course, the physician's knowledge of an individual will dynamically affect clinical decision-making. Further, many important factors that influence the effectiveness of clinical preventive services, such as the benefits of a healthy, caring patient-physician relationship, are not captured by traditional research methods. However, this text uses a clinical epidemiology perspective to summarize what has proven to be effective in primary and secondary prevention, what is known not to work or to work less effectively and what is not known. Unanswered questions for each topic evolve logically into research priorities.

The analytic process utilized by the Task Force involves four major aspects. They are:

- Defining criteria of effectiveness
- Reviewing evidence
- Managing the committee analytic process
- Developing clinical practice guidelines.

Defining Criteria of Effectiveness

Of fundamental importance to effectiveness is whether performing the proposed maneuver is likely to result in more good than harm. Good and harm should be considered broadly. They extend beyond the ability of a maneuver to reduce the incidence or severity of its target condition and include its other effects. As an example, the use of aspirin by asymptomatic men at risk for coronary artery disease might be viewed as effective if it reduced the incidence of myocardial infarction.[7] If, however, long-term aspirin use also increased hemorrhagic complications, the morbidity and mortality associated with non-target conditions (i.e. bleeding) might outweigh the health benefit of reduced coronary artery disease.

At the beginning of the analytic process it is important to lay out a comprehensive list of potential benefits and risks of a maneuver and to adopt explicit analytic methods to ensure that each category of outcomes is evaluated adequately. The smallest size of benefit or risk that is *clinically* (as opposed to statistically) significant also requires clarification.

The strongest evidence that a preventive service is beneficial comes from well-designed studies with adequate follow-up that demonstrate that persons who receive the clinical action experience a significantly better *overall* clinical outcome than those who do not. Unfortunately, there are few such studies to draw upon. Most evaluative studies have examined the effects of prevention on an intermediate outcome. For instance, studies demonstrate the effectiveness of medication in the control of intraocular pressure but not the effect of therapy on the progression of glaucoma.<6,8-9> The analyst must infer (from epidemiologic evidence or separate intervention studies) that an effect on the intermediate outcome will lead to an effect on the target condition – an inference that may not be borne out in many cases.

A useful tool for mapping out the relationship between clinical events, proposed by Battista and Fletcher,<10> is the "causal pathway" to illustrate the sequence of events that must occur for a given maneuver to influence a target condition. For example, the causal pathway for the early detection of hypertension (Fig. 1) illustrates that the most direct evidence of benefit would come from causal link No. 5, studies demonstrating that asymptomatic individuals in whom blood pressure is measured (and then treated) are less likely to suffer the complications of hypertension, such as stroke. In the absence of such evidence it is often possible to infer effectiveness by combining causal links Nos. 1 and 4, or links Nos. 1, 2, and 3.

The causal pathway provides a visual summary of the type of evidence that should be reviewed. The causal pathway for screening tests clarifies the need to evaluate two causal links to infer effectiveness: 1) the ability of the early detection procedure to identify the target condition; and 2) the ability of a treatment intervention to achieve a favourable outcome. As evaluation of screening tests has been a major component of Task Force work, it will be discussed in more detail before turning to the review of evidence. Screening is used primarily in reference to *case-finding*, i.e. the detection of disorders at an asymptomatic stage in individuals who are being seen in the office or clinic for other reasons.

First, the ability of a test to detect early-stage disease requires examination of *sensitivity*, the proportion of persons with the condition who are correctly identified by the screening test, and *specificity*, the proportion of persons without the condition who correctly test negative. A test with inadequate sensitivity means a significant proportion of persons with the disorder will escape detection. For any given sensitivity and specificity, the likelihood that a positive test result indicates disease, depends on the prevalence of the disease in the population of interest. If a disease is rare, the chance of a false positive result increases. Therefore, it is important to determine the *positive* and *negative predictive values* of the test in the population to be screened (the proportion of true positives among the "positive" test results and the proportion of true negatives among the "negative" test results, respectively). For this reason, it is also at times appropriate to screen populations with a higher prevalence of disease (high-risk groups) but not to screen the general population. When prevalence of a condition is high (as in the high-risk population), positive test results are more likely to be accurate.

Persons who are informed of false positive results may experience unnecessary anxiety until the error is corrected.[11] False postive results also lead to unnecessary diagnostic workup, interventions or treatment. This is more of a problem in a relatively healthy population than false negative results but the latter may also lead to a false sense of security, resulting in inadequate attention to risk reduction and delays in seeking medical care when warning symptoms become present.

The second requirement to prove the value of screening, is to demonstrate the added value of early detection – to prove that asymptomatic persons with early-stage disease have a significantly better response to treatment than those who first present with symptoms. A study of appropriate design can show this. However, inferring that this is so based on studies showing better prognosis for individuals treated with early as opposed to late stage disease (particularly those not diagnosed through screening), or only for individuals in a high-risk group, weakens the evidence for screening asymptomatic persons considerably.

Even if all available evidence from experimental studies suggests that a preventive service will achieve a favourable outcome, the procedure may fail to achieve the same beneficial effects under the less controlled conditions of day-to-day clinical practice. Thus, effectiveness may differ from efficacy due to factors related to: 1) the patient population and in particular their compliance, 2) the providers offering care (general practitioners as opposed to researchers with special expertise and a standardized protocol), 3) financial limitations, and 4) logistic limitations of the health care system as a whole.

Beyond discomfort and inconvenience, some tests may also result in physical complications. Examples include colonic perforation during screening sigmoidoscopy[12] and fetal damage during amniocentesis[13] or chorionic villus sampling to screen for congenital birth defects. Although the risk of such complications is often relatively small, even a small risk per screened person can outweigh potential benefits if the target condition is rare in the screened population.

The results of screening tests can influence clinical decisions to perform interventions that are themselves associated with a certain level of risk. For example, data from routine electronic fetal monitoring suggesting fetal distress may prompt a decision to perform caesarean section, an operation associated with a measurable risk of perioperative morbidity and mortality.<14>

The psychological effects of *labelling* are another important complication of the results of screening tests. This is the damage done when we tell someone who feels well that they are sick. For instance, persons diagnosed with hypertension are at increased risk of work absenteeism and other behavioural changes.<15,16> Screening for HIV seropositivity may subject a person to discrimination and prejudice.<17> Forty percent of children whose parents believed they had a cardiac abnormality were found to have restricted daily activities, even though 80% had no clinical evidence of heart disease on careful examination.<18>

All of these factors need to be considered in establishing criteria of effectiveness. After establishing an approach to evaluation, the next step involves identifying the pertinent medical literature and reviewing it in accordance with the established criteria.

Review of Evidence

Literature Retrieval Method

The Task Force usually identifies the medical literature with a computerized search using MEDLINE. The keywords used for each topic and the date of the final search are listed under the Evidence subheading in each of the chapters that follow. The reference list is supplemented by citations obtained from experts and from reviews of bibliographic listings and other sources.

In general, animal investigations and studies that include individuals identified as being ill because they had symptoms are excluded. Evidence based on weak study design is excluded where stronger, more compelling scientific evidence is available. Clinical intervention studies are also given greater prominence than more indirect epidemiologic evidence of causal relationships between risk variables and preventable target conditions.

Documentation of the literature retrieval method is provided to make the review process more accessible to others and to ensure that the scope and pertinence of the literature review can be scrutinized.

Evaluation of Evidence

In evaluating the evidence, data from published reports are examined to determine whether a specific maneuver meets the criteria of effectiveness. The hierarchy of evidence places emphasis on study designs that are less vulnerable to bias and errors of inference, such as randomized controlled trials.

The assessment of quality is not concluded by assigning a study to a particular design category. Poorly-designed randomized controlled trials may provide less persuasive evidence than well-designed non-experimental studies. Thus, all studies must undergo critical appraisal for design strengths and flaws. A detailed review of these issues is beyond the scope of this chapter. However, fundamental concerns include: the presence of blinding, treatment of confounders, statistical power and sample size, population characteristics, a priori specification of hypothesis, data analysis methods and sources of bias including the proportions of persons lost to follow-up.

After the strengths and weaknesses of each individual study have been determined, results must be synthesized to form a comprehensive but usable body of evidence. Meta-analysis is still in a developmental stage<19-24> and currently is not used routinely for this function, but it is seen as a powerful tool for selected situations. The synthesis of multiple studies is usually done by reviewers on a less quantitative basis. The key features of the major studies, such as sample size, and the direction, magnitude and significance of effects are normally presented in a tabular or graphic format for easy comparison. Reviewers identify important patterns in results and examine the role of population characteristics and other confounding variables in accounting for differences in results.

These first two steps enable an assessment of the level of certainty that a maneuver is effective. This approach has been transferred to other situations for evaluation of technologies or non-preventive interventions by individuals or by groups. However, the Task Force itself acts as a whole to facilitate review of evidence in accordance with criteria of effectiveness and in a modified consensus development process to develop practice guidelines. The mechanisms developed by the Task Force to do this are described in the next section.

Managing the Committee Analytic Process

The Task Force has a stable panel of members and engages in a continuous process of revising previous recommendations and addressing new topics. Over the sixteen year history of the Task Force, a gradual turnover of members with varied expertise has been ensured. The Task Force has maintained a mix of clinicians and research methodologists. Family practice, pediatrics, geriatrics and several other specialties are represented.

Topics to be reviewed may arise from challenges from the academic community, ambiguity regarding appropriate current practice, conflict between the recommendations of authoritative bodies, or suggestions from individuals, special interest groups or from government. Topic selection also depends upon publication of new research evidence and the personal expertise of the members. Where resources are limited, members assign priorities by ranking the list of possible topics.

Members are assigned specific topics and each has a mandate to submit background papers to the rest of the committee for discussion. Outside consultants are also asked to work with the Task Force on selected topics. Project support staff has been funded since 1988 by a research grant from the National Health Research Development Program. Staff members work under the direction of the chairman and the Task Force members. Health Canada also funds meetings and travel expenses through the Health Services and Promotions Branch. The Task Force meets 2 or 3 times each year for 1-2 days and all background papers are pre-circulated.

The interchange among expert panelists within the conference room permits the airing of important issues, clarification of ambiguous concepts and careful analysis of evidence and recommendations by the group. The advantages of informal discussion by experts and the process of achieving consensus include the opportunity to deal openly with important issues that are not easily quantified or addressed adequately in a more structured analysis (e.g. ethical issues).

At the same time, the personal opinions individuals bring to the process and familiar human characteristics (e.g. forgetfulness, fatigue, interpersonal conflict) can influence the recommendations that are developed. Consensus conferences have methodological limitations[25-31] and are sometimes criticized because only people with similar views are asked to attend. While the approach of Task Force members to the evaluation of the literature is similar (commitment to the evidence-based approach) and they have developed expertise regarding how the methodolgy works, members of the panel do not always approach the task from the same starting point. Time is taken to reconcile differing points of view. The evidence is presented and deliberated upon until a consensus finally emerges.

It is important to take advantage of the potential strengths of the consensus development process while at the same time adhering to procedural standards and work practices that maintain uniformity and impartiality in the analytic process. These include procedures to achieve adequate documentation, consistency, comprehensiveness, objectivity and adherence to the Task Force methodology.

Developing Clinical Practice Guidelines

The review of evidence of the effectiveness of preventive services serves as the principal basis for clinical practice recommendations. However, the review of the evidence is a conceptually distinct process from the setting of medical policy. Because of the health, economic and social implications of clinical practice guidelines, the scientific evidence must be viewed within the context of the clinical practice and the health care settings to which the recommendations will apply.

As a general rule, the strongest recommendations of the Task Force (A and E Recommendations) are reserved for preventive interventions whose value is supported or negated by high quality evidence (Type I – randomized controlled trials (RCTs)). Type II evidence is of fair quality and generally is associated with B and D Recommendations.

However, other factors come into play as the Task Force considers Canadian practice settings specifically and puts together evidence from various sources. Are the results of studies from the United States, Europe or other developed countries generalizable to Canada? What are the implications in terms of safety, acceptability and cost of clinical procedures to patients and physicians, not only in urban settings but in the variety of practice settings across Canada?

Examples of factors other than evidence that can affect the grade of a recommendation include: limited availability of a particular technology, demonstrated poor average compliance with a procedure and some potential for harm. In such cases the Task Force considers it best to err on the side of caution and not to advocate major changes in accepted practice. On the other hand, in cases where the burden of suffering is overwhelming, the Task Force will tend to be more proactive, since interventions of only minor effectiveness may translate into substantial health benefits for the population as a whole.

The burden of suffering is assessed by considering two factors: first, the impact of the particular condition on the individual, as assessed from the years of life lost, the amount of disability, the pain and discomfort, the cost of treatment and the effect on the individual's family; and, second, the impact on society as assessed from mortality, morbidity and the cost of treatment. Ambiguity in the evidence regarding morbidity and mortality can also lead to more conservative recommendations (tending towards C Recommendations).

Although interventions are generally not recommended when they are linked to an increase in all-cause mortality or morbidity, the absence of a reduction in overall mortality or morbidity is not always a valid basis for recommending against an intervention. Even if the lack of change in a global outcome measure reflects the exchange of one cause of death, or one form of illness, for another, such an outcome may be desirable for patients whose risk preferences favour such an exchange. For example, the suffering that can precede certain causes of death (e.g. stroke) may make their prevention more desirable for some persons than the prevention of more acute causes of death. Bone fractures may be of greater concern to some women considering estrogen replacement therapy than the risk of endometrial cancer. Non-fatal health outcome measures also tend to be more problematic in that they have less uniform definitions and are less precise in terms of impact on burden of suffering.

The "number needed to treat" is another useful tool.<32> Estimates are made of the number of individuals in the population who would have to receive the intervention per case prevented. Interventions with a large "number needed to treat" may not be in the best interest of the population if treatment is associated with significant costs or harmful effects (iatrogenic side effects, labelling, high cost, etc.).

Given the growing concern about health care costs, the Task Force attempts to furnish information about the cost effectiveness of recommended preventive interventions. Where possible, studies that have examined the costs and effects of an intervention are reviewed. However, information of this type is limited and where it does exist questions often arise concerning the appropriateness of study modeling assumptions including criteria of effectiveness and the equivalence of costs and benefits in the Canadian setting. Thus, the Task Force may only be able to describe a procedure or technology in general terms as costly and as a result tend to de-emphasize it.

The Task Force has increased the efficiency of its operations through close collaboration with the U.S. Preventive Services Task Force. On some issues there has been a division of labour (on a topic by topic basis) between the two groups. Several chapters in this Guide have been adapted from reports of the U.S. Task Force. Similarly, the U.S. Preventive Services Task Force will be adapting Canadian reports for the new edition of its Guide. Preliminary draft reports on all topics are exchanged. This allows committee members to proceed more rapidly to formulation of guidelines after careful consideration of the evidence in the local context. In most instances, the two committees have come to the same conclusions but sometimes there are minor differences of opinion regarding the strength of evidence and/or grading of recommendations.

All four recommendations that are graded positively or negatively (A, B, D and E) reflect a strong conviction that all physicians should adapt their practice to these guidelines. A C grade Recommendation means that there is poor or contradictory evidence regarding the intervention and that decision-making must be guided by factors other than the medical scientific evidence. Such interventions lend themselves particularly well to individual adaptation – considering the physician's expertise and the patients' risk profile.

Recognizing the diversity of issues that must be considered in developing sound practice recommendations, the final recommendation is accompanied with a clear and explicit discussion of the underlying rationale. Recommendations and background papers are then distributed to outside experts for peer review and revised appropriately. Detailed Task force technical reports are published in peer-reviewed journals in English (Canadian Medical Association Journal) and in French (*L'Union médicale du Canada*). A full list of reports published to date is included as Appendix A.

Conclusions

Efforts to enhance scientific standards for medical information synthesis and the assessment of effectiveness are combined with a consensus development mechanism in the Task Force approach. Further refinement can be expected in the future to merge these approaches optimally in order to provide more meaningful recommendations and more rigorous accountability for the methods used to develop those recommendations. These efforts will lead ultimately to a more scientific approach to clinical practice decisions and to more effective and efficient use of health care services in general.

Selected References

1. Woolf SH, Battista RN, Anderson GM, *et al*: Assessing the clinical effectiveness of preventive maneuvers: Analytic principles and systematic methods in reviewing evidence and developing clinical practice recommendations. *J Clin Epidemiol* 1990; 43(9): 891-905

2. Report of a Task Force to the Conference of Deputy Ministers of Health (cat no. H39-3/1980E), Health Services and Promotion Branch, Department of National Health and Welfare, Ottawa, 1980

3. Canadian Task Force on the Periodic Health Examination: The periodic health examination: 1989 update part 1, Introduction and Part 2, Early Detection of Colorectal Cancer and Problem Drinking. *Can Med Assoc J* 1989; 141: 209-216

4. Lawrence RS, Mickalide AD: Preventive services in clinical practice: designing the periodic health examination. *JAMA* 1987; 257: 2205-2207

5. Lawrence RS, Mickalide AD, Kamerow DB *et al*: Report of the U.S. Preventive Services Task Force. *JAMA* 1990; 263: 436-437

6. U.S. Preventive Services Task Force: *Guide to clinical preventive services: An assessment of the effectiveness of 169 interventions.* Baltimore, MD: Williams & Wilkins; 1989

7. Steering Committee of the Physicians' Health Study Research Group: Final report on the aspirin component of the ongoing Physicians' Health Study. *N Engl J Med* 1989; 321: 129-135

8. Canadian Task Force on the Periodic Health Examination: The periodic health examination. 1986 update. *Can Med Assoc J* 1986; 134: 721-729

9. Leske MC: The epidemiology of open-angle glaucoma: a review. *Am J Epidemiol* 1983; 118: 166-191

10. Battista RN, Fletcher SW: Making recommendations on preventive practices: methodological issues. In: Battista RN, Lawrence RS (eds.): *Implementing Preventive Services.* New York, Oxford University Press, 1988; 53-67

11. Sorenson JR, Levy HL, Mangione TW, *et al*: Parental response to repeat testing of infants with "false positive" results in a newborn screening program. *Pediatr* 1984; 73: 183-187

12. Nelson RL, Abcarian H, Prasad ML: Iatrogenic perforation of the colon and rectum. *Dis Colon Rectum* 1982; 25: 305-308

13. Campbell TL: Maternal serum alpha-fetoprotein screening: benefits, risks and costs. *J Fam Pract* 1987; 25: 461-467

14. Shy KK, LoGerfo JP, Karp LE: Evaluation of elective repeat cesarean section as a standard of care: an application of decision analysis. *Am J Obstet Gynecol* 1981; 139: 123-129

15. Lefebvre RC, Hursey KG, Carleton RA: Labelling of participants in high blood pressure screening programs. Implications for blood cholesterol screenings. *Arch Intern Med* 1988; 148: 1993-1997

16. MacDonald LA, Sackett DL, Haynes RB *et al*: Labelling in hypertension: a review of the behavioural and psychological consequences. *J Chronic Dis* 1984; 37: 933-942

17. Hermann DHJ: *Torts: Private Lawsuits about AIDS*, Yale U Pr, New Haven, Conn, 1987: 153-172

18. Bergman AB, Stamm SJ: The morbidity of cardiac nondisease in schoolchildren. *N Engl J Med* 1967; 276: 1008-1013

19. Thacker SB: Meta-analysis: A quantitative approach to research integration. *JAMA* 1988; 259: 1685-1689

20. Jenicek M: Meta-analysis in medicine: Where we are and where we want to go. *J Clin Epidemiol* 1989; 42: 35-44

21. L'Abbe KA, Detsky AS, O'Rourke K: Meta-analysis in clinical research. *Ann Intern Med* 1987; 107: 224-233

22. Wittes RE: Problems in the medical interpretation of overviews. *Stat Med* 1987; 6: 269-280

23. Sacks HS, Berrier J, Reitman D *et al*: Meta-analyses of randomized controlled trials. *N Engl J Med* 1987; 316: 450-455

24. Yusuf S: Obtaining medically meaningful answers from an overview of randomized clinical trials. *Stat Med* 1987; 6: 281-294

25. Oliver MF: Consensus or nonsensus conferences on coronary heart disease. *Lancet* 1985; 1(8437): 1087-1089

26. Jacoby I: Evidence and consensus. *JAMA* 1988; 259: 3039

27. Greer AL: The two cultures of biomedicine: Can there be consensus? *JAMA* 1987; 258: 2739-2740

28. Wortman PM, Vinokur A, Sechrest L: Do consensus conferences work? A process evaluation of the NIH Consensus Development Program. *J Health Polit Policy Law* 1988; 13: 469-498

29. Vinokur A, Burnstein E, Sechrest L *et al*: Group decision making by experts: field study of panels evaluating medical technologies. *J Pers Soc Psychol* 1985; 49: 70-84

30. Perry S: The NIH consensus development program: A decade later. *N Engl J Med* 1987; 317: 485-488

31. Institute of Medicine, Council on Health Care Technology: *Consensus Development at the NIH: Improving the Program. Report of a Study by the Committee to Improve the National Institutes of Health Consensus Development Program.* Washington, D.C., National Academy Press, 1990

32. Laupacis A, Sackett DL, Roberts RS: An assessment of clinically useful measures of the consequences of treatment. *New Engl J Med* 1988; 318: 1728-1733

Table 1

Quality of Evidence

I: Evidence obtained from at least one properly randomized controlled trial.

II-1: Evidence obtained from well-designed controlled trials without randomization.

II-2: Evidence obtained from well-designed cohort or case-control analytic studies, preferable from more than one centre or research group.

II-3: Evidence obtained from comparisons between times or places with or without the intervention. Dramatic results in uncontrolled experiments (such as the results of treatment with penicillin in the 1940's) could also be included in this category.

III: Opinions of respected authorities, based on clinical experience, descriptive studies or reports of expert committees.

Classification of Recommendations

A: There is good evidence to support the recommendation that the condition be specifically considered in a periodic health examination.

B: There is fair evidence to support the recommendation that the condition be specifically considered in a periodic health examination.

C: There is poor evidence regarding the inclusion or exclusion of the condition in a periodic health examination, but recommendations may be made on other grounds.

D: There is fair evidence to support the recommendation that the condition be excluded from consideration in a periodic health examination.

E: There is good evidence to support the recommendation that the condition be excluded from consideration in a periodic health examination.

Figure 1

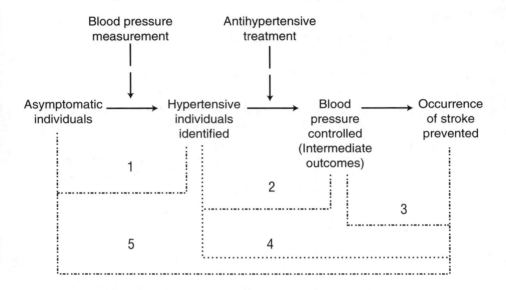

Causal pathways for early detection of hypertension (reprinted with permission from Battista RN, Fletcher SW. Making recommendations on preventive practices: methodological issues. In: Battista RN and Lawrence RS, Eds. *Implementing Preventive Services.* New York: Oxford University Press; 1988: 53-67)

Maneuvers to be Included in Clinical Preventive Health Care

Classified by Age, Strength of Evidence, Target Population and Burden of Suffering

These tables summarize maneuvers reviewed by the Canadian Task Force on the Periodic Health Examination in this text for which the medical evidence documents that benefits outweigh potential harm. They deal with screening and counselling for the asymptomatic individual that would be offered in a clinical setting by physicians, nurses or associated health care workers. The tables exclude evaluation of interventions such as legislation, school-based programs and care provided by dentists. Therapeutic recommendations for individuals who have previously identified conditions (e.g. hypertension) are not included. Previous recommendations made by the Task Force where benefit outweighs harm but that have not been specifically updated for this volume are listed in Appendix B.

Recommendations are summarized by age and gender into subgroups eg. Prenatal/perinatal. The information is displayed with "A Recommendations" for the general population at the top (maneuvers for which there is good evidence for inclusion in a periodic health examination (PHE)). Conditions with a higher burden of suffering are listed first.

The second grouping on each page are "B Recommen-dations" for the general population. (Maneuvers for which there is fair evidence for inclusion in a periodic health examination). Within this category, conditions with a high burden of suffering are again listed first. A subsection of each group of recommendations specifically addresses high-risk populations.

Perinatal Care

CONDITION	MANEUVER	POPULATION	CHAPTER
GOOD EVIDENCE TO INCLUDE IN PHE (A RECOMMENDATIONS):[1]			
Low birth weight/cognitive ability of child	Smoking cessation interventions	Pregnant women	Ch 3
Gastrointestinal and respiratory infection in the newborn	Counselling on breast feeding; peripartum interventions to increase frequency of breast feeding	Pregnant women (or peripartum period)	Ch 22
D (Rh) sensitization	D (Rh) antibody screening and immunoglobulin (D Ig) administration after delivery of D positive infant	Pregnant women	Ch 11
Neural tube defects	Folic acid supplementation	Women capable of becoming pregnant	Ch 7
Bacteriuria in pregnancy	Urine culture	Pregnant women	Ch 9
FAIR EVIDENCE TO INCLUDE IN PHE (B RECOMMENDATIONS):[1]			
Congenital rubella syndrome	Screen, counsel and vaccinate post-partum	Pregnant women	Ch 12
Preeclampsia	Blood pressure measurement	Pregnant women	Ch 13
Fetal alcohol syndrome	Screen and counsel, alcohol consumption	Pregnant women	Ch 5
Chlamydial infection	Smear, culture, or analysis	Pregnant or high-risk women	Ch 60
Perinatal morbidity and mortality	Single prenatal ultrasound	Pregnant women	Ch 1
Neural tube defects	Maternal serum alpha-fetoprotein/ ultrasound, amniocentesis	Pregnant women	Ch 7
Down syndrome	Triple screening and counselling	Pregnant women <35 yrs	Ch 8
Iron deficiency anemia in infants	Counselling parents on breast feeding	Pregnant women (or peripartum period)	Ch 23
High-risk Populations			
D (Rh) sensitization	Repeat D (Rh) antibody screening and immunoglobulin (D Ig) administration	Pregnant women and women undergoing induced abortion or amniocentesis who are antibody negative	Ch 11

[1] See Appendix B for Recommendations not updated since 1979.

Perinatal Care – *Concl'd*

CONDITION	MANEUVER	POPULATION	CHAPTER
D (Rh) sensitization	D (Rh) antibody screening and immunoglobulin (D Ig) administration	After delivery of D positive infant	Ch 11
Down syndrome	Genetic screening and counselling	High-risk pregnant women	Ch 8
Hemoglobinopathies	1) Screen for carrier status (complete blood count and hemoglobin electrophoresis); 2) DNA analysis, fetal tissue sample/counselling	1) High-risk pregnant women; 2) Families, parents confirmed carriers	Ch 20

Neonatal and Well-Baby Care

CONDITION	MANEUVER	POPULATION	CHAPTER
GOOD EVIDENCE TO INCLUDE IN PHE (A RECOMMENDATIONS):[1]			
Immunizable infectious disease	Immunizations, Childhood	Infants and children	Ch 33
Hepatitis B	Immunization	Infants and children	Ch 35
Phenylketonuria	Serum phenylalanine screening	Newborns	Ch 17
Unintentional injury	Counselling on home risk factors, poison control	Parents of infants	Ch 24
Infection	Counselling on breast feeding; peripartum interventions to increase frequency of breast feeding	Pregnant women (or peripartum period)	Ch 22
Congenital hip dislocation	Physical exam, hips	Infants	Ch 24
Ophthalmia neonatorum	Ocular prophylaxis	Newborns	Ch 16
Amblyopia	Eye exam	Infants	Ch 24
Hearing impairment	Hearing exam	Infants	Ch 24
Congenital hypothyroidism	Thyroid-stimulating hormone (TSH) test	Neonates	Ch 18
Night-time crying	Anticipatory guidance on systematic ignoring	Parents of infants distressed by crying	Ch 24
High-risk Populations			
Hemoglobinopathies	Hemoglobin electrophoresis	High-risk neonates	Ch 20
FAIR EVIDENCE TO INCLUDE IN PHE (B RECOMMENDATIONS):[1]			
Iron deficiency anemia in infants	Counselling parents on breast feeding, iron fortified formula, cereal, supplements	Infants	Ch 23
Disorders of physical growth	Serial height, weight, head circumference measurement	Infants	Ch 24
Delayed mental development	Enquire about developmental milestones	Parents of infants	Ch 24

[1] See Appendix B for Recommendations not updated since 1979.

Neonatal and Well-Baby Care – *Concl'd*

CONDITION	MANEUVER	POPULATION	CHAPTER
High-risk Populations			
Iron deficiency anemia	Routine hemoglobin 6-12 mths	High-risk infants	Ch 23
HIV/AIDS	Voluntary HIV antibody screening	Infants of HIV positive women	Ch 58

Preventive Health Care for Children and Adolescents

CONDITION	MANEUVER	POPULATION	CHAPTER
GOOD EVIDENCE TO INCLUDE IN PHE (A RECOMMENDATIONS):[1]			
Tobacco-caused disease	Counselling on smoking cessation	Smokers	Ch 43
Dental caries, periodontal disease	Fluoride, toothpaste or supplement, brushing teeth	General population	Ch 36 Ch 37
Hearing impairment	Noise control and hearing protection	General population	Ch 80
Hepatitis B	Immunization	Children and adolescents	Ch 35
High-risk Populations			
All-cause morbidity and mortality	Referral day care or preschool programs	Disadvantaged children	Ch 32
Child maltreatment	Home visits	High-risk families	Ch 29
Influenza	Amantadine chemoprophylaxis	High-risk or unvaccinated individuals exposed to index case	Ch 61
Tuberculosis	INH prophylaxis	Household contacts and skin test converters	Ch 62
HIV/AIDS, gonorrhea, chlamydia	Screening for sexually transmitted disease	High-risk populations	Ch 58 Ch 59 Ch 60
FAIR EVIDENCE TO INCLUDE IN PHE (B RECOMMENDATIONS):[1]			
MVA injury	Counselling on restraint use and avoidance drinking and driving	General population	Ch 44
Tobacco-caused disease	Counselling to prevent smoking initiation	Children and adolescents	Ch 43
Tobacco-caused disease	Referral to validated cessation program	Smokers	Ch 43
Household and recreational injury	Counselling on home risk factors, poisoning	Children; parents	Ch 28
Vision problems	Visual acuity testing	Preschool children	Ch 27

[1] See Appendix B for Recommendations not updated since 1979.

Preventive Health Care for Children and Adolescents – *Concl'd*

CONDITION	MANEUVER	POPULATION	CHAPTER
Unintended pregnancy; STDs	Counselling, sexual activity, contraception	Adolescents	Ch 46
Congenital rubella syndrome	Screen and vaccinate or universal vaccination	Non-pregnant women of child-bearing age	Ch 12
All-cause mortality and morbidity	Moderate physical activity	General population	Ch 47
Problem drinking	Case finding and counselling	General population	Ch 42
Adverse consequences, children of alcoholics	Children of Alcoholics Screening Test (CAST)	General population	Ch 41
Skin cancer	Counselling, Sun exposure, clothing	General population	Ch 70
High-risk Populations			
Iron deficiency anemia	Routine hemoglobin	Disadvantaged children	Ch 32
Cystic fibrosis (CF)	Sweat test	Siblings of children with CF	Ch 19
Cystic fibrosis	DNA analysis for carrier status	Siblings of children with CF	Ch 19
Lead exposure	Blood lead screening	High-risk children	Ch 25

Preventive Health Care for Adults

CONDITION	MANEUVER	POPULATION	CHAPTER
GOOD EVIDENCE TO INCLUDE IN PHE (A RECOMMENDATIONS):[1]			
Tobacco-caused disease	Counselling on smoking cessation and offer of nicotine replacement therapy	Smokers	Ch 43 Ch 69 Ch 71 Ch 3[2]
Neural tube defects	Folic acid supplementation	Women capable of becoming pregnant	Ch 7[2]
Hearing impairment	Noise control and hearing protection	General population	Ch 80
Breast cancer	Mammography and clinical exam	Women aged 50-69	Ch 65[2]
Dental caries, periodontal disease	Fluoride, toothpaste or supplement, brushing and flossing teeth	General population	Ch 36 Ch 37
High-risk Populations			
HIV/AIDS	Voluntary HIV antibody screening	High-risk populations	Ch 58
Child maltreatment	Home visits	High-risk families	Ch 29
Progressive renal disease	Urine dipstick	Adults with IDDM	Ch 38
Gonorrhea	Gram stain/culture cervical or urethral smear	High-risk groups	Ch 59
Influenza	Amantadine chemoprophylaxis	Individuals exposed to index case	Ch 61
Influenza	Outreach strategies to reach high-risk groups	Specific subgroups (e.g. diabetics, chronic heart disease)	Ch 61
Tuberculosis	Mantoux tuberculin skin test	High-risk groups	Ch 62
Tuberculosis	INH prophylaxis	Household contacts and skin test converters	Ch 62

[1] See Appendix B for Recommendations not updated since 1979.
[2] Maneuvers that are gender-specific

Preventive Health Care for Adults – *Cont'd*

CONDITION	MANEUVER	POPULATION	CHAPTER
FAIR EVIDENCE TO INCLUDE IN PHE (B RECOMMENDATIONS):[1]			
Hypertension	Blood pressure measurement	Adults	Ch 53
MVA injury	Counsel, restraint use	General population	Ch 44
All-cause mortality and morbidity	Moderate physical activity	General population	Ch 47
Tobacco-related disease	Refer to validated cessation programs after cessation advice	Smokers	Ch 43
Diet-related illness	Counselling on adverse nutritional habits	Adults	Ch 49
Problem drinking	Case finding and counselling	General population	Ch 42
Coronary heart disease	General dietary advice on fat and cholesterol	Males 30-69 yrs	Ch 54[2]
Cervical cancer	Papanicolaou smear	Women	Ch 73[2]
Congenital rubella syndrome	Screen and vaccinate or universal vaccination	Non-pregnant women of child-bearing age	Ch 12[2]
Osteoporotic fractures (and side effects)	Counselling, hormone replacement therapy	Perimenopausal women	Ch 52[2]
Gonorrhea	Counselling, Educational materials	General population	Ch 59
Skin cancer	Counselling, sun exposure, clothing	General population	Ch 70
High-risk Populations			
Chlamydial infection	Smear, culture or analysis	High-risk women	Ch 60[2]
Tuberculosis	INH prophylaxis	High-risk sub-groups	Ch 62
Influenza	Immunization, annual	High-risk groups	Ch 61
Colorectal cancer	Colonoscopy	Those with cancer family syndrome	Ch 66

[1] See Appendix B for Recommendations not updated since 1979.
[2] Maneuvers that are gender-specific

Preventive Health Care for Adults – *Concl'd*

CONDITION	MANEUVER	POPULATION	CHAPTER
Diabetic retinopathy	Funduscopy or retinal photography	Diabetics	Ch 78
Lung cancer	Dietary advice on leafy green vegetables and fruit	Smokers	Ch 64
Skin cancer	Physical exam, skin	First degree relative with melanoma	Ch 70

Additional[1] Preventive Health Care for the Elderly

CONDITION	MANEUVER	POPULATION	CHAPTER
GOOD EVIDENCE TO INCLUDE IN PHE (A RECOMMENDATIONS):[2]			
Influenza	Outreach strategies for vaccination	Elderly	Ch 61
High-risk Populations			
Falls/injury	Multidisciplinary post-fall assessment	Elderly	Ch 76
Pneumococcal pneumonia	Immunization	Specific subgroups	Ch 34
FAIR EVIDENCE TO INCLUDE IN PHE (B RECOMMENDATIONS):[2]			
Hypertension	Blood pressure measurement	Elderly	Ch 79
Influenza	Immunization, annual	Elderly	Ch 61
Hearing impairment	Enquiry, whispered voice test or audioscope	Elderly	Ch 80
Diminished visual acuity	Snellen sight card	Elderly	Ch 78

[1] Continue appropriate interventions from adult tables.
[2] See Appendix B for Recommendations not updated since 1979.

Preventive Maneuvers for which there is Evidence that Harm Outweighs Good

Classified by Age and Strength of Evidence

These tables summarize maneuvers reviewed by the Canadian Task Force on the Periodic Health Examination for which medical evidence documents that harm outweighs potential benefit. The tables do not include evaluation of non-clinical interventions such as legislation and school-based programs or care provided by dentists (which are discussed briefly in the text). Therapeutic recommendations for individuals who have previously identified conditions (e.g. hypertension) are not included.

The information concerning recommendations is summarized by age and gender into subgroups, e.g. Prenatal/perinatal. The information is displayed with "E Recommendations" at the top (where there is good evidence to exclude the maneuver from a periodic health examination (PHE)).

The second grouping in each section are "D recommendations" (where there is fair evidence for exclusion of the maneuver from a periodic health examination).

Prenatal Care

CONDITION	MANEUVER	POPULATION	CHAPTER
FAIR EVIDENCE TO EXCLUDE FROM PHE (D RECOMMENDATIONS):			
Low birth weight/Preterm birth	Programs consisting exclusively of social support	High-risk pregnant women	Ch 4
Recurrent herpes simplex type II (progenitalis) infection	Cervical smear, culture; weekly screening	Pregnant women with history, active disease or partner with proven infection	Ch 10
Preterm birth	Home uterine activity monitoring	Low-risk pregnancies	Ch 14
Neonatal morbidity and mortality	Electronic fetal monitoring, intrapartum	Low-risk pregnancies	Ch 15

Neonatal and Well-Baby Care

CONDITION	MANEUVER	POPULATION	CHAPTER
FAIR EVIDENCE TO EXCLUDE FROM PHE (D RECOMMENDATIONS):			
Urinary infection	Urine dipstick	Newborns and infants	Ch 21

Preventive Health Care for Children and Adolescents

CONDITION	MANEUVER	POPULATION	CHAPTER
GOOD EVIDENCE TO EXCLUDE FROM PHE (E RECOMMENDATIONS):			
Urinary tract infection (asymptomatic)	Urine dipstick	Children	Ch 21
Pneumococcal pneumonia	Immunization, one dose of pneumoccal vaccine	Infants and children	Ch 34
FAIR EVIDENCE TO EXCLUDE FROM PHE (D RECOMMENDATIONS):			
Cystic fibrosis	DNA analysis for carrier status	General population	Ch 19
Cystic fibrosis	Sweat test, immunoreactive trypsin and "BM meconium" test	General population	Ch 19
Developmental problems	Denver Developmental Scale	Preschool children	Ch 26
Hearing problems	History, clinical examination	Preschool children	Ch 27
Child maltreatment	Screen for risk of maltreating children	General population	Ch 29
Obesity	Low calorie diet	Pre-adolescent obese children	Ch 30
Periodontal disease	Brushing with electric toothbrush	General population	Ch 37

Preventive Health Care for Adults

CONDITION	MANEUVER	POPULATION	CHAPTER
GOOD EVIDENCE TO EXCLUDE FROM PHE (E RECOMMENDATIONS):			
Tuberculosis	Mantoux tuberculin skin test	General population	Ch 62
Lung cancer	Sputum cytology	General population	Ch 64
FAIR EVIDENCE TO EXCLUDE FROM PHE (D RECOMMENDATIONS):			
Pneumococcal pneumonia	Immunization, one dose	Immunocompromised patients	Ch 34
Progressive renal disease	Urine dipstick	General population	Ch 38
Depression	General Health Questionnaire or Zung Self-rating depression scale	General population	Ch 39
Diabetes mellitus	Blood glucose, fasting	Non-pregnant general population	Ch 50
Osteoporotic fractures	Bone mineral density screening	Women	Ch 52
Carotid Disease/Stroke	Neck auscultation or carotid endarterectomy	General population	Ch 57
Gonorrhea	Gram stain / culture of cervical or urethral smear	General population	Ch 59
Chlamydial infection	Smear, culture or analysis	General population	Ch 60
Cervical cancer	Human papillomavirus screening	Women	Ch 63
Lung cancer	Chest radiography	General population	Ch 64
Breast cancer	Mammography	Women aged 40-49 yrs	Ch 65
Colorectal cancer	Fecal occult blood testing or sigmoidoscopy	Those with cancer family syndrome	Ch 66
Prostate cancer	Prostate specific antigen	Men over age 50 yrs	Ch 67
Prostate cancer	Transrectal ultrasound	Men over age 50 yrs	Ch 67
Bladder cancer	Urine dipstick or cytology	General population	Ch 68
Pancreatic cancer	Abdominal palpation, ultrasound or serologic tumour markers	General population	Ch 71
Ovarian cancer	Pelvic exam, transvaginal ultrasound, CA 125 or combination	Pre- or post-menopausal women	Ch 72
Testicular cancer	Tumour markers	Adolescent and adult males	Ch 74

Preventive Health Care for the Elderly[1]

CONDITION	MANEUVER	POPULATION	CHAPTER
GOOD EVIDENCE TO EXCLUDE FROM PHE (E RECOMMENDATIONS):			
Urinary tract infection (asymptomatic)	Urine dipstick or culture	Elderly, specific subgroups	Ch 81
FAIR EVIDENCE TO EXCLUDE FROM PHE (D RECOMMENDATIONS):			
Urinary infection	Urine dipstick or culture	Elderly, ambulatory men	Ch 81

[1] Continue to exclude appropriate interventions from adult tables.

Recommendations by Strength of Evidence

This table summarizes all the recommendations of the Task Force including evaluation of interventions such as legislation or school-based programs that are not offered in a clinical setting. The recommendations are organized according to strength of evidence for various maneuvers – e.g.

A – There is good evidence to support the recommendation that the condition be specifically considered in a periodic health examination.

B – There is fair evidence to support the recommendation that the condition be specifically considered in a periodic health examination.

C – There is poor evidence regarding the inclusion or exclusion of the condition in a periodic health examination, but recommendations may be made on other grounds.

D – There is fair evidence to support the recommendation that the condition be excluded from consideration in a periodic health examination.

E – There is good evidence to support the recommendation that the condition be excluded from consideration in a periodic health examination

Good Evidence to Include in PHE (A Recommendations)

CONDITION	MANEUVER	POPULATION	CHAPTER
Low birth weight/cognitive ability of child	Smoking cessation interventions	Pregnant women	Ch 3
Neural tube defects	Folic acid supplementation	Women capable of becoming pregnant	Ch 7
Bacteriuria in pregnancy	Urine culture	Pregnant women	Ch 9
D (Rh) sensitization	D (Rh) antibody screening and immunoglobulin (D Ig) administration after delivery of D positive infant	Pregnant women	Ch 11
Ophthalmia neonatorum	Ocular prophylaxis	Newborns	Ch 16
Phenylketonuria	Serum phenylalanine screening	Newborns	Ch 17
Congenital hypothyroidism	Thyroid-stimulating hormone (TSH) test	Neonates	Ch 18
Hemoglobinopathies	Hemoglobin electrophoresis	High-risk neonates	Ch 20
Gastrointestinal and respiratory infection in the newborn	Counselling on breast feeding; peripartum interventions to increase frequency of breast feeding	Pregnant women (or peripartum period)	Ch 22
Accidental injury	Counselling, home risk factors	Parents of infants	Ch 24
Amblyopia	Eye exam	Infants	Ch 24
Congenital hip dislocation	Physical exam, hips	Infants	Ch 24
Hearing impairment	Hearing exam	Infants	Ch 24
Night-time crying	Anticipatory guidance on systematic ignoring	Parents of infants distressed by crying	Ch 24
Household and recreational injury	Public education/Legislation on poison control	General population	Ch 28
Child maltreatment	Home visits	High-risk families	Ch 29
All-cause morbidity and mortality	Day care or preschool programs	Disadvantaged children	Ch 32
Immunizable infectious disease	Immunizations, Childhood	Infants and children	Ch 33
Pneumococcal pneumonia	Immunization	Specific subgroups	Ch 34
Hepatitis B	Immunization	Infants, children and adolescents	Ch 35

Good Evidence to Include in PHE (A Recommendations) – *Concl'd*

CONDITION	MANEUVER	POPULATION	CHAPTER
Dental caries, periodontal disease	Brushing and flossing teeth to apply toothpaste (A) and prevent gingivitis (B) but not cariostatic (C)	General population	Ch 36 Ch 37
Dental caries	Fissure sealants	High-risk children	Ch 36
Dental caries	Community fluoridation, fluoride toothpaste or supplement	General population	Ch 36
Periodontal disease	Flossing teeth	Adults	Ch 37
Progressive renal disease	Urine dipstick	Adults with IDDM	Ch 38
Suicide	Medical treatment for diagnosed depression	High-risk group	Ch 40
Tobacco-caused disease	Counselling, smoking cessation or offer nicotine replacement therapy	Smokers	Ch 43 Ch 69 Ch 71 Ch 3
MVA injury	Legislation, restraint use and control of drinking and driving	General population	Ch 44
Hypertension	Pharmacologic treatment	Adults aged 21-64 yrs with DBP $\geq$ 90 mmHg Elderly, specific subgroups	Ch 53 Ch 79
HIV/AIDS	Voluntary HIV antibody screening	High-risk populations	Ch 58
Gonorrhea	Gram stain/culture cervical or urethral smear	High-risk groups	Ch 59
Influenza	Amantadine chemoprophylaxis	High-risk or unvaccinated individuals exposed to index case	Ch 61
Influenza	Outreach strategies to reach high-risk groups	Specific groups (e.g. diabetics), elderly	Ch 61
Tuberculosis	INH prophylaxis	Household contacts and skin test converters	Ch 62
Tuberculosis	Mantoux tuberculin skin test	High-risk groups	Ch 62
Breast cancer	Mammography and clinical exam	Women aged 50-69 yrs	Ch 65
Falls/injury	Multidisciplinary post-fall assessment	Elderly	Ch 76
Hearing impairment	Noise control and hearing protection	General population	Ch 80

Fair Evidence to Include in PHE (B Recommendations)

CONDITION	MANEUVER	POPULATION	CHAPTER
Perinatal morbidity and mortality	Single prenatal ultrasound, second trimester	Pregnant women	Ch 1
Fetal alcohol syndrome	Screening and Counselling, alcohol consumption	Pregnant women	Ch 5
Neural tube defects	Maternal serum alpha-fetoprotein/ ultrasound, amniocentesis	Pregnant women	Ch 7
Down syndrome	Triple screening and counselling	Pregnant women <35 yrs	Ch 8
Down syndrome	Genetic screening and counselling	High-risk pregnant women	Ch 8
D (Rh) sensitization	Repeat blood test, D (Rh) antibody screening and immunoglobulin (D Ig) administration	Pregnant women who are antibody negative and women undergoing induced abortion or amniocentesis	Ch 11
Congenital rubella syndrome	Screen and vaccinate or universal vaccination	Non-pregnant women of child-bearing age	Ch 12
Congenital rubella syndrome	Screen, counsel and vaccinate post-partum if indicated	Pregnant women	Ch 12
Preeclampsia	Blood pressure measurement	Pregnant women	Ch 13
Cystic fibrosis	DNA analysis for carrier status	Siblings of children with CF	Ch 19
Cystic fibrosis	Sweat test, immunoreactive trypsin and "BM meconium" test	Siblings of children with CF	Ch 19
Hemoglobinopathies	1) Screen for carrier status (complete blood count, hemoglobin and electrophoresis); 2) DNA analysis, fetal tissue sample/ counselling	1) High-risk pregnant women; 2) Families, parents confirmed carriers	Ch 20
Iron deficiency anemia	Routine hemoglobin	High-risk infants, Disadvantaged children	Ch 23 Ch 32
Iron deficiency anemia in infants	Counselling, breast feeding	Pregnant women (or peripartum period)	Ch 23
Iron deficiency anemia in infants	Iron fortified formula, cereal or supplementation	Infants	Ch 23
Disorders of physical growth	Serial height, weight, head circumference measurement	Infants	Ch 24

Fair Evidence to Include in PHE (B Recommendations) – *Cont'd*

CONDITION	MANEUVER	POPULATION	CHAPTER
Delayed mental development	Enquire about developmental milestones	Parents of infants	Ch 24
Lead exposure	Blood lead screening	High-risk children	Ch 25
Vision problems	Visual acuity testing	Preschool children	Ch 27
Household and recreational injury	Counselling on home risk factors, poisoning	Children/parents	Ch 28
Household and recreational injury	Legislation, window and stair guards, smoke detectors	General population	Ch 28
Vehicle-related injury	Legislation, bicycle motorcycle or all terrain vehicle helmet	General population	Ch 28 Ch 44 Ch 45
Household and recreational injury	Public education/Legislation, fire burn and water (tub and swimming) safety	General population	Ch 28
Periodontal disease	Tooth scaling and prophylaxis	General population	Ch 37
Gingivitis	Brushing teeth	General population	Ch 37
Suicide	Physician education, risk recognition and therapy	Physicians	Ch 40
Suicide	Medical treatment, reduction suicidal ideation	High-risk population	Ch 40
Adverse consequences, children of alcoholics	Children of Alcoholics Screening Test (CAST)	General population	Ch 41
Problem drinking	Case finding and counselling	General population	Ch 42
Tobacco-caused disease	Counselling to prevent smoking initiation	Children and adolescents	Ch 43
Tobacco-caused disease	Referral to validated cessation program	Smokers	Ch 43
MVA injury	Counselling on restraint use and avoidance of drinking and driving	General population	Ch 44
Household and recreational injury	Legislation, avoidance of alcohol during water recreation	General population	Ch 45
Unintended pregnancy; STDs	Counselling, sexual activity, contraception	Adolescents	Ch 46
All-cause mortality and morbidity	Moderate physical activity	General population	Ch 47

Fair Evidence to Include in PHE (B Recommendations) – *Concl'd*

CONDITION	MANEUVER	POPULATION	CHAPTER
Diet-related illness	Counselling on adverse nutritional habits	Adults	Ch 49
Osteoporotic fractures (and side effects)	Counselling, hormone replacement therapy	Perimenopausal women	Ch 52
Hypertension	Blood pressure measurement	Adults Elderly	Ch 53 Ch 79
Coronary heart disease	Diet/drug treatment	Males 30-59 yrs with elevated cholesterol or LDL-C	Ch 54
Coronary heart disease	General dietary advice on fat and cholesterol	Males 30-69 yrs	Ch 54
HIV/AIDS	Voluntary HIV antibody screening	Infants of HIV positive women	Ch 58
Gonorrhea	Counselling, Educational materials	General population	Ch 59
Chlamydial infection	Smear, culture or analysis	Pregnant or high-risk women	Ch 60
Influenza	Immunization, annual	High-risk sub-groups and elderly	Ch 61
Tuberculosis	INH prophylaxis	High-risk sub-groups	Ch 62
Lung cancer	Dietary advice on green leafy vegetables and fruit	Smokers	Ch 64
Colorectal cancer	Colonoscopy	Those with cancer family syndrome	Ch 66
Skin cancer	Counselling, sun exposure, clothing	General population	Ch 70
Skin cancer	Physical exam, skin	First degree relative with melanoma	Ch 70
Cervical cancer	Papanicolaou smear	Women	Ch 73
Household and recreational injury	Legislation, safety aides, stairs bathtubs	Elderly	Ch 76
Diabetic retinopathy	Funduscopy or retinal photography	Diabetics	Ch 78
Diminished visual acuity	Snellen sight card	Elderly	Ch 78
Hearing impairment	Enquiry, whispered voice test or audioscope	Elderly	Ch 80

Inconclusive Evidence (C Recommendations)

CONDITION	MANEUVER	POPULATION	CHAPTER
Perinatal morbidity and mortality	Ultrasound, prenatal, serial	Pregnant women	Ch 1
Gestational diabetes mellitus	Blood glucose, fasting/random or glucose challenge test	Pregnant women	Ch 2
Gestational diabetes mellitus	History, risk factors; if positive glucose tolerance test	Pregnant women	Ch 2
Low birth weight/Preterm birth	Multicomponent programs	Pregnant women	Ch 4
Low birth weight/Preterm birth	Diet supplementation	Pregnant women at high risk of undernutrition	Ch 4
Fetal alcohol syndrome	History, questionnaire, interview, clinical judgement/ alcohol consumption	Pregnant women	Ch 5
Low birth weight	Iron supplementation	Pregnant women	Ch 6
Neonatal herpes simplex	Cesarean section	Symptomatic pregnant women	Ch 10
D (Rh) sensitization	Repeat D (Rh) antibody screening and immunoglobulin (D Ig) administration	Women undergoing specific obstetric procedures or complications	Ch 11
Congenital rubella syndrome	Universal vaccination	Young men (living in crowded conditions)	Ch 12
Preeclampsia	Aspirin prophylaxis, low dose	Pregnant women	Ch 13
Preterm birth	Home uterine activity monitoring	High-risk pregnancies	Ch 14
Neonatal morbidity and mortality	Electronic fetal monitoring, intrapartum	High-risk pregnancies	Ch 15
Phenylketonuria	Phenylalanine test	Pregnant women	Ch 17
Hemoglobinopathies	Screening for carrier status & counselling	Non-pregnant adolescents and adults	Ch 20
Iron deficiency anemia	Routine hemoglobin	Infants, general population	Ch 23
Lead exposure	Universal screening (Blood lead level or questionnaire)	General population	Ch 25
Developmental problems	Developmental screening questionnaires	Preschool children	Ch 26

Inconclusive Evidence (C Recommendations) – *Cont'd*

CONDITION	MANEUVER	POPULATION	CHAPTER
Household and recreational injury	Counselling, household and recreational injury (except some home hazards, poisoning for children)	Children, adults, elderly	Ch 28 Ch 45 Ch 76
Child maltreatment	Intensive contact with pediatrician, drop-in centre, parent training	Families with children	Ch 29
Child maltreatment	Sexual abuse, abduction prevention programs	General population	Ch 29
Obesity	Exercise and/or nutrition and behaviour modification	Obese Children	Ch 30
Obesity	Height, weight, skin-fold thickness, BMI, etc	Children	Ch 30
Idiopathic adolescent scoliosis	Physical exam, back	Adolescents	Ch 31
All-cause morbidity and mortality	Office contact or home-based parenting education programs	Disadvantaged children	Ch 32
Pneumococcal pneumonia	Immunization, one dose	Immunocompetent elderly living independently	Ch 34
Dental caries	Counselling, diet or baby bottle	General and high-risk population	Ch 36
Periodontal disease	Brushing and flossing teeth, supervised	High-risk patients	Ch 37
Periodontal disease	Brushing with electric toothbrush	Patients with limited dexterity	Ch 37
Periodontal disease	Flossing teeth	Children	Ch 37
Suicide	Suicide risk evaluation	General population	Ch 40
Suicide	Referral school- or community-based program	High-risk population	Ch 40
Suicide	Hospital admission, discharge home, intensive psycho-social follow-up	Individuals previously attempting suicide	Ch 40
Adverse consequences, children of alcoholics	Routine evaluation; some screening options	General population	Ch 41
Adverse consequences, children of alcoholics	Referral school- or community-based intervention programs	High-risk population	Ch 41
Tobacco-caused disease	Counselling on environmental tobacco smoke	Families with smokers	Ch 43
MVA injury	Counselling, helmet, alcohol use	General population	Ch 44

Inconclusive Evidence (C Recommendations) – *Cont'd*

CONDITION	MANEUVER	POPULATION	CHAPTER
MVA injury	Monitor medical impairment	General population	Ch 44
Household and recreational injury	Public education/Legislation, gun control & use of Heimlich maneuver	General population	Ch 45
Osteoporosis; fractures	Counselling, weight bearing exercise	Pre- and post-menopausal women	Ch 47
All-cause mortality and morbidity	Counselling, physical activity; prevent obesity	General population	Ch 47 Ch 48
All-cause mortality, morbidity	Measure body mass index and treat obesity	General population	Ch 48
Protein/ calorie malnutrition	Protein calorie malnutrition screening	Adults	Ch 49
Thyroid cancer	Neck palpation	Adults	Ch 51
Thyroid disorders	Thyroid stimulating hormone test	Perimenopausal women	Ch 51
Osteoporotic fractures	History and physical examination	Women	Ch 52
Hypertension	Pharmacologic treatment	Adults aged <21 yrs, isolated systolic hypertension, some elderly subgroups	Ch 53 Ch 79
Coronary heart disease	Measurement of blood total cholesterol level	General population with case-finding for males 30-59 yrs	Ch 54
Coronary heart disease	Diet/drug treatment	Individuals with elevated cholesterol or LDL-C except males 30-59 yrs	Ch 54
Coronary heart disease	General dietary advice on fat and cholesterol	General population except males 30-69 yrs	Ch 54
Abdominal aortic aneurysm	Abdominal palpation	General population	Ch 55
Abdominal aortic aneurysm	Abdominal ultrasound	General population	Ch 55
Cardiovascular disease	Acetylsalicylic acid prophylaxis	General population	Ch 56
Carotid disease/ stroke	Antiplatelet therapy	Adults with asymptomatic carotid bruit or stenosis	Ch 57
HIV/AIDS	History, sexual and drug use and counselling	General population	Ch 58
HIV/AIDS	Voluntary HIV antibody screening	General population including pregnant women	Ch 58
Influenza	Immunization, annual	General population <65 yrs	Ch 61

Inconclusive Evidence (C Recommendations) – *Concl'd*

CONDITION	MANEUVER	POPULATION	CHAPTER
Influenza	Rapid diagnostic test	Suspected cases	Ch 61
Tuberculosis	INH prophylaxis	General population aged >35 yrs	Ch 62
Breast cancer	Teach breast self-examination (BSE)	Women	Ch 65
Colorectal cancer	Fecal occult blood testing, sigmoidoscopy or colonoscopy	General population or family history (1 or 2 relatives)	Ch 66
Prostate cancer	Digital rectal examination	Men over age 50 yrs	Ch 67
Bladder cancer	Urine dipstick or cytology	High-risk males >60 yrs	Ch 68
Oral cancer	Physical exam, oral cavity	General population	Ch 69
Skin cancer	Counselling, Skin self-examination	General population	Ch 70
Skin cancer	Counselling, Sun block	General population	Ch 70
Skin cancer	Physical examination, skin	General population	Ch 70
Ovarian cancer	Pelvic exam, transvaginal ultrasound, CA 125 or combination	Pre- or post-menopausal women; family history 1st degree relative	Ch 72
Testicular cancer	Physical exam or self-examination	Adolescent and adult males	Ch 74
Cognitive impairment	Mental status screening	Elderly	Ch 75
Household and recreational injury	Monitor medical impairment	Elderly	Ch 76
Household and recreational injury	Public education, non-flammable fabrics, self-extinguishing cigarettes	Elderly	Ch 76
Elder abuse	Elder abuse questionnaire	Elderly	Ch 77
Age-related macular degeneration	Funduscopy	Elderly	Ch 78
Glaucoma	Funduscopy, tonometry or automated perimetry	Elderly	Ch 78
Urinary infection	Urine dipstick or culture	Elderly, ambulatory women	Ch 81

Fair Evidence to Exclude from PHE (D Recommendations)

CONDITION	MANEUVER	POPULATION	CHAPTER
Low birth weight/Preterm birth	Programs of only social support	High-risk pregnant women	Ch 4
Recurrent herpes simplex type II (progenitalis) infection	Cervical smear, culture; weekly screening	Pregnant women with history, active disease or partner with proven infection	Ch 10
Preterm birth	Home uterine activity monitoring	Low risk pregnancies	Ch 14
Neonatal morbidity and mortality	Electronic fetal monitoring, intrapartum	Low-risk pregnancies	Ch 15
Cystic fibrosis	DNA analysis for carrier status	General population	Ch 19
Cystic fibrosis	Sweat test, immunoreactive trypsin and "BM meconium" test	General population	Ch 19
Urinary infection	Urine dipstick	Newborns and infants	Ch 21
Developmental problems	Denver Developmental Scale	Preschool children	Ch 26
Hearing problems	History, clinical examination	Preschool children	Ch 27
Child maltreatment	Screen for risk of maltreating children	General population	Ch 29
Obesity	Low calorie diet	Pre-adolescent obese children	Ch 30
Pneumococcal pneumonia	Immunization, one dose	Immunocompromised patients	Ch 34
Periodontal disease	Brushing with electric toothbrush	General population	Ch 37
Progressive renal disease	Urine dipstick	General population	Ch 38
Depression	General Health Questionnaire or Zung Self-rating depression scale	General population	Ch 39
Diabetes mellitus	Blood glucose, fasting	Non-pregnant general population	Ch 50
Osteoporotic fractures	Bone mineral density screening	Women	Ch 52
Carotid Disease/Stroke	Neck auscultation or carotid endarterectomy	General population	Ch 57
Gonorrhea	Gram stain / culture of cervical or urethral smear	General population	Ch 59
Chlamydial infection	Smear, culture or analysis	General population	Ch 60

Fair Evidence to Exclude in PHE (D Recommendations) – *Concl'd*

CONDITION	MANEUVER	POPULATION	CHAPTER
Cervical cancer	Human papillomavirus screening	Women	Ch 63
Lung cancer	Chest radiography	General population	Ch 64
Breast cancer	Mammography	Women aged 40-49 yrs	Ch 65
Colorectal cancer	Fecal occult blood testing or sigmoidoscopy	Those with cancer family syndrome	Ch 66
Prostate cancer	Prostate specific antigen	Men over age 50 yrs	Ch 67
Prostate cancer	Transrectal ultrasound	Men over age 50 yrs	Ch 67
Bladder cancer	Urine dipstick or cytology	General population	Ch 68
Pancreatic cancer	Abdominal palpation, ultrasound or serologic tumour markers	General population	Ch 71
Ovarian cancer	Pelvic exam, transvaginal ultrasound, CA 125 or combination	Pre- or post-menopausal women	Ch 72
Testicular cancer	Tumour markers	Adolescent and adult males	Ch 74
Urinary infection	Urine dipstick or culture	Elderly, ambulatory men	Ch 81

Good Evidence to Exclude from PHE (E Recommendations)

CONDITION	MANEUVER	POPULATION	CHAPTER
Urinary tract infection (asymptomatic)	Urine dipstick	Children	Ch 21
Pneumococcal pneumonia	Immunization, one dose	Infants and children	Ch 34
Tuberculosis	Mantoux tuberculin skin test	General population	Ch 62
Lung cancer	Sputum cytology	General population	Ch 64
Urinary tract infection (asymptomatic)	Urine dipstick or culture	Elderly, specific subgroups	Ch 81

Prenatal and Perinatal Preventive Care

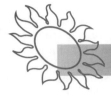

CHAPTER 1

Routine Prenatal Ultrasound Screening

By Geoffrey Anderson

Routine Prenatal Ultrasound Screening

Prepared by Geoffrey Anderson, MD, PhD[1]

Ultrasound examination has been suggested as a prenatal screening tool for various purposes, including the estimation of gestational age, the detection of multiple pregnancies and fetal anomalies, and the identification of intrauterine growth retardation (IUGR). The goal of prenatal ultrasound screening is to reduce the rates of perinatal illness and death from several causes, some of which (e.g., IUGR) are etiologically non-specific. Therefore, the Task Force has reviewed the evidence on the impact of prenatal ultrasound screening on measures of perinatal illness and death rather than on its ability to detect specific abnormalities. Ultrasound is also considered as part of the protocol in screening for neural tube defects (Chapter 7).

Use of Prenatal Ultrasound in Canada

Between 1981/2 and 1989/90, the number of prenatal ultrasound (PNU) services in Ontario and British Columbia more than doubled

The use of perinatal ultrasound has become increasingly common in Canada. Between 1981/82 and 1989/90 the number of prenatal ultrasound (PNU) services in Ontario and British Columbia more than doubled and the rate of PNU per delivery increased from 1.06 to 2.18 in Ontario and from 0.88 to 1.75 in British Columbia.[1] In 1989/90 an average of $160 was spent on PNU per delivery in Ontario and $130 per delivery in British Columbia. This rapid increase in the use and cost of ultrasonography underlines the need for careful assessment of the evidence on the benefits of this procedure.

Maneuver

A single ultrasound examination in the second trimester is used to estimate gestational age and to detect multiple pregnancies and malformations. Two serial examinations (one in the second trimester and one in the third) is used to screen for IUGR and to detect multiple pregnancies and malformations.

Effectiveness of Preventive Intervention

The published trials were separated into two groups. One included four trials that examined the impact of a single ultrasound examination performed in the second trimester.[2-6] The other

---

[1] Senior Scientist, Institute for Clinical Evaluative Sciences in Ontario (ICES) and Associate Professor, Department of Health Administration, University of Toronto, Toronto, Ontario

group included four studies of the impact of serial examinations, one in the second trimester and one in the third.<7-10>

Single Ultrasound Scan

In the first trial<2,3> of this group, a total of 1,621 women underwent an ultrasound examination, including measurement of the biparietal diameter (BPD), at about 16 weeks' gestation. Of these women, 836 were randomly allocated to an experimental group whose ultrasound results were released to the attending physician. The remaining 785 patients were allocated to a control group whose ultrasound results were not released to the attending physician. However, during the trial 30% of the control subjects had their ultrasound results released in response to specific requests from their physician because of clinical concerns. There were eight perinatal deaths in the experimental group and seven in the control group; this difference was not statistically significant. The Apgar score at 1 minute was 7 or less among 172 singleton infants in the experimental group and among 142 singleton infants in the control group; again, this difference was not statistically significant.

The second trial involved 4,997 women with no clinical indication for an ultrasound examination.<4> A total of 2,482 women were randomly assigned to undergo one ultrasound examination and BPD measurement at 15 weeks' gestation (experimental group). The remaining 2,515 women did not have an examination before 19 weeks' gestation (control group). Both groups then received the same antenatal care, including ultrasound examinations later in pregnancy. In the experimental group 32 (1.3%) of the women did not undergo the examination; in the control group 103 (4.1%) had the examination before the 19th week.

The experimental group had 3,068 ultrasound scans, as compared with 1,279 in the control group. Of the women in the control group 68% never underwent ultrasonography. The numbers of prenatal hospital days and hospital admissions were the same in each group. Labour was induced in 41 women in the experimental group and 88 in the control group (p=0.0001).

There were 12 perinatal deaths in each group. In the experimental group eight were in singleton infants and four in twins. In the control group singleton infants accounted for all of the deaths. After the perinatal period but before discharge from hospital there were two additional deaths in each group.

Analysis of the 4,776 singleton births showed no significant difference between the two groups in the proportion of infants with Apgar scores of 7 or less at 1 or at 5 minutes. In each group mechanical ventilation was required at delivery in seven cases and neonatal seizures occurred in four. There was a tendency for fewer babies in the experimental group than in the control group

(231 vs. 275) to be admitted to the neonatal ward; however, this difference was not significant.

Singleton infants in the experimental group were 42 g heavier on average than those in the control group (p=0.008). The average birth weight of infants of nonsmoking women did not differ significantly between the two groups. Infants of smoking women in the experimental group were 75 g heavier on average than those of smoking women in the control group (p=0.013).

The third trial involved 9,310 women from Finland,<5> or about 95% of the pregnant women in the catchment area. A total of 648 women were not followed through to delivery: 569 had a miscarriage, 58 underwent an induced abortion, 17 were found not to be pregnant, and 4 were lost to follow-up.

There were 4,353 deliveries (4,317 of singletons and 72 of twins) in the experimental group. In this group ultrasound screening was done between 16 and 20 weeks' gestation. The BPD was measured, the placenta located and the number of fetuses registered. Most of the 318 women who did not undergo the examination at the study hospital did so elsewhere. In the experimental group 1.6% of the women did not undergo the examination.

In the control group there were 4,309 deliveries (4,271 of singletons and 76 of twins). Although the women were not assigned to undergo an ultrasound examination 77% did so.

The overall perinatal death rate among the infants who were delivered was 4.6 per 1,000 in the experimental group and 9.0 per 1,000 in the control group (p=0.013). In the experimental group 18 singleton babies died (11 were stillborn and 7 died within 1 week after delivery). In the control group 34 singleton babies died (22 were stillborn and 12 died within 1 week after birth). Of the babies that died, only 2 (11%) in the experimental group had major anomalies, as compared with 10 (29%) in the control group. Eleven induced abortions were performed because of the ultrasound findings in the experimental group; there were no such abortions in the control group. There were two deaths in twins in the experimental group and five in the control group.

Among the singleton infants there was no significant difference between the two groups in 1) mean birth weight; 2) proportion of infants with a birth weight of less than 2500 g; 3) mean Apgar score at 1 minute; 4) proportion with an Apgar score of less than 7 at 1 minute; 5) rate of admission to special care unit; and 6) proportion with hospital stay of more than 5 days. The mean birth weight of the twins and the proportion of twins with a birth weight of less than 2500 g did not differ significantly between the two groups; however, all of the twins in the experimental group were detected by 21 weeks' gestation, as compared with 76% of those in the control group (p=0.005).

The difference in the perinatal death rates between the two groups lost its significance when the induced abortions resulting from the ultrasound findings were included as deaths in the analysis. Also, 10 of the "malformations" detected at the ultrasound examination had disappeared by the time of the follow-up examination.

The final study took place in the U.S.[6] The trial involved 915 women at low risk who were randomly allocated to routine prenatal ultrasound screening at 10 to 12 weeks' gestation or routine care. The two groups did not differ significantly in total adverse perinatal outcomes, as measured by the number of perinatal deaths, intensive care admissions and babies with an Apgar score of less than 6 at 5 minutes.

Serial Ultrasonography

The main features of the four trials in this group are summarized in Table 1. The first two trials involved random allocation of patients selected from the general population.[7,8] The third involved random allocation of women who had no clinical indications of IUGR.[9] The most recent trial excluded 60% of the general population.[10]

In the first study[7] three of the infants in the experimental group and eight in the control group died. Of the deaths in the experimental group one was intrauterine and of unexplained cause, and two were due to severe preeclampsia. In the control group four deaths were intrauterine and associated with IUGR, one was due to a severe malformation, and one was of unknown cause; the two postnatal deaths involved a premature twin and an infant with hydrops fetalis. There were no late neonatal deaths in the experimental group and three in the control group. The number of days of pediatric care for malformations due to "overdue pregnancy" (p<0.01) and for hyperbilirubinemia (p<0.05) was significantly lower in the experimental group than in the control group. The significantly fewer hospital admissions in the experimental group (p<0.01) did not result in a difference in the number of days of prenatal care (828 days in the experimental group and 829 in the control group).

There was little description of the causes of perinatal death in the second study.[8] Two of the deaths in the control group involved twins identified through ultrasonography at 24 weeks' gestation. They were delivered 2 weeks later; one was stillborn, and the other died 2 hours postnatally. The distribution of birth weights did not differ significantly between the two groups. Forty-nine of the women in the control group were referred for ultrasonography as part of their routine care. The estimated cost of the screening program was U.S. $250 per pregnancy. Two-thirds of the cost was from the increased use of in-patient services by the experimental group.

The only perinatal death in the third study[9] involved a child born with open spina bifida and microcephaly. The mean birth weight was the same in the two groups. The number of inductions and the delivery methods did not differ significantly between the two groups.

The results of these three smaller trials of serial prenatal ultrasound screening are summarized in Table 2.

The fourth trial was based in 99 obstetrical and family practices in six different American states. A total of 55,744 women registered for the trial, 2,377 were lost before screening and 32,317 were excluded after screening. The major reason for exclusion was because the attending physician indicated that they planned to perform a prenatal ultrasound. The attending physician was not asked to indicate the clinical reason for the proposed ultrasound. The vast majority of the ultrasound exams were performed in one of the 28 laboratories participating in the trial. These laboratories used standardized reporting techniques and scanning equipment. In the screened group, 94% of the women had ultrasound examinations at both 15-22 weeks and 31-35 weeks. Only 2% of the women in the control group had ultrasounds at both of these times. The mean number of ultrasounds in the screened group was 2.2 and the mean number of ultrasounds in the control group was 0.6 with 55% of the group having no prenatal ultrasounds.

The trial used somewhat different outcome measures than the other 3 trials of serial PNU. Three main outcome measures were assessed; 1) perinatal mortality (fetal or neonatal death up to 28 days of age); 2) severe morbidity (including severe intraventricular hemorrhage, seizures, documented sepsis and prolonged use of special care nursery); and 3) moderate morbidity (including use of oxygen for more than 48 hours, nerve injury, short stay in special care nursery). There was no statistically significant difference between the control and screened groups for any of these outcomes (Table 3). There was a total of 52 perinatal deaths in the screened group with 48 of these deaths occurring in singeltons. There was a total of 41 perinatal deaths in the control group with 37 of these deaths occurring in singeltons. There were no statistically significant differences in gestational age at delivery or birth weight between the two groups.

A total of 350 fetuses had at least one major anomaly. Of the 187 fetuses with major anomalies in the ultrasound group 65 (35%) were detected before delivery and 31 (17%) were detected before 24 weeks. Of the 163 fetuses with major anomalies in the control group 18 (11%) were detected before delivery and 8 (5%) were detected before 24 weeks. There were 9 induced abortions for anomalies in the screened group and 5 in the control group.

Systematic Reviews of Trials

The Cochrane Database of Systematic Reviews has published reviews of routine prenatal ultrasound examination in early[11] and late[12] pregnancy. The review of early prenatal ultrasound trials concluded that screening results in early detection of twin pregnancies, a reduced rate of induction of labour, higher birth weights in singeltons and increased rates of abortion for fetal abnormalities, but no statistically significant effects on perinatal mortality or Apgar scores was found. The review of late prenatal ultrasound trials, which did not include the most recent American trial[10], concluded that there was no statistically significant effects of late screening on mortality, morbidity or induction of labour. Another recent meta-analysis, which included the two large studies of single stage screening, concluded that there was no statistically significant effect of screening on live births, although there was a significantly lower perinatal mortality in the screened population.[13]

Recommendations of Others

In Canada, the Federal Task Force on High Risk Pregnancies and Prenatal Record Systems[14] in 1982 stated that "there seems to be very good evidence that ultrasound is a useful adjunct to clinical identification and assessment of intrauterine growth retardation" but that "the use of routine ultrasound without specific indications in pregnancy should be discouraged." The 1984 U.S. National Institutes of Health Consensus Conference on the use of diagnostic ultrasonography during pregnancy[15] concluded that "the data on the clinical efficacy and safety do not allow a recommendation for routine screening at this time." Recently the Society of Obstetrics and Gynecology of Canada recommended the routine use of single PNU in the second trimester.[16] The use of PNU is currently under review by the U.S. Preventive Services Task Force.

Recently the Society of Obstetrics and Gynecology of Canada recommended the routine use of single PNU in the second trimester

Conclusions and Recommendations

Although trials of a single PNU in the second trimester have not shown a statistically significant effect on the rate of live births or Apgar scores, these trials indicate that a single PNU early in pregnancy results in lower rates of induction (presumably through better estimates of gestational age), earlier detection of twin pregnancies, increased birth weight in singeltons and higher rates of therapeutic abortion for fetal abnormalities. Based on these clinical effects there is fair evidence to include a single PNU examination in routine prenatal care (B Recommendation). Trials of serial PNU have not shown any statistically significant effect on perinatal mortality, morbidity or birth weights. Based on this there is poor evidence for the inclusion or exclusion of serial PNU in routine prenatal care (C Recommendation).

Trials of serial PNU have not shown any statistically significant effect on perinatal mortality, morbidity or birth weights

Prenatal ultrasound examination may not only provide the clinician with information on perinatal anomalies and intrauterine problems but may also reassure the expectant mother and provide her with useful information.<17> On the other hand, false positive results can have an adverse psychologic effect on the expectant mother.

Unanswered Questions (Research Agenda)

The benefits and disadvantages of ultrasound examination require further analysis. Such analysis should focus on the impact of the maneuver on fetal survival and perinatal illness rates and should include bi-directional measurement of the psychologic effects of screening on the parents.

Evidence

To identify studies of the effectiveness of routine prenatal ultrasound screening we searched MEDLINE up to October 1993 (with the keywords ultrasonography and randomized controlled trial) for pertinent articles as well as using the references of those articles. Two criteria were used: (a) the study had to have allocated subjects randomly to undergo or not to undergo routine screening and (b) the outcomes had to have included measures of perinatal illness and death.

This review was initiated in October 1993, and based on a previous report.<18> Recommendations were finalized by the Task Force in March 1994.

Selected References

1. Anderson GM: Use of prenatal ultrasound examination in Ontario and British Columbia in the 1980s. *J SOGC* 1994; 16: 1329-1338

2. Bennett MJ, Little G, Dewhurst J, *et al*: Predictive value of ultrasound in early pregnancy: a randomised controlled trial. *Br J Obstet Gynaecol* 1982; 89: 338-341

3. Thacker SB: Quality of controlled clinical trials. The case of imaging ultrasound in obstetrics: a review. *Br J Obstet Gynaecol* 1985; 92: 437-444

4. Waldenstrom U, Axelsson O, Nilsson S, *et al*: Effects of routine one-stage ultrasound screening in pregnancy: a randomised controlled trial. *Lancet* 1988; 2: 585-588

5. Saari-Kemppainen A, Karjalainen O, Ylostalo P, *et al*: Ultrasound screening and perinatal mortality: controlled trial of systematic one-stage screening in pregnancy: The Helsinki Ultrasound Trial. *Lancet* 1990; 336: 387-391

6. Ewigman B, LeFevre M, Hesser J: A randomized trial of routine prenatal ultrasound. *Obstet Gynecol* 1990; 76: 189-194

7. Eik-Nes SH, Okland O, Aure JC, *et al*: Ultrasound screening in pregnancy: a randomised controlled trial. [letter] *Lancet* 1984; 1: 1347

8. Bakketeig LS, Eik-Nes SH, Jacobsen G, *et al*: Randomised controlled trial of ultrasonographic screening in pregnancy. *Lancet* 1984; 2: 207-211

9. Neilson JP, Munjanja SP, Whitfield CR: Screening for small for dates fetuses: a controlled trial. *Br Med J Clin Res Ed* 1984; 289: 1179-1182

10. Ewigman BG, Crane JP, Frigoletto FD, *et al*: Effect of prenatal ultrasound screening on perinatal outcome. RADIUS Study Group. *N Engl J Med* 1993; 329: 821-827

11. Neilson JP: Routine ultrasound in early pregnancy. In: Pregnancy and Childbirth Module (eds. Enkin MW, Keirse MJNC, Renfrew MJ, Neilson JP), "Cochrane Database of Systematic Reviews": Review No. 03872, 9 June 1993. Published through "Cochrane Updates on Disk", Oxford: Update Software, 1994, Disk Issue 1

12. Neilson JP: Routine fetal anthropometry in late pregnancy. In: Pregnancy and Childbirth Module (eds. Enkin MW, Keirse MJNC, Renfrew MJ, Neilson JP), "Cochrane Database of Systematic Reviews": Review No. 03873, 24 March 1993. Published through "Cochrane Updates on Disk", Oxford: Update Software, 1994, Disk Issue 1

13. Bucher HC, Schmidt JG: Does routine ultrasound screening improve outcome in pregnancy? Meta-analysis of various outcome measures. *BMJ* 1993; 307: 13-17

14. *Report of the Federal Task Force on High Risk Pregnancies and Prenatal Records Systems*, Dept of National Health and Welfare, Ottawa, 1982: 25-26

15. Consensus Conference: The use of diagnostic ultrasound imaging during pregnancy. *JAMA* 1984; 252: 669-672

16. Society of Obstetricians and Gynaecologists of Canada Policy Statement: Guidelines for the performance of ultrasound examinations. Obstetrics and Gynaecology, No: 24, October 1993

17. Berwick DM, Weinstein MC: What do patients value? Willingness to pay for ultrasound in normal pregnancy. *Med Care* 1985; 23: 881-893

18. Canadian Task Force on the Periodic Health Examination: The periodic health examination, 1992 update: 2. Routine prenatal ultrasound screening. *Can Med Assoc J* 1992; 147: 627-633

Table 1: Features of trials of routine serial prenatal ultrasound screening[1]

Variable	Eik-Nes et al 1984[7]	Bakketeig et al 1984[8]	Neilson et al 1984[9]	Ewigman et al 1993[10]
Type of population	General	General	Low-risk	Low-risk
Sample size				
Experimental Group	819	510	433	7,812
Control Group	809	499	444	7,718
Interventions				
Experimental Group	Measurement of BPD at 16 weeks and of BPD and AD at 32 weeks	Measurement of BPD at 19 weeks and of BPD and AD at 32 weeks	Measurement of CRL and TA at 24 and 35 weeks	Measurement of placental location, BPD, AC, FL and detailed anatomical survey at 18-20 weeks and at 31-33 weeks
Control Group	Routine care	Routine care	Done, but results not reported to doctor	Routine care

[1] BPD = biparietal diameter, AD = Abdominal diameter, CRL = crown-rump length, TA = trunk area, AC = abdominal circumference, FL = femur length

Table 2: Results of three small trials of routine serial prenatal ultrasound screening[1]

Variable	Eik-Nes et al 1984[7]	Bakketeig et al[2] 1984[8]	Neilson et al 1984[9]
No. (and %) of hospital admissions			
Experimental Group	184 (22.5)	79 (15.5)	43 (9.9)
Control Group	269 (33.2)[3]	46 (9.5)[3]	46 (10.3)
No. (and %) of infants with low Apgar score[4]			
At 1 minute			
Experimental Group	NM	34 (6.9)	37 (9.9)
Control Group	NM	23 (4.9)	40 (9.0)
At 5 minutes			
Experimental Group	NM	15 (3.1)	8 (1.9)
Control Group	NM	9 (1.9)	5 (1.0)
No. (and %) of perinatal deaths			
Experimental Group	3 (0.36)	5 (0.98)	0 (0.00)
Control Group	8 (0.98)	5 (1.00)	1 (0.02)

[1] NM = not measured
[2] Results are given for singleton births only.
[3] $p = 0.05$
[4] Seven or less in study by Bakketeig et al and less than 7 in study by Neilson et al.

Table 3: Results from American Serial Prenatal Ultrasound Trial[10]

Variable	Screened Group N = 7,685 # (%)	Control Group N = 7,596 # (%)
Fetal death	34 (0.4)	23 (0.3)
Neonatal death	18 (0.2)	18 (0.2)
Severe morbidity	99 (1.3)	95 (1.3)
Moderate morbidity	232 (3.0)	237 (3.1)

Routine Prenatal Ultrasound Screening

MANEUVER	EFFECTIVENESS	LEVEL OF EVIDENCE <REF>	RECOMMENDATION
A single ultrasound examination in the second trimester in women without clinical indications	No statistically significant effect of screening on live births or Apgar scores. Screening results in increased birth weight, earlier detection of twins, decreased rates of induction and increased rates of abortion for fetal abnormalities.	Randomized controlled trials<2-6> and meta-analyses<11,13> (I)	Fair evidence to include in periodic health examination (PHE) in normal pregnancies (B)
Serial ultrasound screening in the second and third trimesters in women without clinical indications	No evidence of improved perinatal mortality or morbidity.	Randomized controlled trials<7-10> and meta-analyses<12> (I)	Poor evidence to include in or exclude from PHE in normal pregnancies (C)

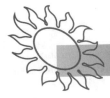
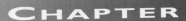

CHAPTER 2

Screening for Gestational Diabetes Mellitus

By Marie-Dominique Beaulieu

Screening for Gestational Diabetes Mellitus

Prepared by Marie-Dominique Beaulieu, MD, MSc, FCFP[1]

The available evidence does not support a recommendation for or against universal screening for gestational diabetes mellitus (GDM). Women have varying degrees of glucose intolerance during pregnancy and a certain proportion will have adverse outcomes. The value of screening is unclear given potential clinical and financial costs. Universal screening with the 50 g glucose challenge test has not been demonstrated to be superior to other tests. Pending the results of ongoing studies on screening test characteristics, factors such as clinical judgement (assessment of risk factors and pregnancy evolution) and available resources should be taken into account in choosing a screening strategy. Women with risk factors for GDM should be carefully followed throughout their pregnancy. Screening for diabetes in non-pregnant adults is addressed in Chapter 50.

Burden of Suffering

Gestational diabetes occurs in about 3% of pregnancies and is associated with perinatal mortality and morbidity

Gestational diabetes, defined as carbohydrate intolerance of variable severity with onset or first recognition during pregnancy, occurs in about 3% of pregnancies. Risk factors for GDM include obesity, history of miscarriage or fetal death, maternal age of 40 years or more, family history of diabetes, history of prematurity, macrosomia, congenital malformation, polyhydramnios, or excessive weight gain. O'Sullivan and Mahan originally restricted the diagnosis to alterations of glucose tolerance during pregnancy that resolved after birth.[1] Using the oral glucose tolerance test (OGTT), women were shown to be at increased risk of overt adult diabetes later in life. Potential flaws in study design (selection bias and confounding) and questions of test validity (reproducibility and obsolescence of blood testing technique) weaken this evidence.

Two case series have shown elevated perinatal loss rates (6.4% vs. 1.5% and 3.2% vs. 0.95%) among those with abnormal as opposed to normal OGTT results. In neither of these studies was there control for confounding.[2,3]

Case series, again not controlling for confounding factors, have reported prevalences of macrosomia among infants born to women with GDM of 12% to 35%.[2-4] GDM is not the only or most important risk factor for macrosomia. In one study with an overall

---

[1] Associate Professor of Family Medicine, University of Montreal, Montreal, Quebec

incidence of macrosomia of 1.7 per 1,000 and where confounding was controlled, the relative risk of macrosomia for GDM was 3.0, as compared with 25.8 and 6.4 per 1,000 for obesity and postmaturity respectively. Indeed, only 5% of infants weighing more than 4,500 g were born to women with GDM.<5> However, macrosomia is clearly associated with increased maternal and neonatal death rates, primary cesarean section for cephalopelvic disproportion and non-progression of labour, brachial plexus paralysis and clavicular fractures. In a series of infants with shoulder dystocia in a community hospital, 5.4% of mothers had GDM.<6>

There is weak and conflicting evidence regarding the association of GDM with an increased risk of congenital anomalies.

Overall, there is evidence of an association between carbohydrate intolerance and adult onset diabetes, macrosomia and perinatal mortality. However, the validity of the initial studies upon which the diagnostic criteria for GDM were established has been questioned.

Maneuver

Many North American authoritative groups have recommended a 1-hour 50 g oral glucose challenge test (OGCT) at about 28 weeks' gestation.<1> Abnormal results are confirmed with a 3-hour 100 g OGTT. GDM is diagnosed if the plasma glucose level equals or exceeds, on two or more occasions, 5.8 mmol/L (fasting), 10.6 mmol/L (1 hour after eating), 9.2 mmol/L (2 hours afterward) and 8.1 mmol/L (3 hours afterward).

The OGCT has reported sensitivity of 79-83% and specificity of 87-93% at plasma glucose cutoff points of 7.8-8.3 mmol/L. However, the OGCT cutoff point and the reproducibility of the OGTT itself over the long and short term have been questioned.

The 50 g 1-hour oral glucose challenge test has been suggested and has sensitivity of 79-83% and specificity of 87-93%

Whom to screen is also debated in relation to yield. Screening women over 30 years of age has been recommended by some since O'Sullivan and coworkers reported an association between adverse outcomes and poor glucose tolerance after excluding women under 25 years old. However, this would miss about half of the women with GDM, and thus some recommend universal screening.

Universal screening with the 50 g 1-hour OGCT is not done in most European countries. The World Health Organization (WHO) uses different diagnostic criteria; the 2-hour 75 g OGTT is the gold standard for both pregnant and nonpregnant adults. The diagnostic cut-off point is lower for pregnant adults (11 mmol/L). GDM is less prevalent if WHO standards are applied to a pregnant population. One randomized study suggests that deciding on treatment using these criteria does not increase adverse outcomes.<7>

Fasting blood glucose levels correlate poorly with the 100 g OGTT and the test can be cumbersome to administer. However, the maintenance of euglycemia after fasting is associated with a low prevalence of perinatal death. Fasting blood glucose has thus been proposed as an alternative screening maneuver.[8,9] Random blood glucose measurement has also been proposed;[10] neither maneuver has been adequately evaluated and their test characteristics are not known.

A study is under way that will compare the sensitivity and specificity of fasting and random blood glucose measurements and measurement of the OGCT in detecting GDM as defined by the OGTT. The study will also compare their value in predicting several perinatal outcomes.

About half of all healthy pregnant women excrete increased amounts of glucose in their urine.[11] Glucose urine measurement[12] and glycohemoglobin have poor sensitivity (30% and 26% respectively).

Effectiveness of Screening and Treatment

Screening's effectiveness in reducing perinatal mortality and morbidity has not been adequately studied

No analytic study has evaluated the impact of screening for GDM on perinatal death and illness. In a recent study[13] involving women who did or did not undergo screening for GDM according to the practices of their obstetricians, screening failed to decrease the rate of macrosomia (10.5% in the unscreened group vs. 11.2% in the screened group) and was associated with more intensive surveillance during pregnancy and a higher rate of primary cesarean section (21.0% vs. 26.7%; p <0.01). However, screened women were more likely to be obese and this is a major threat to the validity of the study.

Observational studies have suggested that the maintenance of euglycemia in women with GDM is associated with a decreased perinatal death rate.[2-4,14] In these studies confounding variables were not taken into account, nor was whether women were identified through universal screening or case-finding. The women studied were all at higher risk of morbidity (at least 2 risk factors for GDM).

Two experimental studies on the effectiveness of treatment of GDM are relevant. The first was conducted by O'Sullivan and coworkers in the late 1950s.[15] All women in the study were first screened with the 1-hour 50 g OGCT. Those with abnormal results and those with two risk factors of GDM then had the OGTT. The 615 women with GDM were randomly allocated to either a routine prenatal care group or an insulin-plus-diet treatment group. The incidence of macrosomia was decreased in the insulin-treated group (3.7% vs. 13.1%) and was comparable to the rate observed in the group of women with normal glucose tolerance (4.3%). No difference in the perinatal death rate was observed. The impact of treatment on the rates of birth trauma and operative delivery was not reported.

In a second experimental study,<16> women at high risk for GDM were offered an OGTT, identifying 72 cases. Treatment allocation was randomized for 52 subjects and the first twenty cases were allocated to the insulin or no treatment groups without randomization. Overall, 27 patients were assigned to receive insulin treatment, 11 a change in diet alone and 34 no treatment. Only 2 of the 11 subjects in the diet-alone group were older than 25 years, as compared with half of those in the two other groups. A significant decrease in macrosomia was noted in the insulin-treated group (7%), as compared with the diet-alone group (36%) and the no-treatment group (50%). One case of Erb's palsy was reported in the diet-alone group. The rate of primary cesarean section, need for forceps delivery and perinatal death rate did not differ significantly between the groups. There was no control of confounding due to maternal weight and postmaturity.

Thus, there is evidence from case series that treatment of GDM can reduce perinatal mortality. However, most women included in these studies were at high risk of GDM and were not necessarily identified through universal screening. Obstetrical practices have also changed considerably since these studies were conducted. There is also evidence from a randomized trial that treatment can reduce macrosomia. However, the benefits to be expected regarding this outcome from a screening program in Canada, even if totally effective, would at the most prevent 50 brachial plexus injuries and 109 clavicular fractures each year. Clavicular fracture is benign, and well over 80% of brachial plexus injuries resolve completely within 3 months.

Management of GDM carries with it the risk of overtreatment. Dietary restrictions may be harmful to the 70% of infants who are not destined to have macrosomia. A significantly higher incidence of small-for-gestational-age infants (20% vs. 11% in the control group) has been reported for women with GDM who maintained a low mean glucose level throughout pregnancy (4.8 mmol/L or less).

The early identification of women at increased risk of diabetes later in life is often thought to be an important outcome of screening for GDM. However, the value of such identification has not been affirmed; screening asymptomatic adults for diabetes mellitus has not been shown to have any benefit. There is a danger of labelling, since 70% of women with GDM will not have overt diabetes and a negative test result does not eliminate risk of diabetes.

Most studies of the potential impact of the treatment of GDM have not included neonatal hypoglycemia as an outcome; there is no evidence regarding prevention of this outcome.

Finally, screening can be costly both for the individual and the health care system.

Recommendations of Others

The U.S. Preventive Services Task Force,[17] as well as the American Diabetes Association and the Canadian Diabetes Association recommends universal screening for GDM in pregnant women, using the 50 g 1-hour OGCT at 28 weeks' gestation.

In 1986, the American College of Obstetricians and Gynecologists recommended screening women older than 30 years of age.[18]

Conclusions and Recommendations

A close examination of all the evidence of the effectiveness of screening for gestational diabetes raises many important questions. The studies that led to the formulation of recommendations to screen all pregnant women with a 50 g OGCT have important limitations. The validity of the diagnostic test itself is questionable. Women included in the studies that have shown potential benefits were generally at an increased risk of GDM and not identified through universal screening. Obstetrical practices have changed drastically in the last 20 years and the potential impact of screening on the perinatal death rate may not be as important as initially expected. The magnitude of the benefit of screening to the incidence of shoulder dystocia and birth trauma is likely to be small, and may not be worth the cost (clinical or financial) of screening.

An alternative to the 1-hour OGCT is the measurement of the blood glucose level after fasting or 2 hours after eating. Although they appear to be physiologically appropriate screening mechanisms, their effectiveness has not been evaluated.

These facts therefore support a cautious approach toward screening all pregnant women with a 1-hour 50 g OGCT, at 28 weeks' gestation. Conversely, women with risk factors for GDM should be carefully followed throughout their pregnancy, even though the effect of minor elevations in the maternal blood glucose level on neonatal health remains to be established.

The quality of available evidence cannot support a recommendation to include universal screening for gestational diabetes; however, a decision on screening must be made on other grounds (C Recommendation). This recommendation applies to the four screening maneuvers currently available.

The Task Force recognizes that women have varying degrees of glucose intolerance during pregnancy and that a certain proportion will have adverse outcomes and could benefit from screening. Universal screening with the 50 g OGCT has not been demonstrated to be superior, yet it can carry considerable costs. Pending the results of ongoing studies on the sensitivity and specificity of other screening maneuvers, factors such as clinical judgement (assessment of risk factors and pregnancy evolution) and available resources should be taken into account in choosing a screening strategy.

Unanswered Questions (Research Agenda)

Further research is needed to establish the relative risk of neonatal and perinatal illness in relation to various degrees of subdiabetic elevations in the maternal blood glucose level.

Evidence

The literature was identified with a MEDLINE search to December 1990 using the following MESH headings: gestational diabetes and macrosomia with the subheadings: diagnosis, prevention and control and screening.

This review was initiated in March 1988 and recommendations were finalized by the Task Force in January 1991. A report with a full reference list was published in February 1992.<19>

Acknowledgements

Assistance was provided by David J.S. Hunter, MB, ChB, Department of Obstetrics and Gynecology, McMaster University Health Sciences Centre, Hamilton, Ontario and David C. Naylor, Md, D Phil, FRCPC, Associate Professor Medicine and Health Administration, University of Toronto, Toronto, Ontario.

Selected References

1. American Diabetes Association, Inc: Gestational diabetes mellitus. *Ann Intern Med* 1986; 105: 461

2. Gyves MT, Podman HM, Little AB *et al*: A modern approach to management of pregnant diabetics: a two year analysis of perinatal outcomes. *Am J Obstet Gynecol* 1977; 128: 606-616

3. Adashi EY, Pinto H, Tyson JE: Impact of maternal euglycemia on fetal outcome in diabetic pregnancy. *Am J Obstet Gynecol* 1979; 133: 268-274

4. Roversi GD, Gargialo M, Nicolini U, *et al*: A new approach to the treatment of diabetic pregnant women. *Am J Obstet Gynecol* 1979; 135: 567-576

5. Spellacy WN, Miller S, Winegar A, *et al*: Macrosomia: maternal characteristics and infant complications. *Obstet Gynecol* 1985; 66: 158-161

6. Boyd ME, Usher RM, McLean FH: Fetal macrosomia: prediction, risks, proposed management. *Obstet Gynecol* 1983; 61: 715-722

7. Li DFH, Wong VC, O'Hoy KMKY, *et al*: Is treatment needed for mild impairment of glucose tolerance in pregnancy? A randomized controlled trial. *Br J Obstet Gynecol* 1987; 94: 851-854

8. Schneider JM, Curet LB: Obstetrical management of the pregnant diabetic. In Depp R, Eschewbach DA, Sciarra JJ (eds): *Gynecology and Obstetrics*, vol 3, Har-Row, New York, 1986

9. Mortensen HB, Molsted-Pedersen L, Kuhl C, *et al*: A screening procedure for diabetes in pregnancy. *Diabete Metab* 1985; 11: 249-253

10. Lind T: Antenatal screening using random blood glucose values. *Diabetes* 1985; 34 (Suppl 2): 17-20

11. Lind T, Anderson J: Does random blood glucose sampling outdate testing for glycosuria in the detection of diabetes during pregnancy? *Br Med J Clin Res Ed* 1984; 289: 1569-1571

12. Bitzen PO, Schersten B: Assessment of laboratory methods for detection of unsuspected diabetes in primary health care. *Scand J Prim Health Care* 1986; 4: 85-95

13. Santini DL, Ales KL: The impact of universal screening for gestational glucose intolerance on outcome of pregnancy. *Surg Gynecol Obstet* 1990; 170: 427-436

14. Coustan DR, Imarah J: Prophylactic insulin treatment of gestational diabetes reduces the incidence of macrosomia, operative delivery and birth trauma. *Am J Obstet Gynecol* 1984; 150: 836-842

15. O'Sullivan JB, Gelliss S, Dandrow RV, *et al*: The potential diabetic and her treatment in pregnancy. *Obstet Gynecol* 1966; 27: 683-689

16. Coustan DR, Lewis SB: Insulin therapy for gestational diabetes. *Obstet Gynecol* 1978; 51: 306-310

17. U.S. Preventive Services Task Force: *Guide to Clinical Preventive Services: an Assessment of the Effectiveness of 169 Interventions*. Williams & Wilkins, Baltimore, Md, 1989: 95-100

18. Management of diabetes mellitus in pregnancy. *Am Coll Obst Gynecol Tech Bull* 1986; 92: 1-2

19. Canadian Task Force on the Periodic Health Examination: The periodic health examination, 1992 update: 1. Screening for gestational diabetes mellitus. *Can Med Assoc J* 1992; 147: 435-443

Screening for Gestational Diabetes Mellitus

MANEUVER	EFFECTIVENESS	LEVEL OF EVIDENCE <REF>	RECOMMENDATION
50 g 1-hour oral glucose challenge test (OGCT) at 28 week's gestation	Effectiveness of universal screening not evaluated. Screening may result in decreased incidence of macrosomia and birth trauma. Important questions persist about the significance of mild elevations in the blood glucose level and the benefit of treatment.	Uncontrolled trial<12> (II-1); cohort study<7> (II-2); case series<8-11> (III)	Poor evidence to include or exclude in periodic health examination of pregnant women (C)
Measurement of fasting and random blood glucose levels	Sensitivity and specificity not properly evaluated. Women with an abnormal fasting glucose level are more likely than others to benefit from intervention.	Case series<2-4> (III)	Poor evidence to include or exclude in periodic health examination of pregnant women (C)
Search for risk factors* at the first visit and test for glycosuria at each visit. If result is positive do fasting, postprandial and oral glucose tolerance tests (OGTTs)	Effectiveness not evaluated.	Expert opinion<5> and case series<6> (III)	Poor evidence to include or exclude in periodic health examination of pregnant women (C)

* Risk factors for gestational diabetes are obesity, history of miscarriage or fetal death, age 40 years or more, family history of diabetes, polyhydramnios, history of premature infant or infant with macrosomia or congenital malformation, pre-eclampsia, excessive weight gain and glycosuria.

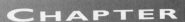

CHAPTER 3

Smoking and Pregnancy

By Susan E. Moner

3

Smoking and Pregnancy

Prepared by Susan E. Moner, MD[1]

Tobacco smoking is associated with adverse pregnancy outcomes which may be preventable through smoking cessation interventions. Advice, multiple component programs, behavioral strategies, repeated contacts, and self-help manuals are effective in decreasing tobacco smoking significantly in pregnant women. Interventions are effective in diverse populations with varying levels of nicotine dependence and at different periods of gestation. A reduction in tobacco use increases birth weight, decreases the incidence of low birth weight infants and is cost effective. Cognitive ability is marginally improved in children of mothers who have not smoked during gestation. Further evaluative research is needed on interventions designed to maintain abstinence. Prevention of tobacco-related illnesses in the non-pregnant population is dealt with in Chapter 43.

Burden of Suffering

Smoking during pregnancy harms both the mother and her developing fetus. Aside from increased morbidity and mortality from cancers, cardiovascular and pulmonary disease in the mother, smoking has been implicated in the etiology of abruptio placenta, placenta previa, spontaneous abortion, premature delivery, and stillbirth. Prenatal smoking is thought to account for about 18% of cases of low birth weight (<2500 g), and also increases risk of shortened gestation, respiratory distress syndrome, and sudden infant death syndrome.

Cigarette smoking is the principal cause of low birth weight in developed countries

Cigarette smoking is the principal cause of low birth weight in developed countries. Intrauterine growth retardation is the most strongly documented adverse effect of smoking during pregnancy. This is a significant public health concern because low birth weight is the most important single determinant of neonatal and infant morbidity and mortality. Retarded fetal growth in the offspring of smokers may be attributable to several factors, including the vasoconstricting properties of nicotine, elevated fetal carboxyhemoglobin and catecholamine levels, fetal tissue hypoxia, reduced delivery of nutritional elements and elevation of heart rate and blood pressure. Even after controlling for alcohol use, socioeconomic status, maternal height, maternal weight and years of education, smoking has been implicated in long-term effects such as poor cognitive performance on achievement tests and decreased physical growth.

---

[1] Spaulding Rehabilitation Hospital, Boston, Massachusetts

In Canada, the incidence of low birth weight in infants of mothers in all age groups declined from 6.6% of 343,000 births in 1971 to 4.6% of 377,00 births in 1989, a 30.3% decline over the 18 year period, comprising mainly birth weights of 1,500 to 2,499 g. The prevalence of birth weights in this range decreased from 5.8% of births in 1971 to 4.0% in 1989, while the prevalence of very low birth weight (<1500 g) remained stable. Most of this decline in low birth weight has been attributed to a decrease in smoking rates in women of reproductive age. The Labour Force Survey Smoking Supplement estimated that smoking rates for Canadian women of reproductive age (15-44 years) declined from 37% in 1972 to 29% in 1986.

Exposure to environmental tobacco smoke (passive smoking) may also have a modest adverse effect on birth weight.[1] Hair concentrations of nicotine and cotinine in women and their newborn infants provide biochemical evidence that infants of smokers and of passive smokers have measurable systemic exposure to cigarette smoke toxins. The clinical significance of this exposure is as yet unclear.

Maneuver

The interventions developed to help pregnant smokers quit that have been evaluated in published research studies include smoking cessation advice, feedback and individual or group counselling.[2] Nicotine replacement therapy has not been adequately studied in pregnant women. Use of such therapy by pregnant women has been advocated by Benowitz[3] because of its benefits as an adjunct to smoking cessation therapy in non-pregnant populations. Nicotine replacement cannot be recommended at present, however, since it could conceivably contribute to adverse effects on the fetus and because its efficacy in pregnant smokers has not yet been established. Interventions aimed at reducing exposure to environmental tobacco smoke have also not been evaluated.

"Smoking Cessation Advice" has been defined as providing health education to tobacco smoking pregnant women to stop smoking.[4-7] The underlying premise has been that if women were aware of the adverse effects of smoking during pregnancy they would stop smoking.[4] Such advice has usually included information about the effects of smoking on the fetus given directly by a physician or midwife, supplemented by a health education booklet. The advantage of this intervention is that it is brief. In the trial reported by Lilley[7] it lasted 10 minutes, and could be given by a physician or midwife, who would ordinarily be in contact with the patient for prenatal care. However, knowledge concerning adverse health effects is necessary but not always sufficient to induce patient compliance.[8] Since addictions are complex behaviours with multifactorial origins, simply giving women information about the ill-effects of smoking and advising

Knowledge concerning adverse health effects is necessary but not always sufficient to induce patient compliance

them to quit without providing the support needed to achieve that goal may not produce the desired result.

"Feedback" implies evaluating patient status prior to the intervention through a carbon monoxide breath sample, a cotinine blood sample, or a fetal ultrasound. Patients are provided with the results of these measures, sometimes with comparative measures in nonsmoking individuals. Health advice is given about how to improve these measures through smoking cessation.

Multiple component intervention programs combine elements of health education, self-help manuals on how to quit smoking, supportive counselling and multiple follow-up contacts. These interventions are more labour intensive than advice, feedback, or group counselling.

Effectiveness of Treatment

It is estimated that 25% to 40% of pregnant women smokers quit smoking without any intervention for at least a brief time upon learning they are pregnant.

Smoking Cessation Advice

There have been several randomized controlled trials[4-7] of smoking cessation advice among pregnant women. Unfortunately, design problems have included small sample size, poor description of the intervention,[5,6] lack of uniform intervention delivery and contamination of treatment and control groups.[6] Follow-up was reported to be 66% to 100%. Outcomes were based on self-report with only one study[5] reporting biochemical verification. Dropouts were omitted from the final analysis in all studies using advice as the intervention. Quit rates (stopping smoking for the remainder of the pregnancy) were consistently higher (but not statistically higher) in the experimental (6-14%) as opposed to the control groups (1-6%).

A 1993 meta-analysis found that advice significantly reduced the proportion of smokers who continued smoking through pregnancy, compared with smokers who received standard antenatal care (odds ratio 0.39; 95% confidence interval (CI): 0.21-0.75).[9]

In primiparas, MacArthur[6] reported that mean birth weight in the intervention group receiving advice was 68 g heavier than that of controls ($p < 0.06$). The author also noted that primiparas in the intervention group were more likely to have received adequate advice. Sixty one percent of primiparas recalled being advised to stop smoking by the obstetrician or by the midwife, compared with only 45% of multiparas. Mean birth weights of multiparas in the two groups were not statistically different.

Feedback

Three trials have used feedback involving serum cotinine levels, carbon monoxide levels, and ultrasound examinations.[10-12] Blood tests and ultrasound are often already part of antenatal care; testing carbon monoxide levels is non-invasive. Thus, minimal additional cost or time was involved. Although these were randomized trials and provided good descriptions of the interventions, design problems included poor follow-up,[10,12] small subject numbers[10,11] and omission of dropouts from analysis. Again, quit rates were higher (but not statistically higher) in the experimental group. One trial was designed to test a self-reported multifactorial lifestyle change which included drinking and other health-related activities as well as smoking. The number of smokers who reported a change in smoking behaviour was low and the results could have been greatly influenced by omission of drop-outs from the analysis.[11] Thus there is insufficient evidence to evaluate the effectiveness of feedback.

Group Counselling

In a group counselling intervention adapted by Loeb et al[13] from the Multiple Risk Factor Intervention Trial, the significance of the results was limited by the fact that only 10% of the treatment group attended all counselling sessions. Experimental and control groups had similar quit rates (15% and 14%, respectively). Two of three trials[14,15] that compared counselling to usual care found significantly increased abstinence rates after the intervention (14% vs. 8%; and 15% vs. 5%). One small trial of women attending a public health clinic[16] found counselling made no difference (21% vs. 23% abstinence during pregnancy) but the usual intervention was clearly very effective. Most studies that compared post-partum recidivism rates between counselling and control groups found higher relapse rates among quitters in the control groups compared to those in the intervention groups. Group counselling thus has had mixed results and should be evaluated further.

Multiple Component Programs

Several trials have evaluated multiple component programs.[17-22] All but two studies[21,22] were randomized trials, and most had over one hundred subjects with 84-98% follow-up. Except for two studies,[18,19] drop-outs were counted as treatment failures.

Quit rates were significantly increased ($p<0.05$) by all behavioral strategy interventions (quit rates, experimental groups 10-27%; control groups 2-9%). Clinically significant birth weight differences were observed, with decreased low (<2500 g) and very low birth weight (<1500 g) in infants of those who quit smoking. One study found a 5.6% incidence of low birth weight in the intervention groups compared with 6.52% incidence in the control groups.<19>

Ershoff,<19> Gillies<22> and Windsor<23> found smoking cessation interventions were cost effective, comparing the cost of hospital delivery in treated versus control groups including the cost of the intervention. Ershoff found a benefit of 2.8 to 1 for the intervention vs. the control group.

A 1993 meta-analysis of behavioral strategies found a significant reduction in the proportion of smokers who continued smoking through pregnancy, compared with standard antenatal care or with personal advice supplemented by written materials (odds ratio 0.30; 95% CI: 0.23-0.38).<24> However, the author concluded that since even the most effective strategies implemented during pregnancy have a limited effect, obstetricians and midwives should also support population strategies towards progressive reduction in cigarette smoking for society as a whole. In a separate analysis of all interventions to reduce smoking in pregnancy, Lumley concluded that smoking cessation interventions result in a small increase in mean birthweight. Effects on preterm birth and perinatal mortality were unclear.

Maternal Smoking After Pregnancy

Postpartum recidivism was high in studies which included post-intervention<4,22> and postpartum assessment.<18-21> Sexton found that three years after completing the trial, 72% of those who quit during pregnancy were smoking again and 91% of those who did not quit during pregnancy were still smoking.

Thus, despite having achieved statistically significant quit rates during pregnancy, these gains were not maintained and would not be assumed to improve the mother's long-term health in the majority of cases. The clinically significant benefit may be limited to the offspring.

Long-term Effects of Maternal Smoking During Pregnancy on Children

Most long-term studies of children whose mothers smoked during pregnancy have focused on growth and neurocognitive ability. Average height and weight of 3-year-old children whose mothers had quit during pregnancy were significantly increased over children of non-quitters (height $p<0.001$, weight $p<0.05$).<25> Whether the differences found, (0.45 kg for weight and 1.13 cm for height) were clinically significant may be open to question.

Several cohort and case-control studies have noted differences in psychometric test results in children of women who smoked during pregnancy and children of non-smokers.<26-33> Sexton and colleagues<26> carried out cognitive testing in the three-year-old offspring of mothers who had quit and in children of women who had continued smoking during pregnancy. The Preschool Version of the Minnesota Child Development Inventory and the McCarthy Scales of Children's Abilities were used as outcome measures. The General Cognitive Index score in children of quitters averaged 5 points higher than in children of non-quitters (p<0.01), even when babies of <2,500 g birth weight were excluded and after controlling for other variables such as socioeconomic status, maternal behaviour, maternal time available to child and child characteristics. Statistically significant differences of one to 3 points were also noted on the McCarthy subscales. McCarthy suggests 15 points between pairs of subscales as a rule of thumb for determining noteworthy differences. Other investigators have reported inconsistent effects of smoking on psychological testing – both 1) significantly lower scores in the smoking group versus the non-smokers and 2) no significant differences between children of smokers and non-smokers. Based on the evidence, one would conclude that smoking during pregnancy may be detrimental to the offspring or at best, smoking has no effect – in no case has smoking been shown to coincide with improved psychometric test scores.

Characteristics of Women Who Quit Smoking During Pregnancy

Women who quit smoking had higher socioeconomic levels, were older, had smoked fewer cigarettes and were better educated

Four percent of women deny smoking even in the face of biochemical evidence to the contrary. To determine how well women who reported quitting smoking prior to pregnancy were able to maintain that status, several authors have studied "spontaneous quitters" (i.e. women who quit smoking in response to pregnancy before the start of prenatal care). In a randomized controlled trial by Quinn, Mullen, and Ershoff,<19,34> spontaneous quitters were defined as women who stated that they had quit smoking since becoming pregnant and had not smoked for at least 24 hours. This group was compared to a group who reported smoking at least seven cigarettes per week prior to pregnancy. Spontaneous quitters and smokers differed significantly in the following respects: 1) Spontaneous quitters had been lighter smokers prior to pregnancy; 2) they were less likely to have another smoker in their household; 3) indicated a stronger belief in the harmful effect of maternal smoking on fetal health; 4) had a history of fewer miscarriages; and 5) had entered prenatal care earlier. Compared to women who maintained cessation as measured by urine cotinine levels, women who relapsed had less confidence in their ability to stay off cigarettes, were more likely to be multigravidas, and believed less strongly in the harmful effects of maternal smoking on fetal health. Other authors have found that women who quit smoking had higher socioeconomic levels, were older, had smoked fewer cigarettes, and were better educated than women who continued smoking.

Recommendations of Others

The Canadian Nurses Association and the U.S. Preventive Services Task Force<35> recommend that pregnant women receive smoking cessation education. The Canadian Medical Association, American College of Physicians, American College of Obstetricians and Gynecologists, and the American Academy of Pediatrics, recommend that physicians encourage smoking cessation. The Royal College of Physicians and Surgeons of Canada recommend that smokers who wish to stop smoking should receive effective help.

Conclusions and Recommendations

Interventions which include advice, multiple components, behavioral strategies, support, multiple contacts, and self-help manuals are effective in significantly decreasing tobacco smoking in pregnant women. Interventions work with diverse populations with different levels of nicotine dependence and at different stages of gestation.

Decrease in tobacco use has a beneficial effect on increasing average birth weight and decreasing the incidence of low birth weight infants. Smoking cessation interventions are cost effective as a result of decreasing the number of low birth weight infants. Cognitive ability is also improved in children of mothers who did not smoke during gestation. Thus, there is good evidence to recommend smoking cessation interventions for all pregnant women who smoke (A Recommendation).

Unanswered Questions (Research Agenda)

More research is needed on interventions to maintain abstinence post-delivery.

Evidence

Information retrieval sources were in consultation with Addiction Research Foundation Library and Fudger Medical Library at Toronto General Hospital using MEDLINE, 1966 to 1993. Key words used include: Smoking, smoking cessation, tobacco; infant, low birth weight, small for gestational age, newborn; birth weight, fetus, growth retardation; abnormalities, brain development; growth, brain growth; psychometrics; child development; pregnancy; prenatal care, exposure, delayed effects; longitudinal studies; evaluation studies.

Science Citation Index, 1990-1992: Author's names in clinical trials.

Expert consultation and review of literature files of: Smoking Cessation Clinic, Community Treatment Research Unit, Addiction Research Foundation Dr. R Frecker. Prevention, Health Promotion, Addiction Research Foundation, M. Pope, and reference sections from articles.

This review was initiated in January 1993 and the recommendations were finalized by the Task Force in June 1993.

Acknowledgements

Funding for this report was provided by Health Canada under the Government of Canada's Brighter Futures Initiatives. The Task Force thanks Helen P. Batty, MD, CCFP, MEd, FCFP, Associate Professor, Department of Family and Community Medicine, University of Toronto, Toronto, Ontario and Douglas M.C. Wilson, MD, CCFP, FCFP, Professor of Family Medicine, McMaster University, Hamilton, Ontario for reviewing the draft report.

Selected References

1. Fortier I, Marcoux S, Brisson J: Passive smoking during pregnancy and the risk of delivering a small-for-gestational-age infant. *Am J Epidemiol* 1994; 139: 294-301

2. Lumley J: Stopping smoking-again. [editorial] *Br J Obstet Gynaecol* 1991; 98: 847-849

3. Benowitz NL: Nicotine replacement therapy during pregnancy. *JAMA* 1991; 266: 3174-3177

4. Baric L, MacArthur C, Sherwood M: A study of health education aspects of smoking in pregnancy. *Int J Health Educ* 1976; 19 (Suppl 2): 1-15

5. Burling T, *et al*: Changes in smoking during pregnancy. Paper presented at the Society for Behavioral Medicine, Philadelphia, PA, May 25, 1984

6. McArthur C, Newton JR, Knox EG: Effect of anti-smoking health education on infant size at birth: a randomized controlled trial. *Br J Obstet Gynaecol* 1987; 94: 295-300

7. Lilley J and Forster DP: A randomized controlled trial of individual counselling of smokers in pregnancy. *Public Health* 1986; 100: 309-315

8. Meichenbaun D, Turk D: Facilitating treatment adherence: a practitioner's guidebook. New York: Plenum, 1987

9. Lumley J: Advice as a strategy for reducing smoking in pregnancy. In Pregnancy and Childbirth Module (eds. Enkin MW, Keirse MJNC, Renfrew MJ, Neilson JP), "Cochrane Database of Systematic Reviews": Review No. 03394, 2 October 1993. Published through "Cochrane Updates on Disk", Oxford: Update Software, 1993, Disk Issue 2

10. Bauman KE, Bryan ES, Dent CW, *et al*: The influence of observing carbon monoxide levels on cigarette smoking by public prenatal patients. *Am J Public Health* 1983; 73: 1089-1091

11. Reading AE, Campbell S, Cox DN, *et al*: Health beliefs and health care behaviours in pregnancy. *Psychol Med* 1982; 12: 379-383

12. Haddow JE, Knight GJ, Kloza EM, *et al*: Cotinine-assisted intervention in pregnancy to reduce smoking and low birth weight delivery. *Br J Obstet Gynaecol* 1991; 98: 859-865

13. Loeb B, *et al*: A randomized trial of smoking intervention during pregnancy. Paper presented to the American Public Health Association Annual Meeting, Dallas, TX, Nov. 15, 1983

14. Windsor RA, Lowe JB, Perkins LL, *et al*: Health education for pregnant smokers: its behavioural impact and cost benefit. *Am J Public Health* 1993; 83: 201-206

15. O'Connor AM, Davies BL, Dulberg CS, *et al*: Effectiveness of a pregnancy smoking cessation program. *JOGNN* 1992; 21: 385-392

16. Petersen L, Handel J, Kotch J, *et al: Smoking reduction during pregnancy by a program of self-help and clinical support.* *Obstet Gynecol* 1992; 79(6): 924-930

17. Windsor RA, Cutler g, Morris J, *et al*: The effectiveness of smoking cessation methods for smokers in public health maternity clinics: a randomized trial. *Am J Public Health* 1985; 75: 1389-1392

18. Sexton M and Hebel JR: A clinical trial of change in maternal smoking and its effect on birth weight. *JAMA* 1984; 251: 911-915

19. Ershoff DH, Quinn VP, Mullen PD, *et al*: Pregnancy and medical cost outcomes of a self-help prenatal smoking cessation program in a HMO. *Public Health Rep* 1990; 105: 340-347

20. Mayer JP, Hawkins B, Todd R: A randomized evaluation of smoking cessation interventions for pregnant women at a WIC clinic. *Am J Public Health* 1990; 80: 76-78

21. Hjalmarson AIM, Hahn L, Svanberg B: Stopping smoking in pregnancy: effect of a self-help manual in controlled trial. *Br J Obstet Gynaecol* 1991; 98: 260-264

22. Gilies PA, *et al*: Successful anti-smoking intervention in pregnancy – behaviour change, "clinical indicators" or both? In Durston B, Jamrozik K (eds): Tobacco and Health 1990, The Global War. Procedings of the Seventh World Conference on Tobacco and Health, 1st-5th April 1990, Perth, Western Australia

23. Windsor RA, Warner KE, Cutter GR: A cost-effectiveness analysis of self-help smoking cessation methods for pregnant women. *Public Health Rep* 1988; 103: 83-88

24. Lumley J: Behavioural strategies for reducing smoking in pregnancy. In Pregnancy and Childbirth Module (eds. Enkin MW, Keirse MJNC, Renfrew MJ, Neilson JP), "Cochrane Database of Systematic Reviews": Review No. 03397, 27 September 1993. Published through "Cochrane Updates on Disk", Oxford: Update Software, 1993, Disk Issue 2

25. Fox NL, Sexton M, Hebel JR: Prenatal exposure to tobacco. Effects on physical growth at age three. *Int J Epidemiol* 1990; 19: 66-71

26. Sexton M, Fox NL, Hebel JR: Prenatal exposure to tobacco. Effects on cognitive functioning at age three. *Int J Epidemiol* 1990; 19: 72-77

27. Fergusson DM, Lloyd M: Smoking during pregnancy and its effects on child cognitive ability from the ages of 8 to 12 years. *Paediatr Perinatal Epidemiol* 1991; 5: 189-200

28. Baghurst PA, Tong SL, Woodward A, *et al*: Effects of maternal smoking upon neuropsychological development in early childhood: importance of taking account of social and environmental factors. *Paediatr Perinatal Epidemiol* 1992; 6: 403-415

29. Makin J, Fried PA, Watkinson B: A comparison of active and passive smoking during pregnancy: long-term effects. *Neurotoxicol Teratol* 1991; 13: 5-12

30. Naeye R, Peters EC: Mental development of children whose mothers smoked during pregnancy. *Obstetr Gynaecol* 1984; 64: 601-607

31. Bauman K, Flewelling RL, LaPrelle J: Parental cigarette smoking and cognitive performance of children. *Health Psychol* 1991; 10: 282-288

32. Rantakallio P, Koiranen M: Neurological handicaps among children whose mothers smoked during pregnancy. *Prev Med* 1987; 16: 597-606

33. Hardy JB and Mellits ED: Does maternal smoking during pregnancy have a long-term effect on the child? *Lancet* 1972; 1332-1336

34. Quinn VP, Mullen PD, Ershoff DH: Women who stop smoking spontaneously prior to prenatal care and predictors of relapse before delivery. *Addict Behav* 1991; 16: 29-40

35. U.S. Preventive Services Task Force: *Guide to Clinical Preventive Services: an Assessment of the Effectiveness of 169 Interventions*. Williams & Wilkins, Baltimore, Md, 1989: 289-292

Smoking and Pregnancy

MANEUVER	EFFECTIVENESS	LEVEL OF EVIDENCE <REF>	RECOMMENDATION
Smoking cessation intervention including advice, multiple component programs and/or behavioral strategies	Smoking cessation interventions improve quit rates.	Randomized controlled trials<14,17-20> and meta-analysis of randomized controlled trials<9,24> (I)	Good evidence to include smoking cessation interventions in the periodic health examination of pregnant women who smoke (A)
	Smoking cessation decreases incidence of low birth weight infants.	Randomized controlled trials<18,19> (I)	
	Smoking cessation interventions are cost effective.	Randomized controlled trials<19,23> (I)	
	Smoking cessation improves cognitive ability in children of mothers who quit smoking during gestation.	Cohort studies<26-33> (II-2)	

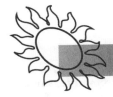

CHAPTER 4

Prevention of Low Birth Weight/Preterm Birth

By Orlando P. da Silva

4

Prevention of Low Birth Weight/Preterm Birth

Prepared by Orlando P. da Silva, MD, FRCPC[1]

Prematurity is defined as gestational age less than 37 completed weeks at birth and low birth weight (LBW), as weight less than 2,500 g. Such infants may be premature, small for gestational age, or both. Social support alone is not effective in improving pregnancy outcome with respect to improving birth weight or gestational age at delivery in high-risk populations. The situation for multicomponent programs is less clear and the Task Force found the evidence available to evaluate them inconclusive. While diet supplementation in the prenatal period in pregnant women at high risk for undernutrition increases birth weight slightly and has been shown to be cost effective in one U.S. study, the evidence regarding its effectiveness in preventing preterm birth or improving fetal and infant survival is also inconclusive. Cessation of smoking in pregnancy is addressed in Chapter 3 and screening for preeclampsia (Chapter 13) do show some benefits with respect to LBW and they are recommended by the Task Force.

Burden of Suffering

Low birth weight is associated with about 75% of early neonatal mortality in both Canada and the U.S

LBW is associated with about 75% of early neonatal mortality in both Canada and the United States. A U.S. study of 349 neonatal deaths found that 83% of deaths were associated with delivery <37 weeks and 66% with delivery <29 weeks. LBW also contributes significantly to infant and childhood morbidity.<1> About 6% of infants born in Canada are of LBW. The cost of care for these babies is very high. The average cost per admission in the United States has been estimated to be over US$ 7,500 per infant. The burden on society is even greater when long-term costs are taken into account.

Cigarette smoking is the most important established risk factor for intrauterine growth retardation

In developed countries, cigarette smoking is the most important established factor with a direct causal impact on the rate of intrauterine growth retardation (defined as birth weight <2500 g and gestational age >37 weeks). Other important factors include poor gestational nutrition, low pre-pregnancy weight, primiparity, female sex and short stature.<1> Although most preterm deliveries are of unknown etiology, cigarette smoking, prior preterm delivery, spontaneous abortion and low pre-pregnancy weight, seem to play an important role in determining the rate of preterm births.<1> The rate

[1] Department of Pediatrics, Division of Neonatology, The University of Western Ontario, St. Joseph's Health Centre, London, Ontario

of LBW deliveries also correlates directly with poverty, social disadvantage<1> and cocaine use.

Maneuver

The prevention of LBW and of preterm births using multicomponent programs was initially implemented in France;<2> programs vary considerably with respect to their components (see Table 1) and target populations. Some strategies are common to most programs, such as staff and patient education concerning the early signs and symptoms of preterm labour and the provision of ready access to health care personnel. All include changes in antenatal care: more frequent visits, longer visits and continuity of care. Most include serial cervical assessment, self-monitoring of uterine contractions and lifestyle modifications. The major feature that distinguishes the French programs from those in North America is their use of home visiting by nurse/midwives.

Effectiveness of Prevention

Several studies have evaluated multicomponent programs using a before-and-after design for both general and high risk patient populations.<2-8> While these studies tend to show significant improvement in preterm delivery rates (from 5.4-6.75% before to 2.4-5.8% after), they have significant methodological limitations (e.g. comparing different patient populations and inadequate controls).

Main et al<9> conducted a randomized trial in Pennsylvania of a preterm prevention program in an indigent, mainly black population of women at high risk for preterm birth. After risk scoring, patients were allocated to either an intervention (n=64) or control group (n=68). The intervention group was followed in a special clinic and received intensive education, frequent clinic visits and easy access to medical staff. The control group received standard care in a separate clinic. The demographic characteristics of the two groups were comparable. Outcomes were not significantly different in the two groups. Deliveries prior to 37 weeks occurred in 25% of the intervention group and 20.6% of the control group. The LBW rate was 21.9% in the study group and 19.1% in the controls.

Mueller-Heubach and colleagues<10> randomized patients after scoring them for risk of preterm labour and delivery. A major component of the study was the training and education of the medical staff in making high-risk patients more aware of the subtle signs and symptoms of preterm labour. All patients were seen in the same clinic. No difference in the rate of preterm birth (20.8% intervention group, 22.1% control group) was found. However, a steady decrease in the rate of premature birth was noted during the study period (statistically lower than historic rates from the same institution).

In a controlled, non-randomized trial in which patients attending a South Carolina Twin Clinic were compared with those attending a normal care high-risk clinic,[11] the intervention included regular evaluation of maternal symptoms and cervical status by a single, certified nurse-midwife, intensive education regarding the prevention of preterm birth, individualized modification of maternal activity, increased attention to nutrition and tracking of clinic non-attenders. There were no inter-group differences in demographic characteristics, adequacy of prenatal care or antepartum complications. Twin Clinic attenders had lower rates of birth weights <1500 g (6% vs. 26%; p<0.0001), neonatal intensive care unit admission (13% vs. 38%; p<0.0001), and perinatal mortality (1% vs. 8%; p<0.0002).

In an evaluation of the West Los Angeles Preterm Birth Prevention Project which served a predominantly Hispanic population, Goldenberg et al,[13] in 8 clinics were randomized to intervention or control groups.[12] High-risk patients were identified by a risk scoring system. Intervention groups received special education, more frequent visits and one of the following bed rest, social work, Provera or placebo (n=1,774). Controls received standard care (n=880). Preterm birth rates were 7.4% in the experimental group and 9.1% in controls (p=0.063). In multiple regression analysis, differences were significant (p<0.05) when preterm risk was taken into account (the experimental group had a lower proportion of Hispanic women, women who had not completed high school, and lower gravidity and parity).

Goldenberg et al,[13] in a prospective, randomized controlled trial in Alabama, evaluated the effectiveness of a program to prevent preterm birth in a predominantly black, low-socioeconomic population. The program consisted of risk scoring, intensive weekly observation including cervical examinations, and education of medical staff and patients about the signs and symptoms of preterm labour. Four hundred and ninety-one high-risk patients were allocated to the intervention group and 478 to the control group. The demographic distribution was similar in both groups, and the two groups received prenatal care at different sites to avoid "contamination". The rate of premature delivery was similar in the intervention and control group (15.9% vs. 14.2%), as was the incidence of LBW (<2,500 g) delivery (12.9% vs. 12.2%).

McLaughlin et al,[14] in a prospective randomized, controlled trial, evaluated the effectiveness of comprehensive prenatal care for low-income women in reducing LBW. Two hundred and seventeen women were assigned to comprehensive care and 211 to standard care. The intervention consisted of care provided by a multidiscliplinary team that included nurse-midwives, social workers, a nutritionist, paraprofessional home visitors, and a psychologist. The team focused on psychosocial support for the mothers, education about self-care, and promotion of healthy behaviours during pregnancy (good nutrition, avoidance of alcohol and drugs, and reduction of smoking). The demographic distribution of both groups was fairly similar, except for a higher percentage of single primiparas in the comprehensive care group (74% vs. 59.2%). The percentage of smokers was not described. The mean birth weight was not significantly different in the two groups. However when the subgroup of primaparas (comprehensive, n=86; standard, n=79) was analyzed separately, mean birth weight was significantly higher in the comprehensive care group (3,233 g vs. 3,089 g).

Heins et al[15] conducted a multicenter randomized controlled trial in South Carolina. They evaluated nurse-midwifery and a comprehensive preterm/LBW prevention program in women identified as being at high risk for LBW deliveries. The intervention, provided by nurse-midwives, included patient education to identify the signs and symptoms of preterm labour, activity counselling based on monitoring of the cervix through frequent visits to the prenatal clinic, stress reduction by enhanced social support, nutrition counselling with emphasis on adequate weight gain, counselling concerning substance abuse and around-the-clock access to medical staff. Women in the control group received standard care by obstetricians. The two groups of patients were seen at different clinic sites. Seven hundred and twenty-eight patients were randomly allocated to the nurse-midwifery intervention and 730 to the control group. The two groups were comparable in terms of race, education, marital status, age, gravidity, and smoking habits. The results showed a LBW rate of 19.0% in the intervention group compared to 20.5% in controls. A subset of the population consisting of black patients with very high-risk scores did show a significant decrease in the incidence of very LBW, when compared to the same population in the control group (odds ratio 0.35, 95% confidence interval (CI): 0.1-0.9).

In summary, randomized multicenter trials evaluating programs at health clinics designed to prevent preterm delivery and/or LBW have shown conflicting results in high-risk populations.

Aspirin for Women At Risk of Pregnancy-induced Hypertension

Meta-analysis of data from randomized controlled trials on the use of low-dose aspirin for the treatment and/or prophylaxis of women at risk for pregnancy-induced hypertension has shown that this intervention significantly reduces the rate of premature deliveries, with no change in perinatal death rate.[16] However, the trials included in the review were too small to provide reliable results. Two recent, large, multicentered trials[17,18] failed to show any benefit on perinatal outcome of low-dose aspirin for the prevention and treatment of pregnancy-induced hypertension (also see preeclampsia, Chapter 13). In an Italian study[17] babies born to women in the

Health clinic programs designed to prevent preterm delivery and/or low birth weight have had contradictory results in high-risk populations

treatment group had a 16 g increase in mean birth weight and a slightly lower rate of premature deliveries (1.7%). In a British study,[18] the average duration of pregnancy was 1 day longer and average birth weight 32 g heavier for babies born to women in the aspirin group compared to those in the placebo group; there was no significant difference in the rate of stillbirths or neonatal deaths. Although the results from the British study were statistically significant, the clinical significance of the differences is questionable. Given the currently available evidence, routine prophylactic or therapeutic administration of low-dose aspirin cannot be recommended for the prevention of LBW or premature delivery in women with pregnancy induced hypertension.

Programs With Greater Emphasis on Social Support

A randomized trial of prenatal nurse visiting was conducted in disadvantaged primiparous women,[19] i.e. teenage mothers, unmarried mothers or mothers of low socioeconomic status. Nurses made home visits to educate parents, enhance informal support, encourage smoking cessation, establish linkages with community services, and emphasize the pregnant woman's personal strengths. One hundred and eighty-nine patients were randomly allocated to the intervention group and 165 to the control group. The mean birth weight in both groups did not differ significantly (3,285 g vs. 3,262 g). The LBW rate was also similar as was the rate of preterm deliveries. However a subset of 21 teenage mothers enrolled in the intervention before mid-gestation had infants with higher birth weights (3,437 g) than did 11 comparable control mothers (2,922 g). This difference was significant ($P<.001$) after adjusting for height, weight, smoking, and length of gestation.

Spencer et al[20] conducted a randomized trial involving 1,227 women at risk for delivering a LBW baby, as identified by a broad risk assessment. The intervention group received home visits by lay workers whose goal was to reduce stress by providing social support. Assistance included acting as a confidante, helping patients obtain state benefits, provision of child care and help with domestic chores. No difference was found in the mean birth weight, or in the proportion of LBW and preterm births in the two groups. A subset of young primiparous women showed a trend toward fewer LBW and preterm babies in the intervention group, but this difference did not reach statistical significance.

Oakley et al,[21] in a randomized controlled trial, evaluated the impact of a social support intervention on pregnancy outcome. Five hundred and nine high-risk, socially disadvantaged women with a previous history of giving birth to a LBW baby, were randomly allocated to receive either a social support intervention in pregnancy in addition to standard care (n=255) or standard care alone (n=254). The intervention consisted of home visiting by the midwives, who provided advice with regards to healthy behaviours, referrals to other health professionals and welfare agencies, a listening service and 24-hour telephone contact. They did not provide any clinical care. The demographic profile of the two groups was comparable. Mean birth weight in the intervention group was only 38 g higher than in the controls. Mothers in the intervention group experienced more vaginal deliveries, and had a positive response to the social experience.

Bryce and coworkers, in Australia,<22> conducted a randomized controlled trial of antenatal social support to prevent preterm birth (defined as gestational age between 20 and 36 weeks at birth) in a population of public and private care patients at high-risk for preterm birth. Women were eligible for the program if they had a previous history of preterm births, LBW, perinatal death, more than two first trimester pregnancy losses, one or more second trimester miscarriages, or antepartum hemorrhage in a previous pregnancy. The patients were randomized by block design prior to obtaining consent, and allocated to control (n=986) or intervention groups (n=981). The control group received standard perinatal care, while the intervention group was offered additional social support provided by midwives. The intervention consisted of frequent home visitation and telephone contact, aimed at providing a listening service, information, advice and material aid as well as acting as a confidante. Clinical care was not provided, except in emergency situations. The patient demographics were similar in both groups. The rate of preterm birth was 12.8% in the intervention group compared to 14.9% in controls. 12.5% of women in the program delivered a LBW infant, compared to 12.9% in the control group. In order to prevent one LBW infant 250 women would have had to receive the intervention. Forty-two women would have had to receive the intervention in order to prevent a single preterm delivery. This study had only 60% power to show a risk reduction greater than 25% in the rate of preterm deliveries in the intervention group.

In a recent, large, multicenter randomized controlled clinical trial of psychosocial support during high-risk pregnancies, Villar et al<23> studied 2,235 patients, in Latin America, randomized to an intervention (n=1,115) or control group (n=1,120). Patients were enrolled in early pregnancy (<22 weeks gestation) if they had one or more of the following risk factors for delivering a LBW infant: previous delivery of a LBW or preterm infant; previous fetal or infant death; maternal age <18 years; body weight ≥50 kg height ≥1.5 meters; low family income; less than three years of primary school; smoking or heavy drinking; and residence apart from the child's father.

The intervention was aimed at increasing social support and reducing stress and anxiety. Either specially trained social workers or obstetrical nurses carried out home visits during weeks 22, 26, 30, and

34 of gestation, with the option of two additional visits. The home visitor provided direct emotional support to the woman and helped her cope with problems related to medical recommendations or prenatal care. In addition, women in the intervention group had 24-hour access to a telephone line in each hospital. No medical care was provided during the home visits.

The control group was provided with the routine prenatal care available at each of the participating institutions. The rate of LBW was 8.7% in the intervention group and 9.4% in the controls. The rate of preterm delivery (<37 weeks) was 11.1% in the intervention group and 12.5% in the control group.

A meta-analysis[24] of trials involving 8,000 women in 9 countries has determined that psychosocial support interventions for at-risk women has not been associated with improvement in any medical outcomes for the index pregnancy.

In summary, the evidence is consistent in showing that social support alone is not effective in overriding the cumulative effects of social and biologic disadvantage in populations at risk for delivering a LBW and/or preterm infant.

Nutritional Supplementation

Over the past two decades a number of intervention studies have evaluated the impact of maternal nutritional supplementation on pregnancy outcome. In the U.S., results of evaluation of the Nutrition Supplementation Programs for Women, Infants, and Children (WIC), have been conflicting. A review of 22 WIC intervention studies by Rush and colleagues in 1988, concluded that the range of reduction in the rate of LBW was approximately 1-2%, while average birth weight increases ranged from 0 to 60 g.[25]

In a cost-benefit analysis of WIC participation in North Carolina,[26] however, a records linkage study indicated that women who received Medicaid benefits and prenatal WIC services had substantially lower rates of low and very LBW than women who received Medicaid but no prenatal WIC. For white women (8.4% vs. 10.8% <2,500 g; p<0.001 and 1.4% vs. 2.5% <1,500 g; p<0.001) and for black women (11.6% vs. 16.9% <2,500 g; p<0.001 and 1.8% vs. 4.1% <1,500 g; p<0.001) the differences were statistically significant. It was estimated that for each $1.00 spent on WIC services, Medicaid savings in costs of newborn medical care were $2.91. For those receiving some prenatal care, longer maternal participation in WIC was also associated with better birth outcomes and lower costs.

The Montreal Diet Dispensary Program was begun in the 1960s in order to improve pregnancy outcome in socially disadvantaged urban women. A recent evaluation of this program reported by Higgins et *al.*[27] in a sibling matched analysis demonstrated an average 107 g increase in the birth rate of the second sibling when the mother had participated in the program during the pregnancy of the second born, but not the first born. The rate of LBW was also significantly decreased among intervention infants when compared to their siblings. These results should be interpreted with caution in view of the study design, and the fact that the Montreal Diet Dispensary Program included social support and suggestions for lifestyle improvements in addition to nutritional supplementation.

In a meta-analysis of randomized trials of balanced protein/energy supplementation in pregnancy,[28] Kramer found that supplementation was associated with a small but significant increase in mean birthweight (weighted mean difference 29.5 g; 95% CI: 0.7-58.3 gm) and a reduction (of borderline statistical significance) in the incidence of small for gestational age births. Mean gestational age was not affected; the available evidence was inadequate to permit conclusions concerning effects on preterm birth, fetal and infant survival, or maternal health.

Thus, specific nutritional supplementation programs have had varying degrees of success in increasing birth weight at term and have led to a small reduction in the incidence of LBW. The clinical significance of this difference is unclear. The wide range of benefit shown in different studies can be attributed to differences in the populations studied, in the supplements used, and in methodological quality of the study design.

Conclusions and Recommendations

There is level I evidence showing that social support alone is not effective in improving pregnancy outcome with regard to birth weight or gestational age at delivery, in high risk patient populations. These programs are not recommended (D Recommendation) to prevent LBW/preterm births. However, their effectiveness in preventing other conditions or problems was not evaluated.

The effectiveness of multicomponent programs in preventing LBW is less clearly defined, since results of randomized controlled trials are conflicting (C Recommendation). The body of information available suggests that they may be effective when applied to a wide population base, but studies conducted to date are methodologically weak, thus definite conclusions are not possible.

Nutritional supplementation has been shown to increase average birth weight, but only slightly. While the clinical significance of this difference can be questioned, the intervention has been shown to cost-effective in at least one U.S. setting. There appear to be no harmful effects but the evidence with regard to improving prevalence of preterm birth, fetal and infant survival and maternal health was inconclusive. Overall, the evidence regarding nutritional supplementation programs for women at high-risk of undernutrition to prevent LBW is inconclusive (C recommendation).

Unanswered Questions (Research Agenda)

A trial to determine whether a comprehensive preterm prevention program decreases the rate of preterm birth and/or LBW in the general population and to determine the cost effectiveness of such programs in Canada, is indicated. Other approaches to prevention of preterm labour and LBW in high-risk women are needed.

Evidence

Articles were retrieved by a computerized search (Cochrane Collaboration Database on Pregnancy and Childbirth and MEDLINE from 1966 to January, 1994, using the following keywords: low birth weight, prematurity, prevention). Content experts were also consulted. Articles that evaluated a single intervention other than nutritional supplementation were excluded (eg. smoking cessation, cerclage, use of tocolytic agents). This review was initiated in January 1993 and recommendations were finalized by the Task Force in April 1994.

Acknowledgements

The Task Force thanks Graham W. Chance, MB, ChB, FRCPC, FRCP(Lond), Professor of Pediatrics and of Obstetrics and Gynecology, University of Western Ontario, London, Ontario and A. Ohlsson, MD, MSc, FRCPC, Associate Professor of Pediatrics, Division of Neonatology, University of Toronto, Toronto, Ontario for their valuable comments.

Selected References

1. Kramer M: Determinants of low birth weight: methodological assessment and meta-analysis. *Bull World Health Organ* 1987; 65: 663-737

2. Papiernik E, Bouyer J, Dreyfus J, *et al*: Prevention of preterm births: a perinatal study in Haguenau, France. *Pediatrics* 1985; 76: 154-158

3. Herron MA, Katz M, Creasy RK: Evaluation of a preterm birth prevention program: preliminary report. *Obstet Gynecol* 1982; 59: 452-456

4. Breart G, Goujard J, Blondel B, *et al*: A comparison of two policies of antenatal supervision for the prevention of prematurity. *Int J Epidemiol* 1981; 10(3): 241-244

5.   Goujon H, Papiernik E, Maine D: The prevention of preterm delivery through prenatal care: an intervention study in Martinique. *Int J Gynaecol Obstet* 1984; 22: 339-343

6.   Meis PJ, Ernest JM, Moore ML, *et al*: Regional program for prevention of premature birth in northwestern North Carolina. *Am J Obstet Gynecol* 1987; 157: 550-556

7.   Konte JM, Creasy RK, Laros RK Jr: California North Coast Preterm Birth Prevention Project. *Obstet Gynecol* 1988; 71: 727-730

8.   Covington DL, Daley JG, Churchill MP, *et al*: The effects of a prematurity prevention program on births to adolescents. *J Adolesc Health Care* 1990; 11: 335-338

9.   Main DM, Gabbe SG, Richardson D, *et al*: Can preterm deliveries be prevented? *Am J Obstet Gynecol* 1985; 151: 892-898

10. Mueller-Heubach E, Reddick D, Barnett B, *et al*: Preterm birth prevention: evaluation of a prospective randomized trial. *Am J Obstet Gynecol* 1989; 160: 1172-1178

11. Ellings JM, Newman RB, Hulsey TC, *et al*: Reduction in very low birth weight deliveries and perinatal mortality in a specialized multidisciplinary twin clinic. *Obstet Gynecol* 1993; 81: 387-391

12. Hobel CJ, Ross MG, Bemis RL, *et al*: The West Los Angeles Preterm Birth Prevention Project. I. Program impact on high-risk women. *Am J Obstet Gynecol* 1994; 170: 54-62

13. Goldenberg RL, Davis RO, Copper RL, *et al*: The Alabama preterm birth prevention project. *Obstet Gynecol* 1990; 75: 933-939

14. McLaughlin FJ, Altemeier WA, Christensen MJ, *et al*: Randomized trial of comprehensive prenatal care for low-income women: effect on infant birth weight. *Pediatrics* 1992; 89: 128-132

15. Heins HC, Nance NW, McCarthy BJ, *et al*: A randomized trial of nurse-midwifery prenatal care to reduce low birth weight. *Obstet Gynecol* 1990; 75: 341-345

16. Collins R: Antiplatelet agents for IUGR and pre-eclampsia. In: Pregnancy and Childbirth Module (eds. Enkin MW, Keirse MJNC, Renfrew Neilson JP), "Cochrane Database of systematic reviews": Review No. 04000, 4 May 1994. Published through "Cochrane Updates on Disk", Oxford, Update Software, 1994, Disk Issue 1

17. Low-dose aspirin in prevention and treatment of intrauterine growth retardation and pregnancy-induced hypertension. Italian study of aspirin in pregnancy. *Lancet* 1993; 341: 396-400

18. CLASP: a randomized trial of low-dose aspirin for the prevention and treatment of pre-eclampsia among 9364 pregnant women. *Lancet* 1994; 343: 619-629

19. Olds DL, Henderson CR Jr, Tatelbaum R, *et al*: Improving the delivery of prenatal care and outcomes of pregnancy: a randomized trial of nurse home visitation. *Pediatrics* 1986; 77: 16-28

20. Spencer B, Thomas H, Morris J: A randomized controlled trial of the provision of a social support service during pregnancy: the South Manchester Family Worker Project. *Br J Obstet Gynecol* 1989; 96: 281-288

21. Oakley A, Rajan L, Grant A: Social support and pregnancy outcome. *Br J Obstet Gynaecol* 1990; 97: 155-162

22. Bryce RL, Stanley FJ, Garner JB: Randomized controlled trial of antenatal social support to prevent preterm birth. *Br J Obstet Gynaecol* 1991; 98: 1001-1008

23. Villar J, Farnot U, Barros F, *et al*: A randomized trial of psychosocial support during high-risk pregnancies. *New Engl J Med* 1992; 327: 1266-1271

24. Hodnett ED: Support from caregivers during at-risk pregnancy. In: Pregnancy and Childbirth Module (eds. Enkin MW, Keirse MJNC, Renfrew Neilson JP), "Cochrane Database of systematic reviews": Review No. 04169, 27 April 1994. Published through "Cochrane Updates on Disk", Oxford: Update Software, 1994, Disk Issue 1

25. Rush D, Sloan NL, Leighton J, *et al*: The National WIC Evaluation: evaluation of the Special Supplementation Food Program For Women, Infants, and Children. vs. Longitudinal study of pregnant women. *Am J Clin Nutr* 1988; 48: 439-483

26. Buescher PA, Larson LC, Nelson MD Jr, *et al*: Prenatal WIC participation can reduce low birth weight and newborn medical costs: a cost-benefit analysis of WIC participation in North Carolina. *J Am Diet Assoc* 1993; 93: 163-166

27. Higgins A, Moxley JE, Pencharz PB, *et al*: Impact of the Higgins Nutrition Intervention Program on birth weight: a within-mother analysis. *J Am Diet Assoc* 1989; 89: 1097-1103

28. Kramer MS: Balanced Protein/energy supplementation in pregnancy. In: Pregnancy and Childbirth Module (eds. Enkin MW, Keirse MJNC, Renfrew Neilson JP), "Cochrane Database of systematic reviews": Review No. 07141, 17 September 1993. Published through "Cochrane Updates on Disk", Oxford: Update Software, 1994, Disk Issue 1

Table 1:   Components of multicomponent prevention programs

Risk assessment

Education
  Staff
  Patients
  Public

Advice
  Reduce paid work
  Reduce housework and child care
  Reduce smoking
  Reduce stress
  Reduce travel, commuting, moving house
  Reduce/stop sexual activity
  Improve nutrition
  Bed rest at home

Self-monitoring of uterine activity

Antenatal care
  Increased frequency of contact
  Continuity of care
  Facilitated access to hospital

Support systems
  Home visiting nurses/midwives
  Home help
  Family help
  Social worker assignment
  Stress management classes

Specific obstetric interventions
  Regular cervical examinations
  Cervical suture
  Bed rest in hospital
  Progestogens
  B-mimetics
  Calcium antagonists

Prevention of Low Birth Weight/Preterm Birth

Maneuver	Effectiveness	Level of Evidence <REF>	Recommendation
Multicomponent education preterm birth/ low birth weight prevention programs	**General Population** Programs have shown some benefits in methodologically weak studies.	Before and after studies<2-8> (II-3)	Inconclusive evidence that programs for the general population or for high-risk pregnant women are effective (C)
	High-risk populations In most studies programs were not effective in improving pregnancy outcome with regards to birth weight or gestational age at delivery; twin clinic showed benefit and improvement of marginal statistical significance in one trial.	Randomized controlled trials<9-15> (I)	
Programs consisting exclusively of social support	Programs were not effective in improving pregnancy outcome.	Randomized controlled trials<19-23> (I)	Fair evidence that programs consisting exclusively of social support for high-risk populations do not prevent preterm birth (D)
Diet supplementation in the prenatal period in pregnant women at high-risk for undernutrition	Average increase in birth weight 29.5 gm. Maternal nutritional supplementation lowered rates of low birth weight for Medicaid recipients and was cost effective.	Meta-analysis of randomized controlled trials<28> (I) Cost-benefit analysis, cohort study<26> (II-2)	Inconclusive evidence regarding diet supplementation in high-risk women to prevent low birth weight (C)

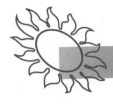

CHAPTER 5

Primary Prevention of Fetal Alcohol Syndrome

By David R. Offord and Deborah L. Craig

Primary Prevention of Fetal Alcohol Syndrome

Prepared by David R. Offord, MD, FRCPC[1] and Deborah L. Craig, MPH[2]

In 1979 the Canadian Task Force on the Periodic Health Examination found there was fair justification for recommending that counselling to reduce alcohol intake in pregnant women should be included in the periodic health examination (B recommendation).<1,2> This was based on evidence that counselling was effective in reducing both the amount of drinking in pregnant women and morbidity in their offspring. The evidence since 1979 supports the original recommendation. Also considered was contraception for alcoholic sexually active women, and, if acceptable, the offer of abortion for pregnant women at high risk.

More general concerns regarding problem drinking have been dealt with in Chapter 42 and are beyond the scope of this report. In brief, however, in 1989<3> and again in this update the Task Force found there was fair evidence that case-finding, counselling and follow-up are effective in managing problem drinking. This volume also contains a separate report on the psychological consequences to children of having alcoholic parents (Chapter 41).

Burden of Suffering

Fetal Alcohol Syndrome (FAS) refers to a constellation of congenital and functional anomalies occurring in children born to alcohol-abusing women. First documented in 1973 by Jones and Smith,<4> FAS has become one of the most actively researched congenital abnormalities in the last two decades.<5> Criteria for defining FAS were standardized by the Fetal Alcohol Study Group<6> and modifications were proposed in 1989 by Sokol and Clarren.<7> FAS is now one of the leading causes of mental retardation. It has been estimated that 50% of FAS victims are mentally retarded and another 30% suffer borderline mental retardation.<8> It is generally accepted that the harmful effects of prenatal alcohol exposure can be plotted on a continuum, with spontaneous abortion at one end, FAS in the middle and subtle behavioral abnormalities at the other end of the scale. FAS represents the severest disabilities caused by maternal alcohol use

---

[1] Professor of Psychiatry, McMaster University, Hamilton, Ontario
[2] Health Care Consultant, Halifax, Nova Scotia

during pregnancy. The term "possible fetal alcohol effects" (FAE) has been introduced to indicate that alcohol is being considered as one of the possible causes of a patient's birth defects, but there are not sufficient features for a firm diagnosis of FAS or strong evidence of an alternative diagnosis.[7]

The accurate determination of the incidence of FAS is difficult primarily because the syndrome is not reliably recognized. It has been reported that between 8% and 11% of child-bearing women in the United States are either problem drinkers or alcoholics. Further, it has been reported that 65% of fetuses are exposed to alcohol prenatally throughout the United States. Between 3% and 10% of pregnant women report patterns of alcohol consumption that have corresponded with harming the fetus.[9] This figure may be low as it is generally accepted that self-reporting of alcohol consumption in women is under-reported due to denial. The precise incidence and prevalence of FAS and FAE are not known in Canada. It is estimated that the incidence rate of FAS is between 1 and 2 per 1,000 live births in the general population. Based on these data, between 400 to 500 Canadian children are born annually with FAS. The incidence of FAS is markedly increased in the native population and in poor, inner-city neighbourhoods, as well as rural, remote villages. The highest reported prevalence of FAS is one child in eight in a native community in British Columbia where all mothers and their offspring were systematically evaluated.[10]

Experts agree that the actual amount of alcohol needed to produce FAS and the precise risk of embryo-fetal damage is largely unknown. It is widely accepted that there is a dose-response relationship, but it is not known how large a dose is needed to cause an injurious effect to the fetus. Investigators[11,12] report that the teratogenicity of alcohol is strictly dose dependent with direct dose-response effects on infant weight, perinatal mortality and soft-tissue malformations.

Lastly, it is known that not all alcoholic women are at risk for giving birth to an alcohol-affected child; genetic and physiologic factors may mediate the risk.[13] Ethnic and cultural factors, family history and tobacco and multiple drug use have been identified as variables that may mediate the risk of morbidity in the offspring of alcoholic mothers.

Maneuver

It is known that, unlike other congenital birth defects, alcohol-related birth defects are preventable. Experts agree that the development of effective screening methodologies to identify women at high risk for heavy alcohol consumption is the key strategy to preventing alcohol-related birth defects. Determining the need for education, counselling and treatment for these patients is dependent

Alcohol-related birth defects are preventable

on recognition of the patient's problem. Identifying high-risk drinkers is difficult for physicians, however. Laboratory tests which might identify biochemical markers of heavy drinking are not available[14] and obtaining an accurate history of maternal alcohol consumption can be complicated by psychological denial.

A number of screening tests for the estimation of alcohol consumption are available. The Michigan Alcoholism Screening Test (MAST) is a 25-question instrument which is extensively utilized for research but is time consuming and thus clinically impractical.[15] The CAGE test is a more recent and effective screening test; it is only four questions long, but has not been studied in pregnancy.[16] Recently, a screening test for the early detection of hazardous and harmful alcohol consumption for use in primary care settings has been developed by the World Health Organization.[17] Again, it has not been specifically tested on pregnant populations.

In 1988, Cyr and Wartman[18] proposed two questions that would improve the practitioner's chances of identifying the alcoholic patient. The questions, "Have you ever had a drinking problem?" combined with "When was your last drink?" had a sensitivity of 91.5%. The researchers recommend the routine incorporation of these two questions into the medical history of the outpatient population to aid in the initial diagnosis of alcoholism.

Sokol and colleagues[19] developed a four-question survey tool to help eliminate denial and under-reporting of heavy drinking by pregnant women. Referred to as the T-ACE, the questionnaire accurately identified 69% of the risk drinkers from a cohort of 971 pregnant women. T-ACE was determined to be superior to other standard questionnaires such as MAST and CAGE for detecting heavy alcohol abuse. Another instrument, a brief Ten Question Drinking History (TQDH) has been incorporated into the Boston City Hospital prenatal clinic record.[20] Reliability has been demonstrated, and the data obtained by obstetrical staff using the TQDH were comparable to those obtained in a more elaborate research interview.

It remains a diagnostic challenge to gain an accurate drinking history from many patients. Laboratory results may prove to be entirely normal though risk-drinking exists. Obtaining a thorough and sensitive history from a possibly evasive and denying patient remains the best technique for identifying risk-drinking.[21] Two points should be kept in mind about screening pregnant women for alcohol intake. It is likely that if the patient screens positive, the response is accurate. However, a negative result on the screen is not necessarily accurate. Second, if the goal is to eliminate all maternal drinking during pregnancy, then the screen simply has to identify any vs. no alcohol intake rather than varying levels of alcohol use.

In the absence of a clearly defined safe threshold for alcohol consumption during pregnancy, experts widely agree that the most conservative approach is best. Therefore, most clinicians advise total abstinence for women who are either considering pregnancy or who are pregnant. This widely accepted recommendation has not gone unchallenged, however. Knupfer[22] has argued that there is no evidence that light drinking is harmful to the fetus and that defects exist in the literature regarding methodologies for categorizing drinking patterns and drawing conclusions from them.

Effectiveness of Prevention

As it is widely accepted that there is no effective treatment for offspring with FAS and FAE, the challenge to physicians and other health care providers lies in the prevention of FAS and FAE through early identification of women who are abusing alcohol and the implementation of treatment interventions with the mother.

Patient Intervention

Several studies have noted the positive benefits of interventions during pregnancy with alcohol-abusing women. Coles and coworkers[23] found that infants of mothers who stopped consuming alcohol in the second trimester displayed less growth retardation and fewer neurobehavioural deficits than neonates of women who continued to drink at the same rate throughout the pregnancy. Other researchers have noted that the risk for intrauterine growth retardation and central nervous system effects decrease in the newborns of mothers who lessen or discontinue their alcohol use during pregnancy.

In one study, alcohol counselling was provided to 85 pregnant women to persuade them to reduce or eliminate their alcohol consumption. Sixty-five percent of the women were able to decrease their alcohol intake by at least 50%. In the total sample, 24% of the offspring had complete FAS, while 26% displayed FAE. Of the women with continuous alcohol consumption, 89% gave birth to neonates with at least one FAE feature compared with only 40% of women who reduced their alcohol intake.[24]

There is evidence that therapeutic interventions in the prenatal clinic setting can be effective in promoting a decrease in alcohol intake, even in high-risk heavy drinkers. Rosett and Weiner[25] reported that 67% of a group of heavy drinkers either decreased or abstained from alcohol use following an intervention of supportive counselling. Larsson[26] reported similar results in that 76% of the women either decreased or eliminated drinking following a minimal intervention which consisted mainly of the provision to the mothers of information about the effects of alcohol consumption during pregnancy. The results of these studies suggest that alcohol-abusing women are responsive to

Alcohol-abusing women are responsive to intervention during pregnancy, possibly more so than at any other time

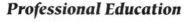

intervention during pregnancy, possibly more so than at any other time.

Professional Education

Clinicians are failing to diagnose alcoholism in at least three of four alcohol-abusing patients

The literature substantiates a lack of awareness among health care providers regarding the range of symptoms associated with FAS and FAE. Many clinicians do not comprehend the ramifications correlated with these diagnoses for the child's development. The diagnosis of alcoholism is often missed as well. Sokol and colleagues[27] have found that clinicians are failing to diagnose alcoholism in at least three of four alcohol-abusing patients. The researchers believe that no other diagnosis is missed as frequently.

There are many reasons why doctors do not routinely ask about alcohol consumption among their pregnant patients. Such explanations include physician bias regarding their own abuse, inadequate training for the task, poor awareness of the problem and its consequences, time restrictions, disinterest, fear of offending the patient, disbelief and denial that FAS occurs in private practice and the view that patients will deny their alcohol use.

Role of the Physician

Several authors stress the importance of the doctor-patient interaction as key in the prevention of alcohol-related birth defects. As many communities have limited resources available to women of child-bearing age, the role of the clinician providing perinatal care becomes even more critical.

Public Prevention Strategies

There are few empirical studies regarding the impact of warning labels on alcohol beverage containers. This is not surprising as Canada does not have legislation requiring warning labels and the U.S. only recently enacted the warning label law in November 1989. However, there is evidence that warning labels can influence behaviour based on studies regarding tobacco, foods and illegal drugs. Further, evidence exists supporting the idea that public educational efforts are effective in modifying behaviour, especially among social drinkers.

Recommendations of Others

The Canadian Medical Association strongly supports all activities that encourage Canadians to reduce their alcohol intake. The Association recommends that the Federal Government prohibit all advertising of alcoholic beverages on radio and television, as well as in printed materials. A Health and Welfare Sub-Committee has recommended to the Minister that the *Food and Drug Act* be amended to require that alcohol beverage containers sold in Canada carry appropriate warning labels alerting consumers that alcohol consumption during pregnancy places the fetus at risk of FAS and FAE. Lastly, the recommendations of American medical organizations are in agreement with those of the Canadian medical community, in that total avoidance of alcohol consumption during pregnancy is the safest course of action. Abstinence of maternal drinking is the official recommendation of the U.S. Surgeon General, the American College of Obstetricians and Gynecologists, the American Council of Science and Health, as well as the American Medical Association Council on Scientific Affairs.

In 1989, the U.S. Preventive Services Task Force recommended that all persons who use alcohol, especially pregnant women, should be encouraged to limit their consumption.<28>

Conclusions and Recommendations

The child born to an alcoholic mother is at risk for the development of craniofacial anomalies, mental retardation and a wide spectrum of developmental delays. There is evidence that counselling is an effective intervention in decreasing both the amount of drinking in pregnant women and morbidity in their offspring.

There is fair justification to support the recommendation that screening and counselling be included in a routine health examination of pregnant women (B Recommendation).

Unanswered Questions (Research Agenda)

The following have been identified as research priorities:

1. Determining the incidence of FAS and FAE in Canada, among the Canadian population in general, as well as in subpopulations known or suspected to be at higher risk for these disorders.

2. Improving the ability of clinicians to identify accurately the drinking patterns of pregnant women.

3. Improving knowledge about fetal and maternal susceptibility to alcohol, time of exposure during pregnancy, effects of varying quantity and concentration of alcohol, patterns of drinking, as well as other dose-response relationships which further define the embryonic and fetal risk.

4. Evaluating promising treatment programs for alcoholic women.

5. Increasing public awareness of the effects on the offspring of maternal alcohol consumption during pregnancy.

6. Determining the effectiveness in high-risk populations (eg., Natives) of counselling to reduce the consumption of alcohol in pregnant women.

Evidence

The literature in this review was identified during a MEDLINE search from 1988 to February 1993, using the following MESH heading: fetal alcohol syndrome. This review was initiated in January 1993 and recommendations were finalized by the Task Force in March 1994.

Acknowledgements

Funding for this report was provided by Health Canada under the Government of Canada's Brighter Futures Initiative. The Task Force thanks Tim Oberlander, MD, FRCPC, Developmental Pediatrician, Assistant Professor of Pediatrics, University of British Columbia, Vancouver, BC; and Sarah Shea, MD, FRCPC, Assistant Professor of Pediatrics, Dalhousie University, Halifax, NS for reviewing the draft chapter.

Selected References

1. Report of the Task Force to the Conference of Deputy Ministers of Health (cat no H39-3/1980E), Health Services and promotion Branch, Department of National Health and Welfare, Ottawa, 1980

2. Canadian Task Force on the Periodic Health Examination: The periodic health examination. *Can Med Assoc J* 1979; 121: 1193-1254

3. Canadian Task Force on the Periodic Health Examination: The periodic health examination: 1989 update part 1, Introduction and part 2, Early detection of colorectal cancer and problem drinking. *Can Med Assoc J* 1989; 141: 205-216

4. Jones KL, Smith DW: Recognition of the fetal alcohol syndrome in early infancy. *Lancet* 1973; 2: 999-1001

5. Abel EL, Welte JW: Publication trends in fetal alcohol, tobacco and narcotic effects. *Drug Alcohol Depend* 1986; 18: 107-114

6. Rosett HL: A clinical perspective of the fetal alcohol syndrome. *Alcohol Clin Exp Res* 1980; 4(2): 119-122

7. Sokol RJ, Clarren SK: Guidelines for use of terminology describing the impact of prenatal alcohol on the offspring. *Alcohol Clin Exp Res* 1989; 13(4): 597-598

8. Report of the Standing Committee on Health and Welfare, Social Affairs, Seniors and the Status of Women, (Proceedings): Foetal Alcohol Syndrome – A Preventable Tragedy: Issue 10, June 1992, p. 2

9. Weiner L, Rosett HL, Mason EA: Training professionals to identify and treat pregnant women who drink heavily. *Alcohol Health Res World* 1985; 10: 32-35

10. Robinson GC, Conry JL, Conry RF: Clinical profile and prevalence of fetal alcohol syndrome in an isolated community in British Columbia. *Can Med Assoc J* 1987; 137: 203-207

11. Sokol RJ: Alcoholism and abnormal outcomes of pregnancy. *Can Med Assoc J* 1981; 125: 143-148

12. Streissguth AP, Landesman-Dweyer S, Martin JC, *et al*: Teratogenic effects of alcohol in human and laboratory animals. *Science* 1980; 209: 535

13. Smith IE, Coles CD: Multilevel intervention for prevention of fetal alcohol syndrome and effects of prenatal alcohol exposure. In Galanter M (ed): Recent Developments in Alcoholism, Vol IX. New York, Plenum Press 1991, 165-182

14. Ernhart CB, Morrow-Tlucak M, Sokol RJ, *et al*: Underreporting of alcohol use in pregnancy. *Alcohol Clin Exp Res* 1988; 12(4): 506-511

15. Sokol RJ, Martier S, Ernhart E: Identification of alcohol abuse in the prenatal clinic. In: Chang NC, Chaott M (eds): Early identification of alcohol abuse. Washington, DC: U.S. Government Printing Office, 1985

16. Ewing JA: Detecting alcoholism. The CAGE questionnaire. *JAMA* 1984; 252: 1905-1907

17. Saunders JB, Aasland OG, Babor TF, *et al*: Development of the alcohol use disorders identification test (AUDIT): WHO Collaborative Project on early detection of persons with harmful alcohol consumption-11. *Addiction* 1993; 88: 791-804

18. Cyr MG, Wartman SA: The effectiveness of routine screening questions in the detection of alcoholism. *JAMA* 1988; 259: 51-54

19. Sokol RJ, Martier SS, Ager JW: The T-ACE questions: practical prenatal detection of risk-drinking. *Am J Obstet Gynecol* 1989; 160(4): 863-870

20. Weiner L, Rosett HL, Edelin KC: Behavioural evaluation of fetal alcohol education for physicians. *Alcohol Clin Exp Res* 1982; 6: 230-233

21. Savitsky J: Early diagnosis and screening. In Barnes H, Aronson MD, Delbanco T (eds): Alcoholism: A guide for the primary care physician. New York: Springer-Verlag 1987; 47-58

22. Knupfer G: Abstaining for foetal health: the fiction that even light drinking is dangerous. *Br J Addict* 1991; 86: 1063-1073

23. Coles CD, Smith I, Fernhoff PM, *et al*: Neonatal neurobehavioral characteristics as correlates of maternal alcohol use during gestation. *Alcohol Clin Exp Res* 1985; 9(5): 454-460

24. Halmesmaki E: Alcohol counselling of 85 pregnant problem drinkers: effect on drinking and fetal outcome. *Br J Obstet Gynaecol* 1988; 95: 243-247

25. Rosett HL, Weiner L: Alcohol and the fetus: a clinical perspective. New York: Oxford University Press, 1984

26.   Larsson G: Prevention of fetal alcohol effects: an antenatal program for early detection of pregnancies at risk. *Acta Obstet Gynecol Scand* 1983; 62: 171-178

27.   Sokol RJ, Miller SI, Martier S: Preventing Fetal Alcohol Effects: A Practical Guide for the Ob/Gyn Physicians and Nurses. Rockville, Md, National Institute on Alcohol Abuse and Alcoholism, 1981

28.   U.S. Preventive Services Task Force: *Guide to Clinical Preventive Health Care: an Assessment of the Effectiveness of 169 Interventions.* Williams & Wilkins, Baltimore, Md, 1989: 277-286

Primary Prevention of Fetal Alcohol Syndrome

MANEUVER	EFFECTIVENESS	LEVEL OF EVIDENCE <REF>	RECOMMENDATION
Screening procedures (self-administered questionnaires, interviews or clinical judgement) used to identify the drinking patterns of pregnant women	Accuracy not known for many procedures which could be used in pregnant population. Ten Question Drinking History (TQDH) is reliable in pregnant women and there is some evidence of validity.	Cohort studies<15-21> (II-2)	Fair evidence to include screening procedures in periodic health examination (B)
Counselling of pregnant women	Counselling reduces consumption of alcohol and morbidity in the offspring (Not established in certain high-risk groups, eg., Native women).	Cohort studies<21-25> (II-2)	Fair evidence to undertake counselling with pregnant women who are consuming alcohol (B)

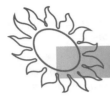

CHAPTER 6

Routine Iron Supplementation during Pregnancy

By John W. Feightner

Routine Iron Supplementation During Pregnancy

Adapted by John W. Feightner, MD, MSc, FCFP[1] from a Review prepared for the U.S. Preventive Services Task Force[2]

There is currently little evidence from published clinical research to suggest that routine iron supplementation during pregnancy improves clinical outcomes for the mother, fetus or newborn. The evidence is insufficient to recommend for or against routine iron supplementation during pregnancy (C Recommendation).

These conclusions apply only to routine iron supplementation and do not pertain to the selection of iron containing foods as part of a healthful pregnancy diet, the use of screening tests to detect anemia during pregnancy, the proper clinical evaluation of the causes of anemia when it is discovered, or the selective use of iron supplements in pregnant women with documented iron deficiency anemia. Prevention of iron deficiency anemia in infants is addressed in Chapter 23.

Because relevant effectiveness data are inadequate, clinicians must use individual judgement in determining how to counsel pregnant women about dietary intake of iron containing foods and iron supplements and in deciding whether and how to screen women for anemia and iron deficiency.

Burden of Suffering

Low hemoglobin concentrations are a normal physiologic response to the expansion in plasma volume that occurs during pregnancy

Both anemia and relative iron deficiency are common during pregnancy. Low hemoglobin concentrations are a normal physiologic response to the expansion in plasma volume that occurs during pregnancy. The normal pattern is for hemoglobin concentrations to fall by about 20 g/L, reaching a nadir in the second trimester, and to return to near pre-pregnancy levels by term.<1> Pregnant women are generally considered to be anemic when hematologic indices fall two or more standard deviations below "normal" levels, although definitions for normal vary. A recent modification of the World Health Organization definition, defines anemia in pregnancy as a hemoglobin concentration (Hgb) below 110 g/L during the first and third

[1] Professor, Department of Family Medicine, McMaster University, Hamilton Ontario
[2] By Steven H. Woolf, MD, MPH, Assistant Clinical Professor, Department of Family Practice, Medical College of Virginia, Richmond, Virgina and Science Advisor, U.S. Preventive Services Task Force, Washington, D.C.

trimesters and below 105 g/L during the second trimester, or an hematocrit less than 32%. In pregnancy, women require a greater amount of iron due to an expanded red blood cell volume, the needs of the fetus and placenta, and blood loss at delivery.

For years mineral and vitamin supplements have been prescribed routinely to pregnant women as a normal part of prenatal care. These supplements are often prescribed as preparations that include 25-65 mg of elemental iron, along with other minerals (e.g., calcium, zinc, magnesium, copper) and vitamins. However, few studies have examined the clinical effectiveness of prenatal vitamin preparations as a group.

Prevalence

The exact prevalence of iron deficiency among pregnant women in Canada is uncertain. In the U.S., data for non-pregnant women from the National Health and Nutrition Examination Survey suggest that about 5-10% of women aged 20 to 44 years are iron deficient. The prevalence in pregnant women is thought to be higher because of the added physiologic demands of pregnancy, but exact data are lacking. Iron deficiency anemia is more common in certain high-risk groups, such as persons of low socioeconomic status or limited education; women with high parity, or those with a history of menorrhagia or multiple gestations; persons with diets that are low in both meat and ascorbic acid; persons who donate blood more than three times per year; adolescents; and persons who use aspirin regularly.

Effects of Anemia and Iron Deficiency on the Mother

Among the postulated risks to the mother are increased fatigue and decreased work performance, cardiovascular stress due to inadequate hemoglobin and low blood oxygen saturation, impaired resistance to infection, and poor tolerance to heavy blood loss and surgical interventions at delivery. There is also a theoretical risk that anemic women are more likely to require blood transfusions (a risk factor for infectious diseases) and emergency caesarean section, but data to support these concerns are lacking.

Although studies of male workers have demonstrated low productivity among iron deficient men, few studies of the health effects of iron deficiency have included women, let alone pregnant women. A Swedish survey of 1,462 women compared the complaints of 82 anemic women (Hgb <120 g/L) with those of non-anemic women and found no difference in the incidence of reported infections, fatigue, sleeping difficulties, headache, or work absenteeism.[2] Anemic women were significantly more likely to report low work productivity than non-anemic women (10% vs. 5%). Physical symptoms of anemia are generally unapparent unless hemoglobin values fall below 70-80 g/L.

Effects of Anemia and Iron Deficiency on the Fetus and Newborn

The postulated risks of iron deficiency on the fetus relate to the impaired delivery of hemoglobin and, thus, of oxygen to the uterus, placenta, and developing fetus.

Cross-sectional and longitudinal observational studies (grade II-2 evidence) in the U.S. and Europe have demonstrated that even mild to moderate anemia can be associated with adverse obstetrical outcomes, including preterm delivery, low birth weight and fetal death.[3,4] However, most of the studies do not control for other factors that can cause low birth weight and prematurity (e.g., poor nutrition, smoking), making it unclear whether anemia and iron deficiency are merely associated with these variables rather than having a direct influence on pregnancy outcomes.

Effects of Anemia and Iron Deficiency on the Developing Child

Another postulated risk of anemia and iron deficiency is that mothers with these conditions may give birth to infants with anemia or iron deficiency and that this may result in abnormal child development if the deficiencies are not corrected early.

Most studies suggest that pregnant women who are iron deficient are no more likely to give birth to iron deficient newborns than women who have adequate iron stores

However, most studies suggest that pregnant women who are iron deficient are no more likely to give birth to iron deficient newborns than women who have adequate iron stores.[5] Nor is there direct evidence that pregnant women who take iron supplements give birth to infants or children with improved mental or psychomotor performance.

Maneuver

The maneuver being evaluated in this review is the routine provision of oral iron supplementation to pregnant women during the prenatal period. Doses provided in the studies reviewed were as high as 100 mg of elemental iron per day. In the clinical setting, iron is often prescribed in combination with other vitamin supplements. The effectiveness of those other supplements is not the subject of this review.

Effectiveness of Prevention and Treatment

The essential clinical question for routine iron supplementation is whether it can reduce the incidence of obstetrical and perinatal complications. Although evidence to date is inconclusive, a large body of data suggests that iron supplements are effective in improving the hematologic indices of the mother. Longitudinal studies in which 30-200 mg of iron were given daily have shown a statistically significant increase (10-17 g/L) in hemoglobin concentration in women taking supplements. However, maternal iron supplements do not appear to have a consistent effect on the hematologic status of the fetus or newborn.

The review by the U.S. Preventive Services Task Force of the evidence for effectiveness focused solely on the ability of iron supplements to improve clinical outcomes in either the mother or newborn (e.g. low birth weight, preterm birth). The biological effectiveness of iron supplements in changing non-clinical outcomes (e.g. hematocrit, hemoglobin, ferritin levels) was not reviewed. This chapter will focus only on studies conducted in industrialized countries.

In a prospective, controlled cohort study in Sweden, Kullander and Kallen collected data on 6,376 women in Malmö in 1963-1965.[6] They found that women who took iron and vitamin supplements were significantly less likely to give birth before 38 weeks (6-9% of births) than women who did not use such supplements (11-13% of births). The birth weight of boys (but not girls) was significantly higher in women who took iron and vitamins than in those who took no supplements. However, without proper control for confounding variables, it is difficult to know whether women who took iron supplements had other characteristics (e.g. healthier lifestyle) that reduced their risk of adverse outcomes. Conversely, a Dutch prospective study indicated no association between low maternal hemoglobin and adverse perinatal outcomes.[7]

The strongest evidence on which to evaluate the effectiveness of routine iron supplementation comes from randomized controlled trials. Most clinical trials of iron supplementation have not demonstrated significant improvements in maternal or neonatal outcomes. Sample sizes in these trials are small, and thus statistical power is generally inadequate to prove that iron supplementation is ineffective. A quasi-experimental study in India reported improved birth weights with supplementation but that may have been confounded by improper randomization.[8] A Scottish randomized controlled trial of 3,600 patients found no difference in the incidence of a wide range of adverse obstetrical outcomes between those receiving iron and those receiving placebo.[9] In a randomized controlled trial with 3,000 women, Hemminki and Rimpela compared routine versus selective iron supplementation.[10] The "routine"

Most clinical trials of iron supplementation have not demonstrated significant improvements in maternal or neonatal outcomes

group was advised to take 100 mg of elemental iron daily beginning by the 17th week of gestation, while the "selective" group was advised to take iron only if certain hematologic parameters were present. Women in the "selective" group were more likely to report poor overall health, to require transfusion and operative delivery, and to have newborns with reduced gestational age at birth. The difference in gestational age was not clinically significant, however, and the authors conjectured that lack of blinding may have contributed to the higher complication rate in the selective group.

Adverse Effects

Iron supplements can cause unpleasant gastrointestinal symptoms (e.g., nausea, constipation), but these usually occur at higher doses than are recommended for routine supplementation. Iron supplements may complicate preexisting gastrointestinal disorders such as ulcerative colitis. Complications of excessive iron storage, including hemochromatosis and hemosiderosis, are possible but very uncommon in women who take only oral (and not parenteral) iron supplements. Finally, a potential hazard of iron supplements is unintentional overdosage by children in the home.

Recommendations of Others

The recommendations of the U.S. Preventive Services Task Force are those outlined in this chapter and, hence, the same as those of the Canadian Task Force.<11>

In 1988, the *U.S. Surgeon General's Report on Nutrition and Health* concluded that iron supplementation is a "reasonable approach" to the prevention of iron deficiency and included pregnant women among the groups that "may need iron supplements." The report also recommended that pregnant women receive laboratory evaluation for anemia and nutritional advice on methods to ensure adequate iron intake and to enhance iron bioavailability from the diet.

In 1989, the U.S. Public Health Service Expert Panel on the Content of Prenatal Care recommended that health promotion activities during routine preconception and prenatal visits should include counselling on vitamin and iron supplementation "on indication", for women at risk. The evidence on which this recommendation was based was classified as "fair." The panel also recommended routine hemoglobin and hematocrit measurements.

In a major report in 1990 on nutrition during pregnancy, the Food and Nutrition Board of the Institute of Medicine recommended routine use of daily iron supplements (30 mg/day) after about the twelfth week of gestation, in conjunction with a well-balanced diet that contains enhancers of iron absorption (ascorbic acid, meat). It also recommended that either hemoglobin or hematocrit should routinely be determined at the first prenatal visit. The report recommended that anemia accompanied by a low serum ferritin concentration should be treated with 60-120 mg of ferrous iron daily until a normal hemoglobin concentration is reached, after which the dose should be lowered to 30 mg daily.

Conclusion and Recommendations

There is currently little evidence from published clinical research to suggest that routine iron supplementation during pregnancy is beneficial in improving clinical outcomes for the mother, fetus or newborn. The evidence is insufficient to recommend for or against routine iron supplementation during pregnancy (C Recommendation).

Although observational data (grade II-2 evidence) suggest that pregnant women with anemia (hemoglobin less than 100 g/L) are at increased risk of preterm birth, low birth weight, or other adverse outcomes, it is unclear from such evidence whether anemia is responsible for these outcomes and whether they can be prevented through iron supplementation. Similarly, it is unclear whether iron supplementation during pregnancy can reduce the incidence of iron deficiency in infants, a condition that has been associated with delayed psychomotor development. Although iron supplementation can improve maternal hematologic indices, controlled clinical trials (grade I and II-1 evidence) have failed to demonstrate that iron supplementation or changes in hematologic indices actually improve clinical outcomes for the mother or newborn.

These conclusions apply only to routine iron supplementation and do not pertain to the selection of iron containing foods as part of a healthful pregnancy diet, the use of screening tests to detect anemia during pregnancy, the proper clinical evaluation of the causes of anemia when it is discovered, or the selective use of iron supplements in pregnant women with documented iron deficiency anemia.

Because relevant effectiveness data are inadequate, clinicians must use individual judgement in determining how to counsel pregnant women about dietary intake of iron-containing foods and iron supplements and in deciding whether and how to screen women for anemia and iron deficiency.

Unanswered Questions

Further research, including randomized controlled trials with adequate sample size and statistical power or carefully performed meta-analyses of existing studies, is needed before definitive conclusions can be reached about the effectiveness or ineffectiveness of routine iron supplementation. Future studies need to address clinical outcomes that are relevant to the health of the mother, fetus, and newborn. Data examining the effects of iron supplementation during pregnancy on long-term pediatric outcomes (e.g., growth, cognitive development, school performance) are currently unavailable and should be a focus of future research. Moreover, there are inadequate data to determine whether giving iron supplements only to pregnant women with documented iron deficiency is less or more cost effective than routine supplementation.

Evidence

The review sought all observational studies and clinical trials published between 1966 and 1991 in the English language literature. Studies were excluded if they did not measure clinical outcomes in either the mother or the newborn. The review was initiated by the Canadian Task Force in April 1993 and the recommendations were finalized in January 1994.

Selected References

1. Institute of Medicine: *Nutrition During Pregnancy Part II: Nutrient Supplements.* Washington, D.C.: National Academy Press, 1990: 272-298

2. Lennartsson J, Bengtsson C, Hallberg L, *et al*: Characteristics of anemic women: the population study of women in Göteborg 1968-1969. *Scand J Haematol* 1979; 22: 17-24

3. Scholl TP, Hediger ML, Fischer RL, *et al*: Anemia vs. iron deficiency: increased risk of preterm delivery in a prospective study. *Am J Clin Nutr* 1992; 55: 985-988

4. Murphy JF, O'Riordan J, Newcombe RG, *et al*: Relation of hemoglobin levels in first and second trimesters to outcome of pregnancy. *Lancet* 1986; 1: 992-994

5. Lao TT, Loong EP, Chin RK, *et al*: Relationship between newborn and maternal iron status and hematological indices. *Biol Neonate* 1991; 60: 303-307

6. Kullander S, Kallen B: A prospective study of drugs and pregnancy. *Acta Obstet Gynecol Scand* 1976; 55: 287-295

7. Knottnerus JA, Delgado LR, Knipschild PG, *et al*: Hematologic parameters and pregnancy outcome: a prospective cohort study in the third trimester. *J Clin Epidemiol* 1990; 43: 461-466

8. Agarwal KN, Agarwal DK, Mishra KP: Impact of anemia prophylaxis in pregnancy on maternal hemoglobin, serum ferritin, and birth weight. *Indian J Med Res* 1991; 95: 277-280

9. Willoughby MLN: An investigation of folic acid requirements in pregnancy. II. *Br J Haematol* 1967; 13: 503-509

10. Hemminki E, Rimpela U: A randomized comparison of routine versus selective iron supplementation during pregnancy. *J Am Coll Nutr* 1991; 10: 3-10

11. U.S. Preventive Services Task Force: Routine iron supplementation during pregnancy: policy statement. *JAMA* 1993; 270: 2846-2848

Routine Iron Supplementation During Pregnancy

MANEUVER	EFFECTIVENESS	LEVEL OF EVIDENCE <REF>	RECOMMENDATION
Routine oral iron supplementation in pregnant women	Mixed results have been reported in terms of pre-term birth and birth weight. Trials have not demonstrated clinically significant benefit but have suffered from methodologic limitations or small sample size.	Cohort and case-control studies<6,7> (II-2) Randomized controlled trials and quasi-randomized controlled trials<8-10> (I;II-1)	There is insufficient evidence to recommend for or against the routine use of oral iron supplements in pregnant women (C)

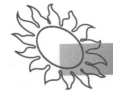

CHAPTER 7

Primary and Secondary Prevention of Neural Tube Defects

By Marie-Dominique Beaulieu
and Brenda L. Beagan

7

Primary and Secondary Prevention of Neural Tube Defects

Prepared by Marie-Dominique Beaulieu, MD, MSc, FCFP[1] and Brenda L. Beagan, MA[2]

In 1979, the Canadian Task Force (CTF) on the Periodic Health Examination,<1> concluded that there was fair evidence to include maternal serum alpha-fetoprotein (MSAFP) measurement as a screening maneuver for neural tube defects (NTD) in the care of pregnant women.

A recent review of published evidence by the CTF<2> confirmed that there is still fair evidence to recommend screening for neural tube defects with MSAFP measurement at 16-18 weeks of gestation in low-risk pregnancies. High resolution ultrasonography performed by a trained radiologist can be an adequate alternative. Women at risk for NTD should be referred directly to specialized services which may include MSAFP screening. All women of child-bearing age considering pregnancy should be advised to increase their intake of folic acid to 0.4 mg per day at least one month before conception and three months after. Pharmaceutical supplementation should be considered if adequate dietary intake is unlikely to be maintained. For high-risk women (women with a previous personal or family history of NTD pregnancy), there is good evidence to recommend folic acid supplementation at a dosage of 4.0 mg/day three months before conception and during the first trimester. This does not replace screening and genetic counselling.

Burden of Suffering

Neural tube defects (NTDs) arise from improper development of the neural tube during embryogenesis. Anencephaly is incompatible with life. Spina bifida can range from mild (spina bifida occulta) to severe (myelomeningocele), and associated morbidity may include paraplegia, bladder and bowel incontinence, and other physical handicaps, as well as possible mental impairment.<3>

The worldwide incidence of fetal NTDs ranges between 1 and 8 per 1,000 births, and varies considerably geographically. In Canada, the incidence of NTD is 1 to 2 per 1,000 births and incidence rates vary regionally, NTD decreasing from east to west. It is estimated to

About 400 to 800 Canadian infants are delivered annually with a NTD

---

[1] Associate Professor Family Medicine, University of Montreal, Montreal, Quebec
[2] Research Associate to the Task Force, 1990-92, Department of Pediatrics, Dalhousie University, Halifax, Nova Scotia

be 4 per 1,000 births in Quebec and 1.6 per 1,000 in British Columbia.<4> Approximately 400 to 800 Canadian infants are delivered annually with a NTD (figure obtained by applying the 1991 birth rate to the prevalence of NTD).

Though 90-95% of NTDs occur in families where there is no previous history of NTD,<3> having a family or obstetric history of NTD places a pregnant woman at a much higher risk. The risk of recurrence for a woman who has had one NTD pregnancy is estimated at about 2-3%, more than 10 times the general population risk.<3>

Maneuver

Primary Prevention: the Role of Folic Acid

Case-control studies have found a protective effect of high maternal red cell folate concentrations, of high maternal dietary folate intake and of peri-conceptional vitamin use in an amount generally less than 1 mg per day. The results of two recent randomized controlled trials (RCTs) have further confirmed the causal association between folic acid and NTD in high-risk as well as in low-risk pregnancies.<5,6>

The daily folic acid allowance recommended for non-pregnant women is 0.17 mg.<7> The mean daily intake of Canadian women is estimated to be around 0.15 mg. On this diet, 10% of them have red cell folates below normal levels.<7> Folate requirement is increased to 0.4 mg/day during pregnancy. Clinical and subclinical folate deficiency is estimated to occur in about 25% of pregnancies in North America and the United Kingdom.<7> Folates are rendered inactive by heat, oxidation, extreme pH and ultraviolet light. Hence folates are likely to be lost during food storage and cooking.

Secondary Prevention: Screening

For screening purposes, MSAFP levels are determined between 16 and 18 weeks of gestation. If MSAFP levels are above 2 multiples of the median (MoM), ultrasonography is performed to confirm the gestational age and to rule out other possible explanations for high MSAFP levels, including multiple gestations, diabetes mellitus, and fetal malformations other than NTD. If MSAFP levels are elevated and ultrasonography provides no explanation, amniocentesis is usually performed for diagnosis.

Sensitivity and specificity of screening MSAFP range respectively between 72% to 91% and 96.2% to 98.7%.<8> The predictive value of a negative test is above 98.96%. In a screening program applied to a low-risk population, the proportion of abnormal screening MSAFP results can be expected to vary between 1.2% and 3.9% of the

Screening MSAFP has a sensitivity of 72-91% and a specificity of 96.2-98.7%

population screened. Only half of these women will have to undergo confirmatory amniocentesis. In most of the large cohort studies on screening programs, there were no terminations of normal pregnancies. However, other investigators have reported false positive rates for amniocentesis of 0.006% to 0.05%.<9> Also note that repeat blood group (D (formerly Rh)) antibody screening is recommended before induced abortion or amniocentesis (see Chapter 11).

The recent improvement in ultrasound diagnosis of NTDs, with specificity and sensitivity approaching 100%, has caused some experts to question the need for amniocentesis in investigating pregnancies with elevated MSAFP and a normal high resolution ultrasonogram.<10>

Effectiveness of Screening and Treatment

Effectiveness of Folic Acid in the Primary Prevention of NTD

Conclusive evidence of the protective effect of folic acid in high risk pregnancies has become available with the publication of the results from an international multicentre randomized double-blind controlled trial.<5> The trial evaluated the effectiveness of 4 mg/day supplementation. NTDs recurred in 6 of 593 (1.0%) pregnancies in which the women were receiving folic acid, and in 21 of 602 (3.5%) pregnancies in which women were not receiving folic acid, for a relative risk of 0.28 (95% confidence interval (CI): 0.12-0.71).

Folic acid supplementation between 0.4-0.8 mg daily reduces the risk of first occurrence of NTD by 40%

Two recent studies have shown that peri-conceptional folic acid supplementation can also decrease by 40% the risk of first occurrence of NTD in low risk pregnancies.<6,11> A randomized double-blind controlled trial showed the efficacy of peri-conceptional multivitamin use containing 0.8 mg/day of folic acid taken at least one month before conception and during the first 12 weeks of pregnancy. The vitamin-supplement group experienced a decreased prevalence of congenital malformations as a whole (13.3 per 1,000 vs. 22.9 per 1,000; p=0.02), and of first occurrence of NTD (no cases of NTD vs. 6; p=0.029).

A 0.4 mg folic acid supplement has been shown to confer a similar protection in a case-controlled study performed in the United States.<11> The authors could not demonstrate that dietary intake alone was as effective, although the test for trend was statistically significant.

Research on the safety and adverse effects of folic acid supplementation is scanty. Physicians should be aware that the 4 mg/day dosage of folic acid may mask the hematologic manifestations of vitamin B12 deficiency without preventing its neurological consequences. Also, it is not known if large doses of folic acid can precipitate convulsions in epileptic women well controlled with phenylhydantoin.

Effectiveness of Screening Programs

There are no randomized controlled trials of screening programs for the early detection of NTDs.

One study has reported on the effectiveness of an alpha-fetoprotein screening program, taking into account the practicalities of implementation.[12] MSAFP screening was offered to all pregnant women who attended antenatal clinics in Mid Glamorgan, South Wales, during the study period (n=15,687). Only 70% actually received screening (n=10,949); most of the others attended too late for screening. Of the 66 NTDs in this series, 12 occurred in the unscreened population, and 54 occurred in the screened group. Eleven out of the latter group were not detected, while another 6 cases were detected but not terminated. Thus, Roberts *et al* concluded that if efficacy is defined as the proportion of NTDs detected and terminated as a consequence of serum-AFP measurements, the efficacy in this study, which had a detection rate of 80%, was 56.1% (37/66) for all open NTDs.

However, termination of pregnancy is not necessarily the only positive outcome of a screening program. There is some evidence that prenatal detection of an NTD may facilitate optimal management of the delivery, thereby reducing subsequent morbidity.[13]

There have been several economic analyses of prenatal NTD screening programs, and they have concluded that screening is cost effective, even in low incidence areas. In Ontario, Tosi and colleagues[14] estimated that there would be a cost-benefit to screening as long as the incidence rate was above 0.7 per 1,000, and MSAFP sensitivity over 61%. Besides some centres in Ontario, Manitoba is the only Canadian province offering an organized MSAFP screening program for low-risk pregnancies.

Recommendations of Others

The Canadian Society of Obstetricians and Gynecologists[4] and the Canadian Centre for Disease Control of the Health Protection Branch[15] recommend that high-risk women should be advised to take 4 mg folic acid daily as soon as they plan to become pregnant. They also recommend that all women of childbearing age who are capable of becoming pregnant should be advised of the options available to them to obtain daily intakes of 0.4 mg of folic acid and be encouraged to meet this goal.

The Canadian College of Medical Geneticists and the Society of Obstetricians and Gynecologists of Canada consider that MSAFP screening is of value in low risk pregnancies when provided in conjunction with access to high quality laboratory, ultrasonography, amniocentesis, abortion, and counselling services. High-risk women should be offered MSAFP screening in conjunction with high resolution ultrasonography and genetic counselling.<4>

In 1989, the U.S. Preventive Services Task Force recommended that amniocentesis for karyotyping be offered to pregnant women aged 35 and older and that MSAFP should be measured on all pregnant women during weeks 16-18 in locations that have adequate counselling and follow-up services; ultrasound was not recommended.<16> These recommendations are currently under review.

Conclusions and Recommendations

Primary Prevention: Folic Acid Supplementation

Folic acid taken one month before and three months after conception is an effective primary prevention maneuver

For women at low risk, there is good to fair evidence that supplementation with folic acid at a dosage between 0.4 mg and 0.8 mg/day reduces the risk of NTD by 40%. To be effective, supplementation should begin at least one month before pregnancy and continue during the first trimester. All women of child-bearing age capable of becoming pregnant should be advised to increase their daily intake of folic acid to the recommended peri-conceptional and pregnancy requirement of 0.4 mg/day. Supplementation appears to be a practical way to achieve this goal (A Recommendation). Preparations containing folic acid only are preferred to avoid the risk of teratogenesis of vitamin A.

For high-risk women, there is good evidence to recommend folic acid supplementation of 4.0 mg/day three months before conception and during the first trimester (A Recommendation). There is a risk that this regimen may precipitate convulsions in women suffering from epilepsy who are controlled by anticonvulsant therapy. These women should be referred to a neurologist for advice.

Secondary Prevention: Prenatal Screening

MSAFP screening at 16-18 weeks of gestation is recommended only if it is part of an organized screening program

There is fair evidence for including screening for neural tube defects in the periodic health examination of low risk pregnant women with maternal serum alpha-fetoprotein measurement at 16-18 weeks of gestation, provided further diagnostic services including amniocentesis and ultrasonography are available, and informed consent is obtained (B Recommendation). Practitioners who have access to high resolution ultrasonography performed by trained radiologists could rely on it as a screening maneuver as long as it is performed between the 16th and the 18th week of gestation.

Women at high risk of NTD should be referred directly to specialized services where appropriate diagnostic services will be

offered to them which may include MSAFP screening
(B Recommendation).

Unanswered Questions (Research Agenda)

Considering the number of individuals to be reached and that
the intervention should begin before pregnancy, there is an urgent
need to evaluate the feasibility and effectiveness of a public health
program of enrichment of commercial food with folic acid. This could
be the most effective strategy to reach the population at risk.

Evidence

A MEDLINE search from 1979 to April 1993 was conducted
using the MESH headings: neural tube defects, prenatal diagnosis, and
prevention and control, with all subheadings. Priority was given to the
highest available levels of evidence according to the CTF's criteria. This
review was initiated in January, 1991 and the recommendations were
finalized by the Task Force in June 1993. A technical report with a full
reference list is available upon request.<2>

Acknowledgements

The Task Force wishes to thank Serge Melançon, MD, Professor
of Pediatrics, University of Montreal, Montreal, Quebec and Chief
geneticist at Hôpital Ste-Justine, Montreal, Quebec, Louis Dallaire, MD,
Professor of Pediatrics, University of Montreal, Montreal, Quebec and
geneticist at Hôpital Ste-Justine, Montreal, Quebec, Members of the
Québec Genetic Screening Network, and Catherine McCourt, MD,
Adjunct Professor, University of Ottawa Laboratory Centre for
Disease Control, Health Canada, Ottawa, Ontario, for their
comments.

Selected References

1. Report of a Task Force to the Conference of Deputy Ministers of
    Health (cat no H39-3/1980E), Health Services and Promotion
    Branch, Department of National Health and Welfare, Ottawa,
    1980

2. Canadian Task Force on the Periodic Health Examination: The
    periodic health examination. 1994 Update: 3. Primary and
    secondary prevention of neural tube defects. *Can Med Assoc J*
    1994; 151: 159-166

3. Cohen FL: Neural tube defects: epidemiology, detection, and
    prevention. *J Obstet Gynecol Neonatal Nurs* 1987; 16: 105-115

4. SOGC Genetic Committee: Recommendations on the use of
    folic acid for the prevention of neural tube defects. *J SOGC*
    1993; March: 41-46

5. MRC Vitamin Study Research Group: Prevention of neural tube defects: Results of the Medical Research Council vitamin study. *Lancet* 1991; 338: 131-137

6. Czeizel AE, Dudas I: Prevention of the first occurrence of neural-tube defects by periconceptional vitamin supplementation. *N Engl J Med* 1992; 327: 1832-1835

7. Nutrition recommendations. The report of the scientific review committee 1990. Minister of Supplies and Services Canada Ottawa 1990, 116-123

8. Crandall BF, Robertson RD, Lebherz TB, *et al*: Maternal serum α-fetoprotein screening for the detection of neural tube defects. *West J Med* 1983: 138: 524-530

9. Milunsky A, Alpert E: Results and benefits of a maternal serum α-fetoprotein screening program. *JAMA* 1984; 252: 1438-1442

10. Nadel AS, Green JK, Holmes LB, *et al*: Absence of need for amniocentesis in patients with elevated levels of maternal serum alpha-fetoprotein and normal ultrasonographic examinations. *New Engl J Med* 1990; 323: 557-561

11. Werler MM, Shapiro S, Mitchel AA: Periconceptional folic acid exposure and risk of occurrence of neural tube defects. *JAMA* 1993; 269: 1257-1261

12. Roberts CJ, Hibbard BM, Elder GH, *et al*: The efficacy of a serum screening service for neural-tube defects: The South Wales experience. *Lancet* 1983; 1: 1315-1318

13. Luthy DA, Wardinsky T, Shurtleff DB, *et al*: Cesarean section before the onset of labor and subsequent motor function in infants with meningomyelocele diagnosed antenatally. *New Engl J Med* 1991; 324: 662-666

14. Tosi LL, Detsky AS, Roye DP, *et al*: When does mass screening for open neural tube defects in low-risk pregnancies result in cost savings? *Can Med Assoc J* 1987; 136: 255-265

15. McCourt C: Primary prevention of neural tube defects: notice from the HPB. *Can Med Assoc J* 1993; 148: 1451

16. U.S. Preventive Services Task Force: *Guide to Clinical Preventive Services: an Assessment of the Effectiveness of 169 Interventions*. Williams & Wilkins, Baltimore, Md, 1989: 225-232

Primary and Secondary Prevention of Neural Tube Defects

MANEUVER	EFFECTIVENESS	LEVEL OF EVIDENCE <REF>	RECOMMENDATION
Periconceptional folic acid supplementation	**High-risk women**: Supplementation with 4 mg folic acid daily during the 3 months before and 3 months after conception reduces the risk of Neural Tube Defect (NTD) recurrence in high-risk women.	Randomized controlled trial<13> (I)	Good evidence to prescribe a 4 mg folic acid supplement daily for women with a previous history of NTD pregnancy (A)*
	Low risk-women: Folic acid supplementation in a daily dose of 0.4 to 0.8 mg taken at least one month before and three months after conception decreases the risk of NTD.	Randomized controlled trial for 0.8 mg<14> (I); case-control study for 0.4 mg<12> (II-2)	Good evidence to advise all women capable of becoming pregnant to increase their consumption of folic acid to 0.4 mg/day. Supplementation appears to be the most effective and practical way to achieve this goal (A)*
Maternal serum alpha-fetoprotein (MSAFP) measurement at 16-18 weeks should be offered to those who may wish to consider interruption of pregnancy with an affected child; elevated levels followed by ultrasonography and amniocentesis if necessary	Screening programs, including the necessary diagnostic services and with termination of affected pregnancies, can significantly reduce the number of children born with NTDs. Up to 90% of open NTDs can be detected. However, there is some risk of terminating unaffected pregnancies.	Cohort studies <27-31,36> (II-2)	Fair evidence to include screening in the periodic health examination of all pregnant women as long as it is part of a quality-controlled program. High resolution ultrasonography may be adequate for low-risk women but MSAFP should be made available to high-risk women (B)

* Folic acid supplementation may provoke convulsions in epileptic women who are controlled by anticonvulsant therapy. It may be prudent to restrict counselling to dietary advice in these women.

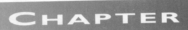

CHAPTER 8

Prenatal Screening and Diagnosis for Down Syndrome Prevention

By Paul Dick

Prenatal Screening and Diagnosis for Down Syndrome Prevention

Prepared by Paul Dick, MDCM, FRCPC[1]

In 1979 the Canadian Task Force on the Periodic Health Examination reviewed the evidence for prenatal diagnosis of Down Syndrome (DS) and concluded that there was fair evidence to offer amniocentesis to pregnant women from high-risk groups, including parents with translocation of chromosome 21, a family history of DS, or maternal age over 35 years.<1> This review will evaluate evidence which has been published recently on the use of the triple marker screen (multiple maternal serum markers), and chorionic villus sampling (CVS) for screening and diagnosis of DS pregnancies.

The logic underlying prenatal screening and diagnosis for DS involves the following assumptions: 1) Screening tests must be reasonably accurate in identifying DS fetuses. Confirmatory diagnostic tests must be highly accurate, with a good safety profile, and available during a period of gestation when pregnancy termination is safe and acceptable and 2) Early detection of DS pregnancies with provision for pregnancy termination provides informed reproductive choice for those who wish to use it.

Burden of Suffering

Down Syndrome, a congenital syndrome associated with chromosomal aneuploidy of all or part of chromosome 21, is the most common pattern of malformation seen in humans, with a median birth incidence rate of 1 per 1,000 births.<2> Clinically important problems include general hypotonia, mental retardation, growth retardation, and a significant risk for congenital malformations, of which a cardiac defect is the most common.<3> Though effective therapies are available for some of the specific malformations and problems associated with DS, there are no proven therapies available for the cognitive deficits.

Literature on DS persons and their families has focused on dysfunctional outcomes. Up to 10% of families are unable or unprepared to cope with a DS child, and many others are affected by maternal depression, and difficulties with marital and sibling relationships.<4-6> Though family functioning may be adversely affected by a DS child, this is not a necessary outcome.<5>

---

[1] Assistant Professor, Department of Pediatrics, University of Toronto, Division of General Pediatrics, The Hospital for Sick Children, Toronto, Ontario

Maneuver

Two approaches are available for prenatal diagnosis of DS: 1) Prenatal diagnosis with amniocentesis or chorionic villus sampling (CVS) offered to women at risk by virtue of their history (previous DS birth, advance maternal age, certain chromosomal rearrangements), and 2) prenatal diagnosis with amniocentesis offered to women identified as at increased risk through the use of screening maneuvers (maternal serum markers, ultrasonography).

Historical Risk Factors

Studies using a variety of methods have consistently demonstrated an increasing risk of DS birth with advancing maternal age (the risk of a DS birth at age 20 being approximately 1 in 1,500, rising to 1 in 30 at 45 years of age).[7-14] Parents carrying chromosome 21 rearrangements are also at an increased risk for DS pregnancies.[15-17] An increased rate of subsequent DS pregnancy has also been reported with parents of previous DS births in the absence of detectable chromosome rearrangements, independent of advancing age.[18-20] Other factors such as paternal age, parental consanguinity, second or third degree DS relationship, environmental radiation, etc. have not been consistently shown to significantly affect the incidence of the DS birth.

Women with advanced maternal age, or a previous history of a DS birth are at a higher risk for a DS pregnancy

Maternal Serum Marker Screening

Maternal serum alpha fetoprotein (AFP), human chorionic gonadotropin (HCG), and unconjugated estriol (uE3) levels have all been shown to be associated with DS gestations. Individually these markers have relatively poor discriminatory power, but the simultaneous use of all three serum markers (Triple Screening) in the second trimester has received much attention recently. Probabilities derived from the individual markers and the maternal age-related risk are used to generate a post-screen probability of a DS fetus for each gestation.[21,22] Women with a post-screen probability that exceeds a certain cut off level (e.g. a 1 in 250 risk, similar to that of risk women age 35 years and over) can be offered amniocentesis.

Four cohort studies have compared the proportion of DS pregnancies identified through Triple Screening with the total number of DS pregnancies (the sum of DS fetuses detected prenatally and those DS pregnancies not detected, but observed as live births through surveillance of regional cytogenetics laboratory results).[23-26] Detection rates ranged from 48-91%, with false positive rates of 3.2-6% respectively. The different risk cutoffs (1 in 190 to 1 in 274) used in the studies account for some of this variation. A positive predictive value of 1.2-1.8% was achieved in the trials among low-risk women without advanced maternal age. Therefore, a woman

Approximately 50% of DS pregnancies in women less than 35 years can be identified with the triple marker screening. Approximately 5% of these women will have a positive screen and will be offered amniocentesis, but only about 2% of these women carry a DS fetus

with a pre-screen risk of 1 in 1,000 who tested positive upon screening would have a post-screen risk of 1 in 56 – 1 in 85 for a DS gestation. This post-screen risk is similar to that of women with advanced age who are currently offered prenatal diagnosis.

A recent descriptive study in women over 35 years of age, reported that using triple marker screening, 90% of DS pregnancies would have been detected with an amniocentesis rate of 25%.[27] The high negative predictive value of the screen in this age group may be helpful to women who wish to exclude the possibilities of a DS fetus but wish to avoid amniocentesis or CVS if possible. At this point there is still insufficient evidence to evaluate offering women over age 35 years only triple marker screening.

Ultrasound Screening

The abnormalities associated with DS (IUGR, hydrops, some cardiac anomalies, etc.) and differences in long bone length and nuchal fold thickness between DS and normal pregnancies that can be observed on ultrasound during the second trimester have recently been reviewed.[28] Only one prospective clinical trial of sonographic screening for DS fetuses has been reported. The sensitivity and positive predictive value of fetal nuchal fold thickening for DS was 75% and 25% respectively (12 out of 16 DS fetuses from a sample of 3,338 women were detected by sonography).[29] As the sample consisted mainly of high-risk women with advanced maternal age or other factors (DS rate of 1/209) the positive predictive value would be significantly lower in lower risk women. The trial did not address important measurement issues. Small differences in technique, equipment or operators may have a substantial impact on screening performance, and the results obtained from a small group of well trained and equipped operators in a research context will not necessarily generalize to widespread use.

Amniocentesis

Second trimester amniocentesis has been demonstrated as extremely accurate and reliable for prenatal diagnosis of DS with a controlled trial, and cohort studies.[30-33]

Chorionic Villus Sampling

Transcervical chorionic villus sampling (CVS) is a first trimester alternative to amniocentesis for diagnosis of chromosomal disorders. Accurate prenatal diagnosis has been obtained in over 99% of high-risk women with CVS with controlled trials vs. amniocentesis,[34-36] and cohort studies.[37-42] Amniocentesis is necessary to clarify the diagnosis, or to obtain a karyotype when CVS fails, as occurs for up to 5% of women. Transabdominal CVS is a new alternative to transcervical CVS and has comparable accuracy.<34,43,44> Placental position and operator experience may best determine the choice of these two procedures. Errors in diagnosis with CVS usually involve sex determination errors from maternal cell contamination, or mosaicism due to karyotypic abnormalities confined to placental tissue.

Pregnancy Termination

Pregnancy termination is sought by the majority of women who have undergone prenatal diagnosis revealing a fetus with DS. First trimester abortion following CVS represents the safest form of termination with serious complications being extremely rare.<45,46> Retained fetal products is common with second trimester abortions, but more serious complications are quite rare.<47,48> Women of unknown or D (Rh negative) bloodgroup undergoing induced abortion or amniocentesis should have repeat blood group antibody screening (see Chapter 11). Screening before CVS or other obstetrical procedures as well as in concert with complications is more controversial.

Effectiveness of Prevention and Treatment

No studies have been performed to prove that those utilizing screening and prenatal diagnosis for DS fetuses have better outcomes compared with those who do not. The goal of prenatal diagnosis is the provision of a safe and efficacious means of identifying pregnancies for those couples who wish to exercise reproductive choice.

Women at high risk for DS gestation, identified either by screening, advanced maternal age, or previous DS birth, can be offered accurate prenatal diagnosis in the second trimester with amniocentesis. Those identified at high risk prior to pregnancy, or during the first trimester can be offered first trimester CVS as an alternative to amniocentesis.

Adverse Effects

Both amniocentesis and CVS are associated with an increased risk of fetal loss. Some studies have suggested a procedure-related loss of up to 0.8% with amniocentesis,<29-32,49> and over 1% to 1.5% with CVS.<34-36> However, the results of the Canadian Multicentre Randomized Trial<36> have shown that the rate of procedure-related loss with amniocentesis can be as low as 0.04% in experienced hands.

The best evidence of risk from CVS has been obtained from randomized controlled trials of CVS versus amniocentesis.<33-36> These consistently show increased fetal loss when compared with amniocentesis, with an estimated procedure-related risk of fetal loss of at least 1% to 1.5%. Inexperience (i.e. the number performed by centre

Amniocentesis and CVS can both accurately diagnose DS fetuses, but carry a small risk of miscarriage. The risk of other fetal injury or neonatal morbidity is still somewhat uncertain, but appears extremely slight

or operator), and the use of trans-cervical CVS rather than trans-abdominal approach appear related to a greater risk of fetal loss in these studies.

Existing trials of amniocentesis and CVS have inadequate sample sizes for detection and statistical testing of rare adverse effects. There have been suggestions of an increase in neonatal respiratory disease following amniocentesis,[30] and an increased risk of fetal limb reduction anomalies with CVS in case-control studies,[50,51] though the significance is unclear. The risk of limb reduction and other anomalies following CVS appears related to gestational age and CVS is discouraged prior to 10 weeks gestation.[52] Severe maternal complications with amniocentesis and CVS are rarely reported.[30-44]

Psychological distress associated with prenatal screening can include the fear of revealing an abnormal pregnancy, and facing a decision about pregnancy continuation, as well as anxiety over possible complications from diagnostic procedures and abortion. Women who have had a positive screening test may have greater distress than those women at the same risk from advanced age.[53,54] Distress is reduced following a diagnostic procedure, with confirmation of a normal pregnancy, but some anxiety related to the false positive test may persist despite reassurance.[55] No studies have addressed the potential for distress experienced by the significant number of women who test positive on the screen, but decline prenatal diagnosis and or pregnancy termination.

There is little available evidence on the long-term psychological implications of having used prenatal screening, diagnosis and termination of abnormal fetuses. Likewise, there is still little evidence about the burden of fear of giving birth to a DS child.

Decision Making in Prenatal Diagnosis

Critical ethical issues are raised by selective abortion for DS pregnancies. Full discussion of these issue is beyond the scope of this review. Society may interpret the offer of diagnosis and termination for DS fetuses as an implicit message that DS is by definition an undesirable state, and DS individuals worthless. Voluntary reproductive services may be promoted, seen, and evaluated by some in eugenic terms. Evolving societal pressures (including economic), may eventually serve to constrain choices, and create a stigma for the family with a DS individual. Diagnostic and preventive services must be aimed at increasing individuals' control. They must be voluntary, not routine or expected, and offered in a value-sensitive fashion with emphasis on reliable information about DS and not just about the procedures.

Utilization of prenatal diagnosis is related both to views on the acceptability of pregnancy termination and the perceived risk of the fetus being abnormal.[56] Health care professionals play an important role in shaping these beliefs and many women feel that the potential for persuasion does exist.<57> The perception of harm or the nature of the disability may play a greater role in the decision than the actual probability of its occurrence.<58-61>

Given the low positive predictive value of a positive screen (1 to 2%) the effectiveness of this maneuver is usually predicated on an intention to proceed with amniocentesis in the event of a positive test, as well as on the couple's understanding of the effect that a DS birth may have. The availability of support (DS societies, etc.) to assist in coping with a DS child, as well as the family's own resources for coping should be considered when assessing the potential impact of a DS birth.

Informed consent for the screen must include details and risks of second trimester amniocentesis and pregnancy termination. A delay in obtaining test results, and in arranging procedures can mean that a women presenting for the triple screen at 16 weeks may not be informed of the result or be able to book an amniocentesis until 18 to 19 weeks gestation, with a further delay in obtaining results and arrangements resulting in termination of pregnancy at or beyond 21 weeks. Some women of advanced maternal age may prefer first trimester CVS for prenatal diagnosis rather than utilizing triple screening which would require second trimester amniocentesis if positive.

Recommendations of Others

The U.S. Preventive Services Task Force,<62> and The Society of Obstetricians and Gynecologists of Canada in association with the Canadian College of Medical Geneticists<63> have all recommended that amniocentesis or CVS be offered to high-risk women with a family history of DS, translocation or advanced maternal age. Other than recognizing their investigational status, no other organizations have addressed the use of multiple maternal serum markers or ultrasonography for DS screening, although the U.S. Preventive Services Task Force recommendation is currently under review. The Cochrane Pregnancy and Childbirth Group has recently reviewed genetic amniocentesis, ultrasound guidance during 2nd trimester amniocentesis, CVS compared with amniocentesis, transabdominal compared with transcervical CVS, and early amniocentesis.<64-68> They concluded that both amniocentesis and CVS are accurate, and that, although amniocentesis has a lower procedure-related fetal loss, the earlier diagnosis obtainable with CVS may make it more desirable for some individuals. Transabdominal CVS has been associated with less procedure-related loss than transcervical CVS.

Conclusions and Recommendations

There is fair evidence to support offering prenatal diagnosis, with CVS or amniocentesis to pregnant women with identified risk factors: advanced maternal age of 35 years or older, a history of previous DS pregnancy, or known carrier status for a chromosomal rearrangement associated with DS (B Recommendation). Fetal loss appears slightly increased with amniocentesis (approximately 0.8% procedure related fetal loss), and CVS (1.0% to 1.5%). The optimal choice of procedure may be influenced by a host of factors. An A Recommendation cannot be made because good evidence is lacking on personal and family outcomes, and the balance of risks and benefits for the group as a whole. However, it is clear that those women at very high risk (e.g. previous DS child, etc.) and who have significant anxiety over this possibility may benefit substantially from prenatal diagnosis.

Triple marker screening in the second trimester with AFP, HCG and uE3 when combined with maternal age-specific risks can offer an approximate 50% risk reduction for low-risk women (less than 35 years), with a false positive rate of approximately 5%. The evidence is derived from cohort studies using amniocentesis as the gold standard in those who screened positive, and follow-up through a regional cytogenetics laboratory in those who screened negative or declined amniocentesis. The results were consistent between trials when accounting for the differing cut-offs chosen. The positive predictive value of a positive screen is similar to, or higher than the age-related risk in women with advanced maternal age (>35 years) who are currently offered prenatal diagnosis, and the number of amniocenteses per DS fetus identified are fewer.

The studies of triple marker screening meet the Task Force criteria for type II evidence.<31> The Task Force concludes that there is fair evidence (B Recommendation) to support offering triple marker screening to women under 35 years of age when a comprehensive screening and prenatal diagnosis program is available (including education, interpretation and follow-up). It should be recognized that triple marker screening is not supported by the same strength of evidence or efficacy when compared with amniocentesis or CVS for advanced maternal age and other risk factors.

The Task Force is concerned with the limited sensitivity of the screening test, the number of women with false positive screens, and the sub-optimal rate of follow-through to amniocentesis noted in the trials. These limitations place a heavy burden on family physicians and obstetricians to provide full information to those couples interested in the screen. Even when a comprehensive screening program is available, many physicians may consider the burden of counselling low-risk women onerous. Screening of maternal serum markers outside of a fully coordinated program is undesirable. Triple marker screening followed by prenatal diagnosis may be offered to women over 35 years of age as an alternative to prenatal diagnosis alone. There is insufficient evidence for the offer of triple marker screening to replace exclusively the offer of prenatal diagnosis with CVS or amniocentesis to women with advanced maternal age.

Informed consent prior to triple marker screening must include: 1) the limitations in screening sensitivity and specificity; 2) the risks and harms associated with prenatal diagnosis and second trimester abortion; and 3) the psychological implications of screening and diagnosis, as well as the implications of having a DS child. Women consenting to the screen must also be aware of the delays inherent in the process and must understand the nature of a 20 week abortion (i.e. induction and delivery of a fetus).

There is a lack of sound evidence to support the use of individual maternal serum markers (such as AFP alone) for DS fetus screening. Maternal serum AFP measurement may be used to screen for neural tube defects (see Chapter 7). The optimal timing for AFP measurement, after 16 weeks, does not overlap with the optimal timing of DS serum marker screening, 15 weeks gestation. Ultrasonographic screening using long bone, and nuchal fold indices is not recommended for DS screening as part of the periodic health examination of pregnant women. Given insufficient evaluation for effectiveness and the concerns regarding measurement reliability and generalizability, there is insufficient evidence to support a recommendation for routinely offering ultrasonographic screening for early diagnosis of DS fetuses.

In these recommendations sole consideration has been given to the prenatal diagnosis of DS. Other chromosomal anomalies are frequently detected during prenatal diagnosis (Turner's syndrome, Trisomy 13, etc.) and many may consider their detection important. Other chromosome anomalies have not been considered independently in these recommendations as the diagnostic issues with CVS and amniocentesis are similar to those with DS, there are few studies directly addressing these anomalies, and screening maneuvers have not been sufficiently evaluated to warrant review at this point. These recommendations do not apply to women who are at risk for non-chromosomal genetic abnormalities.

Unanswered Questions (Research Agenda)

There are a number of outstanding questions about DS prenatal screening and diagnosis. Continued evaluation of the triple screen is necessary. Research is in progress on screening with maternal HCG and AFP (double marker screening) and some experts suggest it should replace triple marker screening. Better age- and race-specific predictive values for triple marker screening are needed to provide confidence for individual estimates within subgroups such as women with significantly advanced maternal age. The value of routine ultrasonography for gestational age determination at the time of triple marker screening requires clarification. The development of a more accurate first-trimester DS screening technique would significantly improve the effectiveness and minimize harms associated with triple marker screening.

The potentially adverse effects of screening and diagnosis require further clarification. Information is needed on the outcomes of women with false positive screening tests, and those with positive screening tests who decline prenatal diagnosis and/or pregnancy termination. Comparison of screening tests followed by prenatal diagnosis vs. prenatal diagnosis alone for women of advanced maternal age or with other risk factors is indicated. The outcome of infants born following prenatal diagnosis requires continued monitoring with special attention to rare events such as limb reduction defects following CVS.

The impact of prenatal screening and diagnosis on societal perceptions of disabled individuals deserves attention. The consequences of DS births and alternatives to screening and diagnosis must be better understood, including the impact of coping skills and supportive interventions on the quality of life in families with handicapped children.

Evidence

The literature was identified with a MEDLINE search, from 1966 to March 1993, using the key words Down Syndrome, prenatal diagnosis, prevention, epidemiology and diagnosis subheadings. The review was initiated in February 1993 and recommendations finalized in March 1994 by the Task Force.

Acknowledgments

The principal author would like to acknowledge the assistance of Dr. William Feldman, and Dr. Elaine Wang in reviewing the evidence, and of Karen Huntley in preparing the manuscript.

Selected References

1. Canadian Task Force on the Periodic Health Examination: The periodic health examination. *Can Med Assoc J* 1979; 121: 1193-1254

2. Adams MM, Erickson JD, Layde PM, *et al*: Down's syndrome. Recent trends in the United States. *JAMA* 1981; 246(7): 758-760

3. Smith DW: Recognizable patterns of human malformation. Philadelphia: Saunders, 1976: 4-6

4. Cnric KA: Families with Down Syndrome: ecological contexts and characteristics. In: Cicchetti D, Beeghly M (eds): *Children with Down Syndrome: a developmental perspective.* Cambridge: Cambridge University Press, 1990: 399-423

5. Carr J: The effect on the family of a severely mentally handicapped child. In: Clarke AM, Clarke ADB, Berg JM (Eds): *Mental deficiency: the changing outlook.* 4th ed London: Methuen, 1985: 512-548

6. Gath A: Down Syndrome children and their families. *Am J Med Genet Suppl* 1990; 7: 314-316

7. Ferguson-Smith MA, Yates JR: Maternal age specific rates for chromosome aberrations and factors influencing them: report of a collaborative European study on 52,965 amniocenteses. *Prenat Diagn* 1984; 4: 5-44

8. Hook EB: Rates of chromosome abnormalities at different maternal ages. *Obstet Gynecol* 1981; 58(3): 282-285

9. Hook EB, Fabia JJ: Frequency of Down syndrome in livebirths by single-year maternal age interval: results of a Massachusetts study. *Teratology* 1978; 17(3): 223-228

10. Trimble BK, Baird PA: Maternal age and Down syndrome: age-specific incidence rates by single-year intervals. *Am J Med Genet* 1978; 2(1): 1-5

11. Sutherland GR, Clisby SR, Bloor G, *et al*: Down's syndrome in South Australia. *Med J Austral* 1979; 2(2): 58-61

12. Koulischer L, Gillerot Y: Down's syndrome in Wallonia (South Belgium), 1971-1978: cytogenetics and incidence. *Hum Genet* 1980; 54(2): 243-250

13. Cuckle HS, Wald NJ: The effect of estimating gestational age by ultrasound cephalometry on the sensitivity of alpha-fetoprotein screening for Down's syndrome. *Br J Obstet Gynaecol* 1987; 94(3): 274-276

14. Hook EB, Topol BB, Cross PK: The natural history of cytogenetically abnormal fetuses detected at midtrimester amniocentesis which are not terminated electively: new data and estimates of the excess and relative risk of late fetal death associated with 47,+21 and some other abnormal karyotypes. *Am J Hum Genet* 1989; 45: 855-861

15. Boue A, Gallano P: A collaborative study of the segregation of inherited chromosome structural rearrangements in 1356 prenatal diagnoses. *Prenat Diagn* 1984; 4: 45-67

16. Stene J: Statistical inference on segregation ratios for D/G translocations, when the families are ascertained in different ways. *Ann Hum Genet* 1970; 34: 93-115

17. Stene J: A statistical segregation analysis of (21q22q)-translocations. *Hum Hered* 1970; 20: 465-472

18. Carter CO, Evans KA: Risk of parents who have had one child with Down's syndrome (mongolism) having another child similarly affected. *Lancet* 1961; ii: 785-787

19. Stene J: Detection of higher recurrance risk for age-dependent chromosome abnormalities with application to Trisomy G_1 (Down syndrome). *Hum Hered* 1970; 20: 112-122

20. Mikkelsen M, Stene J: Previous child with Down's Syndrome and other chromosome aberration. In: Murken JD, Schwinger, SS-R E (Eds): Prenatal Diagnosis: Proceedings of the 3rd European Conference on Prenatal Diagnosis of Genetic Disorders. Stuttgart: Ferdinand Enke, 1979: 22-33

21. Wald NJ, Cuckle HS, Densem JW, *et al*: Maternal serum screening for Down's syndrome in early pregnancy. [published erratum appears in BMJ 1988; 297(6655): 1029] *BMJ* 1988; 297(6653): 883-887

22. Reynolds TM: Software for screening to assess risk of Down's syndrome [letter] *BMJ* 1991; 302(6782): 965

23. Wald NJ, Kennard A, Densem JW, *et al*: Antenatal maternal serum screening for Down's syndrome: results of a demonstration project. *BMJ* 1992; 305(6850): 391-394

24. Cheng EY, Luthy DA, Zebelman AM, *et al*: A prospective evaluation of a second-trimester screening test for fetal Down syndrome using maternal serum alpha-fetoprotein, hCG, and unconjugated estriol. *Obstet Gynecol* 1993; 81(1): 72-77

25. Haddow JE, Palomaki GE, Knight GJ, *et al*: Prenatal screening for Down's syndrome with use of maternal serum markers. *N Engl J Med* 1992; 327(9): 588-593

26. Phillips OP, Elias S, Shulman LP, *et al*: Maternal serum screening for fetal Down syndrome in women less than 35 years of age using alpha-fetoprotein, hCG, and unconjugated estriol: a prospective 2-year study. *Obstet Gynecol* 1992; 80: 353-358

27. Haddow JE, Palomaki GE, Knight GJ, *et al*: Reducing the need for amniocentesis in women 35 years of age or older with serum markers for screening. *New Engl J Med* 1994; 330(16): 1114-1118

28. Lockwood CJ, Lynch L, Berkowitz RL: Ultrasonographic screening for the Down syndrome fetus. *Am J Obstet Gynecol* 1991; 165: 349-352

29. Crane JP, Gray DL: Sonographically measured nuchal skinfold thickness as a screening tool for Down syndrome: results of a prospective clinical trial. *Obstet Gynecol* 1991; 77(4): 533-536

30. Tabor A, Philip J, Madsen M: Randomized controlled trial of genetic amniocentesis in 4606 low-risk women. *Lancet* 1986; 1: 1287-1293

31. NICHD National Registry for Amniocentesis Study Group: Midtrimester amniocentesis for prenatal diagnosis. *JAMA* 1976; 236: 1471-1476

32. MRC Working Party on Amniocentesis: An assessment of the hazard of amniocentesis. *Br J Obstet Gynecol* 1978; 85 (Supp 2): 1-41

33. Simpson N, Dallaire L, Miller JR, *et al*: Prenatal diagnosis of genetic disease in Canada: report of a collaborative study. *Can Med Assoc J* 1976; 23: 739

34. Smidt-Jensen S, Permin M, Philip J, *et al*: Randomized comparison of amniocentesis and transabdominal and transcervical chorionic villus sampling. *Lancet* 1992; 340: 1237-1244

35. MRC Working Party on the Evaluation of Chorionic Villus Sampling, Medical Research Council European Trial of chorion villus sampling. *Lancet* 1991; 337: 1491-1499

36. Lippman A, Darrell J, Tomkins JS, *et al*: Canadian multicentre randomized clinical trial of chorion villus sampling and amniocentesis. Final report. *Prenat Diagn* 1992; 12: 385-476

37. Jahoda M, Piijpers L, Reuss A, *et al*: Evaluation of transcervical chorionic villus sampling with a completed follow-up of 1550 consecutive pregnancies. *Prenat Diagn* 1989; 9: 621-628

38. Leschot NJ, Wolf H, Van-Proolgen-Knegt AC, *et al*: Cytogenetic findings in 1250 chorionic villus samples obtained in the first trimester with clinical follow-up of the first 1,000 pregnancies. *Br J Obstet Gynaecol* 1989; 96: 663-670

39. Brambati B, Oldrini A, Ferrazzi E, *et al*: Chorionic Villus Sampling: an analysis of the obstetric experience of 1,000 cases. *Prenat Diagn* 1987; 7: 157-169

40. Simoni G, Gimelli G, Cuoco C, *et al*: First trimester fetal karyotyping: one thousand diagnoses. *Hum Genet* 1986; 72: 203-209

41. Hogge WA, Schonberg SA, Golbus MS: Chorionic villus sampling: Experience of the first 1,000 cases. *Am J Obstet Gynecol* 1986; 154: 1249-1252

42. Green JE, Dorfmann A, Jones SL, *et al*: Chorionic villus sampling: experience with an initial 940 cases. *Obstet Gynecol* 1988; 71: 208-212

43. Brambati B, Terzian E, Tognoni G: Randomized clinical trial of transabdominal versus transcervical chorionic villus sampling methods. *Prenat Diagn* 1991; 11: 285-293

44. Jackson L, Zachary JM, Fowler SE, *et al*: A randomized comparison of transcervical and transabdominal chorionic-villus sampling. The U.S. National Institute of Child Health and Human Development Chorionic-Villus sampling and Amniocentesis study Group. *N Engl J Med* 1992; 327: 594-598

45. Hakim-Elahi E, Tovell HM, Burnhill MS: Complications of first-trimester abortion: a report of 170,000 cases. *Obstet Gynecol* 1990; 76: 129-135

46. Lawson HW, Atrash HK, Franks AL: Fatal pulmonary embolism during legal induced abortion in the United States from 1972 to 1985. *Am J Obstet Gynecol* 1990; 162: 986-990

47. Harman CR, Fish DG, Tyson JE: Factors influencing morbidity in termination of pregnancy. *Am J Obstet Gynecol* 1981; 139: 333-337

48. Martin MC, Gelfand MM: Mid-trimester abortions: a decade in review. *Can J Surg* 1982; 25: 641-643

49. Tabor A, Philip J, Bang J, *et al*: Needle size and risk of miscarriage after amniocentesis. *Lancet* 1988; 1: 183-184

50. Firth HV, Boyd PA, Chamberlain P, *et al*: Severe limb abnormalities after chorion villus sampling at 56-66 days' gestation. *Lancet* 1991; 337: 762-763

51. Mastroiacovo P, Cavalcanti DP: Limb-reduction defects and chorion villus sampling. *Lancet* 1991; 337: 1091-1092

52. Rodeck, CH: Fetal development after chorionic villus sampling. *Lancet* 1993; 341: 468-469

53. Tunis S, Golbus MS, Copeland KL, *et al*: Patterns of mood states in pregnant women undergoing chorionic villus sampling or amniocentesis. *Am J Med Genet* 1990; 37: 191-199

54. Abuelo DN, Hopmann MR, Barsel-Bowers G, *et al*: Anxiety in women with low maternal serum alpha fetoprotein screening result. *Prenat Diagn* 1991; 11: 381-385

55. Burton BK, Dillard RG, Clark EN: The psychological impact of false positive elevations of maternal serum alpha fetoprotein. *Am J Obstet Gynecol* 1985; 151: 77-82

56. Marteau T, Kidd J, Cook R, *et al*: Perceived risk not actual risk predicts uptake of amniocentesis. *Br J Obstet Gynaecol* 1991; 98: 282-286

57. Sjogren B, Marsk L: Information on prenatal diagnosis at the antenatal clinic. The women's experiences. *Acta Obstet Gynecol Scand* 1989; 68: 35-40

58. Thornton J, Lilford RJ, Howell D: Safety of amniocentesis. [letter] *Lancet* 1986; 2: 225-226

59. Evans M, Bottoms SF, Critchfild GC, *et al*: Parental perceptions of genetic risk: correlation with choice of prenatal diagnostic procedures. *Int J Gynaecol Obstet* 1990; 31: 25-28

60. Ekwo E, Kim J, Gosselink CA: Parental perceptions of the burden of genetic disease. *Am J Med Genet* 1987; 28: 955-963

61. Drugan A, Greb A, Johnson P, *et al*: Determinants of parental decisions to abort for chromosomal abnormalities. *Prenat Diagn* 1990; 10: 483-490

62. U.S. Preventive Services Task Force: *Guide to Clinical Preventive Services: an Assessment of the Effectiveness of 169 Interventions*. Williams & Wilkins, Baltimore, Md, 1989: 225-232

63. Canadian College of Medical Geneticists and Society of Obstetricians and Gynaecologists of Canada: Canadian guidelines for prenatal diagnosis of genetic disorders: An update. *J SOGC* 1993; 15 (Suppl): 15-39

64. Grant AM: Genetic amniocentesis at 16 weeks gestation. In: Pregnancy and Childbirth Module (eds. Enkin MW, Keirse MJNC, Renfrew MJ, Neilson JP), "Cochrane Database of Systematic Reviews": Review No. 04002, 2 April 1992. Published through "Cochrane Updates on Disk", Oxford: Update Software, 1993, Disk Issue 2

65. Grant AM: Chorion villus sampling compared with amniocentesis. In: Pregnancy and Childbirth Module. (eds. Enkin MW, Keirse MJNC, Renfrew MJ, Neilson JP), "Cochrane Database of Systematic Reviews": Review No. 06007, 2 April 1992. Published through "Cochrane Updates on Disk", Oxford: Update Software, 1993, Disk Issue 2

66. Grant AM: Ultrasound guidance during 2nd trimester amniocentesis. In: Pregnancy and Childbirth Module (eds. Enkin MW, Keirse MJNC, Renfrew MJ, Neilson JP), "Cochrane Database of Systematic Reviews": Review No.06588, 30 April 1993. Published through "Cochrane Updates on Disk", Oxford: Update Software, 1993, Disk Issue 2

67. Grant AM: Early amniocentesis vs. chorion villus sampling. In: Pregnancy and Childbirth Module (eds. Enkin MW, Keirse MJNC, Renfrew MJ, Neilson JP), "Cochrane Database of Systematic Reviews": Review No. 07791, 1 October 1993. Published through "Cochrane Updates on Disk", Oxford: Update Software, 1993, Disk Issue 2

68. Grant AM: Transabdominal vs. transcervical CVS. In: Pregnancy and Childbirth Module (eds. Enkin MW, Keirse MJNC, Renfrew MJ, Neilson JP), "Cochrane Database of Systematic Reviews": Review No. 06005, 21 May 1993. Published in "Cochrane Updates on Disk", Oxford: Update Software, 1993, Disk Issue 2

Prenatal Screening and Diagnosis for Down Syndrome Prevention

MANEUVER	EFFECTIVENESS	LEVEL OF EVIDENCE <REF>	RECOMMENDATION
Offer prenatal diagnosis with amniocentesis or chorionic villus sampling (CVS) for: 1) advanced maternal age (35 years or over); 2) previous history of Down Syndrome (DS) birth; or 3) known chromosome anomaly in family associated with risk of DS birth	**RISK IDENTIFICATION** Increased risk of DS birth is well established **PRENATAL DIAGNOSIS** Accurate diagnosis with CVS and amniocentesis Approximate procedure related fetal loss: Amniocentesis: 0.04-0.8%, CVS: 1-1.5%	Cohort studies<7-20> (II-2) Amniocentesis: Randomized controlled trial<30> (I); non-randomized controlled trial<32> (II-1); cohort studies<31,33> (II-2) CVS: Randomized controlled trial<34-36> (I) CVS vs Amnio: Cohort studies<37-44> (II-2)	Fair evidence to include in the periodic health examination (B)
Offer 2nd trimester Triple Marker Screening (maternal serum alpha-fetoprotein/ human chorionic gonadotrophin/ unconjugated estriol (AFP/HCG/uE3)) to pregnant women less than 35 years with education on 1) limited efficacy; 2) 2nd trimester diagnosis and abortion; and 3) psychological implications of screen, as well as of DS birth	**SCREENING** Approximately 50% of 2nd trimester DS pregnancies identified with false positive rate of 5%. Impact of positive screens poorly understood. One fifth of women with positive screens may decline amniocentesis. In women over 35 years of age approximately 90% of DS pregnancies may be identified with an amniocentesis rate of 25%.	Cohort studies<23-26> (II-2) Cross-sectional study<27> (III)	Fair evidence to include in the periodic health examination pregnant women under 35 years of age (B); triple marker screening followed by prenatal diagnosis may be offered as an alternative to prenatal diagnosis alone in women over 35 years

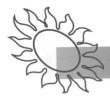

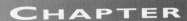

CHAPTER 9

Screening for Asymptomatic Bacteriuria in Pregnancy

By Lindsay E. Nicolle

Screening for Asymptomatic Bacteriuria in Pregnancy

Prepared by Lindsay E. Nicolle, MD[1]

Asymptomatic bacteriuria is common in women and increases in prevalence with age and/or sexual activity. The impact of asymptomatic bacteriuria on pregnancy outcome has been a focus of controversy since the development of quantitative urine culture technique in the mid 1950s allowed clear differentiation of women with bacteriuria from those without. While it is generally accepted that asymptomatic bacteriuria is detrimental to pregnancy, data available to support this contention is limited. Randomized controlled trials and cohort studies have shown that the detection and treatment of asymptomatic bacteriuria can decrease the occurrence of acute pyleonephritis later in pregnancy and decrease the occurrence of intrauterine growth retardation. Asymptomatic bacteriuria in children and in the elderly are addressed in Chapters 21 and 81 respectively.

Burden of Suffering

The prevalence of asymptomatic bacteriuria in pregnancy varies from 4-7% (range 2-11%) and is similar to that observed in non-pregnant women.<1,2> The prevalence is higher among individuals in lower socioeconomic classes, and those with a past history of asymptomatic urinary infection. Increased frequency of screening during pregnancy identifies more cases. Approximately 1-2% of women who are not bacteriuric at initial screening early in pregnancy will develop bacteriuria later in the pregnancy.

There is a high incidence of pyelonephritis occurring later in pregnancy, usually at the end of the second trimester or beginning of the third trimester, in women with asymptomatic bacteriuria identified and not treated early in pregnancy. Initial studies reported 20% to 27% of women with asymptomatic bacteriuria developed pyelonephritis<3,4> compared to 0.4% to 1.2% of those without bacteriuria. A more recent study reported 13% of untreated women with asymptomatic bacteriuria developed pyelonephritis, compared with 0.4% of those with negative screening cultures.<5> Pyelonephritis in pregnancy generally requires hospitalization for treatment and, as with any severe febrile illness in later pregnancy, may be associated with premature labour and delivery. In the pre-antibiotic era 23-54% of

13-27% of women with untreated asymptomatic bacteriuria identified in early pregnancy will develop pyelonephritis later in the pregnancy

---

[1] Associate Professor of Medicine/Medical Microbiology, University of Manitoba, Winnipeg, Manitoba

women with acute pyelonephritis had premature births, and 6% of all premature births were reported to be due to pyelonephritis.[2] In the post-antibiotic era, Gilstrap et al[6] reported 25% of women with intrapartum pyelonephritis delivered low birth weight infants compared to 15% of controls and suggested this was evidence for acute pyelonephritis in pregnancy being associated with pre-term labour.

The association of asymptomatic bacteriuria with other complications of pregnancy including stillbirth, intrauterine growth retardation, and preterm labour in the absence of acute pyelonephritis has been more controversial.[1] However, a review of birth certificate data for the state of Washington for 1980 and 1981 reported that women with urinary infection (UTI) associated pregnancy had a fetal mortality rate 2.4 times greater, low birth rate 2.04 times greater, and prematurity 2.4 times greater than those without urinary infection.[7] Naeye[8] reported observations from the Collaborative Perinatal Study of the U.S. National Institute of Neurological and Communicative Disorders and Stroke which followed 60,000 pregnancies between 1959 and 1966. The perinatal mortality rate was twice as high in women with UTI within 15 days of delivery. The low birth weight associated with urinary infection was due to a contribution of both preterm delivery and fetal growth retardation. Both of these studies included both symptomatic and asymptomatic infections.

In a meta-analysis of 19 studies, Romero et al reported that women with asymptomatic bacteriuria had a 54% higher risk of a low birth weight infant and twice the risk of a pre-term infant compared with non-bacteriuric women.[9] The mechanism by which asymptomatic bacteriuria promotes preterm labour is not clear, but subclinical amnionitis or phospholipid A_2 production by bacteria have been proposed.[1] One study reported that 40% of women with bacteriuria at delivery had post-partum endometritis compared with 2.2% of women without bacteriuria.[10] There is no compelling evidence of an association of asymptomatic bacteriuria with hypertension in pregnancy or of long-term renal damage associated with asymptomatic bacteriuria of pregnancy in the antibiotic era.[1]

Maneuver

The gold standard for screening for asymptomatic bacteriuria is growing bacterial cultures of urine samples from women in early pregnancy (12-16 weeks gestation).

Non-culture methods are not, generally, reliable for the identification of bacteriuria in asymptomatic populations, including pregnant women.[1,11] Routine urinalysis is imprecise for identification of pyuria and other pyuria-based methods, particularly leukocyte-esterase dipstick, are subject to false negatives in bacteriuria without pyuria and false positives with contamination from vaginal secretions. Currently only culture methods can be considered acceptable in pregnancy. The routine use of the standard semi-quantitative culture may be expensive and problems with contamination with vaginal and periurethral flora at collection and overgrowth of organisms when culture is delayed may lead to erroneous results. A dipslide method is substantially less costly, allows immediate inoculation after specimen collection, requires no special equipment for incubation as it may be left at room temperature, and will identify specimens with significant bacteriuria which should be fully analyzed by the laboratory.[1] For women with asymptomatic bacteriuria two consecutive positive specimens are necessary for diagnosis. Thus, for women with a positive dipslide, a second specimen should be forwarded to the laboratory for quantitative culture, identification of organisms, and antimicrobial susceptibility testing.

The optimal timing to obtain specimens to identify women with asymptomatic bacteriuria in pregnancy has been investigated in a number of studies. A specimen obtained at 12-16 weeks will identify 80% of women who will ultimately have asymptomatic bacteriuria during pregnancy.[12] Repeated screening on a monthly basis will identify bacteriuria in only an additional 1-2% of patients. A single urine specimen obtained from 12-16 weeks of pregnancy will identify most women with asymptomatic bacteriuria.

Effectiveness of Prevention and Treatment

Prevention of Acute Pyelonephritis

Studies have consistently reported a decrease in acute pyelonephritis later in pregnancy from 20-30% to 2-4% for women who have been identified with asymptomatic bacteriuria in early pregnancy and treated.[1,3-5] One study, reported in letter form, found no difference in pyelonephritis in treated (3.0%) and untreated (2.5%) women with asymptomatic bacteriuria, but this is at variance with all other reports.[13] However, as 0.5%-1.0% of women with initial negative screening urine cultures will develop pyelonephritis subsequently in pregnancy, only 50-80% of the burden of pyelonephritis in pregnancy is prevented through screening and treatment. One study suggested that screening 4,470 pregnant women with treatment of asymptomatic bacteriuria prevented only 6 cases of pyelonephritis and was likely not cost effective, but no formal cost analysis was provided.[5] Wadland and Plante[14] reported that screening with a single urine specimen in early pregnancy was cost effective as long as the population prevalence of bacteriuria was over 2%.

Prevention of Pre-term Delivery and Low Birth Weight

Early studies of the treatment of asymptomatic bacteriuria generally did not report decreased low birth weight or premature delivery with therapy of asymptomatic bacteriuria.<1> The meta-analysis of Romero et al,<9> however, of 8 clinical trials, reported a relative risk of 0.56, (95% confidence interval 0.43-0.73) for antibiotic treatment of asymptomatic bacteriuria reducing low birth weight. The mechanism by which treatment of asymptomatic bacteriuria prevents low birth weight is not clear. It has been suggested that antibiotic therapy, in fact, eradicates organisms from the cervix and vagina which may be associated with subclinical chorioamnionitis, rather than a direct effect of treatment of urinary infection.<9>

The mechanisms by which treatment of asymptomatic bacteriuria decreases low birth weight or prematurity are unclear

Recommendations of Others

In 1989, the U.S. Preventive Services Task Force<15> recommended periodic testing for asymptomatic bacteriuria for pregnant women. The optimal frequency for urine testing was unknown and therefore left to clinical discretion. Since urine culture is a more accurate screening test then dipstick urinalysis, it was recommended for detecting asymptomatic bacteriuria during pregnancy. This recommendation is currently under review.

Conclusions and Recommendations

Identification and treatment of asymptomatic bacteriuria will lead to a 10-fold decrease in the occurrence of acute pyelonephritis later in pregnancy in women with asymptomatic bacteriuria. Treatment of asymptomatic bacteriuria will also decrease pre-term delivery and low birth weight. A single screening test using a culture method at 12-16 weeks of pregnancy will identify 80% of women with asymptomatic bacteriuria of pregnancy. Screening for and treatment of asymptomatic bacteriuria is likely cost-effective. There is good evidence to recommend screening for asymptomatic bacteriuria in pregnancy (A Recommendation).

Treatment of asymptomatic bacteriuria in pregnant women will lead to a 10-fold decrease in pyelonephritis

Unanswered Questions (Research Agenda)

1. Further studies of optimal screening methods, both nonculture and culture methods, with cost analyses are needed. These should be developed as randomized prospective trials comparing the different methods with endpoints of pregnancy outcomes as well as identification of bacteriuria.

2. The efficacy of screening only targeted high-risk groups such as those with a past history of urinary infection or of lower socioeconomic status compared to screening all pregnant women should be compared.

3. The optimal frequency of screening for recurrent bacteriuria in subjects initially identified with bacteriuria and treated should be determined.

Evidence

The literature was identified with a MEDLINE search to March 1993 using the following MESH headings: urinary tract infections, pregnancy, human, case reports.

This review was initiated in June 1993 and recommendations were finalized by the Task Force in October 1993.

Selected References

1. Patterson TF, Andriole VT: Bacteriuria in pregnancy. *Infect Dis Clin North Am* 1987; 1: 807-822

2. Norden CW, Kass EH: Bacteriuria of pregnancy – a critical appraisal. *Ann Rev Med* 1968; 19: 431-470

3. Little PJ: The incidence of urinary infection in 5,000 pregnant women. *Lancet* 1966; 2(470): 925-928

4. Kincaid-Smith P, Buller M: Bacteriuria in pregnancy. *Lancet* 1965; 1: 395-399

5. Campbell-Brown M, McFadyen IR, Seal DV, *et al*: Is screening for bacteriuria in pregnancy worth while? *Br Med J Clin Res Ed* 1987; 294: 1579-1582

6. Gilstrap LC, Leveno KJ, Cunningham FG, *et al*: Renal infection and pregnancy outcome. *Am J Obstet Gynecol* 1981; 141: 709-716

7. McGrady GA, Daling JR, Peterson DR: Maternal urinary tract infection and adverse fetal outcomes. *Am J Epidemiol* 1985; 121: 377-381

8. Naeye RL: Urinary tract infections and the outcome of pregnancy. *Adv Nephrol Necker Hosp* 1986; 15: 95-102

9. Romero R, Oyarzun E, Mazor M, *et al*: Meta-analysis of the relationship between asymptomatic bacteriuria and preterm delivery/low birth weight. *Obstet Gynecol* 1989; 73: 576-582

10. Monif GRG: Intrapartum bacteriuria and postpartum endometritis. *Obstet Gynecol* 1991; 78: 245-248

11. Mittendorf R, Williams MA, Kass EH: Prevention of preterm delivery and low birth weight associated with asymptomatic bacteriuria. *Clin Infect Dis* 1992; 14: 927-932

12. Stenqvist K, Dahlen-Nilsson I, Lidin-Janson G, *et al*: Bacteriuria in pregnancy: 1. Frequency and risk of acquisition. *Am J Epidemiol* 1989; 129: 372-379

13. Foley ME, Farquharson R, Stronge JM: Is screening for bacteriuria in pregnancy worthwhile? [letter] *Br Med J Clin Res Ed* 1987; 295(6592): 270

14. Wadland WC, Plante DA: Screening for asymptomatic bacteriuria in pregnancy. A decision and cost analysis. *J Fam Pract* 1989; 29: 372-376

15. U.S. Preventive Services Task Force: *Guide to Clinical Preventive Services: an Assessment of the Effectiveness of 169 Interventions*. Williams & Wilkins, Baltimore, Md, 1989: 155-161

Screening for Asymptomatic Bacteriuria in Pregnancy

MANEUVER	EFFECTIVENESS	LEVEL OF EVIDENCE <REF>	RECOMMENDATION
Screening once by culture method for asymptomatic bacteriuria at 12-16 weeks of pregnancy	Pyelonephritis: Identification and treatment of asymptomatic bacteriuria will decrease the subsequent occurrence of pyelonephritis later in pregnancy and may decrease premature labour or delivery associated with acute pyelonephritis.	Controlled trial and cohort studies<1,3-5> (I,II-1)	Good evidence to include in periodic health examination of pregnant women (A)
	Intra-uterine growth retardation: Decreased occurrence of intra-uterine growth retardation.	Randomized controlled trial<9> (I)	
	Other: Decreased occurrence of other negative outcomes including premature labour, stillbirth, and pre-eclampsia.		

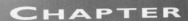

CHAPTER **10**

Prevention
of Neonatal
Herpes Simplex

By Elaine E. L. Wang

Prevention of Neonatal Herpes Simplex

Prepared by Elaine E. L. Wang, MD, CM, FRCPC[1]

Herpes simplex infection in the newborn is thought to be acquired from the mother during passage through an infected birth canal. Experts agree that the infant's exposure to the virus can be prevented by cesarean section if the maternal infection is recognized at the onset of labour and within 4 to 6 hours after rupture of the membranes. However, maternal infection is asymptomatic in 70% of cases. The difficulty in detecting asymptomatic infection has led to the practice of screening women considered to be at high risk (those with a history of recurrent genital infection or active disease during the current pregnancy and those whose sexual partners have proven genital herpes).

However, identification and screening of pregnant women at risk of recurrent infection has not been shown to prevent neonatal death or illness from infection and is not recommended. There is currently no screening strategy for asymptomatic women with no known history of herpes virus exposure, even though the risk of transmission to the newborn is higher in primary infections.

Burden of Suffering

The clinical presentation in 70% of cases of neonatal herpes simplex is skin involvement consisting of cutaneous vesicles. If the cutaneous infection is not treated systemic infection will develop within a week in two-thirds of the infants. The clinical presentation in 20% of cases is major systemic involvement, central nervous system involvement, or both. Less than 10% of babies with neurologic disease develop normally. The overall mortality rate among infants with untreated infection is 65%.

The rising incidence of neonatal herpes simplex has reflected a nationwide increase in the prevalence of herpes simplex. In 1981 the incidence was 12 cases per 100,000 live births, as estimated from a hospital-based study in Washington. In other studies primary infection was responsible for 29-35% of cases. Although both the transmission rate and the attack rate are higher with primary infection, recurrent infection accounts for a greater proportion of the burden of neonatal infection.

---

[1] Associate Professor of Pediatrics and of Preventive Medicine and Biostatistics, University of Toronto, Toronto, Ontario

Maneuver

The target group of women with recurrent infection may be identified through history-taking or detection of herpes simplex virus antibodies by microneutralization. The latter is expensive and unavailable for routine use. Since more than 50% of pregnant women with herpes simplex deliver prematurely, usually between 30 and 37 weeks' gestation, weekly screening is started in the 32nd week of gestation. Women whose most recent culture results or findings at clinical examination were positive for herpes virus undergo cesarean section. Women whose last culture results and findings at clinical examination were negative have vaginal delivery. The decision to do weekly screening depends on the mother's ability to recall previous episodes. Patient recall, however, is not reliable. In one study involving 11 women claiming to be having their first episode of herpes simplex, 5 women had antibodies indicating previous infection. In seroepidemiologic studies of herpes simplex type 2 infection, only 33% of the seropositive patients were aware of previous infection. In another study only 1 of 12 seropositive women indicated a history of disease or of contact with an infected person. A U.S. Centers for Disease Control surveillance study involving 184 cases showed that only 22% of mothers had a history of genital herpes simplex virus (HSV) infection and only 9% had genital lesions at the time of delivery.

The screening test consists of culture of a cervical smear for herpes simplex virus. However, since the results are not available for 3 days, the decision to deliver vaginally or by cesarean section is usually based on the penultimate culture result, which has a very low predictive validity for the presence of infection at the time of delivery. Arvin and associates<1> followed 414 women with a history of recurrent genital herpes. None of 17 women with positive antepartum culture results had positive results at delivery, and 5 of 354 asymptomatic mothers with negative antepartum results had positive results at delivery (sensitivity 0%).

Antepartum cultures have poor sensitivity and specificity for demonstrating viral shedding at delivery

Effectiveness of Prevention and Treatment

Weekly Screening

Since the policy of weekly screening addresses only the problem of recurrent infection, asymptomatic women with primary infection do not benefit at all, yet their infection lasts longer and is more likely to be associated with greater amounts of virus shedding.<2,3> The risk of transmission to the newborn has been estimated to be 50% in cases of primary infection and the probability of clinical disease in the infant (attack rate) 17% to 20%.

Primary maternal infection is associated with a higher transmission rate and more severe neonatal disease than is recurrent infection

Not only is the risk of transmission higher in primary infection, but the outcome is more likely to be severe. Prober and collaborators[4] studied the hypothesis that serologically verified primary infection would be associated with a worse neonatal outcome than that associated with recurrent infection. Through screening of 6,904 mother-infant pairs for both herpes simplex virus antibodies and herpes simplex at delivery they identified infection in 14 women and 3 infants. Two of the three infants were born of the two mothers with primary infection; meningitis developed in one of the two infants at 12 days of age.

Among women with recurrent disease the risk of transmission and clinical disease in the newborn appears to be lower. Of 34 infants inadvertently delivered vaginally from mothers with recurrent infection at the time of delivery and followed up without treatment, all remained asymptomatic. Calculation of the 95% confidence interval within which the mean risk of disease could be expected among these infants resulted in an upper estimate of risk of 8%. A genital lesion consistent with herpes simplex was present in 56% of the mothers, underscoring the importance of careful clinical examination among asymptomatic women.

Decision analysis was used to evaluate 9 strategies for prevention of neonatal HSV (involving physical exam, culture, and antigen testing of all or high-risk women). Physical examination at labour was found to be the optimal strategy given the goal of minimizing the ratio of excess cesarean sections to cases of neonatal HSV infection averted; however, about 30 excess cesarean sections would be performed for each case averted. Strategies involving high-risk women were associated with 36-178 excess cesarean sections per HSV case averted.

The use of cesarean section among symptomatic women only will lead to some missed cases; however, an economic evaluation of the strategy of sequential screening revealed that it would cost US$37 million for each case prevented. A national screening program in the U.S. would prevent 1.8 cases/year.

Recommendations of Others

Because of the limitations of screening only those at high risk, the Committee on Infectious Disease of the American Academy of Pediatrics no longer supports screening.[5]

The Infectious Diseases and Immunization Committee of the Canadian Pediatric Society recommends that all pregnant women be questioned during prenatal visits about any personal history of genital HSV infection or similar history in their sexual partner(s). Signs and symptoms of genital HSV infection should be sought in all women during pregnancy but weekly antepartum cultures for HSV are not recommended, even in women with a history of genital HSV infection.

However, all women should be questioned about recent symptoms and examined carefully for clinical evidence of genital HSV infection on admission for delivery; and all newborn infants whose mothers have genital lesions or a history of infection should be examined/observed.

The U.S. Preventive Services Task Force recommends screening pregnant women with active lesions for genital herpes simplex virus;[6] this recommendation is currently being reviewed.

In December, 1992, the Infectious Disease Society of America (IDSA) recommended that serial viral cultures for women with recurrent infections be abandoned. The IDSA recommended that women with histories of genital herpes should be provided education and reassurance. Assays for detection of HSV antigen or viral cultures should not be performed except to evaluate clinically apparent lesions. While routine samples for cultures were recommended at delivery for women with histories of genital herpes, even in the absence of visible lesions, the lack of established utility for such screening was emphasized. If the patient had active genital herpes when labour occurred (not including active lesions at some distance from the genital tract, e.g. buttock), cesarean section was recommended before membrane rupture or as soon thereafter as possible and viral cultures performed.[7]

Conclusions and Recommendations

Weekly screening among women at high risk for herpes simplex cannot be recommended because 1) it does not address prevention among asymptomatic women with primary infection; 2) history-taking does not adequately identify women at risk of recurrent infection; 3) the predictive validity of the penultimate culture is very poor; 4) the attack rate of recurrent infection is low; and 5) the preventive intervention, cesarean section, is associated with increased maternal morbidity and mortality rates and costs, as compared with vaginal delivery.

A high degree of suspicion of herpes simplex must be maintained since neonatal herpes simplex is usually severe by the time of presentation. Empiric initiation of antiviral therapy should be considered.

Based on fair evidence from well-designed cohort studies, weekly culture for herpes simplex virus should be excluded from the routine prenatal care of women with a history of recurrent herpes simplex (D Recommendation).

A history of genital herpes and clinical evidence of infection at the time of delivery should be sought. If such evidence exists, cesarean section is recommended, particularly if it is known before or within 4 to 6 hours after rupture of the membranes.[5] However, this strategy is based upon expert opinion; there is overall poor evidence

For women with clinical herpes simplex perineal infections, perform cesarean section if membranes have ruptured within 4-6 hours

to include cesarean section in, or exclude it from, routine prepartum care of symptomatic women (C Recommendation).

Unanswered Questions (Research Agenda)

The following have been identified as research priorities:

1. Determining whether cesarean section does more good than harm among women with symptomatic herpes simplex. Evaluating new serologic methods for identifying women at risk for primary infection – that is, seronegative women who are at greater risk of transmitting disease to their infants – in order to allow targeting of investigations in that group.

2. Developing rapid diagnostic tests with adequate sensitivity and specificity for use among asymptomatic women so that interventions can be performed in time to prevent neonatal infection.

3. Evaluating the use of new antiviral agents among pregnant women for the prevention of neonatal herpes simplex.

Evidence

The literature was identified with a MEDLINE search to March, 1993, using the following MESH headings: herpes simplex, pregnancy, and infant, newborn.

This review was initiated in October 1988 and recommendations were finalized by the Task Force in February, 1989. A report with a full reference list was published in December 1989.<8>

Selected References

1. Arvin AM, Hensleigh PA, Prober CG *et al*: Failure of antepartum maternal cultures to predict the infant's risk of exposure to herpes simplex virus at delivery. *N Engl J Med* 1986; 315: 796-800

2. Corey L, Spear PG: Infections with herpes simplex virus (1). *N Engl J Med* 1986; 314: 686-691

3. Corey L, Spear PG: Infections with herpes simplex virus (2). *N Engl J Med* 1986; 314: 686-691

4. Prober CG, Hensleigh PA, Boucher FD, *et al*: Use of routine viral cultures at delivery to identify neonates exposed to herpes simplex virus. *N Engl J Med* 1988; 318: 887-891

5. Committee on Infectious Diseases: *1988 Red Book*, 21st ed, American Academy of Pediatrics, Elk Grove Village, Ill, 1988: 230-239

6. U.S. Preventive Services Task Force: *Guide to Clinical Preventive Services: an Assessment of the Effectiveness of 169 Interventions*, Williams & Wilkins, Baltimore, Md, 1989: 151-154

7. Prober CG, Corey L, Brown ZA, *et al*: The management of pregnancies complicated by genital infections with herpes simplex virus. *Clin Infect Dis* 1992; 15: 1031-1038

8. Canadian Task Force on the Periodic Health Examination: The periodic health examination, 1989 update part 4, Intrapartum electronic fetal monitoring and prevention of neonatal herpes simplex. *Can Med Assoc J* 1989; 141: 1233-1240

Prevention of Neonatal Herpes Simplex

MANEUVER	EFFECTIVENESS	LEVEL OF EVIDENCE <REF>	RECOMMENDATION
Recurrent infection Weekly screening (starting at 32 weeks' gestation); cesarean section among women with positive culture results or findings at clinical examination	Identification and screening of pregnant women at risk of recurrent infection has not been shown to prevent neonatal death and illness from infection.	Screening trial and prospective cohort study<1-4> (II-2)	Fair evidence to exclude from routine prepartum care in high-risk pregnancies* (D)
Symptomatic infection Clinical examination; cesarean section among women with positive findings at clinical examination	Transmission of herpes simplex to newborn can be prevented among women with clinical evidence of genital herpes simplex at delivery.	Expert opinion<5,7> (III)	Poor evidence to include cesarean section in or exclude it from routine prepartum care of symptomatic women (C)

* Women at high risk are those with a history of recurrent herpes simplex or active disease during current pregnancy and those whose sexual partner has proven genital herpes simplex.

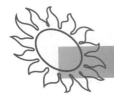

CHAPTER 11

Screening for D (Rh) Sensitization in Pregnancy

By Marie-Dominique Beaulieu

Screening for D (Rh) Sensitization in Pregnancy

Adapted by Marie-Dominique Beaulieu, MD, MSc, FCFP[1] from the report prepared for the U.S. Preventive Services Task Force[2]

In 1979 the Canadian Task Force found good evidence for screening for blood group incompatibility in pregnancy. This review updates the previous recommendation and is based on the recent review of the evidence by the U.S. Preventive Services Task Force for Screening for D (Rh) Incompatibility. We now find that there is good to fair evidence to recommend that all pregnant women should receive D (formerly Rh) blood typing and antibody screening at their first prenatal visit and, if D negative, repeat antibody screening at 24-28 weeks' gestation. Unless the father is known to be D negative, unsensitized D negative women should receive D immunoglobulin (D Ig) at 28-29 weeks' gestation, within 72 hours after delivery of a D positive infant, and after induced abortion or amniocentesis. It may also be prudent to administer D immunoglobulin to unsensitized D negative women after spontaneous abortion, ectopic pregnancy or other obstetrical procedures or complications. The effectiveness of prevention in these situations has never been proven by controlled trials but is inferred considering their similarity with other clinical conditions where prevention has been proven to be effective. There is some controversy on the effectiveness of the administration of D immunoglobulin after chorionic villus sampling (CVS). One study reported results suggesting that it can create adverse effects to the fetus. However these results were preliminary ones and did not control for important confounding variables.

Burden of Suffering

15% of pregnancies in Caucasian Canadians carry the risk of isoimmunization of the fetus

Some degree of fetal-maternal transplacental hemorrhage occurs in 75% of all pregnancies. This phenomenon is not dangerous to the fetus unless there is incompatibility between the mother and her fetus with respect to the D antigen of the red blood cells. D incompatibility exists when a D negative woman is pregnant with a D positive fetus. This occurs in up to 9-10% of pregnancies, depending on race. The incidence in Canadians of caucasian extraction is about 15%, 7% in American blacks, and as low as 1% in North American Indians and

---

[1] Associate Professor, Department of Family Medicine, University of Montreal, Montreal, Quebec

[2] By Carolyn DiGuiseppi, MD, MPH, Science Advisor, U.S. Preventive Services Task Force

Inuit. The majority of fetuses (70%) of D negative women are D positive. About 35,000 D-negative women become pregnant annually. They carry 24,500 D positive fetuses who are at risk of developing D isoimmunization. If no preventive measures are taken, 0.7-1.8% of these women will become isoimmunized antenatally, developing D antibody through exposure to fetal blood; 8-17% will become isoimmunized at delivery, 3-6% after spontaneous or therapeutic abortion, and 2-5% after amniocentesis. Once a woman is isoimmunized, the risk to the fetus increases in subsequent D positive pregnancies because maternal D Ig antibodies are produced earlier in the pregnancy and in greater amount. In isoimmunized D negative women the risk of fetal isoimmunization disease increases with the number of pregnancies.

Once isoimmunization has occurred, the severity of fetal hemolysis varies. In 50% of the cases the fetus is very mildly affected and does not require postpartum treatment. However, without treatment, 25-30% of these offspring will have some degree of hemolytic anemia and hyperbilirubinemia, another 20-25% will be hydropic and many will die either in utero or during the neonatal period.

Since the introduction of routine postpartum prophylaxis in the 1960s, the crude incidence of D isoimmunization in Canada and the United States has fallen from 9.1-10.3 cases to 1.3 cases per 1,000 total births. Hemolytic disease of the fetus or newborn due to D isoimmunization (also called erythroblastosis fetalis) now accounts for only 4-5 deaths per 100,000 births, although this may be an underestimate as early intrauterine deaths are not always reported. However, this decline in fetal and neonatal mortality from D hemolytic disease cannot be attributed exclusively to the effectiveness of primary prevention and early treatment. It has been estimated that 30-40% of the recent decline in disease incidence is attributable to smaller family size, since the incidence of D hemolytic disease increases with increasing birth order. Smaller family size also contributes to the decreasing case fatality rate, since the first affected infant in a family generally has less severe disease. Since the 1940s, the case fatality rate has fallen from about 50% to 2-6%. This decline has also been associated with the introduction of interventions such as amniotic fluid spectrophotometry, exchange transfusion, amniocentesis, intrauterine fetal transfusion, and improved care of both the mother and the premature erythroblastotic infant.

Maneuver

Hemagglutination is the established reference standard for the determination of D blood type. The indirect antiglobulin (Coomb's) test (IAGT) is the reference standard for detecting anti-D antibody in women who have been sensitized to D positive blood. The IAGT will also detect other maternal antibodies that may cause hemolytic disease.

Effectiveness of Screening and Treatment

No therapeutic intervention, with the exception of intravenous serum globulin and plasma exchange, can suppress the isoimmunization process once it is initiated. Primary prevention of D immunization process is therefore the objective. Early detection of D negative blood type in the pregnant woman is of substantial benefit if the patient is not yet isoimmunized and the father is not known to be D negative. Administration of D Immunoglobulin [D Ig, or $Rh_o(D)$ Immune Globulin (Human)] to an unsensitized D negative woman after delivery of a D positive fetus will prevent maternal isoimmunization and consequent hemolytic disease in subsequent D positive offspring. The efficacy of D Ig prophylaxis was demonstrated convincingly in a series of controlled clinical trials in the early 1960s.[1,2] Despite various minor flaws in study design, these trials showed that isoimmunization did not occur in any of the women who received a full dose of D Ig postpartum and who were not sensitized at the time it was administered. These findings led to the introduction in 1968 of routine postpartum prophylaxis following licensure of D Ig.

The most frequent cause of apparent failure of postpartum prophylaxis is antenatal isoimmunization, which happens in 0.7-1.8% of pregnant women at risk. Although sample selection and other design features were not optimal, non-randomized controlled trials have shown that the administration of D Ig at 28 weeks' gestation, when combined with postpartum administration, reduces the incidence of isoimmunization to 0.2% of women at risk.[3-5]

Administration of D immunoglobulin at 28 weeks and within 72 hours post-partum is safe and effective in preventing isoimmunization

Since D isoimmunization during pregnancy is caused by transplacental hemorrhage, the risk of isoimmunization increases whenever such hemorrhage is likely to occur, including after abortion, amniocentesis, chorionic villus sampling (CVS), cordocentesis, ectopic pregnancy, fetal manipulation (e.g. external version procedures) or surgery, antepartum hemorrhage, antepartum fetal death and stillbirth.[6,7] The Task Force makes a number of recommendations which include these procedures in the protocol (see Chapter 7 on neural tube defects, Chapter 8 on Down Syndrome, Chapter 19 on cystic fibrosis and Chapter 46 on unintended teen pregnancy). Studies documenting the effectiveness of D Ig prophylaxis are available for only a few of these indications, however. In a non-randomized trial of D Ig administration after amniocentesis, control Rh-negative women delivering Rh-positive infants were more likely to become isoimmunized than were those receiving D Ig (5.2% vs. 0%), although because of small numbers this difference was not statistically significant. Case series describing D Ig administration after amniocentesis have demonstrated isoimmunization rates as low as

0-0.5%. In a case series of D Ig after termination of pregnancy, the isoimmunization rate was 0.4%,[8] compared to 2.6% among a series of patients who did not receive D Ig described by the same authors.[9]

Some controversy exists concerning the value of D Ig administration after CVS. In the preliminary analysis of a controlled trial planned to evaluate the safety of transcervical CVS compared to transabdominal CVS and amniocentesis,[10] Smidt-Jensen and Philip reported some data on a randomized experiment of D Ig administration in the group allocated to either modality of CVS. All women allocated to amniocentesis received D Ig. Among Rh-negative women delivering Rh-positive infants, similar rates of isoimmunization were seen in both intervention (D Ig after CVS) (2.3%) and control (no D Ig after CVS) (1.1%) groups. Although the women who received D Ig experienced twice as many unintended fetal losses as did controls (6.9% vs. 3.8%), the difference was not statistically significant, possibly due to small sample size. Also, the authors did not control for the effect of the chorionic villus sampling technique. Transabdominal CVS was associated with a lower rate of fetal loss than transcervical CVS. Finally, data were not available for all participants. A full report of this study has yet to be published. Meanwhile, it cannot be considered as evidence of an adverse effect of D Ig administration after CVS and the controversy will persist.

The standard postpartum dose of D Ig (300 μg) contains sufficient anti-D immunoglobulin to prevent sensitization to at least 15 mL of D positive fetal red blood cells (RBCs), or approximately 30 mL of fetal blood; a "minidose" (50 μg) prevents sensitization to 2.5 mL of D positive fetal RBCs. For women with transplacental hemorrhages >30 mL of fetal blood, the risk of D isoimmunization developing after the full post-partum D Ig dose is 30-35%. The incidence of fetal-maternal hemorrhage >30 mL is 0.1-0.7% for all D negative pregnancies, but is 1.7-2.5% after complicated vaginal and cesarian deliveries, and 4.5% after stillbirth. Several methods for detecting excess fetal-maternal hemorrhage are available. Acid elution (Kleihauer-Betke) is both sensitive and specific when done correctly but is subject to substantial laboratory and technological error. Flow cytometry is also highly sensitive and specific, but is technically difficult to perform. The erythrocyte rosette test is simple to perform and highly sensitive (99-100%) for the presence of >15 mL of D positive fetal RBCs, but specificity is low. Positive results must be confirmed by more specific tests such as acid elution and flow cytometry.

In clinical practice, combined antenatal and postnatal prophylaxis will prevent isoimmunization in 96% of women at risk.[5] The remaining cases are due to failure to give D Ig when indicated, administration of an insufficient dose, or treatment failure (i.e., isoimmunization occurring before 28 weeks or transplacental hemorrhage that was too large or occurred too late in pregnancy to be prevented by the standard antepartum dose). Thus, human error causes 22-50% of these cases.<5> Indeed, while clinicians almost always administer D Ig postpartum and after induced abortion, administration rates have been documented to be lower for other obstetric procedures and complications: 81-88% after spontaneous abortion, 36-60% after ectopic pregnancy, 31% after antepartum hemorrhage, and 14% after amniocentesis.

D immunoglobulin has few adverse effects. Some fetuses will become weakly direct-antiglobulin-positive following antenatal administration, but resulting anemia and hyperbilirubinemia in the newborn are very rare.<3> All plasma for D Ig production is screened for infectious diseases as required by the Food and Drug Administration; no cases of HIV infection from D Ig have been reported. The evidence is therefore compelling that early detection and prophylaxis of the unsensitized D negative woman is both safe and effective in preventing isoimmunization and thus in preventing D hemolytic disease.

Early detection is also beneficial for D negative women who are already isoimmunized and are carrying D positive offspring, because early intervention may improve clinical outcome. Decisions to intervene depend on the validity of screening tests in predicting the degree of fetal anemia. Obstetric history, maternal antibody titers and ultrasound are currently used to determine the need for more invasive tests during isoimmunized pregnancies, but in the absence of hydrops none of these reliably distinguishes mild from severe hemolytic disease.<6> Immunologic tests on maternal serum show promise in predicting disease severity. In the third trimester, serial amniotic fluid spectrophotometry has been found to correctly predict disease severity (i.e., cord hemoglobin and need for neonatal therapy) in 94-99% of cases. In the second trimester, however, this test has insufficient sensitivity or specificity for predicting the need for intervention. Determination of fetal hemoglobin and D blood type by ultrasound-guided cordocentesis, which can be performed in the second trimester, quantifies the degree of anemia, can be followed by fetal transfusion if indicated, and allows referral of those with D negative babies to routine care. However, case series have demonstrated complication rates of 2-7% and procedure-related fetal mortality rates of 0.5-1%.<7>

In the presence of severe fetal anemia, early intervention appears to offer substantial improvement in clinical outcome. Current perinatal survival after ultrasound-guided intravascular transfusion at experienced centers is 62-86% for hydropic fetuses and >90% for those without hydrops. Once pulmonary maturity is established, the fetus can be delivered early and exchange transfusion performed with only 1% mortality risk.

Recommendations of Others

In 1989, the U.S. Preventive Services Task Force recommended that all pregnant women should receive ABO/Rh blood typing testing for anti-Rh(D) antibody at their first prenatal visit. Unsensitized Rh-negative women should receive Rh(D) immune globulin (D Ig) at 28-29 weeks' gestation and within 72 hours after delivery, as well as after spontaneous or therapeutic abortion, ectopic pregnancy, amniocentesis, antepartum placental hemorrhage, or a transfusion of Rh-positive blood products.[11]

The Society of Obstetricians and Gynecologists of Canada and the American College of Obstetricians and Gynecologists (ACOG) recommend D blood typing and antibody screening at the first prenatal visit and repeat D antibody screening at 24-28 weeks of pregnancy for D-negative women.[6,12] Both groups recommend offering D Ig to all unsensitized D-negative women at 28 weeks gestation, and to those at increased risk of sensitization because of delivery of a D positive infant, antepartum hemorrhage, spontaneous or induced abortion, amniocentesis, external version procedures or ectopic pregnancy, within 72 hours of the event. They also recommend D Ig administration to unsensitized D-negative women who have CVS, cordocentesis, antepartum fetal death, fetal surgery, or transfusion of D positive blood products, and measuring fetal blood cell levels in the mother when antepartum placental hemorrhage occurs.

Conclusions and Recommendations

There is excellent evidence for the efficacy and effectiveness of blood typing, anti-D antibody screening and postpartum D Ig prophylaxis. Antepartum prophylaxis offers some additional benefit, although some critics have argued that the total impact of antepartum prophylaxis on the incidence of D disease is relatively small. Other studies support the cost effectiveness of antepartum prophylaxis.[5] The cost effectiveness of D Ig after obstetric procedures and complications is unknown.

All pregnant women should receive D blood typing and antibody testing at their first prenatal visit (A Recommendation). D blood typing and antibody screening should also be performed before elective procedures such as amniocentesis and therapeutic abortion (B Recommendation). For purposes of blood typing and prophylaxis, D^u and D positive blood types should be considered equivalent.[6] Unless the father is known to be D negative, a repeat D antibody test should be performed at 24-28 weeks' gestation on all unsensitized D negative women, followed by the administration of a full (300 μg) dose of D Ig if antibody-negative. If a D (or D^u) positive infant is delivered, the dose should be repeated postpartum, preferably within 72 hours after delivery. Unless the father is known to be D negative, all

Detection of D negative blood types at the prenatal first visit, repeated, if D negative, at 28 weeks of gestation and postpartum

unsensitized D negative women should receive a full dose of D Ig after elective abortion (50 µg before 13 weeks) or amniocentesis (B Recommendation). There is currently insufficient evidence to recommend for or against the routine administration of D Ig after other obstetric procedures or complications such as chorionic villus sampling, ectopic pregnancy termination, cordocentesis, fetal surgery or manipulation (including external version), antepartum placental hemorrhage, antepartum fetal death, and stillbirth. It may also be prudent to administer D immunoglobulin to unsensitized D negative women after spontaneous abortion, ectopic pregnancy or other obstetrical procedures or complications (C Recommendation). The effectiveness of prevention in these situations has never been proven by controlled trials but is inferred considering their similarity to other clinical conditions where prevention has been proven to be effective. There is some controversy about the effectiveness of the administration of D immunoglobulin after CVS. One study reported results suggesting that D Ig can create adverse effects to the fetus. However these were preliminary results and lacked control for important confounding variables.

Routine screening for excess maternal hemorrhage is not recommended, because the risk of D isoimmunization from excess hemorrhage is 0.3% for all D negative pregnancies (see above). For women at increased risk for transplacental hemorrhages >30 mL because of antepartum placental hemorrhage, stillbirth, or cesarian or complicated vaginal delivery,<6> the yield from screening is likely to be higher. In these patients, therefore, physicians may wish to test for fetal RBCs in the maternal circulation, using either quantitative methods (acid elution or flow cytometry), or the erythrocyte rosette test with follow-up of positive results by quantitative methods. If transplacental hemorrhage exceeds 30 mL, 20 µg D Ig per 1 mL of fetal red blood cells should be given.<6>

Unanswered Questions (Research Agenda)

The safety and effectiveness of D Ig administration following CVS requires further study.

Evidence

The literature was identified with a MEDLINE search in English for the years 1989 to December 1993, using the following key words: RH-HR blood group system, RH Isoimmunization, immunoglobulins, amniocentesis, ultrasound, blood transfusion intrauterine and erythroblastosis fetalis. This review was initiated in November 1992 and the recommendations finalized by the Task Force in June 1993.

Acknowledgements

The Task Force would like to thank T.F. Baskett, MB, BCh, FRCS, Head, Department of Gynecology, Halifax Infirmary, Halifax, Nova Scotia, Professor, Dalhousie University, Halifax, Nova Scotia for reviewing the draft chapter.

Selected References

1. Chown B, Duff AM, James J, *et al*: Prevention of primary Rh immunization: first report of the Western Canadian Trial, 1966-1968. *Can Med Assoc J* 1969; 100: 1021-1024

2. Pollack W, Gorman JG, Freda VJ, *et al*: Results of clinical trials of RhoGAM in women. *Transfusion* 1968; 8: 151-153

3. Bowman JM, Chown B, Lewis M, *et al*: Rh isoimmunization during pregnancy: antenatal prophylaxis. *Can Med Assoc J* 1978; 118: 623-627

4. Tovey LA, Townley A, Stevenson BJ, *et al*: The Yorkshire antenatal anti-D immunoglobulin trial in primigravidae. *Lancet* 1983; 2: 244-246

5. Trolle B: Prenatal Rh-immune prophylaxis with 300 micrograms immune globulin anti-D in the 28th week of pregnancy. *Acta Obstet Gynecol Scand* 1989; 68: 45-47

6. American College of Obstetricians and Gynecologists: Prevention of D isoimmunization. *ACOG Technical Bulletin No. 147*. Washington, D.C., 1990

7. Daffos F, Capella-Pavlovsky M, Forestier F: Fetal blood sampling during pregnancy with use of a needle guided by ultrasound: a study of 606 consecutive cases. *Am J Obstet Gynecol* 1985; 153: 655-660

8. Simonovits I: Efficiency of anti-D IgG prevention after induced abortion. *Vox Sang* 1974; 26: 361-367

9. Simonovits I, Timar I, Bajtai G: Rate of Rh immunization after induced abortion. *Vox Sang* 1980; 38: 161-164

10. Smidt-Jenson, Philip J: Comparison of transabdominal and transcervical CVS and amniocentesis: sampling success and risk. *Prenat Diagn* 1991; 11: 529-537

11. U.S. Preventive Services Task Force: *Guide to Clinical Preventive Services: an Assessment of the Effectiveness of 169 Interventions*. Williams & Wilkins, Baltimore, Md, 1989: 221-224

12. Society of Obstetricians and Gynaecologists of Canada: The administration of Rh immune globulin. *Bull SOGC* 1980; Vol. I, No.1, Ottawa

Screening for D (Rh) Sensitization in Pregnancy

MANEUVER	EFFECTIVENESS	LEVEL OF EVIDENCE <REF>	RECOMMENDATION
ABO and D (formerly Rh) blood group antibody screening at the first prenatal visit and repeat antibody screening within 72 hours of delivery of a D positive infant	**Intervention** Administration of 300 µg of (D) immunoglobulin (D Ig) IM to unsensitized D negative women within 72 hours of delivery of a D positive newborn prevents sensitization from up to 15 mL of D positive red blood cells.	Randomized controlled trials<1,2> (I)	There is good evidence to support the recommendation for prenatal and antenatal antibody screening (A)
Repeat antibody screening test between the 24-28 weeks of gestation if the mother is negative	Prophylactic administration of 300 µg of D Ig at 28-29 weeks gestation to unsensitized women further reduces the risks of sensitization.	Non-randomized controlled trials<3-5> (II-1)	There is fair evidence to support the recommendation that additional screening be performed at 24-28 weeks gestation (B)
Repeat antibody screening before induced abortion, amniocentesis and other obstetrical complications or procedures in which there is the possibility of fetal bleed	Prophylactic administration of 300 µg D Ig after induced abortion or amniocentesis (50 µg if 13 weeks or less) reduces the incidence of sensitization.	Induced abortion: Case series<8,9> (III) Amniocentesis: Non-randomized controlled trial<7> (II-1)	There is fair evidence to support the recommendation that screening be performed with induced abortion and amniocentesis (B)
	Similar rates of sensitization were found in both intervention and control groups after chorionic villus sampling.	Chorionic Villus Sampling (CVS): Randomized controlled trial<10> (I)	There is poor evidence regarding the inclusion or exclusion of screening with CVS (C)
	No direct evidence for or against use of D Ig with other obstetric procedures and complications although it may be prudent to administer where the possibility of fetal to maternal bleed is anticipated.	Expert Opinion<6,12> (III)	There is poor evidence regarding the inclusion or exclusion of screening for other obstetrical complications, procedures or outcomes (C)

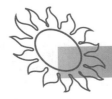

CHAPTER 12

Screening and Vaccinating Adolescents and Adults to Prevent Congenital Rubella Syndrome

By Marie-Dominique Beaulieu

12

Screening and Vaccinating Adolescents and Adults to Prevent Congenital Rubella Syndrome

Adapted by Marie-Dominique Beaulieu, MD, MSc, FCFP[1] from the report prepared for the U.S. Preventive Services Task Force[2]

Screening for rubella immunization status by obtaining proof of vaccination or by serology should be part of the periodic health examination of women of child-bearing age (B Recommendation). Susceptible non-pregnant women should be offered vaccination; susceptible pregnant women should be vaccinated immediately after delivery. An equally acceptable alternative for non-pregnant women of child-bearing age is to offer vaccination against rubella without screening (B Recommendation). There is insufficient evidence to recommend for or against screening or routine vaccination of young men in settings where large numbers of susceptible young adults of both sexes congregate, such as military bases and colleges (C Recommendation). Routine screening or vaccination of young men other than in such settings, or of older men or post-menopausal women, is not recommended.

Burden of Suffering

Rubella is generally a mild illness but when contracted by pregnant women, especially in the first 16 weeks of pregnancy, it frequently causes serious complications including miscarriage, abortion, stillbirth, and congenital rubella syndrome (CRS). The most common manifestations of CRS are hearing loss, developmental delay, growth retardation, and cardiac and ocular defects. The lifetime cost of treating a patient with CRS was estimated in 1985 to exceed 220,000 U.S. dollars.<1>

In 1991, 61.7% of reported cases of rubella infection occurred in adolescent and young adults

Universal childhood immunization was initiated in every province of Canada in the early 1970s. (For current recommendations see Chapter 33). By 1990, reported rubella infection had declined from 30 to 1.5 cases per 100,000 population, and CRS incidence had decreased from 1.7 to 0.01 cases per 100,000 live births.<2> In 1983, however, rubella infection peaked at a rate of 29.8 per 100,000 population. No increase in the rate of CRS was observed.

---

[1] Associate Professor, Department of Family Medicine, University of Montreal, Montreal, Quebec

[2] By Carolyn DiGuiseppi, MD, MPH, Science Advisor, U.S. Preventive Services Task Force, Washington, D.C.

There was also an outbreak of rubella in 1989 in British Columbia. The total number of cases of rubella infection estimated to have occurred in Canada in 1992 was 2,142; a three-fold increase compared to 1991. Males were affected in 72% of the cases. Adolescents and young adults (ages 15-29 years) accounted for 61.7% of the new cases of rubella infection.<2> In 1991, 5 cases of CRS were reported.

Maneuver

Two strategies to prevent CRS are available. One is based on screening for the immunization status of women of child-bearing age, and immunization only of susceptible ones. The other relies on universal vaccination of adolescents and young women.

Screening for rubella susceptibility can be done by serologic tests for antibodies or by obtaining proof of vaccination history. Vaccine trials and cohort studies have shown that most patients with hemagglutination inhibition (HI) antibody are protected from clinical disease.<3,4> However, HI is a labor-intensive test and can be associated with both false positive and false negative results. Enzyme immunoassay and latex agglutination have now replaced HI in most laboratories. Using HI as the comparison standard, these tests have sensitivities of 92-100% and specificities of 71-100%.<5> The apparently low specificities of some newer methods are due to their ability to detect low levels of rubella antibody that are undetectable by HI methods and are therefore reported as false positives. There have been no controlled trials to determine if these low levels confer immunity against wild virus, but other clinical and in vitro evidence suggests that they are protective.<6> These tests therefore appear to be both more accurate and more convenient than HI when performed in laboratories with demonstrated proficiency.

A history of rubella vaccination can identify many individuals who may be protected. Despite a variety of design flaws in some of the available studies, most demonstrate that individuals with a positive history of having received rubella vaccine are significantly more likely to be seropositive (range 82% to 97%) than those without such a history (range 62% to 83%).<7> A positive rubella vaccination history documented by vaccination card, school record, or medical record is more likely to be associated with seropositivity than is an undocumented history. A positive history of rubella infection is substantially less likely to correctly predict rubella immunity than is a positive history of vaccination;<8> therefore, a history of infection should not be used to determine susceptibility.

Screening for immunization status by obtaining proof of vaccination history or serologic testing has a sensitivity between 80% to 100%

Effectiveness of Screening and Treatment

Rubella vaccine, once administered, is efficacious and seropositivity is long lasting.<9> Adverse reactions from the

RA27/3 live attenuated rubella vaccine are generally mild in children. Joint symptoms are common in adults but rarely persist; the incidence of joint symptoms is higher in women than in men and increases with increasing age at vaccination.<4> Vaccination of individuals who are already immune rarely induces the joint symptoms seen upon primary immunization of susceptible individuals.

It is estimated that 6-12% of the young adult population is seronegative.<10> It has been recommended by some authorities that clinicians also direct efforts toward vaccinating susceptible adolescents and young adults, particularly women of childbearing age.<11>Two strategies have been considered: screening for immunization status and vaccination of susceptible women or universal vaccination of adolescent and young adult women.

The new immunization schedule recently approved in Canada (see Chapter 33 on Childhood Immunizations) will result in the systematic vaccination of young women against rubella, since the MMR confers immunity against both conditions. However, it can be expected that full herd immunity will not be conferred to childbearing women before about 15 years.

Screening Followed by Vaccination

Screening followed by immunization of susceptible women or systematic immunization reduces the risk of congenital rubella syndrome

Several factors may reduce the effectiveness of this strategy in preventing CRS. First, the screening test may falsely identify some susceptible individuals as immune. For example, of the 21 CRS cases reported in the U.S. in 1990, 71% of the mothers had a positive serologic test, while 43% gave a history of vaccination.<12> Secondly, people correctly identified as susceptible may not be offered or may not accept the vaccine.

No population studies have evaluated the effectiveness of screening and vaccinating susceptible individuals in reducing the incidence of CRS. Evidence that screening and vaccination can reduce the likelihood of rubella infection was seen in a severe rubella outbreak in Iceland, where identical rates of protection from infection occurred in screened and immunized (98.5%) and in naturally immune (99%) schoolgirls.<13> Evidence for the effectiveness of screening and follow-up vaccination in reducing rubella susceptibility is supplied also by a cohort study from Scotland. Six to seven years after a screening program for schoolgirls took place, 98.7% of girls who had originally been naturally immune had circulating antibodies, compared to 95.1% of those who had been vaccinated as susceptibles and 42.8% of a small group of susceptibles who had refused vaccination.<14> There is thus fair evidence that screening and immunizing susceptible females of child-bearing age reduces both rubella susceptibility and infection, and by inference, CRS.

Universal Vaccination

In addition to protecting those who have not been previously vaccinated, universal vaccination would also potentially eliminate most susceptibility due to primary vaccine failure and waning immunity. In Sweden and Finland, vaccine programs in which all adolescent girls are routinely immunized, as well as all children aged 14-18 months, have been associated with substantially reduced occurrence of both seronegativity and of rubella infection in female compared to male adolescents and adults.<15,16> These data provide fair evidence for routine vaccination of all non-pregnant women of child-bearing age to reduce rubella susceptibility and infection, and therefore CRS.

Pregnancy and Rubella Vaccination

The rubella vaccine is contraindicated during pregnancy because of the theoretical possibility of teratogenicity, although there have been no reported cases of rubella vaccine-related birth defects in the United States after inadvertent vaccination of 321 susceptible pregnant women within 3 months of conception.<3> Because a measurable iatrogenic risk cannot be excluded, vaccination of susceptible women known to be pregnant should be postponed until the postpartum period. Women who are vaccinated should be advised not to become pregnant in the subsequent month. The virus has been isolated in breast milk and in breast fed infants after postpartum vaccination, but no adverse consequences from such exposure have been reported.

Screening and Vaccination in Young Men

In settings where large numbers of young adults are gathered (e.g., military bases and colleges), outbreaks of rubella are not uncommon and males and females are infected at similar rates.<2> Rubella screening or routine vaccination of young men in such settings might reduce the risk of spreading rubella to susceptible pregnant women. There is weak evidence from before-after studies that universal rubella screening and follow-up vaccination of military recruits is effective in preventing rubella infection and eliminating epidemic rubella.<17> There is no direct evidence that either screening or routine vaccination of males in these settings reduces CRS. For young men not living in such settings, no evidence at all was found supporting either screening or routine vaccination in reducing susceptibility infection or CRS.

Recommendations of Others

The Canadian Immunization Guide <18> recommends that rubella vaccine should be given to all female adolescents and women of child-bearing age unless they have either laboratory evidence of detectable antibody or documented evidence of having received vaccine. Susceptibility should be determined by serological testing whenever possible. The Guide also considers that serologic testing for rubella antibody should be a routine procedure during prenatal care. Recommendations from a January, 1994 meeting sponsored by the Laboratory Center for Disease Control on rubella and mumps should become available in 1994.

In 1989, the U.S. Preventive Services Task Force recommended that serologic testing for rubella antibodies should be performed at the first clinical encounter with all pregnant and non-pregnant women of child-bearing age lacking evidence of immunity. They also recommended that susceptible non-pregnant women who agree not to become pregnant for three months should be vaccinated and that susceptible pregnant women should not be vaccinated until immediately after delivery. These recommendations are currently under review.[19]

Conclusions and Recommendations

When administered to children, the current rubella vaccine is efficacious in the induction of rubella immunity and in the prevention of rubella infection and CRS. The added coverage provided by the two MMR vaccinations many will receive during childhood to meet current recommendations for measles immunization (see Chapter 33) should eliminate most primary vaccine failures and increase the rate of primary immunization among women of child-bearing age. Therefore, the incidence of CRS will probably decline as the current cohort of highly immunized female children and adolescents enters its child-bearing years.

In the intervening years, however, many women of child-bearing age will remain susceptible to rubella infection. Universal screening and follow-up vaccination of susceptible females would reduce rubella susceptibility, infections, and CRS; however, the effectiveness of this strategy in the clinical setting may be limited by incomplete screening, imperfect screening tests and failure to vaccinate susceptibles. Routine vaccination of all women of child-bearing age, without screening, also appears to be effective in reducing rubella infections, and avoids the problem of noncompliance with return visits, but results in vaccination of many women who are already immune. Because the adverse effects of vaccinating immune individuals appears to be minimal, cost and convenience are likely to be the determining factors in deciding which strategy should be used.

There is fair evidence to support screening for rubella immunity in the periodic health examination of women of child-bearing age, either by serologic testing or by eliciting a history of vaccination. A documented history of vaccination is more accurate than an undocumented history. All susceptible non-pregnant women of child-bearing age should be offered vaccination (B Recommendation). Susceptible pregnant women should be vaccinated in the immediate postpartum period (B Recommendation). There is also fair evidence to support offering routine vaccination to all women of child-bearing age, without screening by history or serology (B Recommendation). The decision of which strategy to use should be tailored to the individual clinician's practice population, depending on the availability of vaccination records, the reliability of the vaccination history, the rate of immunity, the cost of serologic testing, and the cost and likelihood of follow-up vaccination for susceptible individuals identified by serologic testing. There is insufficient evidence to recommend for or against routine vaccination of young men in settings where large numbers of susceptible young adults of both sexes congregate, such as military bases and colleges, in order to prevent CRS (C Recommendation).

Unanswered Questions (Research Agenda)

There is a need to study the costs and the benefits of alternative primary prevention strategies in various Canadian settings.

Evidence

The literature was identified with a MEDLINE search in the English language for the years of 1989 to 1993, using the following key words: rubella vaccine, adverse effects and rubella. This review was initiated in October 1993 and the recommendations finalized by the Task Force in January 1994.

Acknowledgements

The Task Force would like to thank Dr. Robert Pless, Field Epidemiologist, Laboratory Centre for Disease Control, Childhood Immunization Division, Ottawa, Ontario for his assistance.

Selected References

1. Orenstein WA, Bart KJ, Hinman AR, *et al*: The opportunity and obligation to eliminate rubella from the United States. *JAMA* 1984; 251: 1988-1994

2. Health and Welfare Canada: *Notifiable Diseases Annual Summary*. Ottawa: Minister of National Health & Welfare 1991: 63-64

3. Cradock-Watson JE: Laboratory diagnosis of rubella: past, present and future. *Epidemiol Infect* 1991; 107: 1-15

4. Best JM: Rubella vaccines: past, present and future. *Epidemiol Infect* 1991; 107: 17-30

5. Field PR, Ho DW, Cunningham AL: Evaluation of rubella immune status by three commercial enzyme-linked immunosorbent assays. *J Clin Microbiol* 1988; 26: 990-994

6. Kleeman KT, Kiefer DJ, Halbert SP: Rubella antibodies detected by several commercial immunoassays in hemagglutination inhibition-negative sera. *J Clin Microbiol* 1983; 1131-1137

7. Orenstein WA, Herrman KL, Holmgreen P, *et al*: Prevalence of rubella antibodies in Massachusetts schoolchildren. *Am J Epidemiol* 1986; 124: 290-298

8. Dales LG, Chin J: Public health implications of rubella antibody levels in California. *Am J Public Health* 1982; 72: 167-172

9. Enders g, Nickerl U: Rubella vaccination: persistence of antibodies for 14-17 years and immune status of women with and without vaccination history. *Immun Infect* 1988; 16: 58-64

10. Murray DL, Lynch MA: Determination of immune status to measles, rubella, and varicella-zoster viruses among medical students: assessment of historical information. *Am J Public Health* 1988; 78: 836-838

11. Centers for Disease Control: Rubella prevention: recommendations of the Immunization Practices Advisory Committee (ACIP). *MMWR* 1990; 39(RR-15): 1-18

12. Lee SH, Ewert DP, Frederick PD, *et al*: Resurgence of congenital rubella syndrome in the 1990s. Report on missed opportunities and failed prevention policies among women of childbearing age. *JAMA* 1992; 267: 2616-2620

13. Rafnar B: Rubella immunization of teenage girls in Iceland and follow-up after a severe rubella epidemic. *Bull WHO* 1982; 60: 141-146

14. Zealley H, Edmond E: Rubella screening and immunization of schoolgirls: results six to seven years after vaccination. *Br Med J* 1982; 284: 382-384

15. Bottiger M, Christenson B, Romanus V, *et al*: Swedish experience of two dose vaccination programme aiming at eliminating measles, mumps, and rubella. *Br Med J (Clin Res Ed)* 1987; 295: 1264-1267

16. Ukkonen P, von Bonsdorff C-H: Rubella immunity and morbidity: effects of vaccination in Finland. *Scand J Infect Dis* 1988; 20: 255-259

17. Crawford GE, Gremillion DH: Epidemic measles and rubella in Air Force recruits: impact of immunization. *J Infect Dis* 1981; 144: 403-410

18. Health Canada. *Canadian Immunization Guide. 4th ed.* Ottawa, 1993 (Cat No. H41-8/1993E)

19. U.S. Preventive Services Task Force: *Guide to Clinical Preventive Services: an Assessment of the Effectiveness of 169 Interventions.* Williams & Wilkins, Baltimore, Md, 1989: 215-219

Screening and Vaccinating Adolescents and Adults to Prevent Congenital Rubella Syndrome

MANEUVER	EFFECTIVENESS	LEVEL OF EVIDENCE <REF>	RECOMMENDATION
Screening for immunization status followed by vaccination*			
Screening for immunization status (serology or proof of vaccination) and immunization of women at risk	Screening for immunization status and vaccination of women at risk can increase seropositivity rates to 95%.	Cohort studies <12-14> (II)	Fair evidence to include in the periodic health examination of women of child-bearing age (B)
Screening for serologic proof of immunization in pregnant women and counselling of seronegative women	No studies have evaluated the effectiveness of this strategy. Knowledge of the serologic status of pregnant women is considered important to counsel/document new infection.	Expert opinion <3> (III)	Fair evidence to include in the periodic health examination of pregnant women (B)
Universal vaccination*			
Universal vaccination of adolescent and young women independently of prior knowledge of immunization	Confers immunity without significant adverse effects. Universal immunization of adolescent and young women is an effective alternative to screening followed by immunization and may be less expensive.	Cohort studies <15,16> (II)	Fair evidence to include in the periodic health examination of women of child-bearing age (B)
Universal vaccination of young men in settings where large number of people gathered	The only cohort study used a less immunogenic vaccine than the one used in women's studies.	Cohort study (methodologic problems) <17> (II)	Lack of evidence to include or exclude in the periodic health examination of young men gathered in large settings (C)

* The decision of which strategy to use should be tailored to the individual clinician's practice population, depending on the availability of vaccination records, the rate of immunity, the cost of serologic testing and of follow-up vaccination for susceptible people.

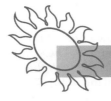

CHAPTER 13

Prevention of Preeclampsia

By Marie-Dominique Beaulieu

Prevention of Preeclampsia

Adapted by Marie-Dominique Beaulieu, MD, MSc, FCFP[1] from
the report prepared for the U.S. Preventive Services Task Force[2]

*Blood pressure (BP) measurement should be part of the
periodic health examinations of all pregnant women. The
technique for BP measurement should be consistent, with the
patient always in the same position (B Recommendation). There
is no evidence to recommend low dose aspirin prophylaxis as a
primary preventive measure in women at low risk of developing
preeclampsia. Low dose aspirin prophylaxis can be considered in
women at high risk of preeclampsia and intra-uterine growth
retardation (IUGR) (C Recommendation).*

Burden of Suffering

Hypertension is the most common medical complication of
pregnancy, occurring in 6-8% of all pregnancies.<1,2> It is seen in a
group of disorders that include preeclampsia-eclampsia, latent or
chronic essential hypertension, a variety of renal diseases, and
transient gestational hypertension.

Preeclampsia/eclampsia
syndrome is the
second leading cause
of maternal death

Preeclampsia, once called toxemia of pregnancy, is the most
dangerous of these disorders, occurring in about 2.6% of pregnancies.
Women with preeclampsia are at increased risk for abruptio placenta,
acute renal failure, cerebral hemorrhage, disseminated intravascular
coagulation, pulmonary edema, circulatory collapse, and eclampsia.

The fetus may become hypoxic, increasing risk of low
birthweight, premature delivery, or perinatal death.<3> Women who
suffered from preeclampsia are not at increased risk of developing
chronic hypertension.

Risk factors for preeclampsia and eclampsia include black
ancestry, nulliparity or first pregnancy with the actual partner, multiple
gestations, chronic hypertension or diabetes, a family history of
eclampsia or preeclampsia and possibly obesity.<4>

Although definitions differ, many define preeclampsia as acute
hypertension presenting after the 20th week of gestation accompanied
by abnormal edema and/or proteinuria (more than 0.3 g/24h), or
both.<5> BP over 140/90, or a rise of 15 mmHg or 30 mmHg above

---

[1] Associate Professor, Department of Family Medicine, University of Montreal,
Montreal, Quebec
[2] By Michelle Berlin, MD, MPH, Assistant Professor of Obstetrics & Gynecology,
University of Pennsylvania Medical Center, Philadelphia, Pennsylvania and A.
Eugene Washington, MD, MSc, Co-director, Center for Reproductive Health
Policy Research, University of California School of Medicine, San Francisco,
California

the usual diastolic and systolic BP respectively, is considered abnormal. The appearance of edema and proteinuria alone is unreliable because edema is common in normal pregnancies.<6> BP levels should be normalized 6 weeks post-partum.

Transient gestational hypertension is defined as acute onset of hypertension in pregnancy or the early puerperium without proteinuria or abnormal edema and resolving within 10 days after delivery.<2> Chronic hypertension that had been latent prior to the pregnancy may become evident during gestation. Pregnant women with chronic hypertension are also at increased risk for stillbirth, neonatal death, and other fetal complications, but the risk is much lower than that of women with preeclampsia. Women with transient or latent chronic hypertension are more likely to develop chronic hypertension in later years.<4,5>

Maneuver

Two preventive maneuvers are considered. Screening for early signs of preeclampsia followed by appropriate clinical interventions has been for a long time the only strategy available. Recently, low dose aspirin prophylaxis has been evaluated as a primary prevention maneuver in low-risk and high-risk pregnancies.

Low Dose Aspirin Prophylaxis

Endothelial dysfunction caused by the systemic effects of decreased placental blood flow is postulated to be the pathophysiologic mechanism for preeclampsia. Compared to women with normal pregnancies, women with preeclampsia have a relative excess of thromboxane A2 compared to prostacyclin. It has been hypothesized that the correction of the thromboxane: prostacyclin ratio by aspirin could prevent preeclampsia and its complications. The aspirin dosage proposed varies between 60 to 150 mg per day and has been initiated between 13 to 26 weeks of pregnancy, in different studies.<7-9>

Screening for Early Signs of Preeclampsia

Much research has been done to identify screening tests that would predict the risk of developing preeclampsia before the classical triad of symptoms appears. The validity of proposed tests is difficult to evaluate due to the absence of a gold standard to confirm the diagnosis. Glomerular endotheliosis, the renal lesion characteristic of preeclampsia, is present in only 54% of patients who meet the clinical criteria for the disease,<10> and is not specific for preeclampsia. For practical reasons, most studies of potential screening tests for preeclampsia have relied on clinical criteria to confirm the diagnosis.

Measurable proteinuria usually occurs late in the course of the illness and therefore is not useful for early detection.<2> However, screening for bacteriuria in pregnancy is recommended at 12 to 16 weeks (see Chapter 9). In a prospective study of women between 24 and 34 weeks of gestation, a urine albumin concentration ≥11 mcg/L had a sensitivity of 50% in predicting subsequent preeclampsia.<11> The conventional dipstick test is unreliable in detecting the moderate and highly variable elevations in albumin that occur early in the course of preeclampsia but it can help ascertain the diagnosis when it is present.<12>

Other screening tests that have been suggested, include the angiotensin II infusion test and the supine pressor "rollover" examination, but these have also been found to be unsuitable, as the former is impractical and the latter lacks adequate sensitivity, specificity and positive predictive value.<1,12>

To be valid, the blood pressure must be measured in a consistent manner at each visit

BP measurement remains the cornerstone of early diagnosis, although it has limitations. First, there are the usual sources of measurement errors associated with sphygmomanometry. In addition, maternal posture can affect BP in pregnant women significantly.<12> The results can be erroneous, for example, if BP is measured with the woman in the supine position. Most important, a single elevated BP reading is neither diagnostic of nor a reliable predictor of preeclampsia.

Absence of the normal decline in BP that occurs in the middle trimester or an increase in BP during the second trimester may be an early indicator of increased risk for preeclampsia.<3,13> Some experts recommend using the middle trimester mean arterial pressure (MAP), defined as ((2 x diastolic BP) + systolic BP)/3 as a screening test.<3> Studies indicate that a middle trimester MAP above 90 mmHg has a sensitivity of 61-71% and a specificity of 62-74% in predicting preeclampsia.<3,14>

Effectiveness of Prevention and Treatment

Low Dose Aspirin Prophylaxis

The effectiveness of prophylactic acetylsalicylic acid (ASA) at doses ranging between 60 and 150 mg has been the object of some randomized controlled trials. Most were conducted in women at high risk for preeclampsia. All showed that low-dose aspirin can effectively reduce pregnancy-induced hypertension and preeclampsia and IUGR associated with the conditions. The decrease in the incidence of preeclampsia was not, however, associated with a decrease in neonatal mortality but the cesarian section rate was significantly lower in the aspirin group in two studies.<8,9>

A large randomized controlled trial was conducted recently in 3,135 low-risk nulliparous women.<7> In this trial 60 mg of ASA was effective in reducing preeclampsia incidence from 6.3% to 4.6% but was associated with a statistically significant increase in abruptio placenta which was not observed in a much larger study (CLASP).<15> The beneficial effect of ASA was observed only in women whose BP was >120 mmHg at recruitment.<7>

Screening for Preeclampsia Followed by Early Intervention

Delivery is the only specific, definitive treatment of preeclampsia. However, early detection of hypertension during pregnancy permits clinical monitoring and prompt therapeutic intervention should severe preeclampsia or eclampsia develop. Although some studies support the use of bedrest, pharmacologic agents, and early delivery of the fetus to prevent complications, there is little conclusive evidence that these measures improve outcome.<12,16,17> A randomized controlled trial found that antihypertensive therapy and hospitalization, when compared with hospitalization alone, did not improve maternal or fetal outcome.<18> There have been no clinical trials to determine whether hypertensive women treated early in pregnancy have a better prognosis than those who are not detected early. Nonetheless, most obstetrical experts believe, based on clinical experience, that early detection and preventive non-pharmacologic treatment of preeclampsia may be beneficial to both mother and fetus.<1,6,18,19> This view is based in part on inferences drawn from the apparent effectiveness of regular prenatal care in reducing the risk of preeclampsia-eclampsia. Studies conducted as early as the 1940s suggested an inverse relationship between the extent of prenatal care and the incidence of eclampsia, perhaps reflecting a beneficial effect due to early detection.<20> These findings do not provide direct evidence, however, that improved outcome is due solely to BP measurement itself, rather than to other components of prenatal care or to the characteristics of women who receive regular prenatal care.

Recommendations of Others

The Canadian and American Colleges of Obstetricians and Gynecologists recommend BP measurements at the initial visit, every 4 weeks until 28 weeks' gestation, every 2-3 weeks until 36 weeks' gestation, and weekly thereafter.<21,22>

In 1989, the U.S. Preventive Services Task Force recommended that all pregnant women should receive systolic and diastolic blood pressure measurements at the first prenatal visit and periodically until delivery or throughout the three trimesters.<23>

Conclusions and Recommendations

There is no evidence to recommend universal low-dose ASA prophylaxis in nulliparous women (C Recommendation). Although there is grade I evidence of its capacity to reduce the incidence of preeclampsia, it has not been shown to decrease neonatal mortality, and has been associated with adverse outcome in some studies. The safety of aspirin prophylaxis must be carefully evaluated. However, this treatment may be considered for women at high risk for the condition.

To date, the only readily available screening strategy for preeclampsia is the early detection of an abnormal BP trend over time. A diagnosis of preeclampsia should not be made solely on the presence of elevated BP. There is no experimental evidence that these efforts will result in reduced maternal or perinatal morbidity and mortality. However, there is grade II-2 evidence that regular prenatal care is associated with a reduced incidence of preeclampsia.

Blood pressure should be measured at each prenatal visit. There is insufficient data to recommend routine aspirin prophylaxis

Systolic and diastolic pressures should be measured on all obstetric patients at the first prenatal visit and periodically throughout the remainder of pregnancy (B Recommendation). The optimal frequency for measuring BP in pregnant women has not been determined and is therefore left to clinical discretion. The collection of reliable BP data requires consistent use of correct technique and a cuff of appropriate size encircling at least 2/3 of the upper arm length. The patient should consistently be in the same position, and the BP should be measured in the sitting position, after the patient's arm has rested at heart level for 5 minutes.<5> For additional guidelines, see Chapter 53 on Screening for Hypertension.

Further diagnostic evaluation and clinical monitoring, including frequent BP monitoring and urinalysis, are indicated if BP does not decrease normally during the third trimester, if the diastolic pressure increases 15 mmHg above baseline or the systolic pressure increases 30 mmHg above baseline, or if the BP exceeds 140/90. Medical interventions upon the suspicion of a diagnosis of preeclampsia must include hospital admission to substantiate the diagnosis and its severity.

Unanswered Questions Research Agenda

The following have been identified as research priorities:

1. The identification of biologic markers to predict early detection of preeclampsia.

2. The identification of women likely to benefit from prophylactic aspirin prophylaxis.

Evidence

The literature was identified with a MEDLINE search in the English language for the years 1966 to July 1993 using the following key words: preeclampsia, prevention and control. The review was initiated by the Task Force in December 1993 and the Recommendations finalized in January 1994.

Acknowledgements

We would like to thank Jean-Marie Moutquin, MD, FRCPC, Professor, Department of Obstetrics and Gynecology, Université Laval, Québec City, Québec, for reviewing this chapter.

Selected References

1. DeVoe SJ, O'Shaughnessy R: Clinical manifestations and diagnosis of pregnancy-induced hypertension. *Clin Obstet Gynecol* 1984; 27: 836-853

2. Chesley LC: History and epidemiology of preeclampsia-eclampsia. *Clin Obstet Gynecol* 1984; 27: 801-820

3. Page EW, Christanson R: The impact of mean arterial pressure in the middle trimester upon the outcome of pregnancy. *Am J Obstet Gynecol* 1976; 125: 740-746

4. Roberts JM, Redman CW: Pre-eclampsia: more than pregnancy-induced hypertension. *Lancet* 1993; 341: 1447-1451

5. National High Blood Pressure Education Working Group Report on High Blood Pressure in Pregnancy. *Am J Obstet Gynecol* 1990; 163: 1691-1712

6. Wallenburg HCS: Detecting hypertensive disorders of pregnancy. In: Chalmers I, Enkin M, Kierse, ed: Effective care in pregnancy and childbirth. Oxford: Oxford University Press, 1989; 382-402

7. Sibai BM, Caritis SN, Thom E, *et al*: Prevention of preeclampsia with low-dose aspirin in healthy, nulliparous pregnant women. *N Engl J Med* 1993; 329: 1213-1218

8. Beaufils M, Donsimoni R, Uzan S, *et al*: Prevention of pre-eclampsia by early antiplatelet therapy. *Lancet* 1985; 840-842

9. Benigni A, Gregorini G, Frusca T, *et al*: Effect of low-dose aspirin on fetal and maternal generation of thromboxane by platelets in women at risk for pregnancy-induced hypertension. *N Engl J Med* 1989; 321: 357-362

10. Fisher KA, Luger A, Spargo BH, *et al*: Hypertension in pregnancy: clinical-pathological correlations and remote prognosis. *Medicine-Baltimore* 1981; 60: 267-276

11. Rodriguez MH, Masaki DI, Mestman J, *et al*: Calcium/creatinine ration and microalbuminuria in the prediction of preeclampsia. *Am J Obstet Gynecol* 1988; 159: 1452-1455

12. Sibai BM: Pitfalls in diagnosis and management of preeclampsia. *Am J Obstet Gynecol* 1988; 159: 1-5

13. Fallis NE, Langford HG: Relation of second trimester blood pressure to toxemia of pregnancy in the primigravid patient. *Am J Obstet Gynecol* 1963; 87: 123-125

14. Moutquin JM, Rainville C, Giroux L, *et al*: A prospective study of blood pressure in pregnancy: prediction of preeclampsia. *Am J Obstet Gynecol* 1985; 151: 191-196

15. CLASP Collaborative Group: CLASP: a randomized controlled trial of low-dose aspirin for the prevention and treatment of pre-eclampsia among 9364 pregnant women. *Lancet* 1994; 343: 619-629

16. Mathews DD, Shuttleworth TP, Hamilton EFB: Modern trends in management of non-albminuric hypertension in late pregnancy. *Br Med J* 1978; 2: 623-625

17. Gilstrap LC, Cunningham FG, Whalley PG: Management of pregnancy-induced hypertension in the nulliparous patient remote from term. *Semin Perinatol* 1978; 2: 73

18. Sibai BM, Gonzalez AR, Mabie WC, *et al*: A comparison of labetalol plus hospitalization versus hospitalization alone in the management of preeclampsia remote from term. *Obstet Gynecol* 1987; 70: 323-327

19. Redman CW, Roberts JM: Management of pre-eclampsia. *Lancet* 1993; 341: 1451-1454

20. Cunningham FG, Lindheimer MD: Hypertension in pregnancy. *N Engl J Med* 1992; 326: 927-932

21. Chelsey LC: Eclampsia at the Margaret Hague Maternity Hospital. *Bull Marg Hague Hosp* 1953; 6: 2-11

22. American College of Obstetricians and Gynecologists. Standards for obstetric-gynecologic services, 6th ed. Washington, D.C.: *American College of Obstetricians and Gynecologists,* 1985: 17-18

23. The Society of Obstetricians and Gynaecologists of Canada: Guidelines for prenatal care in Canada – 1984. *Bulletin* 1984; 6(4): 1

24. U.S. Preventive Services Task Force: *Guide to Clinical Preventive Services: an Assessment of the Effectiveness of 169 Interventions.* Williams & Wilkins, Baltimore, Md, 1989: 95-103

Prevention of Preeclampsia

MANEUVER	EFFECTIVENESS	LEVEL OF EVIDENCE <REF>	RECOMMENDATION
Routine prenatal care with blood pressure measurement	Early detection and non-specific preventive treatment is beneficial to the mother and fetus.	Cohort studies <16,17,21> (II-2); expert opinion <1,6,19,20> (III)	There is fair evidence to recommend screening for preeclampsia in the periodic examination of all pregnant women (B)
Low-dose (60-150 mg per day) aspirin in nulliparous women with/without risk factors of preeclampsia	Low-dose aspirin reduces incidence of preeclampsia and intra-uterine growth retardation but has been associated with increased risks of complications in some studies without impact on neonatal mortality and morbidity.	Randomized controlled trials<7-9,15> (I)	There is insufficient evidence to recommend for or against low-dose aspirin in women with/without risk factors of preeclampsia (C)

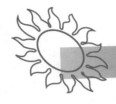

CHAPTER 14

The Use of Home Uterine Activity Monitoring to Prevent Preterm Birth

By Geoffrey Anderson

14

The Use of Home Uterine Activity Monitoring to Prevent Preterm Birth

Adapted by Geoffrey Anderson, MD, PhD,[1] from the report written for the U.S. Preventive Services Task Force[2]

This review of the evidence for the use of home uterine activity monitoring (HUAM) in the prevention of preterm birth is based on the U.S. Preventive Services Task Force review of the subject.<1> The review identified 6 randomized trials of HUAM screening and subsequent therapeutic interventions that reported perinatal outcomes. There are no controlled trials of home uterine activity monitoring (HUAM) in pregnancies with no risk factors for preterm labour. All of the trials included populations of women at high risk for preterm labour.

The Canadian Task Force concurs with the U.S. Preventive Services Task Force that the lack of evidence of benefit of HUAM in normal pregnancies suggests that this maneuver not be included in the management of normal pregnancies (D Recommendation).

The results of 6 randomized controlled trials of HUAM screening in women with high risk of preterm labour have been published. Four of these indicated some positive effects of HUAM screening. However, the design of two studies made it difficult to separate the effects of HUAM from other components of the experimental intervention. The two other studies which indicated positive effects of HUAM screening used controversial techniques in the statistical analysis of the trial results. Although HUAM screening of high risk pregnancies may be a promising technique for the prevention of preterm birth, currently there is insufficient evidence of clinical effectiveness to recommend for or against its routine use as a screening maneuver. (C Recommendation)

[1] Senior Scientist, Institute for Clinical Evaluative Sciences in Ontario (ICES); Associate Professor, Department of Health Administration, University of Toronto, Toronto, Ontario

[2] By Steven H. Woolf, MD, MPH, Science Advisor, U.S. Preventive Services Task Force, Washington, D.C. and Assistant Clinical Professor, Dept. of Family Practice, Medical College of Virginia, Richmond, Virginia

Burden of Suffering

Birth before 36 or 37 weeks of gestation is defined as preterm birth.<2> The incidence of preterm birth is about 6 percent of total deliveries in Canada.<2,3> Such births account for 75-85% percent of perinatal mortality, and about 10-15% percent of survivors having major handicaps.<2,3>

Maneuver

Home uterine activity monitoring (HUAM) involves the collection of data on uterine contractions using a tocodynamometer. The home tocodynamometer consists of a pressure sensor held against the abdomen by a belt and a recording/storage device that is carried by a belt or hung from the shoulder. Uterine activity is typically recorded by the patient for one hour, twice daily, while performing routine activities. The stored data are transmitted via telephone to a practitioner, where a receiving device prints out data. Patients are often contacted by, or have access to, personnel who can address monitoring problems.

Home uterine activity monitoring (HUAM) involves the collection of data on uterine contractions using a tocodynamometer

Effectiveness of Prevention and Treatment

The goal of HUAM screening is to detect preterm labour at a stage that will allow for intervention to prevent preterm delivery. A range of therapies are available to prevent preterm labour. The most effective therapies include the use of tocolytic drugs.<3>

This review of the evidence on the impact of HUAM screening excludes studies that solely examine the value of HUAM in detecting preterm labour and is limited to studies that examine the impact of programs that combine detection of preterm labour using HUAM and the treatment of preterm labour with tocolytic agents.

The design of most trials of HUAM is similar. High-risk patients are selected on the basis of a history of prior preterm deliveries, multiple gestations, uterine anomalies, or other risk factors. Patients receive initial training and are instructed to monitor their contractions at home two to four times each day and to transmit stored data daily via telephone to receiving tocographs. Study personnel are available by telephone, sometimes on a 24-hour basis, to answer patient inquiries. If the patient detects more than four contractions per hour or other specified symptoms, she monitors contractions for an additional hour while lying on her side and taking fluids. If the symptoms persist, the patient is evaluated in hospital. If preterm labour does not resolve with rest and hydration, tocolytic therapy is begun. Long-term tocolysis, if instituted, is generally discontinued at 35-37 weeks. Patients are usually examined every one to two weeks. Monitoring is discontinued at 36-37 weeks. Preterm labour is defined by persistent uterine

The goal of HUAM screening is to detect preterm labour and allow for interventions to prevent preterm delivery

contractions and cervical change, and preterm delivery is usually defined as a delivery before 36 completed gestational weeks.

Morrison et al (1987)<4> assigned 69 out of 75 eligible high-risk patients to a study group that received HUAM, education, and self-palpation instructions or a control group that received education and self-palpation instructions only. Although monitored women were contacted daily, subjects in the control group were contacted by telephone twice each week.

There was no difference between groups in the incidence of preterm labour or in the gestational age at which preterm labour was diagnosed. Among women who developed preterm labour, there were statistically significant differences between groups in the incidence of cervical dilation of 3 cm or more, cervical effacement of greater than 50%, and rupture of membranes. A greater proportion of monitored cases were eligible for long-term tocolysis. The time gained in utero was an average of four weeks longer in the monitored group, and the proportion that reached a gestational age of 36 weeks was also significantly greater. Clinical outcomes in newborns were reported in a separate paper.<5> The authors reported a significantly lower overall number of complications in the monitored group than in controls.

Study and control groups differed in the intensity of nursing follow-up; women in the study group received daily telephone calls from study nurses, whereas women in the control group were contacted twice each week.

Iams et al<6> randomly assigned 157 high-risk women at 20-34 weeks gestation to a study group that received HUAM, education and self-palpation instructions only. In contrast to the previous study, women in the control group were contacted at least five times each week, daily on weekdays and as needed on weekends. Fifteen women dropped out of the study after randomization. There were no statistically significant differences between groups in the incidence of preterm labour, preterm deliveries, gestational age at delivery, or mean birth weight. Clinical outcomes in the newborn were not measured.

In 1988, Iams et al (1988)<7> published a subsequent report based on additional 152 subjects enrolled in the second year of the study, providing a total sample of 309 patients over two years. Twenty-eight subjects in the second year dropped out after randomization. Over the two-year period, the authors again found no significant differences between groups in preterm labour and delivery rates, mean birth weight, or gestational age at delivery.

The statistical power of this study, even with the larger sample, has been questioned by some critics but this has since been refuted by the authors.<8> Other criticisms include the lack of a standardized definition for preterm labour, the failure of some physicians in the study to continue tocolysis beyond 35 weeks, inadequate randomization, and the administration of prophylactic tocolytics by some physicians.<9>

In a multicentre study, Hill et al (1990)<10> randomly assigned 299 high-risk women at 20 to 34 weeks gestation to a study group that received daily HUAM, education, and daily nursing contacts or to a control group that received education and self-palpation instructions. Women in the control group were advised to contact their physicians for certain symptoms and did not receive frequent nursing contacts. Fifty-four women (18%) were excluded from the study following randomization. There was no significant difference between the groups in the incidence of preterm labour. The monitored group had significantly fewer cases of cervical dilation beyond 2 cm and delivery within 48 hours of the first labour episode (18% vs. 37%). Term delivery was achieved by more women in the monitored group than in the control group. Clinical outcomes in the newborn were not measured.

Women in the study group were contacted daily, whereas women in the control group were not contacted regularly. High attrition and exclusion rates may also have influenced the results.

Dyson et al (1991)<11> provided education, self-palpation instructions, and HUAM to 251 high-risk women in California and then randomized them to two groups. Both groups transmitted monitor data, but data transmitted by women in the control group were not analyzed or used in patient management. Patients were unaware of their group assignments. Results from both groups were compared to data from a non-randomly selected "standard care" group, consisting of 143 women with similar risk factors who were cared for in the 30 month period before the study. All patients were contacted five days per week. Outcomes were reported separately for singleton and multiple gestations.

For singleton gestations, the incidence of preterm births was lower in the control group than in the standard care group, but the rate of preterm births in the monitored group did not differ significantly from outcomes in the control group. Among women who developed preterm labour before 34 weeks, outcomes were poorer in the standard care group than in the monitored and control groups.

In twin gestations, the incidence of preterm birth was significantly lower in the monitored and control groups than in the standard care group. There were also significantly lower rates of neonatal death, intensive care nursery admission, and respiratory distress syndrome in the control group than in the standard care group. All neonatal outcomes were significantly better in the monitored group than in the standard care group. The monitored group had significantly lower rates than controls in the incidence of birth weight less than 1,500 g, intensive care nursery admission, and length of hospital stay.

This study benefitted from a large sample size and an innovative design that attempted to separate the effects of HUAM from those of nursing contact. Unfortunately, overall results were not reported to determine whether monitored women as a group, including those with singleton and twin gestations experienced better outcomes than women in the control group. Significant results for women with twin gestations were reported for three out of eight clinical outcomes, but the calculations of statistical significance were based on different denominators. Although calculations for the singleton group used the number of women as the denominator, calculations for twin gestations used the number of newborns as the denominator. This doubling of the denominator increased the apparent degrees of freedom, thereby achieving statistical significance. The use of newborns as the denominator for twin gestations is of concern because newborns were not the unit of analysis in the study and because twin gestations are not independent variables.

In a multicentre study, Mou et al (1991)<12> randomly assigned 377 of 509 eligible high-risk women at 23-30 weeks gestation to a study group that received HUAM, education, and self-palpation instructions or to a control group that received education and self-palpation instructions. The 132 women who were not enrolled (26% of the eligible sample) failed to participate because they refused, because consent was not requested, or because they lacked a telephone. Women in the control group were not contacted by study personnel, and personnel who contacted women in the study group were instructed to report the number of contractions but not to ask questions or provide medical advice.

There was no significant difference between groups in the incidence of preterm labour or in the gestational age at the diagnosis of preterm labour. Although clinical outcomes were examined, cervical dilation was the primary end point of the study. When the number of women who developed preterm labour was used as the denominator, mean cervical dilation was significantly similar in the monitored group (1.4 cm) than in the control group (2.5 cm). The proportion with cervical dilation less than 2 cm, time gained in utero after diagnosis of preterm labour, and mean gestational age at delivery were also significantly greater in monitored women than in controls. Among a subset of singleton gestations (see below), newborns from monitored pregnancies had significantly greater birth weight (2,934 g vs. 2,329 g) and required fewer days of neonatal intensive care (50 vs. 324 days), oxygen therapy (0 vs. 68 days), and mechanical ventilation (0 vs. 54 days) than newborns from unmonitored pregnancies.

The randomization did not include 132 (26%) of the 509 eligible women, and about 11% of the randomized sample were subsequently excluded. Of the remaining 334 women, 252 women who did not develop preterm labour (67% of the randomized sample) were not included in the overall calculations. The major findings of the study were drawn from the remaining 82 women who developed preterm labour. In this group, monitoring was associated with a significantly smaller cervical dilation at the onset of labour, but it is unclear whether this difference in dilation resulted in improved clinical outcome for the newborns. Although significant differences between the groups were reported for gestational age at delivery, birth weight, neonatal intensive care, and respiratory therapy, the calculations were based on a subset of the 82 women, excluding 19 (23%) cases that involved twin gestations and medically indicated preterm deliveries.

In a French study, Blondel et al (1992)[13] randomly assigned 94 high-risk women to a study group that received HUAM and daily midwife contact or to a control group that received home visits by a community health nurse once or twice each week. The monitoring device standards, and organization of home care were similar to those used in the U.S. studies. The patients were at 24-34 weeks gestation and were recruited from four public maternity units.

The investigators found no difference between groups in the rate of hospital admission for threatened preterm labour. There were no statistically significant differences between groups in the incidence of preterm births before 37 weeks or of birth weight less than 2,500 g. No other clinical outcomes were measured.

Summary of Evidence for Benefits

Four of the published studies indicate at least some perinatal benefit in the group receiving the intervention involving HUAM recording and reporting.

Although this evidence suggests at least some perinatal benefit from HUAM screening there are important conceptual or methodological problems with each of the positive trials.[4,5,10-12] In two of the earlier studies[4,5,10] the experimental and control groups differed not only in the use of HUAM, but also in the level and intensity of contact with nursing staff. This makes it difficult at a conceptual level to determine if the difference in observed outcomes is the result of HUAM screening or nursing contact. The two latter trials[11,12] that have positive results do not have a problem with defining HUAM as the intervention, but involve the use of controversial statistical analysis techniques.

The evidence suggests some perinatal benefit from HUAM screening but there are important methodological problems with the positive trials

Cost

Currently, HUAM is available from Tokos Medical Corporation. The firm reports that it would charge about $90 per day per patient for HUAM in Canada.[14] This would include the costs of the tocodynamometer and the nursing services. Costs for 1 to 12 weeks of monitoring would be between $630 and $7,560. An American study of the cost-benefit of HUAM in high-risk patients indicated a net saving due to the lower treatment costs in a screening group.<15>

Recommendations of Others

The U.S. Preventive Services Task Force recommend against the use of HUAM screening in normal pregnancies (D Recommendation). They found insufficient evidence of clinical effectiveness to recommend for or against HUAM as a screening test in high-risk pregnancies (C Recommendation).<1> The British Columbia Office of Health Technology Assessment concluded that "currently available data do not support the adoption of this new technology, even for selective use in high-risk patients".<14>

At this time the Society of Obstetricians and Gynaecologists of Canada has not made an official statement on guidelines for the use of HUAM.

Conclusions and Recommendations

The prevention of preterm birth by early detection and treatment of preterm labour is a promising approach to the reduction of prenatal mortality and morbidity. The effect of HUAM in screening normal pregnancies for the development of preterm labour has not been examined in randomized controlled trials. There have been six trials of HUAM monitoring and tocolytic therapy in high-risk pregnancies. Four of these trials indicated some positive effects of these detection and treatment programs but there are conceptual or methodological problems with each of these trials.

HUAM screening could cost between $600 and $7,000 per monitored pregnancy. Given the high cost of this maneuver and the lack of any experimental evidence of its benefits in normal pregnancies, its routine use in normal pregnancies cannot be justified at this time (D Recommendation). The problems with existing trials in high-risk pregnancies means that there is inconclusive evidence regarding the inclusion or exclusion of HUAM in the high-risk population (C Recommendation).

Unanswered Questions (Research Agenda)

There is the need for a well designed and analyzed trial of HUAM in high-risk pregnancies. This should be accompanied by an analysis of the cost effectiveness of HUAM in Canada.

Evidence

The literature was identified with a MEDLINE search from the literature after 1983 in the English language. MESH keywords included: monitoring, physiologic, home care services, fetal monitoring and home.

This review was initiated in March 1993 and recommendations finalized by the Task Force in June 1993. For a complete reference list please see reference 1.

Selected References

1. U.S. Preventive Services Task Force: Home uterine activity monitoring for preterm labour: Review article. *JAMA* 1993; 270: 369-370

2. Moutquin JM, Pepiernik E: Can we lower the rate of preterm birth? *Bull SOGC* 1990; September: 19-20

3. Maternal Fetal Medicine Committee: Preterm labour Investigation and Management. *Bull SOGC* 1988; January/February: 13-15

4. Morrison JC, Martin JN Jr., Martin RW, *et al*: Prevention of preterm birth by ambulatory assessment of uterine activity: a randomized study. *Am J Obstet Gyencol* 1987; 156: 536-543

5. Morrison JC, Martin JN Jr, Martin RW, *et al*: A program of uterine activity monitoring and its effect on neonatal morbidity. *J Perinatol* 1988; 8: 228-231

6. Iams JD, Johnson FF, O'Shaughnessy RW, *et al*: A prospective random trial of home uterine activity monitoring in pregnancies at increased risk of preterm labour. *Am J Obstet Gynecol* 1987; 157: 638-643

7. Iams JD, Johnson FF, O'Shaughnessy RW, *et al*: A prospective random trial of home uterine activity monitoring in pregnancies at increased risk of preterm labour. Part II. *Am J Obstet Gynecol* 1988; 159: 595-603

8. Katz M: Home uterine activity monitoring. [letter] *Am J Obstet Gynecol* 1988; 159: 787-789

9. Newman RB: Randomized trial of home uterine activity monitoring. [letter] *Am J Obstet Gynecol* 1988; 159: 1308-1309

10. Hill WC, Fleming AD, Martin RW, *et al*: Home uterine activity monitoring is associated with a reduction in preterm birth. *Obstet Gynecol* 1990; 76: 13S-18S

11. Dyson DC, Crites YM, Ray DA, *et al*: Prevention of preterm birth in high-risk patients: the role of education and provider contact versus home uterine monitoring. *Am J Obstet Gynecol* 1991; 164: 756-762

12. Mou SM, Sunderji SG, Gall S, *et al*: Multicenter randomized clinical trial of home uterine activity monitoring for detection of preterm labour. *Am J Obstet Gynecol* 1991; 165: 858-866

13. Blondel B, Breart G, Berthoux Y, *et al*: Home uterine activity monitoring in France: a randomized controlled trial. *Am J Obstet Gynecol* 1992; 167: 424-429

14. Green CJ, Sheps SB, Friesen KD, *et al*: Home uterine activity monitoring: A review of the scientific evidence. British Columbia Office of Health Technology Assessment Discussion Paper Series (BCOHTA 92:2), 1992: 1-49

15. Kosasa TS, Abou-Sayf FK, Li-Ma G, *et al*: Evaluation of the cost-effectiveness of home monitoring of uterine contractions. *Obstet Gynecol* 1990; 76(1 suppl): 71S-75S

The Use of Home Uterine Activity Monitoring to Prevent Preterm Birth

MANEUVER	EFFECTIVENESS	LEVEL OF EVIDENCE <REF>	RECOMMENDATION
Screening for preterm labour with home uterine activity (HUAM) monitor in pregnancies with risk factors*	Improved outcomes for women at high risk are unclear due to design limitations.	Randomized controlled trials<4-7,10-13> (I)	Insufficient evidence to recommend for or against HUAM as a screening test for preterm labour in high-risk* pregnancies (C)
Routine screening for preterm labour with HUAM in normal pregnancies	There have been no controlled trials of HUAM in normal pregnancies and costs have been incompletely evaluated in published research.	Expert opinion<1,14> (III)	Given the costs of HUAM and the lack of research evidence on benefits, there is fair evidence to exclude HUAM screening in low-risk pregnancies (D)

* High-risk pregnancies include: prior preterm deliveries, multiple gestations, uterine anomalies, or other risk factors

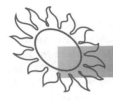

 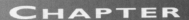 **15**

Intrapartum Electronic Fetal Monitoring

By Geoffrey Anderson

Intrapartum Electronic Fetal Monitoring

Prepared by Geoffrey Anderson, MD, PhD[1]

The widespread, increased use of electronic fetal monitoring (EFM) prompted the Task Force in 1989 to examine the evidence regarding the effectiveness of this procedure in the prevention of intrapartum asphyxia and its consequences. At that time there was inconclusive evidence regarding its use in high-risk pregnancies and fair evidence to exclude EFM from routine intrapartum care in low-risk pregnancies. The individual trials justifying this position were reviewed together with new meta-analyses. This resulted in no change in the recommendations of the Task Force.

Burden of Suffering

The rate of perinatal complications and death in Canada has declined steadily over the last 20 years. Early and accurate identification of fetal distress with EFM permits medical or obstetric intervention that may reduce the frequency and severity of adverse outcomes due to asphyxia.

The reported incidence of fetal distress has been increasing rapidly in recent years. In Ontario the recorded incidence of fetal distress increased from 2.4 per 100 deliveries in 1979 to 6.4 per 100 deliveries in 1987.<1>

Maneuver

Monitoring can be done either externally, with sensors placed on the mother's abdomen, or internally, with an electrode attached to the fetal scalp. Sampling of blood from the fetal scalp and monitoring of uterine contraction pressure by placement of a sensor in the uterine cavity are adjuncts to internal monitoring.

Effectiveness of EFM

Changes in fetal heart rate may be related to fetal hypoxia. However, the effects of EFM on health outcomes depends not only on this relation but also on the sensitivity and specificity of EFM, the prevalence of hypoxia and the availability of effective therapeutic interventions. Evidence on the link between fetal hypoxia and changes in fetal heart rate alone does not provide clinicians with a useful guide

[1] Senior Scientist, Institute for Clinical Evaluative Sciences in Ontario (ICES); Associate Professor, Department of Health Administration, University of Toronto, Toronto, Ontario

to the appropriate use of EFM. The recommendations presented here are based on studies of the effects of EFM on fetal outcome and cesarean section rates.

The Task Force attributes the highest grade of quality to evidence from randomized controlled trials. Eight such trials were identified;<2-9> unfortunately, the total sample sizes for most of the trials were small, and only two had sufficiently large samples to detect important differences in perinatal death rates.<8-9>

All of the eight randomized controlled trials had inclusion or exclusion rules that defined the study populations as either high- or low-risk. Four of the trials examined the effects of EFM in high-risk populations (Table 1)<2-5> and four in low-risk populations (Table 2).<6-9> The technique for EFM was not stated explicitly in the report of one trial,<9> but internal monitoring was used in all the others. The method used in the control groups involved active clinical monitoring by nursing and medical staff. In four studies<3-6> auscultation of the fetal heart was done every 15 minutes in the first stage of labour and at least every 5 minutes in the second stage. In the Dublin trial<8> the heart was auscultated at least every 15 minutes in the first stage and between all contractions in the second stage. In three trials the monitoring technique in the control group was not explicitly defined.<2,7,9>

In the randomized controlled trials involving high-risk pregnancies there were no statistically significant differences in mortality rates between the EFM and clinically monitored groups,<2-6> but this is not surprising given the small sample sizes. One study showed possible benefits of EFM in terms of the measurement of cord blood gas levels and the identification of neurologic signs;<2> however, the authors pointed out that EFM was part of an intensive care strategy that included other specialized services. None of the studies showed statistically significant differences in Apgar scores between the study and control groups. The only consistent statistically significant effect was an increase in the rates of cesarean section and other operative deliveries in the EFM groups.

Two of the small randomized controlled trials that compared EFM with clinical monitoring in low-risk pregnancies showed no significant effect of monitoring on fetal outcomes.<6,7> One trial showed a statistically significant increase in the cesarean section rate<6> and the other an increase in the rate of other operative deliveries<7> in the EFM group.

The Dublin trial<8> was performed on a broadly defined population of 12,964 low-risk women – only 5.7% of the eligible women were excluded because they were considered to be at high risk on the basis of meconium staining or other grounds. Except for an increase in the rate of operative deliveries other than cesarean section and a possible decrease in the rate of neurologic signs there were no

The recommendations presented here are based on studies of the effects of EFM on fetal outcome and cesarean section rates

statistically significant differences between the EFM and the control groups. More babies in the control group than in the EFM group had neonatal seizures. Long-term follow-up of all infants with neonatal seizures showed no differences in outcome between the two groups: three infants in each group showed clearly abnormal neurologic signs at follow-up one year later.

Obstetric practices in the Dublin institution differed from North American practices, as evidenced by the low baseline rate for cesarean section (2.3% in Dublin versus almost 20% in Canada<1>). Given these differences it may be difficult to extrapolate the results of the Dublin trial to the situation in North America.

There was no significant effect of universal monitoring in low-risk pregnancies other than an increased cesarean section rate

Leveno and colleagues,<9> in studying the use of EFM in low-risk pregnancies, allocated patients to either universal or selective EFM depending on the month of admission. The two study groups were similar in ethnic background, age, parity, level of prenatal care received and birth weight. During the selective months the use of EFM was limited to high-risk pregnancies (37% of the total pregnancies), and during the universal months EFM was used in as many cases as possible (79%). Other than the degree of monitoring, the standards of obstetric care did not vary in the alternate study months. There was no significant effect of universal monitoring other than an increased cesarean section rate. A post-hoc analysis of the outcomes in the low-risk group showed similar results. Interestingly, there seemed to be evidence of an increased cesarean section rate specifically for fetal distress in this group.

Systematic Review

The Cochrane Database of Systematic Reviews has produced 4 reviews of EFM.<10-13> These reviews concluded that EFM did not provide any benefit in terms of Apgar scores, admission to special care nursery or perinatal death. The only observed benefit of EFM was a decreased incidence of neonatal seizures. The reviews also concluded that EFM resulted in higher cesarean section rates and higher rates of maternal infection.

Recommendations of Others

The Task Force on Predictors of Fetal Distress supported the use of EFM in high-risk but not necessarily in low-risk pregnancies.<14> In 1982 the Federal Task Force on High Risk Pregnancies and Prenatal Record Systems stated that there was no acceptable evidence to indicate any beneficial effects of EFM in low-risk pregnancies.<15> The recommendations of the U.S. Preventive Services Task Force on screening for fetal distress are currently under review.

Conclusions and Recommendations

The recommendations pertain to the choice between EFM and active clinical monitoring, not between EFM and no monitoring. Active clinical monitoring requires that trained staff are available.

In high-risk pregnancies there is little sound scientific evidence to support the choice of EFM over intermittent auscultation (at least once every 15 minutes in the first stage of labour and at least once every 5 minutes in the second stage). This does not mean that EFM may not be beneficial in high-risk pregnancies; there is simply insufficient evidence for recommending the exclusion or inclusion of EFM rather than active clinical monitoring in all high-risk pregnancies (C Recommendation). High-risk categories include low gestational age, high maternal age, placenta or cord problems, meconium in the amniotic fluid, hypertension, proteinuria, malpresentation, poor outcome in previous pregnancies and medical complications.

In high-risk pregnancies there is little sound scientific evidence to support the choice of EFM over intermittent auscultation

There is fair evidence to exclude EFM from routine intrapartum care in low-risk pregnancies (D Recommendation) because studies have consistently shown no benefit in reducing the risk of perinatal complications and death, whereas they have shown an increased rate of cesarean section and other operative procedures among those monitored. Since the operative procedures are associated with a high risk of maternal complications and increased costs, the routine use of EFM could increase the risk and costs.

Unanswered Questions (Research Agenda)

Determining the appropriate role for EFM with the use of a trial large enough to detect clinically significant differences in fetal outcomes in high-risk pregnancies.

Evidence

The literature was identified with a MEDLINE search for the years 1988 to October, 1993 using the MESH heading, fetal monitoring and publication type, randomized controlled trial.

This review was initiated in October, 1993, and based on a previous report.<16> Recommendations were finalized by the Task Force in March, 1994.

Selected References

1. Anderson G, Lomas J: Recent trends in cesarean section rates in Ontario. *Can Med Assoc J* 1989; 141: 1049-1053

2. Renou P, Chang A, Anderson I, *et al*: Controlled trial of fetal intensive care. *Am J Obstet Gynecol* 1976; 126: 470-476

3. Haverkamp AD, Thompson HE, McFee JG, *et al*: The evaluation of continuous fetal heart rate monitoring in high risk pregnancy. *Am J Obstet Gynecol* 1976; 125: 310-320

4. Haverkamp AD, Orleans M, Langendoerfer S, *et al*: A controlled trial of the differential effects of intrapartum fetal monitoring. *Am J Obstet Gynecol* 1979; 134: 399-412

5. Luthy DA, Shy KK, vanBelle G, *et al*: A randomized trial of electronic fetal monitoring in preterm labor. *Obstet Gynecol* 1987; 69: 687-695

6. Kelso IM, Parson RJ, Lawrence GF, *et al*: An assessment of continuous fetal heart rate monitoring in labor. *Am J Obstet Gynecol* 1978; 131: 526-532

7. Wood C, Renou P, Oats J, *et al*: A controlled trial of fetal heart rate monitoring in a low risk obstetric population. *Am J Obstet Gynecol* 1981; 141: 527-534

8. MacDonald D, Grant A, Sheridan-Pereira M, *et al*: The Dublin randomized controlled trial of intrapartum fetal heart rate monitoring. *Am J Obstet Gynecol* 1985; 152: 524-539

9. Leveno KJ, Cunningham FG, Nelson S, *et al*: A prospective comparison of selective and universal electronic fetal monitoring in 34,995 pregnancies. *N Engl J Med* 1986; 315: 615-619

10. Grant AM: EFM vs. intermittent auscultation in labour. In: Pregnancy and Childbirth Module (eds. Enkin MW, Keirse MJNC, Renfrew MJ, Neilson JP), "Cochrane Database of Systematic Reviews": Review No. 03884, 4 May 1994. Published through "Cochrane Updates on Disk", Oxford: Update Software, 1994, Disk Issue 1

11. Grant AM: EFM + scalp sampling vs. intermittent auscultation in labour. In: Pregnancy and Childbirth Module (eds. Enkin MW, Keirse MJNC, Renfrew MJ, Neilson JP), "Cochrane Database of Systematic Reviews": Review No. 03297, 4 May 1994. Published through "Cochrane Updates on Disk", Oxford: Update Software, 1994, Disk Issue 1

12. Grant AM: Liberal vs. restrictive use of EFM in labour (all labours). In: Pregnancy and Childbirth Module (eds. Enkin MW, Keirse MJNC, Renfrew MJ, Neilson JP), "Cochrane Database of Systematic Reviews": Review No. 03885, 8 April 1994. Published through "Cochrane Updates on Disk", Oxford: Update Software, 1994, Disk Issue 1

13. Grant AM: Liberal vs. restrictive use of EFM in labour (low-risk labours). In: Pregnancy and Childbirth Module (eds. Enkin MW, Keirse MJNC, Renfrew MJ, Neilson JP), "Cochrane Database of Systematic Reviews": Review No. 03886, 8 April 1994. Published through "Cochrane Updates on Disk", Oxford: Update Software, 1994, Disk Issue 1

14. Task Force on Predictors of Fetal Distress: Consensus Development Conference of the National Institute of Child Health and Human Development. *Clin Pediatr* 1979; 18: 585-598

15.   *Report of the Federal Task Force on High Risk Pregnancies and Prenatal Record Systems.* Publications Unit, Health Services and Promotion Branch, Department of National Health and Welfare, Ottawa, 1982: 26

16.   Canadian Task Force on the Periodic Health Examination: The periodic health examination: 1989 update part 4, Intrapartum electronic fetal monitoring and prevention of neonatal herpes simplex. *Can Med Assoc J* 1989; 141: 1233-1240

Table 1: Characteristics of Randomized Controlled Trials for High Risk Pregnancies

Trial[REF]	Renou et al.[2]	Haverkamp et al.[3]	Haverkamp et al.[4]	Luthy et al.[5]
Trial Characteristics				
Total pregnancies (n)	350	483	360	246
Total perinatal deaths	2	3	3	35
Neonatal deaths	1	1	3	n/a
Postneonatal deaths	n/a	n/a	5	n/a
Neurological signs	15	4	4	14
Comparison of EFM to Routine Care[1]				
Perinatal mortality	n.s.	n.s.	n.s.	n.s.
Post neonatal mortality	n/a	n/a	n.s.	n/a
Caesarean section rate	higher	higher	higher	n.s.
Operative deliveries	n.s.	higher	higher	n.s.
Apgar scores	n.s.	n.s.	n.s.	n.s.
Cord blood pH	better	n.s.	n.s.	n.s.
Neurological signs	better	n.s.	n.s.	n.s.

[1] n.s. indicates no significant difference; n/a is not available and higher or better are statistically significant differences at $p<0.05$.

Table 2: Characteristics of Randomized Controlled Trials for Low Risk Pregnancies

Trial[REF]	Kelso et al.[6]	Wood et al.[7]	MacDonald et al.[8]	Leveno et al.[9][1]
Trial Characteristics				
Total pregnancies (n)	504	890	12,964	14,618
Total perinatal deaths	1	1	n/a	n/a
Intrapartum Deaths	0	0	2	0
Neonatal Deaths	1	1	12	9
Neurological Signs	n/a	4	66	4
Comparison of EFM to Routine Care[2]				
Perinatal mortality	n.s.	n.s.	n/a	n.s.
Intrapartum mortality	n.s.	n.s.	n.s.	n.s.
Caesarean section rate	higher	n.s.	n.s.	higher
Operative deliveries	n.s.	higher	higher	n/a
Apgar scores	n.s.	n.s.	n.s.	n.s.
Cord blood pH	n.s.	n.s.	n.s.	n/a
Neurological signs	n.s.	n.s.	n.s.	n.s.

[1] Post hoc analysis of low risk subgroup by Leveno et al.[9]
[2] n.s. indicates no significant difference; n/a is not available and higher or better are statistically significant differences at $p<0.05$.

Intrapartum Electronic Fetal Monitoring

MANEUVER	EFFECTIVENESS	LEVEL OF EVIDENCE <REF>	RECOMMENDATION
Electronic fetal monitoring (EFM) in high-risk* pregnancies	Neonatal morbidity and mortality rates have not been definitively shown to be reduced with the use of EFM over intermittent auscultation. An increase in the rates of cesarean section has been associated with EFM.	Randomized controlled trials<2-5> (I)	Weak evidence for either inclusion in or exclusion from the periodic health examination (C)
EFM in low-risk pregnancies	The use of EFM as compared with intermittent auscultation has not been shown to reduce neonatal morbidity or mortality rates but has been associated with increased rates of cesarean section and maternal infection.	Randomized controlled trials<6-9> (I)	Fair evidence to exclude from routine intrapartum care (D)

* High-risk categories include: low gestational age, high maternal age, placenta or cord problems, meconium in the amniotic fluid, hypertension, proteinuria, malpresentation, poor outcome in previous pregnancies and medical complications.

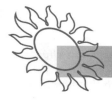

CHAPTER 16

Prophylaxis for Gonococcal and Chlamydial Ophthalmia Neonatorum

By Richard B. Goldbloom

16

Prophylaxis for Gonococcal and Chlamydial Ophthalmia Neonatorum

Prepared by Richard B. Goldbloom, MD, FRCPC[1]

The term ophthalmia neonatorum applies in this chapter to acute conjunctivitis in the newborn from any cause. In 1979, the Canadian Task Force on the Periodic Health Examination concluded that there was good evidence to support prophylaxis with routine instillation of 1% silver nitrate solution into each eye at birth. Several important developments have occurred over the subsequent years: 1) Other antibiotics, notably tetracycline and erythromycin, have been evaluated as alternative agents for the prevention of gonococcal and chlamydial ophthalmia neonatorum; 2) The importance of Chlamydia trachomatis as a cause of neonatal conjunctivitis has been recognized; and 3) Concern has been expressed regarding the transient chemical conjunctivitis that may occur following instillation of the silver nitrate solution and the possibility that this complication will interfere with parent-infant attachment ("bonding"). The evidence does not demonstrate the superiority of any one prophylactic agent and in 1992<1> the Task Force recommended the use of 1% silver nitrate solution, 1% tetracycline ointment or 0.5% erythromycin ointment, primarily to prevent gonococcal ophthalmia.

Separate chapters were prepared on screening for gonorrhea (Chapter 59) and Chlamydial infection (Chapter 60).

Burden of Suffering

In the absence of preventive measures it is estimated that gonococcal ophthalmia neonatorum will develop in approximately 28% of infants born to women with gonorrhea. Gonococcal conjunctivitis is usually severe, and *N. gonorrhoeae* can penetrate the intact corneal epithelium and cause microbial keratitis, ulceration and perforation. Maternal gonococcal infection is particularly common in developing countries, where penicillin-resistant gonococci account for up to 60% of the strains isolated. Infection in such women is often asymptomatic. Since 1981 the rate of reported gonorrhea in Canada (about 230 per 100,000) has been steadily decreasing: in 1989 there were 19,110 cases (73 cases per 100,000); 8,421 of the cases involved women aged 15 to 59 years. The number of reported cases of penicillinase-producing *Neisseria gonorrhoeae* (PPNG) infection increased from 591 in 1988 to 1,046 in 1989; 92% were reported in Ontario and Quebec.

---

[1] Professor of Pediatrics, Dalhousie University, Halifax, Nova Scotia

In 1989 the Laboratory Centre for Disease Control, Ottawa, received reports of 55,186 cases of chlamydial infection across Canada (excluding British Columbia and the Yukon Territory). In 1989-90 women aged 15 to 39 years accounted for 34,802 of the cases of genital chlamydial infection (excluding British Columbia and the Northwest Territories). Although chlamydial infection became nationally notifiable in 1990, reporting practices may vary between provinces and territories. More than 4 million cases of chlamydial infection occur each year in the U.S., and 155,000 infants are born to women with cervical infection. At a community health centre in Montreal, 7.1% of women presenting for a routine gynecologic examination were found to have *C. trachomatis* infection. Chlamydial infection can cause pseudomembranous or membranous conjunctivitis in the newborn that may result in conjunctival scarring and corneal infiltrates. The recorded risk of conjunctivitis in infants born to women with *C. trachomatis* infection has varied from 18% to 50%.

> At a community health centre, 7.1% of women having routine gynecologic examinations tested positive for *C. trachomatis* infection

In descending order of frequency, the infectious causes of ophthalmia neonatorum are *C. trachomatis*, *Staphylococcus*, *N. gonorrhoeae*, *Streptococcus*, *Hemophilus* and, rarely, herpes simplex virus, molluscum contagiosum virus and papilloma virus.

Maneuver

Instillation of 1% silver nitrate solution or antibiotic ointment (0.5% erythromycin or 1% tetracycline) into the conjunctival sac of the newborn soon after birth.

Effectiveness of Prevention

Gonococcal Ophthalmia

The establishment of legal requirements for silver nitrate prophylaxis was followed by a dramatic reduction in the incidence of blindness due to gonococcal ophthalmia neonatorum.[2,3] Other agents have been evaluated in controlled trials of varying design.

In a prospective controlled clinical trial Lund and associates[4] compared the effectiveness of 1% silver nitrate solution and 0.5% erythromycin ointment in the obstetric units of three hospitals in Capetown, South Africa. In the 13 months before the trial began, when ocular prophylaxis was not practised, the incidence of gonococcal ophthalmia neonatorum in the study area was 273 per 100,000 live births. Twenty-eight cases of gonococcal ophthalmia neonatorum were diagnosed among 24,575 births during the 13-month pretrial period, as compared with only five cases among 23,883 births during the 12 months after the prophylaxis was introduced (p<0.001). Four of the five infected infants had inadvertently not received prophylaxis. During the same two periods the incidence rates of gonococcal ophthalmia neonatorum in three midwife obstetric units that did not practise ocular prophylaxis were unchanged (39 cases in the pretrial period vs. 38 in the trial period).

In a prospective clinical trial,[5] the efficacy of prophylaxis with silver nitrate drops, tetracycline ointment and erythromycin ointment were compared among 12,431 infants born during the study period. Treatment was changed monthly. Gonococcal ophthalmia neonatorum occurred in one infant in the silver nitrate group, three in the tetracycline group and four in the erythromycin group; these differences were not statistically significant. Seven mothers of these eight infants had received no prenatal care, and five were drug abusers. The respective risks of gonococcal ophthalmia neonatorum after prophylactic treatment were 0.03%, 0.07% and 0.1%.

Laga and colleagues[2] compared the efficacy of 1% silver nitrate drops and 1% tetracycline ointment in a controlled trial involving 2,732 newborns in Kenya. The prevalence rate of intrapartum gonococcal infection was 6.4%; the frequency of multiresistant strains was high. The drugs were alternated every week for 15 months and were administered within 30 minutes after birth. To evaluate the protective efficacy of the two regimens mother-infant transmission rates were compared with those observed in a cohort study at the same hospital before prophylaxis was given at birth. After the silver nitrate and tetracycline prophylaxis the prevalence rates of gonococcal ophthalmia neonatorum were 0.4% and 0.1% respectively (difference not statistically significant). Attack rates in newborns exposed to *N. gonorrhoeae* at birth were 7.0% among those who received the silver nitrate and 3.0% among those who received the tetracycline (95% confidence interval: 3.4% to 11.4%). Thus, compared with the rates among the historical controls, the incidence of gonococcal ophthalmia neonatorum was 83% lower among infants treated with silver nitrate and 93% lower among those treated with tetracycline. Two factors may have contributed to the higher attack rates in the silver nitrate group. First, three of the five cases of infection occurred during the first week of the study, before nurses were fully familiar with the technique for applying the silver nitrate drops. Second, a substantial number of patients were lost to follow-up: 31% by day 7 and 57% by day 28.

In summary, the available evidence indicates that 1% silver nitrate solution, 1% tetracycline ointment and 0.5% erythromycin ointment have comparable efficacy in preventing gonococcal infection. On the basis of cost estimates and the attack rates reported in the Kenyan trial, tetracycline is more cost-effective than silver nitrate. Unfortunately, the only costs considered were those of the antibiotics used in prophylaxis and treatment. Given this limitation as well as the differences in 1) the price and availability of antibiotics or silver nitrate

1% silver nitrate solution, 1% tetracycline ointment and 0.5% erythromycin ointment have comparable efficacy in preventing gonococcal infection

ampoules; and 2) the prevalence of gonococcal infection and PPNG strains, these results cannot be generalized to Canada.

Chlamydial Ophthalmia Neonatorum

The evidence supporting the efficacy of any of the currently available agents (silver nitrate, erythromycin or tetracycline) in preventing chlamydial ophthalmia neonatorum is conflicting and inconclusive.<2,5-7>

Chemical Conjunctivitis Due to Prophylaxis

Randomized clinical trials have shown that the use of silver nitrate in the delivery room decreases eye openness and inhibits visual responses within the first hour after birth. A comparison of times and places indicated that the use of single-dose wax ampoules reduced the accidental instillation of high concentrations of silver nitrate solution (as a result of evaporation of water). However, in a large case series, silver nitrate instillation (by ampoule, with or without rinsing) within the first hour after birth caused conjunctivitis in 90% of infants between 3 to 6 hours of age; the ocular reaction subsided within 24 hours in most cases. Topically applied antibiotics resulted in chemical conjunctivitis in less than 10% of cases and compared with silver nitrate have been associated with a 2.5 to 12-fold reduction in the incidence of such ocular reactions. This finding is consistent with the results of controlled trials, but its clinical significance has not been determined. The possibility that chemical conjunctivitis after silver nitrate prophylaxis might impair parent-infant bonding, by interfering with eye contact, was one of the main reasons for introducing a topical antibiotic ointment. This led to widespread abandonment of silver nitrate prophylaxis in the 1980s in favour of the more expensive antibiotic ointments.

In a randomized clinical trial Butterfield, Emde and Svejda<8> compared the effect on bonding of silver nitrate prophylaxis given immediately after birth and 1 hour after birth. Although mothers in the first group noted diminished eye openness it did not alter their baby-focused attention or prevent their pleasure and excitement in the initial encounter. For fathers the increased eye openness associated with delayed prophylaxis appeared to encourage more affectionate attention. These observations suggested that there might be some merit in delaying silver nitrate prophylaxis for a short time after birth but did not indicate any significant effect on ultimate parent-infant attachment.

Prenatal Maternal Screening

The availability of effective ocular prophylaxis for gonococcal ophthalmia neonatorum does not diminish the importance of prenatal

For chlamydial ophthalmia, prenatal screening currently appears to offer better prospects for prevention than topical ocular prophylaxis

screening for and appropriate treatment of maternal gonorrheal and chlamydial infection (see Chapters 59 and 60). Indeed, several Western countries depend on universal prenatal care and contact tracing rather than on ocular prophylaxis to prevent gonorrheal ophthalmia. In the case of chlamydial ophthalmia, prenatal screening currently appears to offer better prospects for prevention than topical ocular prophylaxis in the newborn.

The ideal prophylactic agent would be both nontoxic and highly effective in preventing gonococcal, chlamydial and nongonococcal, nonchlamydial ophthalmia neonatorum. Since gonococcal ophthalmia poses the greatest threat to a child's vision it is generally believed that the principal goal of ocular prophylaxis should be the prevention of gonococcal infection.

Recommendations of Others

The American Academy of Pediatrics and the U.S. Centers for Disease Control (CDC) recommend administering ointment or drops containing tetracycline or erythromycin, or 1% silver nitrate solution, to the eyes of all infants shortly after birth. The CDC and the American College of Obstetricians and Gynecologists recommend obtaining endocervical cultures for N. gonorrheae in all pregnant women during their first prenatal visit; a second culture is recommended late in the third trimester for women at high risk of acquiring sexually transmitted diseases.

The U.S. Preventive Services Task Force has recommended that endocervical culture for gonorrhea be performed at the first prenatal visit in all pregnant women in high-risk categories.<9> Further, an ophthalmic antibiotic (erythromycin 0.5% or tetracycline 1% ophthalmic ointment) should be applied topically to the eyes of all newborns immediately after birth.

Conclusions and Recommendations

Prenatal screening for gonorrheal and chlamydial infections, particularly among high-risk women, should play a major role in the prevention of ophthalmia neonatorum.

There is good evidence to support the use of universal ocular prophylaxis for gonococcal ophthalmia, at least in the absence of universal prenatal screening for gonorrhea. Prophylaxis should be administered as soon as possible (within 1 hour) after birth; 1% silver nitrate solution, 1% tetracycline ointment and 0.5% erythromycin ointment are approximately comparable in efficacy.

The occurrence of transient chemical conjunctivitis in some infants after silver nitrate prophylaxis is a minor disadvantage. The risk can be reduced to some degree through the use of single-dose ampoules. Alternatively, tetracycline or erythromycin ointment can be used. Additional considerations in choosing a prophylactic agent are individual preference, cost and the theoretic possibility that chemical conjunctivitis due to silver nitrate prophylaxis might adversely affect parent-infant bonding.

There is poor evidence to support the use of neonatal ocular prophylaxis with any agent for chlamydial ophthalmia neonatorum.

Unanswered Questions (Research Agenda)

The ideal form of topical prophylaxis would be equally effective in preventing both gonococcal and chlamydial ophthalmia, free of side effects such as chemical conjunctivitis and no more expensive than silver nitrate. The search for agents that fulfil these criteria is a worthwhile objective for future research.

Evidence

The literature was identified with a MEDLINE search up to September 1991, using the following MESH heading: ophthalmia neonatorum.

This review was initiated in March 1990 and recommendations were finalized by the Task Force in September 1990. A report with a full reference list was published in November 1992 (see reference #1 below).

Acknowledgements

The Task Force thanks Alexander C. Allen, MD, FAAP, FRCPC, Peds., Professor of Pediatrics and of Obstetrics and Gynaecology, Dalhousie University, Halifax, NS; Robert A. Bortolussi, MD, FRCPC, Associate Professor of Pediatrics, Dalhousie University, Halifax, NS; Scott A. Halperin, MD, FRCPC, Peds., Associate Professor of Pediatrics and of Microbiology, Dalhousie University, Halifax, NS; and Michael J. Vincer, MD, FRCPC, Peds., Assistant Professor of Pediatrics, Dalhousie University, Halifax, NS, for reviewing the draft chapter and providing useful comments.

Selected References

1. Canadian Task Force on the Periodic Health Examination: The periodic health examination, 1992 update: 4. Prophylaxis for gonococcal and chlamydial ophthalmia neonatorum. *Can Med Assoc J* 1992; 147: 1449-1454

2. Laga M, Plummer FA, Piot P, *et al*: Prophylaxis of gonococcal and chlamydial ophthalmia neonatorum. A comparison of silver nitrate and tetracycline. *N Engl J Med* 1988; 318: 653-657

3. Laga M, Meheus A, Piot P: Epidemiology and control of gonococcal ophthalmia neonatorum. *Bull World Health Organ* 1989; 67: 471-477

4. Lund RJ, Kibel MA, Knight GJ, *et al*: Prophylaxis against gonococcal ophthalmia neonatorum. A prospective study. *S Afr Med J* 1987; 72: 620-622

5. Hammerschlag MR, Cummings C, Roblin PM, *et al*: Efficacy of neonatal ocular prophylaxis for the prevention of chlamydial and gonococcal conjunctivitis. *N Engl J Med* 1989; 320: 769-772

6. Hammerschlag MR, Chandler JW, Alexander ER, *et al*: Erythromycin ointment for ocular prophylaxis of neonatal chlamydial infection. *JAMA* 1980; 244: 2291-2293

7. Bell TA, Sandstrom KI, Gravett MG, *et al*: Comparison of ophthalmic silver nitrate solution and erythromycin ointment for prevention of natally acquired *Chlamydia trachomatis. Sex Transm Dis* 1987; 14: 195-200

8. Butterfield PM, Emde RN, Svejda MJ: Does the early application of silver nitrate impair maternal attachment? *Pediatrics* 1981; 67: 737-738

9. U.S. Preventive Services Task Force: *Guide to Clinical Preventive Services: an Assessment of the Effectiveness of 169 Interventions*. Williams & Wilkins, Baltimore, Md, 1989: 147-150

Prophylaxis for Gonococcal and Chlamydial Ophthalmia Neonatorum

MANEUVER	EFFECTIVENESS	LEVEL OF EVIDENCE <REF>	RECOMMENDATION
Universal ocular prophylaxis within 1 hr after birth with 1% silver nitrate solution, 1% tetracycline ointment or 0.5% erythromycin ointment (single-dose ampoules recommended for all agents)	**Gonococcal infection:** Dramatic reduction in incidence of gonococcal ophthalmia and blindness.	Comparison of times and places<2-5> (II-3)	Good evidence to recommend ocular prophylaxis in newborns (A)
	Prophylactic agents have comparable efficacy.	Controlled trials<2,5> (II-1)	
	Chlamydial infection: Prophylactic agents have comparable efficacy, but evidence for efficacy of any agent is inconclusive.	Randomized controlled trials<2,5,7> (I)	
	Immediate as opposed to delayed silver nitrate prophylaxis does not significantly affect parent-infant bonding.	Randomized controlled trial<8> (I)	

Pediatric Preventive Care

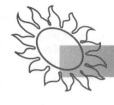

CHAPTER 17

Screening for Phenylketonuria

By William Feldman

17

Screening for Phenylketonuria

Adapted by William Feldman, MD, FRCPC,[1] from a report prepared for the U.S. Preventive Services Task Force[2]

There is good evidence for universal newborn screening and treatment for phenylketonuria (PKU). (A Recommendation) Since such programs have been implemented, mental handicap due to PKU has virtually disappeared. Screening for PKU is recommended for all newborns prior to discharge from the nursery. Infants who are tested before 24 hours of age should receive a repeat screening test between 2-7 days of age. There is insufficient evidence to recommend for or against prenatal screening for maternal PKU. (C Recommendation)

Burden of Suffering

Phenylketonuria is an inborn error of phenylalanine metabolism that occurs in 1 out of every 12,000 births in North America.<1> In the absence of treatment during infancy, most persons with this disorder develop severe, irreversible mental retardation. Many also experience neurobehavioral symptoms such as seizures, tremors, gait disorders, athetoid movements, and psychotic episodes with behaviors resembling autism.<2> These clinical manifestations of PKU have rarely developed in children born after the mid-1960s, when routine screening was legislated and early treatment for PKU became common. This has resulted in a cohort of healthy phenylketonuric women have entered childbearing age. If dietary restriction of phenylalanine is not maintained during pregnancy, these women are at increased risk of giving birth to a child with mental retardation, microcephaly, congenital heart disease, and low birthweight.<3> The incidence of this maternal PKU syndrome is 1 out of every 30,000-40,000 pregnancies.<4> In the absence of dietary control in women with PKU who become pregnant, it has been estimated that exposure of the fetus to the teratogenic effects of maternal hyperphenylalaninemia could result in an increase in the incidence of PKU-related mental retardation to the level seen before PKU screening was established.<5>

[1] Professor of Pediatrics and of Preventive Medicine and Biostatistics, University of Toronto, Toronto, Ontario
[2] By Robert Baldwin, MD, Post-Doctoral Fellow, Johns Hopkins University, Department of Pediatrics, Baltimore, Maryland and Modena E.H. Wilson, MD, MPH, Associate Professor, Department of Pediatrics, Johns Hopkins University, Baltimore, Maryland

Efficacy of Screening Tests

Blood phenylalanine determination by the Guthrie test has been the principal screening test for PKU for three decades.<6> Although well-designed evaluations of the sensitivity and specificity of the Guthrie test have never been performed,<5> sensitivity estimates and international experience with its use in millions of newborns suggests that false negative results are rare. Most missed cases of PKU do not appear to be due to false negative results of the screening tests, but rather to submission of an inadequate sample, clerical error involving the sample, infants who have failed to have a blood specimen drawn for screening, e.g. as a result of early discharge, or failure to follow up positive results. Fluorometric assays, that can detect differences in blood phenylalanine levels as low as 6 μmol/L (0.1 mg/dl), are alternative forms of testing that also offer excellent sensitivity.<5> False positive and false negative results can occur in PKU screening. In certain situations and population conditions, the ratio of false positives to true positives is as high as 32 to 1.<5> Although false positives have been viewed for many years as less important than false negative results because they can be corrected easily by repeating the test, it should be noted that recalling patients for a second PKU test generates significant parental anxiety.

The sensitivity of the Guthrie test is influenced by the age of the newborn when the sample is obtained. The current trend toward early discharge from the nursery (resulting in PKU screening being performed as early as 1 to 2 days of age) has raised concerns that test results obtained during this early period may be inaccurate. This is because the blood level of phenylalanine in affected neonates is typically normal at birth, and with the initiation of protein feedings, increases progressively during the first days of life. Using the conventional cutoff of 240 μmol/L (4 mg/dL), diagnostic levels of phenylalanine may not be present in some phenylketonuric newborns tested in the first 24 hours of life. Prospective, longitudinal evaluations of serum phenylalanine levels in infants known to be at risk for PKU have demonstrated a variable rate of false negative results when screening has occurred within the first 24 hours of life.<7,8> False negative rates ranged from 2% to 31% for the first day of life, but decreased to 0.6%-2% on the second day and to 0.3% on the third day.<5,7,8> Current rates may be lower due to the participation of many labs in a voluntary proficiency program run by the Centers for Disease Control. Fluorometric assays, provide more precise measurements of blood phenylanine levels than the Guthrie test and lower false negative rates as well.<5> Two additional solutions designed to improve sensitivity – repeat testing of all newborns after early discharge and lowering the cutoff value to reduce the false negative rate – have encountered criticism for several reasons. Repeat testing would have low yield and cost effectiveness;<9,10> it has been estimated that detecting even one case of PKU in this manner would

The current trend toward early discharge from the nursery (resulting in PKU screening being performed as early as 1 to 2 days of age) has raised concerns that test results obtained during this early period may be inaccurate

require performing an additional 600,000 to perhaps 6 million tests.<5> Lowering the cutoff value, on the other hand, improves sensitivity at the expense of specificity, thereby increasing the ratio of false positives to true positives.<5> As of 1990, eight of the fifty-two screening programs in the U.S. use a cutoff level of 120 µmol/L (2 mg/dl). The majority of labs continue to use a cutoff of 240 µmol/L (4 mg/dl) or greater.

The development of a cloned phenylalanine hydroxylase gene probe has made possible the prenatal diagnosis of phenylketonuria in families with previously affected children by analyzing DNA isolated from cultured amniotic cells or samples of chorionic villi. Through the use of the polymerase chain reaction, thirty-one alleles of the phenylalanine hydroxylase gene have been identified. This may eventually permit the screening of the general population for carriers of these alleles, thereby detecting at-risk families prior to the birth of an affected child.

Routine screening of pregnant women for maternal PKU has been recommended as a means of preventing fetal complications.<1,4> This disorder is rare in the general population, however, and as a result of screening programs, many women with PKU are aware of their diagnosis. As the cohort of women born before implementation of routine newborn screening move out of their childbearing years, the yield from screening all pregnant women should be very low. In Massachusetts, routine screening of cord blood for 10 years detected only 22 mothers with previously undiagnosed hyperphenylalaninemia.<1,11>

Effectiveness of Prevention and Treatment

Since dietary phenylalanine restriction was introduced over 95% of children with PKU have developed normal or near normal intelligence

Before treatment with dietary phenylalanine restriction became common in the early 1960s, severe mental retardation was a common outcome in children with PKU. A review in 1953 reported that 85% of patients had an intelligence quotient (IQ) less than 40, and 37% had IQ scores below 10; less than 1% had scores above 70.<2> Since dietary phenylalanine restriction was introduced, however, over 95% of children with PKU have developed normal or near normal intelligence.<12-15> A large longitudinal study has reported a mean IQ of 100 in children followed to age twelve years<16> and other reports show that adolescent and young adult patients are functioning well in society.<17> Although the efficacy of dietary treatment has never been proven in a properly designed controlled trial, the contrast between children receiving dietary treatment and historical controls provides compelling evidence of its effectiveness. This prompted most Western governments to require routine neonatal screening as early as the late 1960s.

It is essential that phenylalanine restriction be instituted in early infancy to prevent the irreversible effects of PKU.<12,14,18>

Traditionally, strict adherence to the diet was recommended for the first four to eight years of life after which it was felt that liberalization of protein intake could occur without damage to the developed central nervous system.<12,14,18> Recent data, however, suggest that discontinuation of the diet may result in some deterioration of cognitive functioning, leading many to recommend continuation of the diet through adolescence and into adulthood.<19,20,21> Even if such precautions are taken, dietary treatment may not offer full protection from subtle effects of PKU. Intelligence scores in treated persons with PKU, although often in the normal range for the general population, are somewhat lower than those of siblings and parents,<12> and mild psychological deficits, such as perceptual motor dysfunction, and attention and academic difficulties have been reported. For more information on screening for abnormal mental development, see Chapter 24.

Early detection of maternal PKU in pregnant women may also be beneficial. The incidence of maternal PKU is increasing with the growing number of healthy phenylketonuric females now entering childbearing age. Maternal hyperphenylalaninemia can produce teratogenic effects, even on normal fetuses who have not inherited PKU. If the mother does not follow a restricted phenylalanine diet during pregnancy, there is an overwhelming risk of birth of an abnormal child. This risk appears to increase as the average maternal levels of phenylalanine during pregnancy increase.<22,23> Over 90% of these children will have mental retardation, 75% microcephaly, 40-50% intrauterine growth retardation, and 10-25% other birth defects.<3,4> Uncertainties exist, however, as to whether these outcomes can be prevented by instituting treatment with dietary phenylalanine restriction.<3,24> Although some pregnant women under treatment have given birth to normal children, a number of investigators,<24-28> have found that dietary intervention fails to prevent fetal damage. Many believe dietary restrictions must be instituted prior to conception to be effective.<1,3,26-28> There are also concerns that the low phenylalanine diet may produce deficiencies in calories, protein, and other nutrients needed for proper fetal growth.<4,24> A major study examining the health effects of such diets during pregnancy is currently under way.

Maternal hyperphenylalaninemia can produce teratogenic effects, even on normal fetuses who have not inherited PKU

Recommendations of Others

In 1989, the U.S. Preventive Services Task Force recommended screening for all newborns prior to discharge from the nursery, repeat screening for infants discharged prior to 24 hours between 7-14 days and recommended against prenatal screening for maternal PKU.<29>

While there are no federal guidelines for metabolic programs, every Canadian province and U.S. state has mandated routine screening services for all newborns. Individual states vary regarding participation requirements with participation in three jurisdictions (District of Columbia, Maryland, and North Carolina) being completely voluntary. All Canadian provinces have universal screening programs. The American Academy of Pediatrics (AAP) and the American Academy of Family Physicians (AAFP) recommend that a capillary blood specimen be obtained from every neonate before leaving the nursery and as close as possible to discharge. Premature infants and those being treated for illness should be tested on or near the seventh day. The AAP recommends that infants who are tested before 24 hours of age receive a repeat screening test at 1 to 2 weeks of age. The AAP also recommends that if appropriate screening results cannot be documented for a patient transferring into a practice, the physician should obtain a specimen for screening, even if the patient is beyond the neonatal period. Routine prenatal screening for maternal PKU has been advocated by some authors, but most groups, including the AAP and the American College of Obstetricians and Gynecologists, have not recommended this approach due to concerns about cost-effectiveness.[4,10]

Conclusions and Recommendations

A capillary blood test for phenylalanine level is recommended for all newborns before discharge from the nursery (A Recommendation). Infants who were tested in the first 24 hours of age should receive a repeat screening test at 2 – 7 days of age. We recommend earlier re-screening than the U.S. Task Force because it is felt that the earlier a diagnosis is established and therapy is begun, the better the outcome. Premature infants and those with illnesses should be tested at or near 7 days of age. All parents should be adequately informed regarding the indications for testing and the interpretation of PKU test results, including the probability of false positives and false negatives. There is no evidence to recommend for or against routine prenatal screening for maternal PKU (C Recommendation). We differ from the U.S. Task Force which recommends against routine prenatal screening because there is no clear evidence either in favour of or against such a policy.

Unanswered Questions (Research Agenda)

The following have been identified as research priorities:

1. If chemical tests such as the fluorometric test are found to have better measurement and predictive properties than the Guthrie test when done within the first 24 hours of life, can follow-up testing be safely eliminated in infants discharged within that time period?

2. Controlled clinical trials of varying protein, mineral and vitamin diets given before conception or early in pregnancy to women with PKU are required to answer questions regarding routine prenatal or preconception screening of females of child bearing age.

Evidence

The literature was identified with a MEDLINE search using the MESH headings phenylketonuria, culminating in January 1993. This review was initiated in August 1993 and the recommendations of the Canadian Task Force were finalized in October, 1993.

Acknowledgements

The Task Force is grateful to William B. Hanley, MD, FRCPC, Director, PKU Program, Division Clinical Genetics, Hospital for Sick Children, Toronto, Ontario and Professor, University of Toronto, Toronto, Ontario for his helpful contributions and Kent Dooley, PhD, BSc, Director, Depts of Pathology and Laboratory Medicine, Izaak Walton Killam Hospital, Halifax, Nova Scotia for reviewing the chapter.

Selected References

1. Waisbren SE, Doherty LB, Baily IV, *et al*: The New England Maternal PKU Project: identification of at-risk women. *Am J Public Health* 1988; 78: 789-792

2. Jervis GA: Phenylpyruvic oligophrenia (phenylketonuria). *Res Publ Assoc Res Nerv Ment Dis* 1953; 33: 259-282

3. Lenke RR, Levy HL: Maternal phenylketonuria and hyperphenylalaninemia: an international survey of the outcome of untreated and treated pregnancies. *N Engl J Med* 1980; 303: 1202-1208

4. Hanley WB, Clarke JT, Schoonheyt W: Maternal phenylketonuria (PKU) – a review. *Clin Biochem* 1987; 20: 149-156

5. Kirkman HN, Carroll CL, Moore EG, *et al*: Fifteen-year experience with screening for phenylketonuria with an automated fluorometric method. *Am J Hum Genet* 1982; 34: 743-752

6. Guthrie R, Susi A: A simple phenylalanine method for detecting phenylketonuria in large populations of newborn infants. *Pediatrics* 1963; 32: 338-343

7. Meryash DL, Levy HL, Guthrie R, *et al*: Prospective study of early neonatal screening for phenylketonuria. *N Engl J Med* 1981; 304: 294-296

8. Doherty LB, Rohr FJ, Levy HL: Detection of phenylketonuria in the very early newborn blood specimen. *Pediatrics* 1991; 87: 240-244

9. Schneider AJ: Newborn phenylalanine/tyrosine metabolism. Implications for screening for phenylketonuria. *Am J Dis Child* 1983; 137: 427-432

10. Hanley WB: (personal communication), September 1993

11. Levy HL, Waisbren SE: Effects of untreated maternal phenylketonuria and hyperphenylalaninemia on the fetus. *N Engl J Med* 1983; 309: 1269-1274

12. Berman PW, Waisman HA, Graham FK: Intelligence in treated phenylketonuric children: a developmental study. *Child Develop* 1966; 37: 731-747

13. Hudson FP, Mordaunt VL, Leahy I: Evaluation of treatment begun in first three months of life in 184 cases of phenylketonuria. *Arch Dis Child* 1970; 45: 5-12

14. Williamson ML, Koch R, Azen C, *et al*: Correlates of intelligence test results in treated phenylketonuric children. *Pediatrics* 1981; 68: 161-167

15. Hsia DY: Phenylketonuria 1967. *Dev Med Child Neurol* 1967; 9: 531-540

16. Azen CG, Koch R, Friedman EG, *et al*: Intellectual development in 12-year old children treated for phenylketonuria. *Am J Dis Child* 1991; 145: 35-39

17. Koch R, Yusin M, Fishler K: Successful adjustment to society by adults with phenylketonuria. *J Inherit Metab Dis* 1985; 8: 209-211

18. Holtzman NA, Kronmal RA, van Doorninck W, *et al*: Effect of age at loss of dietary control on intellectual performance and behaviours of children with phenylketonuria. *N Engl J Med* 1986; 314: 593-598

19. Seashore MR, Friedman E, Novelly R, *et al*: Loss of intellectual function in children with phenylketonuria after relaxation of dietary phenylalanine restriction. *Pediatrics* 1985; 75: 226-232

20. Thompson AJ, Smith I, Brenton D, *et al*: Neurological deterioration in young adults with phenylketonuria. *Lancet* 1990; 336: 602-605

21. Smith I, Beasley MG, Wolff OH, *et al*: Behavior disturbance in 8-year-old children with early treated phenylketonuria. Report from the MRC/DHHS Phenylketonuria Register. *J Pediatr* 1988: 403-408

22. Platt LD, Koch R, Azen C, *et al*: Maternal phenylketonuria collaborative study, obstetric aspects and outcome: the first 6 years. *Am J Obstet Gynecol* 1992; 166: 1150-1162

23. Matalon R, Michals K, Azen C, *et al*: Maternal PKU collaborative study: the effect of nutrient intake on pregnancy outcome. *J Inherit Metab Dis* 1991; 14: 371-374

24. Lenke RR, Levy HL: Maternal phenylketonuria: results of dietary therapy. *Am J Obstet Gynecol* 1982; 142: 548-553

25. Murphy D, Saul I, Kirby M: Maternal PKU and phenylalanine-restricted diet. Studies of 7 pregnancies and of offsprings produced. *Ir J Med Sci* 1985; 154: 66-70

26. Scott TM, Fyfe WM, Hart DM: Maternal phenylketonuria: abnormal baby despite low phenylalanine diet during pregnancy. *Arch Dis Child* 1980; 55: 634-637

27. Koch R, Hanley W, Levy H, *et al*: A preliminary report of the collaborative study of maternal phenylketonuria in the United States and Canada. *J Inherit Metab Dis* 1990; 13: 641-650

28. Smith I, Glossop J, Beasley M: Fetal damage due to maternal phenylketonuria: effects of dietary treatment and maternal phenylalanine concentrations around the time of conception. *J Inherit Metab Dis* 1990; 13: 651-657

29. U.S. Preventive Services Task Force: *Guide to Clinical Preventive Services: an Assessment of the Effectiveness of 169 Interventions.* Williams & Wilkins, Baltimore, Md, 1989: 115-119

Screening for Phenylketonuria

MANEUVER	EFFECTIVENESS	LEVEL OF EVIDENCE <REF>	RECOMMENDATION
Newborn screening by automated blood phenylalanine prior to discharge from the nursery. Infants tested before 24 hours of age should receive a repeat screening test between 2-7 days of age	Guthrie test has high sensitivity and an acceptable false-positive rate; fluorometric assays have a higher sensitivity.	Case series<5,6> (III)	There is good evidence for newborn screening for PKU (A)
	False negative rates from 2-31% have been reported for testing within the first 24 hours after birth.	Case series<5,7,8> (III)	
	Burden of suffering is great and dietary treatment with low phenylalanine diet has had a dramatic effect on morbidity (pre-treatment era mean intelligence quotient (IQ) of ≤40 to a post-treatment era mean IQ of ≥100).	Dramatic differences between times and places<6,12-18> (I); case series<2> (III)	
Screening pregnant women by automated blood phenylalanine for phenylketonuria (PKU) to prevent intrauterine damage to the fetus	The incidence of undiagnosed maternal PKU is low.	Case series <1,11> (III);	There is no evidence to recommend for or against screening pregnant women for undiagnosed PKU (C)
	In women with undiagnosed mild PKU, fetus may be damaged by excess dietary phenylalanine.	Expert opinion <4,10> (III)	
	No universal maternal PKU screening program has been implemented or evaluated.		
	Some investigators have not found maternal diet beneficial Low protein diet required may have negative effects on fetus.	Cohort<22> (II-2); case series <4,24-28> (III)	
	Diet may need to be started prior to conception.	Expert opinion <1,3,22,23,26-28> (III)	

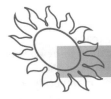

CHAPTER 18

Screening for Congenital Hypothyroidism

By Marie-Dominique Beaulieu

Screening for Congenital Hypothyroidism

Prepared by Marie-Dominique Beaulieu, MD, MSc, FCFP[1]

The Canadian Task Force on the Periodic Health Examination concludes that there is good evidence to recommend screening for congenital hypothyroidism in newborns between 2 and 6 days of life. The maneuver consists of the measurement of thyroid-stimulating hormone (TSH) levels in a dried capillary blood sample, usually taken from the newborn's heel. Thyroxine (T4) level is measured if necessary. This recommendation is unchanged from that made by the Task Force in 1990,<1> except that, reflecting current thinking regarding test characteristics, TSH is now considered the primary screening test followed by T4, if necessary (previous recommendation T4 followed by TSH).

Burden of Suffering

Congenital hypothyroidism occurs in 1 per 4,000 live births. Intellectual deficits develop in 65% of the cases without early treatment

The incidence of congenital hypothyroidism ranges between 1 per 4,000 to 1 per 3,500 live births<2> and can be as high as 1 per 141 live births among infants with Down syndrome.<3> Before screening was available, the age at diagnosis ranged from 1 week to 5 years or more. The intelligence quotient (IQ) of 65% of patients with congenital hypothyroidism was below 85 (borderline intellectual functioning or lower), and in 19% it was below 15 (profound mental retardation).<4> It is estimated that about 30% of infants with delayed diagnosis would qualify for institutional care. Children whose mothers ingested iodides, propylthiouracil or radioactive iodine or had circulating antithyroid antibodies are at high risk for congenital hypothyroidism.

Maneuver

All industrialized countries now have well organized screening programs for congenital hypothyroidism. Most screening programs in Canada and in Europe use a two-step laboratory approach where TSH is measured first and T4 in borderline cases. However, many programs in the United States measure T4 first. The recall rate for T4 averages 1.1% with a positive predictive value of 2.4%.

Blood samples from the heel are collected on filter paper, ideally 3 to 6 days after birth, and tested for TSH concentration. TSH levels after the first 24 hours of life can be as high as 20 mIU/ml, thus increasing the number of false positive results. For this reason,

---

[1] Associate Professor of Family Medicine, University of Montreal, Montreal, Quebec

newborns leaving the hospital in their first 24 hours of life are usually not tested.

The cut-off point for hypothyroidism is defined according to the daily standard deviation of test results rather than by a predetermined concentration. Since the laboratory method and the size of the blood spot influence the TSH and T4 levels each program must define its own standards and reference values. If the TSH level falls within normal limits the T4 concentration is measured with another blood spot on the filter paper. The recall rate with TSH testing averages 0.05%. At this rate, two infants are recalled for testing for every case detected. The sensitivity of the combined maneuver is about 95%.

Cases of primary, congenital hypothyroidism or about 5% of all cases of congenital hypothyroidism cannot be identified with the TSH screening approach.[5]

Effectiveness of Screening and Treatment

The first evidence of the benefits of screening for congenital hypothyroidism in Canada came with publication of the one-year follow-up data from the Quebec Screening Program.[6]

The mean IQ of affected infants less than 12 months of age was greater than 100, and did not differ from that of control subjects. Both the Quebec screening program and the New England Congenital Hypothyroidism Collaborative have published five-year follow-up data on children screened at birth.[7,8] The children who had been treated for congenital hypothyroidism were comparable to matched controls on all developmental scales. In the Quebec program, the IQ of the children treated for congenital hypothyroidism was within normal limits for children of their age, though the average IQ was statistically lower than that of the control group (105 vs. 110).[7]

Follow-up data up to 12 years after screening have recently been published.[9] The IQ and developmental scores of the hypothyroid children were still within normal limits. The degree of fetal hypothyroidism at birth influenced the final outcome.

The fact that most hypothyroid infants identified at birth by screening have intellectual and psychomotor development in the normal range, constitutes a dramatic improvement over the outcomes in children previously diagnosed later in life.

Screening and early treatment dramatically decrease the morbidity associated with congenital hypothyroidism

Recommendations of Others

Few Canadian organisations have issued recommendations on screening for thyroid diseases. The U.S. Preventive Services Task Force has recommended universal screening for congenital hypothyroidism.[10]

Conclusions and Recommendations

The dramatic change in the natural history of congenital hypothyroidism since the advent of screening warrants a grade A Recommendation, even in the absence of a randomized controlled trial. Thus, there is good evidence to recommend routine testing of all neonates.

Screening for congenital hypothyroidism is generally carried out by hospitals and is therefore outside the control of most individual physicians. Nonetheless, primary care physicians should make sure that all infants who are born at home or discharged from hospital within 24 hours after birth are tested for hypothyroidism within 7 days after birth. It is better to obtain a specimen within 24 hours than no specimen at all.

Newborns born at home or discharged within the first 24 hours of life must be tested within the first 7 days of life

Evidence

Since the last review of the Task Force on thyroid diseases was published in 1990, a MEDLINE search between 1989 and 1993 was conducted. The search was done using congenital hypothyroidism with screening and prevention and control. Only original articles were considered. The search yielded few new articles. Priority was given to the highest levels of evidence according to the Task Force methodology. This review was initiated in February 1993 updating a report published in 1990.<1> Recommendations were finalized by the Task Force in January 1994.

Selected References

1. Canadian Task Force on the Periodic Health Examination: Periodic health examination, 1990 update: 1. Early detection of hyperthyroidism and hypothyroidism in adults and screening of newborns for congenital hypothyroidism. *Can Med Assoc J* 1990; 142: 955-961

2. Fisher DA, Dussault JH, Foley TP, *et al*: Screening for congenital hypothyroidism: results of screening one million North American infants. *J Pedriatr* 1979; 94: 700-705

3. Postellon DC, Abdallah A: Congenital hypothyroidism: diagnosis, treatment, and prognosis. *Compr Ther* 1986; 12: 67-71

4. Klein RZ: Infantile hypothyroidism then and now: the results of neonatal screening. *Curr Probl Pediatr* 1985; 15: 1-58

5. Dussault JH, Morissette J, Letarte J, *et al*: Modification of a screening program for neonatal hypothyroidism. *J Pediatr* 1978; 92: 274-277

6. Glorieux J, Dussault JH, Letarte J, *et al*: Preliminary results on the mental development of hypothyroid infants detected by the Quebec Screening Program. *J Pediatr* 1983; 102: 19-22

7. Glorieux J, Dussault JH, Morissette J, *et al*: Follow-up at ages 5 and 7 years on mental development in children detected by the Quebec Screening Program. *J Pediatr* 1985; 107: 913-915

8. New England Congenital Hypothyroidism Collaborative: Effects of neonatal screening for hypothyroidism: prevention of mental retardation by treatment before clinical manifestations. *Lancet* 1981; 2: 1095-1098

9. Glorieux J, Dussault J, Van Vliet G: Intellectual development at age 12 years of children with congenital hypothyroidism diagnosed by neonatal screening. *J Pediatr* 1992; 121: 581-584

10. U.S. Preventive Services Task Force: *Guide to Clinical Preventive Services: an Assessment of the Effectiveness of 169 Interventions.* Williams & Wilkins, Baltimore, Md, 1989: 105-110

Screening for Congenital Hypothyroidism

MANEUVER	EFFECTIVENESS	LEVEL OF EVIDENCE <REF>	RECOMMENDATION
Measurement of thyroid-stimulating hormone (TSH) level in dried capillary blood sample in first week of life; measurement of thyroxine (T4) level if necessary	Routine screening programs are effective in detecting preclinical hypothyroidism; early treatment radically modifies the mental development of affected infants.	Dramatic outcome improvements in prospective cohort studies<2-9> (II-2)	Good evidence to ensure routine TSH testing among all* neonates (A)

* Infants delivered at home or leaving the nursery within 48 hours may escape screening and must be reached otherwise.

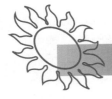

CHAPTER 19

Screening
for
Cystic
Fibrosis

By William Feldman

Screening for Cystic Fibrosis

Prepared by William Feldman, MD, FRCPC[1]

The genetic mutation (ΔF_{508}) will identify about 50% of people homozygous for cystic fibrosis (CF) and about 70% of carriers; approximately 225 other mutations have been found, but to date a simple, inexpensive way of identifying all the mutations in a heterogeneous population has not been readily available. The sweat test is difficult to do before 4-8 weeks of age, and the positive predictive validity of the immunoreactive trypsin test is very low. The meconium albumin test has very low sensitivity. In addition, there is good evidence that early diagnosis is not associated with clinically improved outcomes measured between 1 and 4 years of age. Thus, screening for CF is not recommended except for siblings of children with CF.

Burden of Suffering

In a recent Canadian study the incidence of CF was reported to be 1 in 2,927 live births; there may have been a decrease due to earlier diagnosis and genetic counselling. The disease is transmitted in an autosomal recessive manner, and it is estimated that about 5% of the general population carry the gene.

The triad of chronic obstructive pulmonary disease, pancreatic exocrine deficiency and abnormally high sweat electrolyte concentrations is present in most patients. Many of the clinical and pathological findings are thought to be attributable to a generalized defect in mucus secretion due to an abnormality in the chloride channel. The genetic defect is believed to produce an abnormal protein as a component of the chloride channel gate at the cell surface.

In 1985 the median age at the time of death from CF was 24 years. Pulmonary complications usually dominate the course of the disease, although clinical manifestations may not appear until weeks, months or years of age. Bronchiectasis is present in most patients by the end of the second year of life. Lung infections due to *Staphylococcus aureus* and *Pseudomonas aeruginosa* are extremely common and cause additional lung damage. In patients with advanced lung disease frequent complications include pneumothorax, hemoptysis and cor pulmonale. Chronic nasal congestion due to hyperactive mucus-secreting glands, nasal polyps and sinus disease are common.

Gastrointestinal manifestations result from loss of pancreatic enzyme activity and consequent intestinal malabsorption, primarily of

---

[1] Professor of Pediatrics and of Preventive Medicine and Biostatistics, University of Toronto, Toronto, Ontario

fats and proteins. Significant loss of exocrine pancreatic activity is seen in about 80% of patients. Malabsorption with consequent malnutrition can lead to poor weight gain, lack of subcutaneous fat and muscle tissue, and delayed puberty. Other complications include late intestinal obstruction, gastroesophageal reflux, vitamin and mineral deficiencies, hypoproteinemia and edema, salt loss, biliary cirrhosis, portal hypertension, male infertility and reduced female fertility. The psychologic impact on the child and the family can be significant, especially in severe cases that progress rapidly in spite of treatment.

Social class appears to be an important factor in the longevity of children with CF: the higher the social class, the later the age at death. It is possible that families of higher social class are better able to cope with the many stresses and activities necessary in complying with a difficult treatment regimen.

The financial burden is considerable. Each year nearly 40% of patients with CF are hospitalized for at least 1 week. These episodes and the cost of outpatient medical care have an effect on the health care delivery system that is out of proportion to the number of patients with CF.

Maneuver

The gold standard against which CF screening tests are measured is the sweat chloride test. There would be no need for other screening tests if sufficient sweat could be obtained from newborns, but even after stimulating localized sweating by administering pilocarpine into the skin it is often impossible to collect sufficient sweat for accurate analysis. The sweat test is also time-consuming and expensive for routine mass screening.

As a result, newborn screening programs have relied on other tests. The "BM meconium test" identifies infants with high albumin content in their stool resulting from pancreatic insufficiency but it has very low sensitivity.[1]

An advantage to any newborn screening test would be to combine it with tests for phenylketonuria and congenital hypothyroidism already widely done by means of a dried blood spot on filter paper. The immunoreactive trypsin (IRT) test can be performed in this manner and thus would be relatively inexpensive as part of a mass screening program. Unfortunately, the positive predictive value of the test is only 1-7%.[2,3] A false positive rate of 93-99% could and likely does generate considerable anxiety, which may be long-lasting.[2]

In an attempt to diagnose CF prenatally, amniotic fluid alkaline phosphatase isoenzymes have been studied; they were abnormal in 9 of 10 proven cases of CF, but the predictive value of a positive test result was only 50%.<4> If termination of pregnancy is one possible outcome, the positive predictive value should be much higher.

Because of the problems with the measurement properties of CF screening tests the recent identification of the genetic mutation responsible for about 70% of CF carriers (ΔF_{508}) has generated considerable excitement. Using the polymerase chain reaction, mutations in the CF gene can be detected in minute quantities of blood. Automation will make neonatal or heterozygote screening possible using the dried blood spot on filter paper already used for other screening programs.

The identification of many individually rare cystic fibrosis mutations has dampened enthusiasm for DNA analysis

Initially the discoverers of the CF gene were quite optimistic that the mutation(s) responsible for the other 30% of CF carriers would soon be found. However, the identification of many individually rare mutations rather than a small number of common mutations has dampened enthusiasm somewhat and will make carrier testing more difficult.<5>

In spite of this unexpected problem and the lower frequency of ΔF_{508} in some ethnic populations (30% to 50%) there is still great potential in the area of screening. Screening the relatives of individuals with CF has excellent sensitivity, since the specific mutation involved can be identified.<6> However, this screening approach has not been evaluated.

Effectiveness of Screening and Treatment

Several cohort studies of screened and unscreened subjects have suggested that people identified with CF in the presymptomatic phase do better than those in whom a diagnosis is made because of symptoms. In one study<7> done in the Netherlands, 88% of screened children but only 60% of unscreened children were still alive at age 11 years (p=0.045). The screening method used was determination of the albumin content of meconium. The number of false-negative test results was large. Although screening was done between 1973 and 1979, only patients surviving until 1980 were included in the follow-up. Before 1980, 4 of 22 screened and 5 of 24 unscreened children had died.

In an earlier study by the same group, screened children were found to have better clinical scores at age 8 years than did unscreened children with CF, but the differences in chest radiographs, heights and weights were not statistically significant.<8> The only selection factor for screening was the willingness of the hospital, maternity ward or regional maternity service to cooperate in the screening and follow-up program. Thus volunteer bias makes interpretation of the results difficult.

An Australian study compared hospital admissions of 40 children identified at birth by screening with the IRT test and 56 children born in the 3 years before screening began.<9> Unscreened patients without meconium ileus had spent a mean of 27 days in hospital because of CF-related illness in the first 2 years of life, whereas screened patients had spent a mean of 4 days. The authors noted that the control and screened groups may not have been comparable, that there may have been changes in hospital admission policies during the study and that there may have been significant changes in outpatient therapy.

In another Australian study, involving 23 unscreened children born between 1980 and 1983 and 28 children born between 1983 and 1985 and screened at birth with the IRT test, the screened children were found to have had fewer chest infections and to have gained more weight during the first 2 years of life.<10> The difference in mean weight between the screened and unscreened groups was significantly different at 6 months (7.0 vs. 6.3 kg, p=0.001) but not at 12 and 24 months. Hospital admissions were not significantly more frequent in the unscreened group. The authors acknowledged that the two groups may not have been comparable: the screened group may have included mildly affected children who might have done well even without therapy, and the unscreened group may have included only those with disease severe enough to have been diagnosed in the first 2 years of life.

Finally, authors of a recent controlled newborn screening study using the IRT reported no differences between 1- to 4-year-old children identified either at birth, or later, when symptoms developed, with regard to height and weight, chest radiographs, CF-specific quality-of-life scores, and hematologic and biochemical laboratory tests.<11>

1- to 4-year-old children had similar therapeutic outcomes whether identified by newborn screening or later, when symptoms developed

The treatment of CF is complex, costly and time-consuming. Most children with CF in the developed world are followed in CF clinics which are typically multidisciplinary, involving physicians, nurses, social workers, nutritionists and physiotherapists. There have been no randomized controlled trials comparing outcomes of children with CF treated in multidisciplinary clinics and those treated by physicians alone.

Treatment is directed at improving nutrition through the use of replacement pancreatic enzymes and vitamins, as well as a high-energy, high-protein and liberal-fat diet. For those not responding to this approach, enteral supplementation by nightly nasogastric, gastrostomy or jejunostomy infusion of high-energy diets has been used. Pulmonary treatment includes antibiotic therapy, either maintained continuously or reserved for exacerbations, and chest physiotherapy consisting of postural drainage, percussion, vibration and assisted coughing.

Which components of this complex regimen are responsible for the striking increase in longevity over the last 30 years is unknown, but it is likely that improved antibiotic and nutritional therapy is mainly responsible. It is very unlikely that the increase in survival is due to the identification in recent years of mild cases that would not have been identified previously. Again, it is still not clear that initiation of this regimen in the presymptomatic phase is beneficial.

On the other hand, there have been a number of randomized controlled trials involving individual components of treatment, principally antibiotic and nutritional therapy, showing progressive improvement in outcome.<12-17> One study showed that for mild to moderate episodes antibiotic therapy added nothing to the benefits derived from nutritional support and bronchodilator and oxygen therapy as needed.<18> The sample was too small to detect any difference of less than 30% between the groups (for α=0.05 and β=0.2). A recent review of therapy with inhaled antibiotics concluded that, until additional well-controlled trials are completed, routine aerosol administration of antibiotics to patients with CF is not warranted because of cost, potential side effects and the propensity for organisms to become resistant to antibiotics.<19>

With regard to treatment of the nutritional deficiency secondary to pancreatic insufficiency, randomized controlled trials comparing different forms of pancreatic enzyme replacements have shown significant decreases in symptoms and improvements in fat absorption and weight with newer enzyme formulations.<15,16> Supplementary enteral feeding has also been shown to increase weight among those who were malnourished at the beginning of therapy.<17> The long-term clinical benefit of physiotherapy for CF is not conclusively established.<20,21>

Recently a small randomized double-blind study of an inhaled sodium-channel blocker, amiloride, showed less deterioration of pulmonary function and less sputum viscosity among treated patients.<22> Exciting research involving gene transfer into respiratory cells employing a recombinant adenovirus vector requires further evaluation.<23>

Exciting research involving gene transfer into respiratory cells employing a recombinant adenovirus vector requires further evaluation

Recommendations of Others

The American Society of Human Genetics reached consensus that carrier testing should be offered to couples in which either partner has a close relative with CF. At the time (Nov. 13, 1989) it was felt to be premature to undertake population screening or carrier testing of pregnant women. Such screening would miss about 30% of carriers. The statement did not address the issue of newborn screening.

The participants of the *National Institutes of Health Workshop on Population Screening for the Cystic Fibrosis Gene*<5> concluded that, unlike carrier testing through DNA analysis in the general population, carrier testing in families in which the disease has occurred is nearly 100% informative. Carrier testing should therefore be offered to all individuals and couples with a family history of CF. This statement also did not address the issue of newborn screening.

The Research Advisory and Medical Advisory Committee of the Cystic Fibrosis Research Trust in Britain has invited pilot projects on CF heterozygote screening based in general practitioners' offices as well as in hospital clinics. Hospital clinics have already been used to screen for neural tube defects and the expected detection rate for CF is comparable at approximately at 70%.

A recent statement of the U.S. Office of Technology Assessment does not offer a judgement on the appropriateness of routine CF carrier screening.<24>

Conclusions and Recommendations

There is fair evidence not to perform universal newborn screening for CF by DNA analysis or other tests, based on the poor positive predictive value of the sweat, IRT and "BM meconium" tests and the fact that the recently discovered genetic mutation (ΔF_{508}) characterizes only about 50% of people homozygous for CF and about 70% of carriers (D recommendation).

Similarly, there is fair evidence not to screen the general population for heterozygote status (D recommendation). Siblings of children with CF should have a sweat test after 4 to 6 weeks of age (B recommendation). First-degree relatives of children with CF should be screened by DNA analysis for carrier status (B recommendation).

Unanswered Questions (Research Agenda)

The following have been identified as research priorities:

1. Continuation of studies of DNA analysis for those mutations responsible for the 30% of carriers who lack the recently discovered mutation.

2. Continuation of studies designed to make screening for CF less costly, such as the use of dried blood spot specimens and polymerase chain reactions.

3. Randomized controlled trials of neonatal screening to see if earlier diagnosis makes a difference, once the technology for mass screening is available and the measurement properties of the DNA analysis are acceptable.

4. Cost-benefit and psychosocial studies of neonatal and general population screening.

5. Gene transfer studies to determine clinical effectiveness.

Evidence

A MEDLINE search to November 1993 using the MESH headings: cystic fibrosis, screening, and human, was undertaken. The review was initiated in September 1993 and the recommendation finalized by the Task Force in January 1994. A report with a full reference list was published in 1991.<25>

Selected References

1. Naylor EW: Recent developments in neonatal screening. *Semin Perinatol* 1985; 9: 232-249

2. Ryley HC, Deam SM, Williams J, *et al*: Neonatal screening for cystic fibrosis in Wales and the West Midlands: 1. Evaluation of immunoreactive trypsin test. *J Clin Pathol* 1988; 41: 726-729

3. Edminson PD, Michalsen H, Aagenaeso, *et al*: Screening for cystic fibrosis among newborns in Norway by measurement of serum/plasma trypsin-like immunoreactivity. Results of a 2 1/2-year pilot project. *Scand J Gastroenterol Suppl* 1988; 143: 13-18

4. Brock DJ: Amniotic fluid alkaline phosphatase isoenzymes in early prenatal diagnosis of cystic fibrosis. *Lancet* 1983; 2: 941-943

5. Statement from the National Institutes of Health workshop on population screening for the cystic fibrosis gene. *N Engl J Med* 1990; 323: 70-71

6. Wilfond BS, Fost N: The cystic fibrosis gene: medical and social implications for heterozygote detection. *JAMA* 1990; 263: 2777-2783

7. Dankert-Roelse JE, te Meerman GJ, Martijn A, *et al*: Survival and clinical outcome in patients with cystic fibrosis, with or without neonatal screening. *J Pediatr* 1989; 114: 362-367

8. Dankert-Roelse JE: Screening for cystic fibrosis. A comparative study. *Acta Paediatr Scand* 1987; 76: 209-214

9. Wilcken B, Chalmers G: Reduced morbidity in patients with cystic fibrosis detected by neonatal screening. *Lancet* 1985; 2: 1319-1321

10. Bowling F, Cleghorn G, Chester A, *et al*: Neonatal screening for cystic fibrosis. *Arch Dis Child* 1988; 63: 196-198

11. Chatfield S, Owen G, Ryley HC, *et al*: Neonatal screening for cystic fibrosis in Wales and the West Midlands: clinical assessment after five years of screening. *Arch Dis Child* 1991; 66: 29-33

12. Bosso JA, Black PG, Matsen JM: Ciprofloxacin versus tobramycin plus azlocillin in pulmonary exacerbations in adult patients with cystic fibrosis. *Am J Med* 1987; 82(4A): 180-184

13. Hodson ME, Roberts CM, Butland RJA, *et al*: Oral ciprofloxacin compared with conventional intravenous treatment for *Pseudomonas aeruginosa* infection in adults with cystic fibrosis. *Lancet* 1987; 1: 235-237

14. Huang NN, Palmer J, Keith H, *et al*: Comparative efficacy and tolerance study of azlocillin and carbenicillin in patients with cystic fibrosis: a double blind study. *J Antimicrob Chemother* 1983; 11 (Suppl B): 205-214

15. Petersen W, Heilmann C, Garne S: Pancreatic enzyme supplementation as acid-resistant microspheres versus enteric-coated granules in cystic fibrosis. A double placebo-controlled cross-over study. *Acta Paediatr Scand* 1987; 76: 66-69

16. Beverley DW, Kelleher J, MacDonald A, *et al*: Comparison of four pancreatic extracts in cystic fibrosis. *Arch Dis Child* 1987; 62: 564-568

17. Shepherd RW, Holt TL, Cleghorn G, *et al*: Short-term nutritional supplementation during management of pulmonary exacerbations in cystic fibrosis: a controlled study, including effects of protein turnover. *Am J Clin Nutr* 1988; 48: 235-239

18. Gold R, Carpenter S, Heurter H, *et al*: Randomized trial of ceftazidime versus placebo in the management of acute respiratory exacerbations in patients with cystic fibrosis. *J Pediatr* 1987; 111: 907-913

19. MacLusky I, Levinson H, Gold R, *et al*: Inhaled antibiotics in cystic fibrosis: Is there a therapeutic effect? *J Pediatr* 1986; 108: 861-865

20. Desmond KJ, Schwenk WF, Thomas E, *et al*: Immediate and long-term effects of chest physiotherapy in patients with cystic fibrosis. *J Pediatr* 1983; 103: 538-542

21. Reisman JJ, Rivington-Law B, Corey M, *et al*: Role of conventional physiotherapy in cystic fibrosis. *J Pediatr* 1988; 113: 632-636

22. Knowles MR, Church NL, Waltner WE, *et al*: A pilot study of aerosolized amiloride for the treatment of lung disease in cystic fibrosis. *N Engl J Med* 1990; 322: 1189-1194

23. Healy, B: The pace of human gene transfer research quickens. *JAMA* 1993; 269(5): 567

24. Nishimi R: Cystic fibrosis and DNA tests – The implications of carrier screening. *JAMA* 1993; 269(15): 1921

25. Canadian Task Force on the Periodic Health Examination: The periodic health examination, 1991 update: 4. Screening for cystic fibrosis. *Can Med Assoc J* 1991; 145: 629-635

Screening for Cystic Fibrosis

MANEUVER	EFFECTIVENESS	LEVEL OF EVIDENCE <REF>	RECOMMENDATION
Sweat test, immunoreactive trypsin and "BM meconium" tests	Positive results in newborns have poor predictive value.	Cohort studies <1-4> (II-2)	Fair evidence not to perform universal newborn screening (D)
	The benefits of treatment before 4 to 6 weeks of age have not been established.	Randomized controlled trial<11> (I); cohort studies <7-10> (II-2)	
Sweat test at 4 to 6 weeks of age	Early diagnosis of cystic fibrosis (CF) may benefit treatment outcome.	Cohort studies <7-10> (II-2)	Fair evidence to test siblings of children with CF for the diagnosis of CF (B)
DNA analysis in newborns for case-finding or subsequently to determine carrier status	ΔF_{508} characterizes only about 50% of homozygotes and about 70% of carriers, and the benefits of treatment before 4 to 6 weeks of age have not been established.	Cohort studies <6> (II-2)	Fair evidence not to perform universal screening (D)
DNA analysis matching mutation with that in child who has CF	Test characteristics are superior (sensitivity may approach 100%) in the high-risk population since the mutation is known.	Expert opinion<6> (III)	Fair evidence to screen siblings of children with CF for carrier status (B)

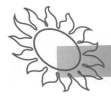

CHAPTER 20

Screening for Hemoglobinopathies in Canada

By Richard B. Goldbloom

Screening for Hemoglobinopathies in Canada

Adapted by Richard B. Goldbloom, OC, MD, FRCPC[1] from
materials prepared for the U.S. Preventive Services Task Force[2]

In its 1979 report, the Canadian Task Force on the Periodic Health Examination reviewed the available evidence and concluded that there was no scientific evidence to support screening for thalassemia in the general population, but that there was fair evidence to support screening of people of Asian, African, and Mediterranean ancestry.<1> This chapter updates the earlier report in the light of further publications and technological advances and extends its scope to consider screening for other hemoglobinopathies, including sickle cell disease.

Based on this updated review the Task Force concludes that 1) there is fair evidence to support selective prenatal screening of pregnant women from high risk groups (African, Mediterranean, Middle Eastern, East Indian, Hispanic and Southeast Asian ancestry) (B Recommendation); 2) there is fair evidence to offer DNA analysis of amniotic fluid or chorionic villus samples when both parents have established positive carrier status (B Recommendation); 3) there is good evidence to recommend screening to identify high-risk neonates (A Recommendation). Whether such screening should be applied universally or targeted to identified high risk groups should depend on the demographics of the population being screened; 4) there is insufficient evidence to recommend for or against screening and counselling non-pregnant adolescents and adults for carrier status (C Recommendation). All screening efforts must be accompanied by comprehensive counselling and treatment services.

Burden of Suffering

The Thalassemias

The thalassemias are hereditary conditions due to mutations causing decreased or absent production of the α-globin or β-globin chains of hemoglobin. β-thalassemia major occurs in individuals

---

[1] Professor of Pediatrics, Dalhousie University, Halifax, Nova Scotia
[2] By John S. Andrews, MD, Instructor, Department of Pediatrics, Johns Hopkins University, Baltimore, Maryland and Modena E.H. Wilson, MD, MPH, Associate Professor of Pediatrics, Johns Hopkins University, Baltimore, Maryland

homozygous for a genetic defect in β-globin synthesis. Infants with β-thalassemia are usually born healthy and may remain so for as long as 2-3 years. They then develop severe anemia, requiring regular transfusions and later, iron chelation therapy. Affected individuals usually die in the third decade of life. The cost of treatment is very high, estimated at $30,000 per year, over 30-35 years or almost $1 million per patient. Parents of affected children experience considerable stress as a result of this chronic health problem and its treatment. Individuals who are heterozygous for either type of thalassemia may experience mild, hypochromic anemia but are otherwise healthy and asymptomatic.

The β-thalassemias occur among individuals of East Indian, Mediterranean, African, Middle Eastern, Southeast Asian or Hispanic origin, and the proportion of such individuals in the Canadian population is increasing. For example, among Ontario's population of approximately 10 million, about 20% are of African, Southeast Asian, Mediterranean or Middle Eastern ancestry – all groups in which the incidence of hemoglobinopathies is relatively high. Over 130 β-thalassemia mutations have been described.

α-thalassemias result from deletions in 1 or more of the 4 genes responsible for α-globin synthesis. They are common in persons of Southeast Asian descent, but also occur in persons of African and Mediterranean origin. Fetuses with a 4-gene deletion develop hydrops fetalis secondary to severe anemia and die before or soon after birth.

Mothers of these infants are at risk for toxemia during pregnancy, for operative delivery, and for post-partum hemorrhage. The three-gene deletion is referred to as Hemoglobin H disease and affects about 1% of Southeast Asians. Persons with Hemoglobin H disease experience chronic hemolytic anemia that is exacerbated by exposure to oxidants and may require transfusion. Persons with a two-gene deletion have microcytic red blood cells and occasionally mild anemia. The one-gene deletion is a "silent" carrier state. These latter two conditions are often called α-thalassemia trait. The exact prevalence of α-thalassemia is uncertain, but is estimated to be 5-30% among African-Americans, and 15-30% among Southeast Asians.

Hemoglobin E trait is the third most common hemoglobin disorder in the world and the most frequent in Southeast Asia, where its prevalence is estimated to be 30%. Although Hemoglobin E trait is associated with no morbidity, the offspring of individuals who carry this hemoglobin variant may exhibit thalassemia major (hemoglobin E/β-thalassemia) if the other parent has β-thalassemia trait and contributes that gene. This combination is the most common cause of transfusion-dependent thalassemia in areas of Southeast Asia.

Sickle Cell Disease

The Sickle Cell Association of Ontario estimates the black population of Canada at about 700,000, and growing. The carrier frequency of the sickle gene is cited at 1 in 10 in the U.S. The carrier rate may be higher in Canada, where the black population is composed largely of individuals of Caribbean (carrier rate 10-14%) and African origin (carrier rate 20-25% in West Africa). Based on various assumptions, it has been estimated that as many as 67 black infants affected with sickle cell disease may be born annually in Canada. This figure does not take into account other population groups, e.g. East Indian, Middle Eastern and Mediterranean in which the sickle gene is also represented with considerable frequency. In the United States, 1 of every 150 African-American families is at risk of giving birth to a child with sickle cell disease (about 3,000 pregnancies per year).

Mortality in sickle cell disease peaks at 1-3 years of age, chiefly due to Streptococcus pneumoniae

Mortality in patients with sickle cell disease peaks between 1 and 3 years of age, chiefly due to sepsis caused by *Streptococcus pneumoniae*, estimated to occur in a frequency of 8 episodes per 100 person-years of observation in affected children under 3 years of age.

After infancy, patients with sickle cell disease are usually anemic and may experience painful crises and other complications, including acute chest syndrome, strokes, splenic and renal dysfunction, bone and joint symptoms, priapism, ischemic ulcers, cholecystitis and hepatic dysfunction associated with cholelithiasis.

Less severe but similar symptoms may be experienced by persons heterozygous for hemoglobin-S and hemoglobin-C (Hb SC) and those heterozygous for hemoglobin-S and β-thalassemia (HbS/β-thal). It has recently been reported that individuals with sickle cell trait have increased susceptibility to death from exertional heat illness during military training. Otherwise, morbidity for such individuals has been considered to be negligible.

Maneuver

Determination of the mean corpuscular volume (MCV) as part of a complete blood count (CBC) provides a primary indicator for the presence of α- or β-thalassemia trait (carrier state).[2] Carriers of either trait have microcytosis (MCV <80 fL) and hypochromia. Carriers of β-thalassemia usually have an elevated concentration of HbA2 (>3.5%), with or without an elevated concentration of HbF (>1.5%), as determined by hemoglobin electrophoresis. By contrast, α-thalassemia carriers have normal hemoglobin electrophoresis.

Blood for screening for carrier states is collected in heparinized tubes. For newborn screening, capillary blood is collected on filter paper (Guthrie paper blotter). Cellulose acetate electrophoresis, or thin layer isoelectric focusing are the preferred screening tests for hemoglobin disorders. Cellulose acetate electrophoresis is not specific for HbS if used alone. Citrate agar electrophoresis is used by many laboratories to confirm the presence of abnormal hemoglobins detected by another technique. High-performance liquid chromatography (HPLC) is a newer technique that offers higher resolution than 2-tier electrophoresis.

In over two million automated HPLC screening tests carried out in California between 1990 and 1993, only 1 false positive and 1 false negative test have been recorded (unpublished report). Newer techniques, employing monoclonal antibodies and recombinant DNA technology may be used more widely in the future.

Electrophoresis is highly specific in the detection of certain hemoglobin disorders, such as sickle cell disease. In one study, all 138 children with hemoglobin S identified in screening 2,976 African-american newborns were found to have a sickling disorder when retested at age 3-5 years.<3> Another study of 131 infants detected by screening found only nine instances in which the sickling disorder required reclassification and no instance in which a child originally diagnosed as having sickle cell disease was found to have sickle cell trait.<4> Ten years' experience with universal screening of Colorado newborns (528,711) using filter paper specimens and two-tier hemoglobin electrophoresis was recently reported.<5> Fifty infants with sickle cell diseases (HbSS, HbSC, HbS/α-thal) and 27 infants with other hemoglobin disorders were identified. Initial screening failed to identify 4 infants with sickle cell disease, but three of these were diagnosed on routine follow-up testing of infants suspected of having sickle cell trait. There were 32 false positive results, 27 of whom were confirmed to have a hemoglobinopathy trait on follow-up testing. The remaining 5 had normal hemoglobin.<5>

Electrophoresis is highly specific in the detection of certain hemoglobin disorders, such as sickle cell disease

The yield in screening pregnant women for hemoglobin disorders depends on the risk profile of the population being tested. In one study, electrophoresis in combination with a complete blood count was performed on 298 African-American and Southeast Asian prenatal patients. Ninety-four women (31.5%) had a hemoglobin disorder (including sickle cell disease, sickle cell trait, hemoglobin E, α-thalassemia trait, β-thalassemia trait, hemoglobin H, and hemoglobin C).<6> In a larger study in a different community, similar tests were performed on 6,641 prenatal patients selected without regard to race or ethnic origin.<7> One hundred eighty-five women (3%) had sickle cell trait, 68 (1%) had hemoglobin C, 30 (0.5%) had β-thalassemia trait, and 17 (0.3%) had other disorders (hemoglobin E, α-thalassemia trait, hemoglobin H, hemoglobin E/β-thalassemia disease). These results were obtained by combining electrophoresis with red cell indices. When low mean corpuscular volume (MCV) has been used as the only screening test to detect thalassemia, the yield has been 0.3-0.5%.

Prenatal diagnosis of sickle cell disease and other hemoglobinopathies in the fetus has been aided by advances in techniques of obtaining and analyzing specimens. Early tests involved the analysis of fetal blood obtained by fetoscopy or placental aspiration.[8] Recent genetic advances, however, have provided a safer[9] and more practical method in which amniocytes are obtained by amniocentesis and chromosomal mutations are identified directly through recombinant DNA technology. These techniques are highly accurate in detecting sickle cell disease and certain forms of thalassemia.[8-12] Their principal disadvantage, however, is that amniocentesis cannot be performed safely until about 16 weeks' gestation, thus delaying diagnosis and potential intervention until late in the second trimester. Chorionic villus sampling (CVS) is a means of obtaining tissue for DNA analysis as early as 8-10 weeks of gestation and is an established technique for prenatal diagnosis.[13,14] Several centers now offer the option of "early amniocentesis" (done several weeks earlier than conventional amniocentesis) as an alternative to CVS. Amniocentesis or CVS are part of the screening protocols for Down Syndrome (Chapter 8) and neural tube defects (Chapter 8).

Effectiveness of Early Detection and Treatment

Newborns with sickle cell disease benefit from early detection through early institution of penicillin prophylaxis to prevent pneumococcal sepsis

Screening for hemoglobin disorders is usually considered for two target populations: neonates, and adults of reproductive age. Newborns with sickle cell disease benefit from early detection through early institution of penicillin prophylaxis to prevent pneumococcal sepsis. A multi-center, randomized, double-blind, placebo-controlled trial demonstrated that the administration of prophylactic oral penicillin to infants and young children with sickle cell disease reduced the incidence of pneumococcal septicemia by 84%.[15] Other benefits of identifying newborns with sickle cell disease include prompt clinical intervention for infection or splenic sequestration crises and education of caretakers about the signs and symptoms of illness in these children. A seven-year longitudinal study reported lower mortality in children with sickle cell disease identified in the newborn period than in children diagnosed after 3 months of age (2% vs. 8%), but the investigators did not account for confounding variables in the control group.[16] A briefer longitudinal study (8-20 months) reported no deaths in 131 newborns detected through screening.[4] In the experience described above, 47 of the 50 newborns with sickle cell disease identified through screening remained in the study area beyond 6 months of age. None of the 47 died during the period of observation.[5] In addition to the health benefits to affected infants, neonatal screening carries the added benefit of identifying at-risk couples, thereby providing the opportunity for genetic counselling regarding options for future pregnancies. Screening of older children and adolescents is designed to detect carriers with sickle cell trait, β-thalassemia trait, and other hemoglobin disorders that often escape detection during the first years of life. Although heterozygotes rarely suffer clinically significant effects, their carrier status has direct implications for their offspring. Identification of carriers before childbearing permits genetic counselling about partner selection and the availability of diagnostic tests in the event of pregnancy. There is some evidence that individuals who receive certain forms of counselling retain this information and may encourage other individuals, such as their partners, to be tested.[7,17-19] A prospective study of 142 persons screened for β-thalassemia trait found that 62 (43%) encouraged other persons to be screened.[17] Compared with controls, those who had received counselling demonstrated significantly better understanding of thalassemia when tested immediately after the session. There is no direct evidence, however, that individual genetic counselling by itself significantly alters reproductive behavior or the incidence of births of infants with hemoglobin disorders.[20]

Detection of carrier status during pregnancy can provide prospective parents with the option of testing the fetus for a hemoglobinopathy. If the test is positive, they have the time to discuss continuation of the pregnancy and to plan optimal care for their newborn. Parents appear to act on this genetic information. About 70% of pregnant women who were identified as β-thalassemia carriers and received counselling referred their partners for testing. Among couples at risk for sickle cell disease, about 60% consent to amniocentesis.[7] If sickle cell disease is diagnosed in the fetus, about 50% of parents elect therapeutic abortion.[11,21] In a recent study, in Rochester, N.Y., 18,907 samples from pregnant women were screened for abnormal hemoglobin including thalassemia and hemoglobin S. In 810 (4.3%), an abnormal hemoglobin was identified. Sixty-six percent occurred in mothers unaware that they carried an abnormal hemoglobin, and 80% occurred in mothers unaware that they were at risk for giving birth to a child with a serious hematologic disorder. Eighty-six percent of mothers who received counselling said they wanted their partner tested and 55% of partners were tested. Seventy-seven pregnancies were identified as being at high risk because the partner also was a carrier of an abnormal hemoglobin. Of these 77 pregnancies, the gestation was too advanced for prenatal diagnosis in 12 cases and the condition for which the pregnancy was at risk was too mild for this service to be offered in 12 others. Prenatal diagnosis was offered in the remaining 53 pregnancies and accepted by 25 couples (47%). Of 18 amniocenteses performed, 14 were at risk for sickling disorders and the remaining 4 for the Hb H disease or Hb H with Hb E trait. Five fetuses were found to have clinically significant hemoglobinopathies and one of these pregnancies was terminated.[22] A comparison of the distribution of hemoglobinopathies detected in the Rochester, N.Y. study with screening results reported from Hamilton, Ontario[23] shows significant differences in the spectrum of abnormalities detected.

Those differences may reflect different ethnic mixes in Canada and the U.S. or may be partly due to ascertainment bias since most referrals in the Hamilton study were for investigation of low MCV.

Hemoglobinopathy	Rochester (Rowley 1991)[7]	Hamilton (Ali & Lafferty 1992)[23]
Hb S trait	474 (58.5%)	847 (10.7%)
Hb C trait	150 (18.5%)	230 (2.9%)
β-thalassemia trait	92 (11.4%)	4,497 (56.7%)
Hb E trait	37 (4.6%)	149 (1.9%)
Hb D or G trait	17 (2.1%)	49 (0.6%)
δβ-thal trait	6 (0.7%)	191 (2.4%)
α-thalassemia trait	3 (0.4%)	1,248 (15.7%)
Others	31 (3.8%)	724 (9.1%)
TOTALS	810 (100%)	7,935 (100%)

There is evidence from some European communities with a high prevalence of β-thalassemia that the birth rate of affected infants declined significantly following the implementation of routine prenatal screening,[8,24,25] and other data suggest a similar trend in some North American communities that have introduced community education and testing for thalassemia. This decline may reflect more than one factor, possibly including 1) a general decline in birth rate; 2) termination of pregnancies with affected fetuses; and 3) "at risk" couples choosing not to have children.

Since hemoglobinopathies occur among all ethnic and racial groups, efforts at targeting specific high-risk groups for newborn screening inevitably miss some affected individuals due to difficulties in properly assigning race or ethnic origin in the newborn nursery. In one study of 528,711 newborns, parental race, as requested on a screening form, was found to be inaccurate or incomplete in 30% of cases.[5] Proponents of selective screening of high-risk populations emphasize that, especially in geographic areas with a small population at risk, cost effectiveness is compromised and considerable expense incurred in screening large numbers of low-risk newborns to identify the rare individuals with sickle cell disease or other uncommon hemoglobin disorders. Studies supporting this argument have compared universal screening to no screening, not to targeted screening. Recent research that accounts for the additional procedural and administrative costs of targeted screening suggests that universal screening may be the more cost effective alternative to targeted screening.

There has been considerable debate over the value of sickle screening and screening for other hemoglobinopathies in persons of reproductive age. Critics cite evidence that sickle cell screening programs in the past have failed to educate patients and the public adequately about the significant differences between sickle cell trait and sickle cell disease. This has resulted in unnecessary anxiety for carriers and inappropriate labelling by insurers and employers. In addition, there is no evidence that counselling, however comprehensive, will be remembered throughout the individual's reproductive life, influence partner selection, alter use of prenatal testing, or ultimately reduce the rate of births of affected children. Proponents argue that these outcomes should not be used as measures of effectiveness since the goal of genetic counselling is to facilitate informed decision making by prospective parents. In this regard, clinicians are responsible for making the individual aware of the diagnosis, the risk to future offspring, and the recommended methods to reduce that risk, regardless of the strength of the evidence that such counselling reduces the number of affected offspring.

Recommendations of Others

The U.S. Preventive Services Task Force recommendations are currently under review. Universal screening of newborns for sickle cell disease, regardless of race or ethnic origin, has been recommended in the U.S. by the National Institutes of Health Consensus Development Conference on Newborn Screening for Sickle Cell Disease and other hemoglobinopathies. In April, 1993, the Agency for Health Care Policy and Research (a division of the U.S. Department of Health and Human Services) published its Clinical Practice Guidelines on screening, diagnosis and management of sickle cell disease in newborns and infants, recommending universal screening of newborns for sickle cell disease. Screening of infants from high-risk groups has been recommended by the World Health Organization and the British Society of Haematology. Newborn screening for sickle cell disease, coupled with comprehensive counselling, is advocated in the medical literature[3] and is currently universal in 34 states.[4]

Screening of older children and young adults is not universally recommended. Some U.S. states require sickle cell screening of school children, but many medical authorities have advised against this practice.

In Canada, thalassemia screening programs for carrier detection and prenatal diagnosis targeted at known high-risk groups, are currently available in Montreal, Quebec and in Hamilton, Ontario, though large communities at risk are present elsewhere in Canada. Hemoglobinopathy DNA referral diagnostic laboratories are available in Calgary, Hamilton and Montreal, where prenatal diagnosis from chorionic villus sampling or amniocentesis is also available. In Hamilton,

Ontario, the Regional Hemoglobinopathy Reference Laboratory investigates several thousand cases each year. Over a 20-year period, this laboratory has tested over 38,000 samples, referred because of an abnormal CBC (hypochromia, microcytosis or mild anemia). Of these 38,000 referrals, more than 7,300 were carriers of hemoglobin variants or thalassemia, showing that the spectrum of hemoglobinopathies in Canada differs significantly from that of the U.S.

Conclusions and Recommendations

A family and genetic history should be obtained from all patients of Mediterranean, African, Middle Eastern, East Indian, Hispanic or Asian ancestry who may become parents (B Recommendation). Screening for sickle cell hemoglobin and other hemoglobin variants should be performed at the first prenatal visit for all pregnant women from racial and ethnic groups known to be at increased risk for hemoglobinopathies (Asian, African and Mediterranean).

In all neonates from high risk ethnic groups, newborn screening for hemoglobinopathies is recommended, using dried filter paper blood spots (A Recommendation). Cellulose acetate electrophoresis or thin layer isoelectric focusing are currently the preferred screening tests, with citrate agar electrophoresis or high-performance liquid chromatography in a reference laboratory for confirmation. These methods may be superseded by more rapid and accurate techniques in future.

Unanswered Questions (Research Agenda)

1. Further studies are needed to determine the effectiveness and cost-effectiveness of screening non-pregnant adolescents and adults for carrier status.

2. The impact of individual genetic counselling on reproductive behavior requires further study.

3. The criteria for universal as opposed to selective screening for hemoglobinopathies need further definition.

Evidence

The literature was identified with a MEDLINE search in the English language literature for the years 1989 to 1993, using the following key words: anemia, hemoglobinopathies, sickle cell, thalassemia, ethnic groups (Ep). This review was initiated in January 1993 and approved by the Task Force in March 1994.

Acknowledgements

The Task Force wishes to thank Dr. John S. Waye, Co-Director, Provincial Hemoglobinopathy DNA Diagnostic Laboratory, McMaster University Medical Centre, Hamilton, Ontario for his assistance and valuable review of this document.

Selected References

1. Canadian Task Force on the Periodic Health Examination: The periodic health examination. *Can Med Assoc J* 1979; 121: 1193-1254

2. Chui DHK, Waye JS, Chitayat, *et al*: Screening for thalassemia and sickle hemoglobin. *Can J Ob Gyn Wom Hlth Care* 1993; 5(3): 453-457

3. Kramer MS, Rooks Y, Johnston D, *et al*: Accuracy of cord blood screening for sickle hemoglobinopathies: three- to five-year follow-up. *JAMA* 1979; 241: 485-486

4. Grover R, Shahidi S, Fisher B, *et al*: Current sickle cell screening program for newborns in New York City, 1979-1980. *Am J Public Health* 1983; 73: 249-251

5. Githens JH, Lane PA, McCurdy RS, *et al*: Newborn screening in Colorado: the first ten years. *AJDC* 1990; 144: 466-470

6. Stein J, Berg C, Jones JA, *et al*: A screening protocol for a prenatal population at risk for inherited hemoglobin disorders: results of its application to a group of Southeast Asians and blacks. *Am J Obstet Gynecol* 1984; 150: 333-341

7. Rowley PT, Loader S, Walden ME: Toward providing parents the option of avoiding the birth of the first child with Cooley's anemia: response to hemoglobinopathy screening and counseling during pregnancy. *Ann NY Acad Sci* 1986; 445: 408-416

8. Alter BP: Advances in the prenatal diagnosis of hematologic diseases. *Blood* 1984; 64: 329-340

9. Kazazian HH Jr, Boehm CD, Dowling CE: Prenatal diagnosis of hemoglobinopathies by DNA analysis. *Ann NY Acad Sci* 1985; 445: 337-348

10. Weatherall DJ, Mold J, Thein SL, *et al*: Prenatal diagnosis of the common hemoglobin disorders. *J Med Genet* 1985; 22: 422-430

11. Boehm CD, Antonarakis SE, Phillips JA III, *et al*: Prenatal diagnosis using DNA polymorphisms: report on 95 pregnancies at risk for sickle-cell disease or beta-thalassemia. *N Engl J Med* 1983; 308: 1054-1058

12. Orkin SH: Prenatal diagnosis of hemoglobin disorders by DNA analysis. *Blood* 1984; 63: 249-253

13. Goosens M, Dumez Y, Kaplan L, et al: Prenatal diagnosis of sickle-cell anemia in the first trimester of pregnancy. *N Engl J Med* 1983; 309: 831-833

14. Old JM, Fitches A, Heath C, et al: First-trimester fetal diagnosis for hemoglobinopathies: report on 200 cases. *Lancet* 1986; 2: 763-767

15. Gaston MH, Verter JI, Woods G, et al: Prophylaxis with oral penicillin in children with sickle cell anemia: a randomized trial. *N Engl J Med* 1986; 314: 1593-1599

16. Vichinsky E, Hurst D, Earles A, et al: Newborn screening for sickle cell disease: effect on mortality. *Pediatrics* 1988; 81: 749-755

17. Lipkin M, Fisher L, Rowley PT, et al: Genetic counseling of asymptomatic carriers in a primary care setting: the effectiveness of screening and counseling for beta-thalassemia trait. *Ann Intern Med* 1986; 105: 115-123

18. Whitten CF, Thomas JF, Nishiura EN: Sickle cell trait counseling: evaluation of counselors and counselees. *Am J Hum Genet* 1981; 33: 802-816

19. Scriver CR, Bardanis M, Cartier L, et al: Beta-thalassemia disease prevention: genetic medicine applied. *Am J Hum Genet* 1984; 36: 1024-1038

20. Rucknagel DL: A decade of screening in the hemoglobinopathies: is a national program to prevent sickle cell anemia possible? *Am J Ped Hem Onc* 1983; 5: 373-377

21. Driscoll MC, Lerner N, Anyane-Yeboa K, et al: Prenatal diagnosis of sickle hemoglobinopathies: the experience of the Columbia University Comprehensive Center for Sickle Cell Disease. *Am J Hum Genet* 1987; 40: 548-558

22. Rowley PT, Loader S, Sutera CJ, et al: Prenatal screening for hemoglobinopathies: I. A prospective regional trial. *Am J Hum Genet* 1991; 48: 439-446

23. Ali M, Lafferty J: The clinical significance of hemoglobinopathies in the Hamilton region: a twenty-year review. *Clin Invest Med* 1992; 15(5): 401-405

24. Cao A, Rosatelli C, Galanello R, et al: The prevention of thalassemia in Sardinia. *Clin Gen* 1989; 36: 277-285

25. Cao A, Rosatelli C, Galanello R: Population-based genetic screening. *Curr Opin Gen Dev* 1991; 1: 48-53

Screening for Hemoglobinopathies in Canada

MANEUVER	EFFECTIVENESS	LEVEL OF EVIDENCE <REF>	RECOMMENDATION
Screening for Carrier Status - Pregnant Women*			
Complete blood count (CBC) for identification of hypochromia and microcytosis (MCV <80 fL) followed by hemoglobin electrophoresis when iron deficiency ruled out; cellulose acetate electrophoresis or thin layer isoelectric focusing of blood sample with citrate agar electrophoresis for confirmation (High performance liquid chromatography (HPLC) offers higher resolution)	Tests sensitive and highly specific but yield depends on risk profile.	Cohort and cross-sectional studies <6,7,17> (II-2) Expert opinion<2> (III)	Fair evidence to recommend screening for hemoglobinopathies in high-risk** pregnant women (B)
	50-55% refer partners for testing and 60% subsequently consent to amniocentesis for sickle cell disease. Uptake rates are higher for the thalassemias.	Cross-sectional studies<6,22> (II-2); expert opinion <23,24> (III)	
Prenatal Screening and Counselling*			
DNA analysis of tissue sample (amniocentesis or chorionic villus sampling) after confirming positive carrier status of both partners	Technology is highly accurate and available through referral to diagnostic centers.	Case-series and expert opinion<2,8-12> (III)	Fair evidence to offer prenatal screening and counselling to families with positive carrier status (B)
	47-60% of parents consent to procedure and 20-50% consent to therapeutic abortion of affected fetus with sickle cell. Rates are higher for the thalassemias.	Cross-sectional studies<7,22> (II-2); case-series <17-21> (III)	
	Decline in prevalence of ß-thalassemia in European communities with screening programs.	Comparison of times and places <8,23,24> (II-3)	

*   All screening must be accompanied by counselling.

** High-risk individuals include all patients of Mediterranean, African, East Indian, Middle Eastern, Hispanic or Asian ancestry and those with a family history of disease.

(Continued on next page)

Screening for Hemoglobinopathies in Canada (concl'd)

MANEUVER	EFFECTIVENESS	LEVEL OF EVIDENCE <REF>	RECOMMENDATION
Neonatal Screening			
Testing of dried capillary blood samples collected on filter paper: Cellulose acetate electrophoresis or thin layer isoelectric focusing, citrate agar electrophoresis liquid chromatography for confirmation (high performance liquid chromatography (HPLC) offers higher resolution)	Tests sensitive and highly specific for Hb Sickle. Prophylactic oral penicillin to infants and young children with sickle cell anemia reduced pneumococcal septicemia 84%. Mortality may also be reduced.	Cohort studies <3-5,16> (II-2) Randomized controlled trials<15> (I)	Good evidence to recommend for high-risk** neonates (A)
Screening for Carrier Status - Non-Pregnant Adolescents and Adults and Counselling*			
CBC for identification of hypochromia and microcytosis (MCV <80 fL) followed by hemoglobin electrophoresis (as described above) when iron deficiency ruled out	Tests sensitive and highly specific. Individuals who receive counselling may encourage partners to be treated; no evidence regarding reproductive behavior or use of prenatal testing. Potential for labelling by insurers and employers and unnecessary anxiety for carriers.	Cohort and cross-sectional studies <6,7> (II-2); expert opinion<2> (III) Controlled trial <17> (II-1); case-series <7,18,19,23,24> (III)	Insufficient evidence to recommend for or against universal screening for non-pregnant adolescents and adults for carrier status (C)

*   All screening must be accompanied by counselling.

** High-risk individuals for sickle cell disease include all patients of African ancestry.

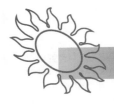

CHAPTER 21

Screening for Urinary Infection in Asymptomatic Infants and Children

By Michael B.H. Smith

Screening for Urinary Infection in Asymptomatic Infants and Children

Prepared by Michael B.H. Smith, MB BCh, CCFP, FRCPC[1]

The aim of a pediatric urine screening program is early detection of silent infections which if left untreated, progress to develop irreversible renal disease. It has been assumed that asymptomatic bacteriuria (ABU) represented the beginning of urinary tract disease and that early detection and antimicrobial therapy could avert serious renal disease. Unfortunately the significance of ABU is poorly understood. In particular, its relationship to urinary tract infection (UTI), reflux nephropathy and endstage renal disease (ESRD) is unknown.

In its last statement in 1979, the Canadian Task Force on the Periodic Health Examination did not recommend screening for urinary infection in asymptomatic children. Since that time, there have been several important developments in this area. There has been a dramatic improvement in urinalysis technology with the use of leucocyte esterase and nitrite testing by dipstick. In addition, several long-term follow-up studies on the treatment of children with ABU have been reported. Therefore, the value of periodic screening urinalysis in asymptomatic children was re-examined. Other reviews have been prepared on screening urinalysis in pregnant women (Chapter 9) and in the elderly (Chapter 81).

Burden of Suffering

There are four interrelated areas in the prevention of infection related renal disease.

Asymptomatic or Covert Bacteriuria

Asymptomatic bacteriuria (ABU) indicates a significant bacterial count present in the urine (usually 10^5 or 10^4 colony forming units (CFUs) per ml) in an individual without symptoms of a urinary infection. It has also been termed covert bacteriuria as many children on specific questioning have minor symptoms such as frequency, urgency, dysuria or bed-wetting.<1> The prevalence of ABU varies with gender and age (see Table 1) as well as socioeconomic status and race. A weakness of many published prevalence studies is contamination – symptomatic individuals are also included.

---

[1] Lecturer in Pediatrics, Dalhousie University, Halifax, Nova Scotia

Table 1:   Prevalence of asymptomatic bacteriuria by age/sex<2>

	Male	Female
Preterm infants		2.9-9.8%
Term infants	2.7%	0-1%
Preschool	0.2%	0.8%
School age (4-11 yrs)	–	1.8%
School age/adolescence (5-20 yrs)	0.026%	1.1-2.4%

ABU responds to antibiotics<2> but reinfection is common, especially in girls and during puberty. Certain girls end up prone to periods of infected urine in adult life and may be at risk for pyelonephritis during pregnancy.<3> The majority, however, enjoy good health in long-term follow-up.<4>

Urinary Tract Infections

UTIs are among the more common illnesses of childhood and affect the entire age range. UTIs can be potentially fatal in the neonatal period because of associated septicemia and meningitis. In later childhood, urinary infections are responsible for less severe illness but in rare situations progress to reflux nephropathy (chronic pyelonephritis), hypertension and ESRD. Generally, UTIs are more common in girls except in the first year of life. Winberg calculated that the risk of developing symptomatic infections before age 11 years, was 3% for girls and 1.1% for boys.<5> Oral antibiotic treatment usually produces prompt resolution of symptoms. Intravenous therapy is usually necessary in young infants and in those with suspected pyelonephritis. Host factors associated with an increased likelihood of infection include female sex, vesicoureteral reflux, urinary tract obstruction, constipation, a family history of UTIs and possibly lack of circumcision. Some women may have more UTIs because the infecting microorganism adheres more effectively to the periurethral mucosa.<4>

The exact prevalence of urinary infections is unknown for several reasons. First, the infections may be subclinical or the clinical signs vague and non-specific. Second, collection techniques are prone to errors especially in the younger patient. Third, antibiotics are often given to the febrile child for other purposes eradicating the silent infection. As a result of these problems the relationship of symptomatic UTI and ABU is unknown. Some investigators have divided ABU into primary and secondary to distinguish those infections that arise de novo from those that follow previous urinary infections. The significance of primary and secondary ABU is unknown.<6> It is possible that ABU may represent a transiently positive culture much like the bacteremia following dental manipulation.

Reflux Nephropathy and Vesicoureteral Reflux

Reflux nephropathy is defined as renal scarring associated with vesicoureteral reflux (VUR). This consists of calyceal clubbing or deformity with overlying corticomedullary scarring.[7] It results from the abnormal regurgitation of urine back to the kidneys. Its relationship to UTI remains unclear. Up to 30-50% of children with UTI will have VUR detected at first presentation. One third of this group will have unilateral reflux nephropathy. An even smaller subset of this third will have bilateral reflux nephropathy but only a few of these will progress to end stage renal disease (ESRD).[7] Reflux nephropathy is thought to be the cause in 10% of individuals with ESRD.[8] The vast majority (over 80%) of VUR is transient and resolves spontaneously. Hypertension does not appear to be a complication of primary VUR and UTI.[9] Despite this reassurance, careful follow up is recommended.[10]

End Stage Renal Disease

ESRD is a term indicating less than 10% of normal renal function and the clinical need for regular dialysis or renal transplantation to maintain life. It is a devastating disease with multiple effects including hypertension, growth failure and bone deformities. Affected children require complex, time-consuming and costly care. The incidence of ESRD increases with age. In early childhood the cause is related to a structural abnormality of the renal tract whereas in older children, acquired renal disease predominates. Pyelonephritis and malfunction of the urinary tract is the etiology of 22.5% of children with renal failure.[11] (For further discussion of ESRD in older age groups, see Chapter 38).

Clearly, there is a spectrum of urinary tract disease of which only a very few will progress to ESRD. The major challenge therefore is to detect those that progress so that early intervention can preserve renal function and improve outcome.

Maneuver

Urine culture is the gold standard for the diagnosis of urinary tract infection. The standard is defined based on the colony count (10^5 CFUs/ml or 10^4 CFUs/ml) and the number of consecutive cultures (one vs. two vs. three) required.

The current screening tests are dipstick methods (incorporating leucocyte esterase (LE) and nitrite level) and direct microscopy. The dipstick test has the advantages of speed, low cost and that limited technical expertise is required. The LE test detects esterases released from degraded white blood cells (WBC). It is therefore an indirect measure of WBCs whose presence is induced by urinary bacteria. The nitrite test detects nitrites produced by urinary bacteria – usually limited to gram-negative organisms. Because both reactions require a concentrated urine, an early morning urine specimen is preferable. Conversely, microscopic examination of urine for WBCs and bacteria provides direct evidence of their presence, but there are varying standards and techniques.[12] Specimens have been assessed uncentrifuged and centrifuged as well as stained and unstained. WBCs have been counted per high power field and in others per cubic milliliter. With these variations in technique, it is not surprising that there have been inconsistencies in those studies evaluating the microscopic examination of urine.

Several recent studies have evaluated the individual components of urinalysis and compared them with the results of bacterial cultures in pediatric populations.[13-18] Dipstick testing has been found to be no better than urine microscopy and both techniques have only modest sensitivities and specificities (around 80%) when compared to quantitative culture.[12,19] One consistent result is the high negative predictive value (>95%). This may reflect the low prevalence of UTIs (4-14.8%) in these studies (which included some symptomatic individuals). In the asymptomatic population it is likely that the negative predictive value would exceed 99% for both sexes.[19] A high negative predictive value is extremely useful as it helps to decide which urine samples to culture and which to discard.

Debate continues regarding the best age at which to test a child. Theoretically, younger children and infants should be the best candidates for screening on the assumption that such screening would avert early renal scar formation. Unfortunately, the younger child is also the most difficult from whom to obtain a "clean" specimen. Adhesive polyethylene bag specimens remain the kindest choice but have an unacceptable contamination rate. When compared with suprapubic aspiration of urine, bag specimens indicate true bladder bacteriuria in only 7.5% of specimens.[20] Straight catheterization and suprapubic aspiration of the bladder are options when a UTI is highly suspected.

The cost of screening is significant. Using a hypothetical cohort of 100,000 children and the current prevalence of ABU, Kemper and Avner estimated the costs of urine screening and cultures would exceed $2.9 million.[19] These charges did not include physician costs, medications, diagnostic imaging and days lost from work or school. Additional hidden costs of screening may include the psychological effects of labelling,[21] and the morbidity and discomfort associated with investigations.[22]

Effectiveness of Screening and Treatment

Several studies have examined the natural history of ABU in infants and children and in individuals with renal abnormalities.

Infants presenting with fever should have a urinalysis and culture performed even if there is an identifiable focus of infection

The epidemiology of bacteriuria in infants has been studied by a group of Swedish investigators.[23,24] All newborns in a defined geographic area had screening urinalysis performed, with follow-up cultures and radiological imaging performed when bacteriuria was found. Of the 3,581 infants, bacteriuria was found in 2.5% of boys and 0.9% of girls (total n=50). No major malformations were found on urography and only 11% had reflux of minor degree. No treatment was given to infants if they were asymptomatic and had a C-reactive protein <20 mg/L. Two infants developed symptoms of pyelonephritis and were treated without complication. Two infants had minor renal anomalies on radiography and were given antibiotics. Regular follow-up urine testing showed that the bacteriuria cleared spontaneously in 72% and with antibiotics (given for other reasons) in 16%. In others it persisted without symptoms. Follow-up urography in most of the children with ABU at 3 years showed no renal damage. Symptomatic UTIs were also examined in this cohort of young infants and were seen in 1.1-1.2%. Overlap between the symptomatic and asymptomatic groups was very small with only two infants with ABU developing symptoms of UTI and pyelonephritis within two weeks of the initial testing. Among the infants with symptomatic UTI, 12% had major abnormalities (agenesis of the kidney, uretero-pelvic stenosis, >grade 3 VUR) detected by urography. It was concluded that infants with ABU are at low risk of renal damage, but the appearance of any symptoms suggestive of a UTI should prompt a thorough assessment.[23]

Healthy infants without symptoms do not require a screening urine test performed

In another cohort study, 1,617 healthy infants under age 23 months were studied for asymptomatic and symptomatic UTI and followed for five years.[25] ABU was found in 1.8% of female infants and 0.5% of males. VUR was present in 46% of the infants with ABU and was associated with recurrent infections for a longer period of time. Despite this abnormality, early treatment of these infants resulted in a good prognosis with subsequent improvement of the imaging studies and a decreased number of infections. The screening of asymptomatic infants detected 5/1,617 (0.3%) with high risk lesions (such as obstructive uropathy, vesicoureteral junction ectopia and deformity). Of these five infants, all had infections within one to three years and two eventually required surgery. If there had been no screening program, these infants would have eventually presented with signs of UTI and it was argued that screening detected the lesions earlier and possibly improved the prognosis. This was not established by this study. To do this would require urine screening of all infants with follow-up imaging studies in those with ABU. This would mean that approximately 1-2% of all children would require imaging studies to detect a very small number of abnormalities. In general, it appears that infants with ABU are at very low risk group for subsequent renal damage.

In older children with ABU, some silent infections may persist for many years while others resolve spontaneously.[26] Further reinfections may follow or be eradicated by antibiotics prescribed for other reasons. Symptomatic urinary infections develop in 10% and pyelonephritis in less than 5% of children with ABU and this may be associated with a change in the bacterial isolates.<2,27> Without underlying renal abnormalities, the bacterial isolates will tend to remain stable for a number of years.<28> If given antimicrobial treatment, the bacterial isolates change and there is no change in the rate of UTIs and the risk of pyelonephritis is increased. Three randomized, controlled trials of antibiotic treatment of ABU have shown no improvement in outcome.<29-31> All of these studies were performed on schoolgirls over age 5 years because of the high prevalence of ABU in this group. They were followed clinically with frequent urine cultures and radiological imaging for one to four years. In all of these studies antibiotic treatment did not affect the rate of symptomatic recurrences including pyelonephritis. Follow-up imaging of both treated and untreated patients showed no difference in renal growth, clearance of VUR or renal scarring. Ideally, a longer period of follow-up would be desirable but the information from these studies presents a very reassuring natural history. Furthermore, long-term antibiotic treatment carries its own side effects and compliance is difficult to achieve. Therefore, urine screening for the purpose of identifying and treating ABU cannot be recommended based on the current evidence.

Healthy schoolgirls with ABU do not require antibiotic treatment

Healthy schoolgirls do not require urine infection screening

Vesicoureteral reflux (VUR) is found in 11-46% of infants and prepubertal children who have ABU.<6,25,32> In children who present with symptomatic UTIs, 18-50% will have VUR.<6,32> A four-year follow-up study of ABU in schoolgirls showed that treatment had no effect on the disappearance of VUR.<31> Renal abnormalities are found in 1.37% of infants and 0.5% of schoolchildren who are considered normal.<33,34> In infants with ABU, renal abnormalities (including VUR, scars as well as congenital abnormalities) were seen in 14% of female and 3% of male infants.<23> These children might have been detected outside the screening program as their symptoms developed. In children with ABU, 28% had radiological evidence of VUR and/pyelonephritis.<29> In this controlled trial of therapy there was no significant difference in outcome even in individuals with abnormal renal tracts. Furthermore, treatment of children with renal scarring may be harmful. In Hansson's retrospective review of 26 girls with ABU and scarring, of those who were treated (12/26) 3 developed pyelonephritis compared with none in the untreated group.<28> Therefore, even in what is considered a high-risk group, screening to enable early treatment cannot be recommended.

No studies have addressed the other issues related to screening for urinary tract disease. An abnormal urine test usually mandates further testing and often leads to radiological imaging with its associated discomfort, risks and costs.

Recommendations of Others

Periodic urinalysis is recommended by the American Academy of Pediatrics.<35,36> The U.S. Preventive Services Task Force recommendation is currently under review.

Conclusions and Recommendations

A review of the evidence for screening urinalysis in children has not shown an improvement in outcome after early diagnosis and treatment. This problem highlights our lack of understanding of the normal bacteriological and mechanical maturation of the urinary tract. Screening urinalysis detects what may be a normal phenomenon in some infants and children and which, for the vast majority, results in no significant clinical problems. For the small minority that progress to true infections, symptoms bring the patient to medical attention whereupon appropriate testing is performed. In this situation, a high index of suspicion for UTI is necessary especially in the younger age groups.

There is fair evidence that urinalysis screening should not be performed on healthy infants for the purpose of detecting bacteriuria and renal abnormalities (D Recommendation). There is good evidence that urinalysis screening should not be performed on healthy children for the purpose of detecting bacteriuria (E Recommendation).

Unanswered Questions (Research Agenda)

The following have been identified as research priorities:

1. The clinical significance of primary and secondary ABU requires clarification.

2. The value of radiological investigation of all children with ABU and UTI needs to be studied.

3. The cost-benefit and psychosocial effects of UTI screening on children.

Evidence

The medical literature was identified using the MEDLINE bibliographic database (Jan 1978-Sep 1993). The Medical Subject Headings used included: urinary tract infections, mass screening, child, asymptomatic, epidemiology, bacteriuria, prognosis and prevention. In addition, relevant studies were obtained from reference lists from these published studies. The review was initiated in January 1993 and the recommendations finalized by the Task Force in October 1994.

Selected References

1. Savage DCL, Wilson MI, McHardy M, et al: Covert bacteriuria of childhood. A clinical and epidemiological study. Arch Dis Child 1973; 48: 8-20

2. Lindberg U, Claesson I, Hanson LA, et al: Asymptomatic bacteriuria in schoolgirls. VIII. Clinical course during a 3 year follow up. J Pediatr 1978; 92: 194-199

3. Sacks SH, Verrier Jones K, Roberts R, et al: Effect of symptomless bacteriuria in childhood on subsequent pregnancy. Lancet 1987; 2(8566): 991-994

4. Verrier Jones K, Asscher AW: Urinary Tract Infection and Vesicoureteral Reflux. In: Edelmann CM Jr (ed): Pediatric Kidney Disease. Boston: Little, Brown and Company, 1992; 827-916

5. Winberg J, Bergstrom T, Jacobsson B: Morbidity, age and sex distribution, recurrences and renal scarring in symptomatic urinary tract infection in childhood. Kidney Int Suppl 1975; Suppl 4: S101-S106

6. Jodal U: The natural history of bacteriuria in childhood. Infect Dis Clin North Am 1987; 1: 713-729

7. Lerner GR, Fleischmann LE, Perlmutter AD: Reflux nephropathy. Pediatr Clin North Am 1987; 34: 747-770

8. Chantler C, Carter JE, Bewick M, et al: 10 years' experience with regular haemodialysis and renal transplantation. Arch Dis Child 1980; 55: 435-445

9. Wolfish NM, Delbrouck NF, Shanon A, et al: Prevalence of hypertension in children with primary vesicoureteral reflux. J Pediatr 1993; 123: 559-563

10. Arant BS Jr: Medical management of mild and moderate vesicoureteral reflux: follow-up studies of infants and young children. A preliminary report of the Southwest Pediatric Nephrology Study Group. J Urol 1992; 148(5 Pt 2): 1683-1687

11. Gruskin AB, Baluarte HJ, Dabbagh S: Hemodialysis and Peritoneal Dialysis. In: Edelmann CM Jr (ed): Pediatric Kidney Disease. Boston: Little, Brown and Company, 1992; 827-916

12. Lohr JA: Use of routine urinalysis in making a presumptive diagnosis of urinary tract infection in children. Pediatr Infect Dis J 1991; 10: 646-650

13. Cannon HJ Jr, Goetz ES, Hamoudi AC, et al: Rapid screening and microbiologic processing of pediatric urine specimens. Diagn Microbiol Infect Dis 1986; 4: 11-17

14. Marsik FJ, Owens D, Lewandowski J: Use of the leukocyte esterase and nitrite tests to determine the need for culturing urine specimens from a pediatric and adolescent population. Diagn Microbiol Infect Dis 1986; 4: 181-183

15. Goldsmith BM, Campos JM: Comparison of urine dipstick, microscopy, and culture for the detection of bacteriuria in children. Clin Pediatr Phila 1990; 29: 214-218

16. Shaw KN, Hexter D, McGowan KL, *et al*: Clinical evaluation of a rapid screening test for urinary tract infections in children. *J Pediatr* 1991; 118: 733-736

17. Weinberg AG, Gan VN: Urine screen for bacteriuria in symptomatic pediatric outpatients. *Pediatr Infect Dis J* 1991; 10: 651-654

18. Lohr JA, Portilla MG, Geuder TG, *et al*: Making a presumptive diagnosis of urinary tract infection by using a urinalysis performed in an on-site laboratory. *J Pediatr* 1993; 122: 22-25

19. Kemper KJ, Avner ED: The case against screening urinalyses for asymptomatic bacteriuria in children. *Am J Dis Child* 1992; 146: 343-346

20. Burns MW, Burns JL, Krieger JN: Pediatric urinary tract infection. Diagnosis, classification, and significance. *Pediatr Clin North Am* 1987; 34: 1111-1120

21. Bergman AB, Stamm SJ: The morbidity of cardiac nondisease in schoolchildren. *N Engl J Med* 1967; 276: 1008-1013

22. Feldman W: How serious are the adverse effects of screening? *J Gen Intern Med* 1990; 5(suppl): S50-S53

23. Wettergren B, Hellstrom M, Stokland E, *et al*: Six year follow up of infants with bacteriuria on screening. *BMJ* 1990; 301(6756): 845-848

24. Wettergren B, Jodal U, Jonasson G: Epidemiology of bacteriuria during the first year of life. *Acta Paediatr Scand* 1985; 74: 925-933

25. Siegel SR, Siegel B, Sokoloff BZ, *et al*: Urinary infection in infants and preschool children. Five-year follow-up. *Am J Dis Child* 1980; 134: 369-372

26. Olling S, Jones KV, MacKenzie R, *et al*: A four year follow up of schoolgirls with untreated covert bacteriuria: bacteriological aspects. *Clin Nephrol* 1981; 16: 169-171

27. Newcastle Covert Bacteriuria Research Group: Covert bacteriuria in school girls in Newcastle upon Tyne: a 5-year follow-up. *Arch Dis Child* 1981; 56: 585-592

28. Hansson S, Jodal U, Noren L, *et al*: Untreated bacteriuria in asymptomatic girls with renal scarring. *Pediatrics* 1989; 84: 964-968

29. Savage DCL, Howie G, Adler K, *et al*: Controlled trial of therapy in covert bacteriuria in childhood. *Lancet* 1975; 1(7903): 358-361

30. Lindberg U: Asymptomatic bacteriuria in school girls. V. The clinical course and response to treatment. *Acta Paediatr Scand* 1975; 64: 718-724

31. Cardiff-Oxford Bacteriuria Study Group: Sequelae of covert bacteriuria in schoolgirls. A four-year follow-up study. *Lancet* 1978; 1(8070): 889-893

32. Mininberg DT: Preventing complications of vesicoureteral reflux. *Conn Med* 1986; 50(10): 659-665

33. Steinhart JM, Kuhn JP, Eisenberg B, *et al*: Ultrasound screening of healthy infants for urinary tract abnormalities. *Pediatrics* 1988; 82: 609-614

34. Sheih CP, Liu MB, Hung CS, *et al*: Renal abnormalities in schoolchildren. *Pediatr* 1989; 84: 1086-1090

35. Committee on Standards of Child Health Care: Standards of Child Health Care. 3rd ed. Evanston Ill: American Academy of Pediatrics, 1977: 9-36

36. Guidelines for Health Supervision II. Evanston Ill: American Academy of Pediatric, 1988: 155-159

Screening for Urinary Infection in Asymptomatic Infants and Children

MANEUVER	EFFECTIVENESS	LEVEL OF EVIDENCE <REF>	RECOMMENDATION
Dipstick urinalysis (with nitrite and leucocyte esterase tests) on healthy newborns and infants	Sensitivity and specificy around 80%. Screening detects asymptomatic bacteriuria which often resolves spontaneously. The number of clinically significant abnormalities detected is small. Non treatment has resulted in good outcomes.	Cohort studies <12-17,22-24> (II-I)	Fair evidence to exclude from periodic health examination of healthy infants (D)
Dipstick urinalysis (with nitrite and leucocyte esterase tests) on healthy children	Sensitivity and specificy around 80%. Asymptomatic bacteriuria may be detected by screening but treatment with antibiotics does not improve outcome.	Cohort studies <12-17> (II-2) Randomized controlled trials<28-30> (I)	Good evidence to exclude from periodic health examination of healthy children (E)

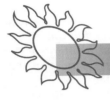

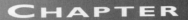

CHAPTER

22

Breast
Feeding

By Elaine E.L. Wang

22

Breast Feeding

Prepared by Elaine E. L. Wang, MD, CM, FRCPC[1]

There is good evidence that breast feeding reduces the rate of gastrointestinal and respiratory infections and that this effect is found even in developed countries. In addition, in infants who have a family history of atopy, breast feeding in conjunction with restricted maternal diet during pregnancy and lactation may reduce the incidence of atopic illness in their children. Finally, numerous case-control studies have observed that those with insulin-dependent diabetes were either not breast fed or were breast fed for a shorter duration than controls without the disease.

There is good evidence for implementation of a number of peripartum maneuvers such as rooming-in of newborns with their mothers, early and frequent physical contact, and banning of the provision of commercial samples to encourage the duration of breast feeding. Both antepartum and postpartum counselling prolong breast feeding duration. The effect of supplemental bottles of formula or water on duration of breast feeding remains unclear.

Burden of Suffering

For the purpose of this paper, breast feeding refers to exclusive breast feeding unless otherwise stated. Rates of breast feeding in one-week-old infants in the U.S. increased from 29% in 1955 to 52% in 1989.<1> This increase, however, reached a peak in 1982 when 62% of infants were breast fed at age one week. This pattern is matched by rates of breast feeding at 5-6 months which rose from 5% in 1971 to 28% in 1984 and fell to 18% in 1989. Certain groups are at greater risk of not breast feeding, including young mothers and those in lower socioeconomic groups, particularly those receiving social insurance benefits.<2> Data from the Ross Database on breast feeding in Canada show overall rates of breast feeding initiation of 75% among 3 cohorts born in 1991 and 1992 (personal communication, Anne Dumas, Manager, Nutrition Services, Ross Laboratories). Fifty-four percent and 30% were still breast feeding at 3 and 6 months of age, respectively. Lower rates were observed in Quebec and the Maritimes and higher rates in British Columbia.

[1] Associate Professor of Pediatrics and of Preventive Medicine and Biostatistics, University of Toronto, Toronto, Ontario

Effectiveness of Breast Feeding in Prevention of Adverse Outcomes

Infections

In their critical review of the literature, Bauchner and colleagues<3> concluded that there was no definitive evidence in developed countries that breast feeding reduced infections, since those studies of the highest methodologic quality did not find any differences. Since that review, three cohort studies have met the stringent methodologic requirements set forth by these authors.

In a British study,<4> 750 mother-infant pairs were seen at home on thirteen occasions during the first 24 months of life. Health visitors administered a questionnaire detailing feeding method as well as illness history in the intervening period between visits. Maternal education, maternal age, and smoking history, which were the only factors predicting infections were included in a multiple regression model. Breast feeding for a period beyond thirteen weeks was independently protective for gastrointestinal infections, and to a lesser extent, respiratory infections. Four percent of 227 infants who were breast feeding at this time vs. 15.7% of infants who were bottle feeding had experienced a gastrointestinal infection. A significantly lower proportion had been hospitalized for their infection – 2% of those breast feeding more than 13 weeks vs. 7.7% of those who never breast fed had been hospitalized in the first year. Twenty-six percent of breast vs. 37% of bottle feeding infants experienced respiratory infections. A similar reduction in respiratory illness hospitalizations was observed but the difference did not reach statistical significance. The effect of breast feeding persisted beyond the period of breast feeding and occurred despite supplementation.

In another cohort study conducted in Denmark, monthly questionnaires were sent to the home for self-administration to ascertain feeding methods and infections.<5> 500 patients were enrolled, but only 44% were followed for the full 12 months of the study. No protection against infection was afforded by breast feeding in this study. This may have been due to a lower overall rate of infection in this largely middle-class population, the inclusion of partial along with exclusive breast feeding in the breast feeding group, the use of self-administered monthly questionnaires, or incomplete follow-up of patients.

Compared with exclusive or supplementary bottle feeding, exclusive breast feeding for four months or more was found in the third study to protect against both acute and recurrent otitis media.<6> Healthy infants enrolled at birth were followed for the occurrence of acute and recurrent otitis media diagnosed by their physicians during the first year of life. Infants exclusively breast fed during the first 4 months of life had a 0.72 and 0.54 odds of developing acute and recurrent otitis media respectively, compared with those who were exclusively bottle fed or received breast milk for less than 6 months. A dose-response effect was observed in that infants who received supplementation in addition to breast feeding had intermediate infection rates.

In summary, two well-conducted cohort studies provide evidence supporting protection against gastroenteric and respiratory infections and otitis media. Thus, there is grade II-2 evidence in support of protection against infection through breast feeding.

Breast feeding is associated with fewer infections and in certain populations may reduce atopy and insulin-dependent diabetes

Atopy

The studies which relate breast feeding to protection against atopic disease are not of high quality. Kramer critically reviewed the literature up to 1986 and concluded that methodologic limitations of the available studies prevented conclusions about any protective effect of breast feeding.[7] Notably, women who belong to higher socioeconomic classes have higher rates of atopic children and are more likely to breast feed, so the bias would be to reduce observed benefits for breast feeding if adjustment for social class did not take place.[7] Similarly, concerns regarding atopy in their offspring may cause more atopic women to breast feed, also reducing benefits observed from breast feeding in research studies.

Several cohort studies and a single randomized controlled trial in preterm infants have not found any significant benefit of breast feeding compared with bottle feeding on the onset of atopy.[8-10] However, in those at increased risk of atopy as defined by a positive family history or positive cord immunoglobulin E (IgE), breast feeding may prevent atopy.[11] Similarly in a subgroup of 160 preterm infants involved in a randomized trial comparing breast milk with two lactose-based formulas, there was a 3.6 fold odds of atopy in those receiving formula.[10]

One cohort study and two trials of maternal dietary restriction in conjunction with breast feeding also observed benefit in those receiving the intervention.[12-14] Because of the lack of blinding in the cohort study, its conclusions are limited. However, there was a halving of the incidence of atopy in the two trials in the treatment arm compared with the control arm. It is not possible to separate the relative contribution of antenatal dietary restriction from the effect of avoidance of certain foods during lactation to the outcome. In addition, problems with the dietary restriction resulted in low compliance in one of the studies and only those who complied with the intervention were included in the final analysis.[14]

In summary, breast feeding does not appear to alter the development of atopy in the general population. However, poor study power and short duration of breast feeding in some studies weaken the evidence. One cohort study and several trials have suggested that restricting maternal diets during breast feeding may reduce the incidence of atopy in their children. Thus, exclusion of various foods from the diet of breast feeding mothers may be useful in a subpopulation at increased risk of atopy (positive family history or markers such as increased cord IgE).

Insulin-dependent Diabetes Mellitus

Numerous case-control studies have observed either a lower frequency or shorter duration of breast feeding in patients developing diabetes compared with population or sibling controls. This protection from diabetes through breast feeding has been shown even after adjusting for differences in potential confounders such as socioeconomic status. This effect may be due to immunologic properties of breast milk or alternatively to delayed exposure to cow's milk.[15] One group hypothesized that antibody directed to a component of bovine serum albumin not found in human or murine albumin cross-reacts with a pancreatic beta-cell receptor.[16] They observed significantly higher levels of this antibody among newly diagnosed diabetics compared with an age-, gender- and region-matched control group.[16]

Thus, there is fair evidence to support the role of breast feeding in preventing diabetes, particularly in a subgroup with genetic markers indicating an increased risk of diabetes.[17,18] For more information on diabetes mellitus consult Chapters 2 and 50 (pregnant and non-pregnant adults, respectively).

Growth and Development

Studies with limited power have reported no difference in either skin fold thickness or weights in infants fed different formulas compared with breast milk. However, a cohort study of infants matched for family socioeconomic status, ethnicity, birth weight, gender, and time of introduction of solids reported a significantly higher mean weight in the first eighteen months among those receiving formula. Whether this difference suggests that formula-fed infants are overweight or that breast-feeding protects against subsequent obesity is unclear. It is, therefore, not possible to conclude which is the better diet since the most desirable outcomes have not been defined.

Studies examining maternal bonding (parent-infant attachment) and breast feeding are inconclusive since they do not adjust for major confounders that affect choice of feeding method and bonding. Cohort studies linking breast milk feeding to increased intelligence quotients also need replication. However, some evidence of this type including the benefits of breast feeding are included in the next Chapter on iron deficiency anemia in infants (Chapter 23).

Efficacy of Interventions to Encourage Breast Feeding

In a meta-analysis Renfrew[19] found that, based on two studies of antenatal breast feeding education, the odds of discontinuing breast feeding at one to two months was significantly reduced at 0.2. A single trial of antenatal breast feeding classes versus individual teaching did not show any consistent differences in breast feeding.[20] In a meta-analysis of six trials, a significant benefit was observed for postnatal support.[21] The pooled odds ratio of 0.75 (95% confidence interval (CI): 0.62-0.91) for stopping breast feeding before 8-12 weeks despite differences in the nature of this support.

A randomized controlled trial involving primiparas has observed prolonged duration of breast feeding from a median of 77 days in a control group allowed to nurse four to six hours after delivery and every 4 hours thereafter to 182 days in the group who breast fed within 10 minutes of delivery and every two hours thereafter.[22] A group receiving only early initiation appeared to have a longer duration of breast feeding than a group with delayed onset but frequent breast feeding in the peripartum period. In a Canadian randomized trial of early contact compared with the control group, 9 of 15 mothers who had early contact with their infants were still exclusively nursing their infants compared with 3 of 15 control mothers (Fisher's exact test, $p<0.001$).[23] Two other studies also indicate that early contact prolongs breast feeding – the first used systematic allocation based on birth week and the second used true random allocation.[24,25] Although the direction of improvement was towards the early contact group, the differences did not reach statistical significance, possibly because only a small number of subjects had complete follow-up. Another randomized trial of 78 subjects did not observe a benefit of early mother-infant contact on duration of breast feeding.[26] However, randomization was not successful since more women intending to breast feed were in the group receiving early contact vs. routine contact, the population involved advantaged women who were already likely to breast feed and might therefore show less improvement with the intervention, and follow-up involved only 50 subjects thus severely limiting power. Combining the data from all studies of early contact compared with a control group shows a significant increase in breast feeding as measured at the different observation periods.

Another potential method for increasing breast feeding is the avoidance of bottle supplementation. There are two theories as to why bottle supplementation may discourage breast feeding. The first is that bottle feeding is mechanically easier than breast feeding. The second is that the perception that their milk supply is inadequate may be reinforced in mothers who observe their infants nursing from a bottle. However, conflicting results have been reported from a cohort study, a quasi-experimental study and a randomized trial. Differences in patient population and intervention make the evidence regarding bottle supplementation difficult to interpret.

Two well designed randomized trials suggest that provision of formula samples prior to discharge reduces the proportion of infants still being breast fed at either three or four months after discharge.<27,28> In both studies, using a Cox analysis, the effect of providing formula samples was seen within two months of birth.

From these studies, one can conclude that peripartum practices that enhance breast feeding include unrestricted contact between mother and baby following delivery, encouragement of demand feeding, and avoidance of giving formula samples to parents at discharge. However, there is poor compliance with these practices in English and Canadian maternity hospitals.<29,30>

Peripartum practices (e.g. early frequent mother-baby contact, demand feeding, avoidance of giving formula samples) promote breast feeding

Care must be taken to ensure hydration in breast fed babies since breast feeding leads to greater weight loss during the early postnatal period compared with bottle feeding, presumably due to inadequate fluid intake. Dehydration coupled with inadequate stooling may result in jaundice.

Viruses, including cytomegaloviruses (CMV), hepatitis B, HIV, and HTLV-1, have been isolated from breast milk and may cause infections in the newborn. The significance of breast milk transmission of CMV during the neonatal period is unclear. With universal immunization against hepatitis B, the incremental increase in transmission of this virus is likely to be minimal. However, the threat of HIV infection has led to discouragement of breast feeding by HIV-infected mothers in developed countries. It would be reasonable to consider maternal screening programs for HIV infection (as discussed in Chapter 58).

Guilt or other negative impacts may occur in women who are being told that 'breast is best' but are unable to either initiate or sustain breast feeding. Of women who had discontinued breast feeding prior to 12 weeks, two-thirds admitted feeling upset or guilty at having stopped.<31>

Recommendations of Others

Both the American Academy of Pediatrics and the Canadian Pediatric Society have recommended breast feeding as the preferred mode of infant feeding.<32> Their recommendations include public education programs, encouragement of breast feeding during prenatal care as well as on maternity wards, and examination of feasibility of breast feeding in day care centres adjacent to places of work.

The World Health Organization and UNICEF have developed explicit guidelines to encourage breast feeding around the world.<33> They incorporate the peripartum practices described above.

Conclusions and Recommendations

There is level II-2 evidence indicating that breast feeding will reduce morbidity related to infectious illnesses in developed countries. In subgroups at high risk of atopy, randomized trials suggest that breast feeding in conjunction with restriction of the mother's diet during pregnancy and lactation may reduce the incidence of atopy in the baby. Case-control studies have observed a higher incidence of lack of breast feeding or shorter duration of breast feeding in patients with insulin-dependent diabetes mellitus compared with controls. Given the evidence for benefit of breast feeding in the prevention of several adverse outcomes and that this is the strongest evidence that can ethically be obtaining for causation, breast feeding should be recommended as the preferred method of infant feeding. Based on meta-analysis of randomized trials of counselling, there is good evidence to support antenatal and postnatal counselling (A Recommendation).

Trials dealing with the peripartum environment also support a recommendation for early frequent contact and rooming-in privileges as well as banning provision of free formula samples (A Recommendation). The evidence for avoidance of bottle supplementation in the peripartum period is contradictory and inconclusive.

Unanswered Questions (Research Agenda)

The following have been identified as research priorities:

1. Randomized trials to enhance breast feeding with illness serving as the primary outcome.

2. Observations that breast milk may confer increased intelligence on preterm recipients should be studied by others. In addition, prospective studies of breast feeding in families with a history of insulin-dependent diabetes mellitus are needed.

3. More precise information about the ideal duration of breast feeding is required as well as the need for exclusivity of breast feeding, since many women are currently discontinuing breast feeding prior to six months because of return to work. Since the studies on the effect of supplementation on duration of breast feeding are contradictory, more information on this issue may be gained from studies of mixed feeding practices.

4. Future studies should also examine the usefulness of brochures in transmitting breast feeding information. One recent study sampled breast feeding reading materials and found the materials wanting in a number of respects. Materials from commercial sources, in particular were more inaccurate and conveyed a more negative attitude toward breast feeding than those produced by non-profit organizations.

Evidence

A MEDLINE search to December 1993, was performed using the MESH terms breast feeding, and counselling, infections, allergy, nutrition, or infant development. References were searched for further relevant references. Only studies conducted in developed countries with clinical outcomes rather than those with immunologic or biochemical measurements were included. Review of the evidence also focused on studies published after that summarized in two critical reviews of the literature on the role of breast feeding in reducing infections[7] or atopy.[8]

This review was initiated in June 1993 and recommendations were finalized by the Task Force in January 1994.

Acknowledgements

The Task Force thanks Michael S. Kramer, MD, Peds (P.Q.), Professor of Pediatrics and of Epidemiology and Biostatistics, McGill University, Montreal, Quebec; Ms. Marie Labrèche, Reg N, Program Officer, Family and Child Health, Health Promotion Directorate, Health Canada, Ottawa, Ontario; and Stanley H. Zlotkin, MD, PhD, FRCPC (Peds), Associate Professor of Pediatrics and Nutritional Sciences, University of Toronto, Toronto, Ontario for reviewing the draft report. Funding for this report was provided by Health Canada under the Government of Canada's Brighter Futures Initiative.

Selected References

1. Hoekelman RA: Highs and lows in breast-feeding rates. *Pediatr Ann* 1992; 21: 615-617

2. Ryan AS, Rush D, Krieger FW, *et al*: Recent declines in breast-feeding in the United States, 1984 through 1989. *Pediatrics* 1991; 88: 719-727

3. Bauchner H, Leventhal JM, Shapiro ED: Studies of breast-feeding and infections. How good is the evidence? *JAMA* 1986; 256: 887-892

4. Howie PW, Forsyth JS, Ogston SA, *et al*: Protective effect of breast feeding against infection. *BMJ* 1990; 300: 11-16

5. Rubin DH, Leventhal JM, Krasilnikoff PA, *et al*: Relationship between infant feeding and infectious illness: a prospective study of infants during the first year of life. *Pediatrics* 1990; 85: 464-471

6. Duncan B, Ey J, Holberg CJ, *et al*: Exclusive breast-feeding for at least 4 months protects against otitis media. *Pediatrics* 1993; 91: 867-872

7. Kramer MS: Does breast feeding help protect against atopic disease? Biology, methodology, and a golden jubilee of controversy. *J Pediatr* 1988; 112: 181-190

8. Savilahti E, Tainio V-M, Salmenpera L, *et al*: Prolonged exclusive breast feeding and heredity as determinants in infantile atopy. *Arch Dis Child* 1987; 62: 269-273

9. Midwinter RE, Morris AF, Colley JR: Infant feeding and atopy. *Arch Dis Child* 1987; 62: 965-967

10. Lucas A, Brooke OG, Morley R, *et al*: Early diet of preterm infants and development of allergic or atopic disease: randomised prospective study. *BMJ* 1990; 300: 837-840

11. Burr ML, Limb ES, Maguire MJ, *et al*: Infant feeding, wheezing, and allergy: a prospective study. *Arch Dis Child* 1993; 68: 724-728

12. Hattevig G, Kjellman B, Sigurs N, *et al*: The effect of maternal avoidance of eggs, cow's milk and fish during lactation upon allergic manifestations in infants. *Clin Exp Allergy* 1989; 19: 27-32

13. Chandra RK, Puri S, Suraiya C, *et al*: Influence of maternal food antigen avoidance during pregnancy and lactation on incidence of atopic eczema in infants. *Clin Allergy* 1986; 16: 563-569

14. Zeiger RS, Heller S, Mellon MH, *et al*: Effect of combined maternal and infant food-allergen avoidance on development of atopy in early infancy: a randomized study. *J Allergy Clin Immunol* 1989; 84: 72-89

15. Bjorksten B: Breast feeding and atopic dermatitis. *Allergy* 1989; 44 (Suppl 9): 129-134

16. Karjalainen J, Martin JM, Knip M, *et al*: A bovine albumin peptide as a possible trigger of insulin-dependent diabetes mellitus. *N Engl J Med* 1992; 327: 302-307

17. Kostraba JN, Cruickshanks KJ, Lawler-Heavner J, *et al*: Early exposure to cow's milk and solid foods in infancy, genetic predisposition, and risk of IDDM. *Diabetes* 1993; 42: 288-295

18. Bognetti E, Meschi F, Malavasi C, *et al*: HLA antigens in Italian type 1 diabetic patients: role of DR3/DR4 antigens and breast feeding in the onset of the disease. *Acta Diabetol* 1992; 28: 229-232

19. Renfrew MJ: Antenatal breastfeeding education. In: Pregnancy and Childbirth Module (eds. Enkin MW, Keirse MJNC, Renfrew MJ, Neilson JP), "Cochrane Database of Systematic Reviews": Review No. 04171. Published through "Cochrane Updates on Disk", Oxford: Update Software, 1993, Disk Issue 2

20. Renfrew MJ: Antenatal breastfeeding classes vs individual teaching. In: Pregnancy and Childbirth Module (eds. Enkin MW, Keirse MJNC, Renfrew MJ, Neilson JP), "Cochrane Database of Systemic Reviews": Review No. 07144. Published through "Cochrane Updates on Disk", Oxford: Update Software, 1993, Disk Issue 2

21. Renfrew MJ: Postnatal support for breastfeeding mothers. In: Pregnancy and Childbirth Module (eds. Enkin MW, Keirse MJNC, Renfrew MJ, Neilson JP), "Cochrane Database of Systemic Reviews": Review No. 04173. Published through "Cochrane Updates on Disk", Oxford: Update Software, 1993, Disk Issue 2

22. Salariya EM, Easton PM, Cater JI: Duration of breast-feeding after early initiation and frequent feeding. *Lancet* 1978; ii: 1141-1143

23. Thomson ME, Hartsock TG, Larson C: The importance of immediate postnatal contact: Its effect on breastfeeding. *Can Fam Physician* 1979; 25: 1374-1378

24. Cohen SA: Postpartum teaching and the subsequent use of milk supplements. *Birth Fam J* 1980; 7: 163-167

25. de Chateau P, Winberg J: Immediate postpartum suckling contact and duration of breastfeeding. *J Mat Child Health* 1978; 3: 392-395

26. Taylor PM, Maloni JA, Taylor FH, *et al*: II. Extra early mother-infant contact and duration of breast-feeding. *Acta Paediatr Scand Suppl* 1985; 316: 15-22

27. Bergevin Y, Dougherty C, Kramer MS: Do infant formula samples shorten the duration of breast-feeding? *Lancet* 1983; 1: 1148-1151

28. Frank DA, Wirtz SJ, Sorenson JR, *et al*: Commercial discharge packs and breast-feeding counseling: effects on infant- feeding practices in a randomised trial. *Pediatrics* 1987; 80: 845-854

29. Garforth S, Garcia J: Breast feeding policies in practice – 'no wonder they get confused.' *Midwifery* 1989; 5: 75-83

30. Houston MJR, Field PA: Practices and policies in the initiation of breastfeeding. *J Obstet Gynecol Neonatal Nurs* 1988; 17: 418-424

31. Houston M, Howie P, McNeilly A: Nursing mirror midwifery forum. 2. Breast feeding. *Nurs Mirror* 1983; 156: i-ix

32. Nutrition Committee of the Canadian Pediatric Society and The Committee on Nutrition of the American Academy of Pediatrics: Breast-feeding. A commentary in celebration of the International Year of the Child, 1979. *Pediatrics* 1978; 62: 591-601

33. Jolly R: Breastfeeding and health care services. *Int J Gynaecol Obstet* 1990; 31 (Suppl 1): 7-9

Breast Feeding

MANEUVER	EFFECTIVENESS	LEVEL OF EVIDENCE <REF>	RECOMMENDATION
Counselling regarding breast feeding	Breast feeding (vs. formula feeding) reduces gastrointestinal and respiratory infections.	Cohort studies<4-6> (II-2)	Good evidence to counsel women regarding breast feeding (A)
	Counselling increases breast feeding rates; both antepartum and postpartum counselling prolong breast feeding duration.	Meta-analysis of randomized controlled trials<19-21> (I)	
Peripartum interventions: Early, frequent mother-infant contact, rooming in, banning provision of free formula samples	Peripartum interventions increase breast feeding rates.	Randomized controlled trials<22-28> (I)	Good evidence to implement peripartum interventions that promote breast feeding (A)

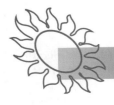

CHAPTER 23

Prevention of Iron Deficiency Anemia in Infants

By John W. Feightner

Prevention of Iron Deficiency Anemia in Infants

Prepared by John W. Feightner, MD, MSc, FCFP[1]

In 1979, the Canadian Task Force on the Periodic Health Examination concluded that there was poor justification for the inclusion of screening for iron deficiency anemia (IDA) in the periodic health examination, though particular attention was considered warranted for higher risk groups.<1> This position, a C Recommendation, was based on the lack of Level I evidence on the value of treatment of all but the most severe iron deficiency.

Since then, several well-designed trials have provided additional evidence concerning the consequences of iron deficiency; the strongest evidence for an association between IDA and clinical outcomes comes from studies of infants and children, while for other groups the issue is even more controversial. The screening tests are reasonably sensitive and specific, particularly when used in combination, and there is convincing evidence that treatment – both food fortification and supplementation – is effective in reversing anemia and iron deficiency. The evidence concerning whether the reversal of iron deficiency corrects the cognitive, behavioral, and physical consequences of the deficiency is equivocal, at best.

This review does not address the issue of IDA in pregnancy. (see Chapter 6)

Burden of Suffering

Prevalence

In North America, the prevalence of iron deficiency anemia has been declining over the last three decades

In North America, the prevalence of IDA has been declining over the last two to three decades. Recent U.S. statistics indicate a rate of 0.2% among men and 2.6% in menstruating women. Estimates of prevalence, particularly in high-risk groups, are affected by the varying definitions used for IDA among the available studies.

In Canada, the overall prevalence of IDA in infants and young children has declined significantly and in the normal population is not considered a major health issue. However, a number of high-risk groups have been identified recently in Canadian studies.

---

[1] Professor of Family Medicine, McMaster University, Hamilton, Ontario

While there have been some ethnic associations with IDA, the major risk factors are related to low socioeconomic status. Specific high risk groups include the following:

Low Socioeconomic Status

A Montreal study evaluating children at one year of age in the 5 poorest health districts found 15% had hemoglobin below 105 g/L and 27% below 110 g/L.[2] In a 1991 Ottawa study, 8.2% of children from families of low socioeconomic status had hemoglobin levels <110 g/L.[3]

Chinese Population

A study evaluating iron deficiency in a Chinese population identified iron deficiency in 4.1% of the children and within this group the mean hemoglobin was 91 g/L.[4]

Aboriginal Children

Forty-three percent of infants in one aboriginal community had hemoglobin levels <110 g/L.

Infants of Low Birth Weight

A relationship exists between low birth weight and iron deficiency.

Consumption of Whole Cow's Milk

The risk of iron deficiency and IDA appears to be greater in infants fed whole cow's milk (WCM) during the first year of life. One study found that in infants fed WCM starting at six months of age, 25% had a hemoglobin below 110 g/L compared to 11% for infants fed iron fortified formula over the same age range.[5] There is conflicting evidence regarding the etiology of this phenomenon, but the main postulated mechanisms include the fact that WCM is a poor source of iron, and the possibility of decreased iron intake in alternate forms is associated with poor absorption and bioavailability.

Clinical Impact

In infants iron deficiency is most prevalent between six and 24 months of age, a time of rapid brain growth and psychomotor development. A deficiency of iron at this stage in development has the potential for severe consequences both in terms of cognitive function as well as psychomotor development and behaviour. While it is postulated that iron deficiency even before the appearance of anemia may have an affect on brain function, the evidence is more limited.

While the evidence is strongly suggestive of a causal relationship between IDA and deficiency in cognition and psychomotor development, it falls short of confirming a causal relationship. Many of the studies which have evaluated a casual relationship as well as those which have looked at the benefits of intervention have relied solely on laboratory outcome measures such as hemoglobin. Those which have focused on clinical outcomes for infants have primarily used the Bayley Scales which have two components, a mental development index and a psychomotor development index. Some studies have used IQ tests and other tests of cognition. While some studies have shown an association between IDA and decreased cognitive function and decreased psychomotor development, there is conflicting data regarding subsequent improvement with therapy.

The issue of causal relationship is important in determining what degree of confidence to place in studies which only use hematologic laboratory indices as measures of outcome. This review will give primary weighting to studies using clinical outcomes. However, where the clinical question is relevant and the only available data from well designed studies is expressed in terms of laboratory outcome, these studies will also be reviewed.

There are data which suggests IDA may also have a primary affect on infant behaviour. Such studies indicate that IDA may be associated with increased irritability and fussiness and with decreased attention.

Iron deficiency anemia may be associated with increased irritability and fussiness and with decreased attention

Studies focusing on children and adults have suggested an association between IDA and cognition as well as strength, work capacity and endurance. In adults, those studies focusing on relationship to muscle strength have primarily demonstrated a relationship only to maximal performance and have not shown an association between IDA and normal daily activity. One study evaluating the productivity of rubber plantation workers in Indonesia suggested that iron deficiency may be associated with decreased endurance and, hence, decreased productivity.

Maneuver

There are essentially two approaches to dealing with IDA, particularly in infants. The first is to embark on early detection efforts to identify anemic infants and subsequently, embark on a course of iron therapy. The alternate approach is one of primary prevention wherein all infants in a population are provided iron fortified formula or cereal in an attempt to prevent the occurrence of anemia. In this section only the early detection efforts will be reviewed.

There are several tests available for the diagnosis of iron deficiency and IDA. However, from the perspective of early detection, only a limited number of tests can realistically be considered. Historically, the most commonly used laboratory test, clinically and in research studies, has been the hemoglobin level. Hematocrit has been used to some degree in the past and more recently serum ferritin has been used for the early detection of iron deficiency.

The gold standard against which most early detection tests are evaluated is the evaluation of iron stores in a patient's bone marrow.

Serum Ferritin

Studies evaluating the test characteristics of serum ferritin have largely been conducted in adults. While the results vary, the best estimates for serum ferritin levels <12 ug/L indicate a sensitivity of 86% and a specificity of 92%.[6]

Hemoglobin

Again, estimates of the sensitivity and specificity vary depending on the study. However, in a key study using bone marrow as the gold standard in an adult population, the hemoglobin was found to have a sensitivity of 8% and a specificity of 97%.[6] A study which used response to therapy and achieving a hemoglobin level over 133 g/L found a sensitivity of 66% and a specificity of 65%.[7]

The test performance of hemoglobin as a screening test has clear performance limitations which must be considered if early detection of iron deficiency is to be used as the main approach to dealing with IDA in infants. This will be discussed later.

Effectiveness of Prevention and Treatment

The problem of IDA (in infants) can be addressed through primary prevention efforts or through the secondary prevention efforts of early detection and subsequent therapy. Primary prevention has the potential of providing benefit to a whole population and preventing the onset of IDA. This assumes that the strategies for ensuring adequate iron intake are available and affordable for all infants and that such interventions are effective in preventing IDA. Early detection has the potential of focusing efforts only on those who have definitely been identified as having IDA. The success of this approach depends both on being able to accurately identify individuals with anemia and on proof that subsequent therapy is effective. Complete success would assume that all infants would be screened or that high-risk infants could be accurately identified for screening.

Potentially, primary prevention can benefit the entire population and prevent the onset of iron deficiency anemia

Fortification of Formula and Cereal

The evidence for the benefit of iron fortification, comes from studies evaluating programs aimed at large populations as well as from randomized controlled trials with more carefully defined study populations. Unfortunately, these studies have not evaluated clinical outcomes.

Population studies have primarily focused on the impact in the U.S. of the "WIC Program", which provides iron fortified formula and cereals to low income families, primarily in urban settings. These studies have compared hemoglobin in a cross section sample of children before the implementation of the program, with a similar group of children selected for evaluation some years after the implementation of the program. One such study indicated that the percentage of children with the hemoglobin <99 g/L changed from 23% before the program in 1971 to 1% in 1984, some years after the program had been implemented.<8> While these results can be attributed at least in part to the benefits of the program, there are likely several confounding factors which are at work as well. Evidence to support the fact that all of this improvement is not the result of the program's iron fortification comes from studies which have indicated a significant decrease in anemic children screened prior to entry to the WIC Program in 1975 compared to children screened in 1985 but also before entering the program. The percentage of anemic children dropped from 7.8% to 2.9% from 1975 to 1985 even before these children were entered into the program providing iron fortified formula in cereal.<9>

The strongest evidence comes from two randomized controlled trials and one non-randomized trial evaluating infant formula in infant cereal.

Walter and colleagues demonstrated the benefits of iron fortified formula as well as iron fortified cereal.<10> Each was successful in preventing anemia in infants whether they were weaned from the breast prior to four months of age or whether the iron fortified cereal was added after four months of age and with continued breast-feeding.

In the early weaned group, anemia rates at eight months of age were 6% for iron fortified cereal, 4.5% for iron fortified formula, and 20% in those receiving no iron fortified products. In the breast-fed group, the rate of anemia at eight months of age was 3.5% in those receiving iron fortified cereal compared to 15% for those breast-fed only.

Zlotkin and co-authors, in a study of infants six to 12 months of age, found that in infants fed iron fortified cereal the percentage of infants with ferritin values <10 ug/L or hemoglobin <110 g/L was 22%

compared to 48% in a control group receiving non-iron fortified cereal.<11>

Similarly, Pazarro and co-workers in a non-randomized trial, demonstrated that children receiving iron fortified formula had a lower rate of anemia (0.6%) than a comparison group fed cow's milk (15%).<12>

Once again, none of these studies measured outcomes in terms of cognitive function or psycho motor development.

Supplementation

While iron supplementation provided through drops or iron fortified cereal is not currently a common practice in North America, two randomized controlled trials have demonstrated the effectiveness of iron supplementation in infants.<13,14>

Breast-feeding

There is limited evidence regarding the benefits of breast-feeding in reducing anemia in infants. While the evidence is limited, there is a plausible biologic argument. Iron in human milk has a relatively higher bio-availability. However, there is only a small absolute amount absorbed. What data do exist suggest that the likelihood of anemia can be reduced by breast-feeding, although, not to levels that match those of children who are breast-fed plus receive iron fortified cereal after the age of four to six months, nor compared to those children who have received iron fortified formula and subsequently, iron fortified cereal.<3,12>

Effectiveness of Treatment

Secondary prevention efforts rely on the early detection of IDA in infants and the implementation of therapy in those identified as anemic. Four randomized trials have evaluated the impact on cognitive function and psychomotor development of iron therapy provided to infants identified as having IDA. All studies have been conducted in Chile, Indonesia, or Central America.

Three studies failed to show the benefit of oral iron therapy.<15,16,17> Two of these studies provided a relatively short course of iron therapy (six to ten days) while one provided therapy of up to three months and still showed no benefit. A five year follow-up of one study group showed that there was no delayed benefit of iron therapy and that children with IDA in infancy still had lower mental and motor function at school entry.<18> These findings have raised concerns that one possible explanation is that lasting damage has occurred before the IDA was discovered and treated.

In a more recent study, Idjradinata and Pollit (1993) demonstrated a significant improvement in cognitive function and psychomotor development with four months of oral therapy in infants aged 12-18 months.<19> In infants with IDA, the treatment group showed a significantly greater improvement in mean hemoglobin and in serum transferrin. On the Bayley Scales, there was a 20 point improvement in mental development scores and a 14 point improvement in motor development scores, with no significant improvement in the placebo group. While the results of this trial are important, it is unclear why they differ from the findings of the other three studies.

Recommendations of Others

The Nutrition Committee of the Canadian Pediatrics Society has recently published a position statement on meeting the iron needs of infants and young children (Nutrition Committee, Canadian Pediatrics Society, 1991).<20> These recommendations support the use of iron-fortified formula for non-breast-fed infants as well as the use of iron-fortified infant cereals and other iron rich foods for all term infants. For premature infants the recommendations are that iron supplements should be started by at least eight weeks of age and continued until the first birthday. The recommendations do not include a specific statement regarding screening of children either in the general population or for high-risk groups.

In 1989, the U.S. Preventive Services Task Force recommended that screening should be offered once to all infants, and that parents should be encouraged to include iron enriched foods in the diet of infants. This recommendation is currently under review.<21>

The American Academy of Pediatrics recommends at least one measurement of hemoglobin or hematocrit in infancy, and at least one at ages 1-4, 5-12, and 14-20.

Conclusions and Recommendations

In Canada, IDA in infants is most appropriately considered as both a socioeconomic as well as a nutritional problem. The prevalence (and, hence, the risk for newborns) in identifiable high-risk groups is significant. However, in the general population, the risk is relatively low. Both of these realities influence how existing data might be converted to recommendations for clinical policy.

General Population

With a low prevalence of IDA in infants in the general population, the inaccuracy of hemoglobin measurement, and the conflicting evidence for iron therapy, there is insufficient evidence to recommend the inclusion of routine early detection of anemia by hemoglobin measurement between ages six and 12 months (C Recommendation).

For the general population it is recommended that physicians encourage breast-feeding for at least six months and the introduction of iron fortified formula and/or cereal after six months of age (B Recommendation). It should be noted that the Task Force strongly recommends breast-feeding for other reasons (A Recommendation; see Chapter 22). For children weaned from the breast early or who are not breast-fed from birth, iron fortified formula followed by iron fortified cereal at a later age should be recommended. Whole cow's milk should be avoided, certainly before nine months of age and perhaps until after 12 months.

High-risk Groups

This approach can be a difficult one for families of lower socioeconomic status because the cost of iron fortified formulas and cereals may be beyond their means. This is even more problematic if nutritional habits and/or income preclude the provision of iron enriched foods and foods rich in ascorbic acid. For infants of all high-risk groups, it is recommended that physicians take particular care to determine the nutritional intake and consider a hemoglobin measurement between ages six and 12 months, perhaps optimally at nine months of age (B Recommendation).

A hemoglobin measurement in any infant between ages six and 12 months of age where there is a suspicion of poor iron and general nutritional intake is prudent even if the child is not from a high-risk group. While serum ferritin has not been evaluated as a screening test, it measures poor iron stores and allows the identification of iron deficiency prior to the development of anemia. It may be considered as an additional test in selected infants.

Unanswered Questions (Research Agenda)

Randomized controlled trials evaluating the impact of iron fortified formula and cereal on clinical outcomes are a high priority. Studies evaluating clinical outcomes of strategies to prevent and/or treat IDA in high risk groups, including the evaluation of early detection measures are likewise of high priority.

Evidence

The evidence in this review was identified using a MEDLINE search with the key words: anemia, hypochromic for the years 1984 to October 1993. The review was initiated in June 1991 and recommendations were finalized by the Task Force in February 1994.

Selected References

1. Canadian Task Force on the Periodic Health Examination: The periodic health examination. *Can Med Assoc J* 1979; 121: 1193-1254

2. Lehmann F, Gray-Donald K, Mongeon M, *et al*: Iron deficiency anemia in 1-year-old children of disadvantaged families in Montreal. *Can Med Assoc J* 1992; 146: 1571-1577

3. Greene-Finestone L, Feldman W, Heick H, *et al*: Prevalence and risk factors of iron depletion and iron deficiency anemia among infants in Ottawa-Carlton. *Can Diet Assoc J* 1991; 52: 20-23

4. Chan-Yip A, Gray-Donald K: Prevalence of iron deficiency among Chinese children aged 6 to 36 months in Montreal. *Can Med Assoc J* 1987; 136: 373-378

5. Tunnessen WW Jr, Oski FA: Consequences of starting whole cow milk at 6 months of age. *J Pediatr* 1987; 111: 813-816

6. Rybo E: Diagnosis of iron deficiency. *Scand J Hemotol Suppl* 1985; 43: 5-39

7. Freire WB: Hemoglobin as a predictor of response to iron therapy and its use in screening and prevalence estimates. *Am J Clin Nutr* 1989; 50: 1442-1449

8. Vazquez-Seoane P, Windom R, Pearson HA: Disappearance of iron deficiency anemia in high-risk population given supplemental iron. *N Engl J Med* 1985; 313: 1239-1240

9. Yip R, Binkin NJ, Fleshood L, *et al*: Declining prevalence of anemia among low-income children in the United States. *JAMA* 1987; 258: 1619-1623

10. Walter T, Dallman PR, Pizarro F, *et al*: Effectiveness of iron-fortified infant cereal in prevention of iron deficiency anemia. *Pediatrics* 1993; 91: 976-982

11. Zlotkin SH, Beaton GH, Tanaka P, *et al*: Double-blind trial of iron fortification of infant cereals: effect on growth and hemotologic status. *Pediatric Research* 1993; 33: (abstract no.113a)

12. Pizarro F, Yip R, Dallman PR, *et al*: Iron status with different infant feeding regimens: relevance to screening and prevention of iron deficiency. *J Pediatr* 1991; 118: 687-692

13. Smith AW, Hendrickse RG, Harrison C, *et al*: Iron deficiency anemia and its response to oral iron: report of a study in rural Gambian children treated at home by their mothers. *Ann Trop Paediatr* 1989; 9: 6-16

14. Chwang LC, Soemantri AG, Pollitt E: Iron supplementation and physical growth of rural Indonesian children. *Am J Clin Nutr* 1988; 47: 496-501

15. Lozoff B, Brittenham GM, Viteri FE, *et al*: The effects of short-term oral iron therapy on developmental deficits of iron-deficient anemic infants. *J Pediat* 1982; 100: 351-357

16. Lozoff B, Brittenham GM, Wolf AW, *et al*: Iron deficiency anemia and iron therapy effects on infants developmental test performance. *Pediatrics* 1987; 79: 981-995

17. Walter T, DeAndraca I, Chadud P, *et al*: Iron deficiency anemia: adverse effects on infant psychomotor development. *Pediatrics* 1989; 84: 7-17

18. Lozoff B, Jimenez E, Wolf AW: Long-term developmental outcomes of infants with iron deficiency. *N Engl J Med* 1991; 325: 687-694

19. Idjradinata P, Pollitt E: Reversal of developmental delays in iron-deficient anemic infants treated with iron. *Lancet* 1993; 341: 1-4

20. National Committee, Canadian Pediatrics Society: Meeting the iron needs of infants and young children: an update. *Can Med Assoc J* 1991; 144: 1451-1453

21. U.S. Preventive Services Task Force: *Guide to Clinical Preventive Services: an Assessment of the Effectiveness of 169 Interventions.* Williams & Wilkins, Baltimore, Md, 1989: 163-167

Prevention of Iron Deficiency Anemia in Infants

MANEUVER	EFFECTIVENESS	LEVEL OF EVIDENCE <REF>	RECOMMENDATION
Iron fortified formula (if not breast-feeding)	Use of fortified formula lowers rates of iron deficiency anemia (IDA). Studies measuring clinical outcomes have not been conducted.	Randomized controlled trial<10> (I); quasi-randomized trial<12> (II-1)	There is fair evidence to recommend fortified formula for non-breast-fed infants (B)
Iron fortified cereal	Lower IDA rates, for infants consuming iron fortified cereal compared to placebo, after the age of 4-6 months. Studies measuring clinical outcomes have not been conducted.	Randomized controlled trials<10,11> (I)	There is fair evidence to recommend iron fortified cereal for infants beginning at 4-6 months of age (B)
Breast-feeding	Decrease in iron deficiency in breast-fed infants compared to infants fed cows milk (but not as low as the prevalence in those fed iron fortified formula).	Quasi-randomized study<12> (II-1)	There is fair evidence to recommend breast-feeding in newborn infants to lower the risk of iron deficiency anemia* (B); however, infants breast-fed beyond 6 months of age benefit from iron fortified cereal to prevent the development of IDA
	Decreased IDA in breast-fed infants; breast-feeding has been recommended on other grounds as well.*	Cohort analytic study<3> (II-3)	
Iron Supplementation	Two trials have demonstrated the benefit of iron oral supplements in infants. In North American the use of iron fortified formula and cereal is more widely used and may be more feasible.	Randomized controlled trials<13,14> (I)	There is fair evidence to recommend iron supplementation in infancy but iron fortified formula and cereal may be more feasible in most settings (B)

* **There is good evidence to recommend breast feeding for other reasons (A recommendation for preventing infection; see Chapter 22).**

(Continued on next page)

Prevention of Iron Deficiency Anemia in Infants (concl'd)

MANEUVER	EFFECTIVENESS	LEVEL OF EVIDENCE <REF>	RECOMMENDATION
Routine Hemoglobin measurement at 6-12 months	Conflicting evidence from randomized controlled trials evaluating clinical outcomes. Three studies showed no benefit from therapy; one recent study demonstrated improvement in both cognitive and motor development.	Randomized controlled trials<15-19> (I)	Conflicting and insufficient evidence to recommend the inclusion or the exclusion of routine hemoglobin determination in normal-risk infants (C); on the basis of a higher prevalence in certain risk groups** and a greater likelihood of inability to consume iron fortified products, there is fair evidence to recommend a routine hemoglobin measurement for high-risk infants (B)

** High-risk infants include: infants of families of low socioeconomic status, Chinese or aboriginal ethnic origin, low birth weight (<2,500 grams) or fed only whole cow's milk during the first year of life.

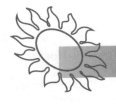

CHAPTER 24

Well-Baby Care in the First 2 Years of Life

By William Feldman

Well-Baby Care in the First 2 Years of Life

Prepared by William Feldman, MD, FRCPC[1]

In 1990, the Canadian Task Force on the Periodic Health Examination reviewed the evidence on various elements of well-baby care<1> and found good evidence for immunization against diphtheria, measles, mumps, pertussis, poliomyelitis, rubella and tetanus and Hemophilus influenzae type B (HIB) infection during well-baby examinations (A Recommendation). Since that time the effectiveness of immunization against hepatitis B infection has been established. The subject of childhood immunization, however, is dealt with in a separate section and will not be covered here. (See section on Immunization of Children and Adults.) In its 1979 report, the Task Force found fair evidence to support inclusion of clinical examination for disorders of physical growth (serial measurement of height and weight) in the periodic health examination of well infants and children (B Recommendation). This recommendation is brought forward without evaluation of new evidence. In 1990, the Task Force concluded that there was good evidence to support counselling to reduce injury risk factors in the home, as well as anticipatory guidance for night-time crying. The subject of risk reduction is also dealt with in Chapter 28 on Prevention of Household and Recreational Injuries in Children. On the basis of good detection maneuvers, effective treatment, and the alleviation of the burden of suffering, an A Recommendation was given to certain components of the physical examination, specifically examination of the hips, the eyes, and of hearing during well-baby care in the first year of life. New evidence relating to screening for congenital hip disease<2,3> and deafness<4> has been published and is reviewed here. We also found fair evidence that enquiring about developmental milestones may lead to effective environmental stimulation in infants with developmental delay caused by environmental deprivation (B Recommendation) and no evidence that screening for potential child abuse is effective (C Recommendation). The subject of prevention of child abuse is currently reviewed in Chapter 29 on Primary Prevention of Child Maltreatment which reviews this topic in detail. For recommendations on various other issues in pediatric preventive health care see the section on Pediatric Preventive Care.

---

[1] Professor of Pediatrics and of Preventive Medicine and Biostatics, University of Toronto, Toronto, Ontario

Burden of Suffering

The goals of visits for well-baby care are 1) to immunize, 2) to provide parents with reassurance and counselling on safety, nutrition and behavioral problems; and 3) to identify and treat physical, developmental and parenting problems.

Unintentional Injury

Trauma is the leading cause of death among children over 1 year of age. In developed countries injuries cause at least four times more childhood deaths than any disease. The leading cause of death among Canadian children is motor vehicle accidents; this is followed in descending order by drowning, burns, choking and falls. The morbidity rate is also considerable, although the true rate is impossible to ascertain since only in-patient data are gathered systematically. Disfigurement, disability, developmental delay and emotional problems are major sequelae of accidental injuries to children.

Trauma is the leading cause of death among children over 1 year of age

Sleep Problems

Night-time awakening and crying in children beyond the age when infants require night-time feeding occurs in at least 20% of children in the first few years.<5>

Hearing Problems

Severe bilateral congenital deafness is found in 1 of every 2,000 newborns. If profound hearing loss is not identified within the first year of life the likelihood that the child will have intelligible speech and attain educational standards commensurate with intellectual ability will be greatly reduced.

Amblyopia

The prevalence of amblyopia depends on the criterion used to measure it. If a corrected visual acuity of 6/12 (20/40) or worse is used, 2% of the population is affected.

Congenital Hip Dislocation

Controversy exists regarding the incidence of congenital hip dislocation, estimates varying from 2 to 50 per 1,000 live births.<6> These wide differences in estimates of incidence may be explained by differences in the infants' ages at examination, in the thoroughness and skill of the examiners and by racial differences. The higher prevalence observed in the neonatal period is likely due to the transient laxity of ligaments during the first few weeks of life. Over diagnosis presents certain risks. First, a proportion of subluxatable hips become stable spontaneously during the first year of life. In addition, over-aggressive abduction treatment may be harmful, leading to avascular necrosis of the femoral head.

Developmental Delay

Mental retardation, defined for statistical purposes as an intelligence quotient at least two standard deviations below the mean as determined by a standard test of intelligence, occurs by definition in 2% to 3% of children.

Parenting Problems and Child Maltreatment

The true incidence of parenting problems leading to child abuse in the first 2 years of life is unknown since it is not known what proportion of cases are reported. In the United States the estimated prevalence of maltreatment is 1% to 2% among children under 18 years of age. The outcomes of such maltreatment include death, disfigurement, disability, developmental delay and emotional problems. (See Chapter 29 on Primary Prevention of Child Maltreatment)

Maneuver

During the era in which healthy newborns were kept in hospital for 5-7 days the Task Force recommended six well-baby visits for healthy term infants born to primiparous women (one within the first month and then at 2, 4, 6, 12 and 18 months) to include 1) an assessment of growth and development as well as parenting skills; 2) counselling on nutrition, safety and common problems such as night-time crying; 3) physical examination, particularly for hearing impairment (parents were asked about their concerns regarding the infant's hearing, and the response to the clap test is noted), strabismus (as determined through the cover test and the light reflex test) and congenital anomalies such as hip dislocation (as determined through the Ortolani test); and 4) immunization.[1]

Since the recent shift to early discharge of healthy full-term newborns at 1-3 days after birth from the previous discharge policy of 5-7 days of age, the optimum timing of the first well-baby visit has not been established in terms of effectiveness. Previously, problems such as feeding difficulties, jaundice, etc., were usually dealt with while infants were still in hospital. Now, such problems may arise after the baby has been discharged. For these reasons a well-baby visit during the first week or two may well be advisable for primiparous as well as multiparous women, although the effectiveness of this schedule has not been examined through clinical research studies.

With regard to screening for hearing, a recent National Institute of Health Consensus Statement on early identification of hearing impairment in infants and young children recommended universal screening by 3 months of age using auditory brainstem responses (ABR) or evoked otoacoustic emissions (OCE). The statement acknowledges a high false positive rate using either technique and that much of the evidence is descriptive. There are no randomized trials supporting the benefits of early identification and intervention[4]; until there is better evidence that universal screening using ABR or OCE is superior to enquiring of parents and the clap test in long-term outcome, the latter approaches continue to be recommended.

Counselling on safety should include a recommendation to maintain the temperature in the hot water heater at less than 54.46°C (120°F), to safety-proof cupboards and drawers containing medicines, cleaners and solvents, to put up gates across stairways and to prevent access to sharp objects or electric outlets.

Counselling on safety should include a recommendation to maintain the temperature in the hot water heater at less than 54.4°C (120°F)

Anticipatory guidance for persistent night-time crying involves enquiring at the 6-month visit whether the infant is sleeping through the night and, if not, whether this is distressing to the parents. If so, systematic ignoring is recommended.

Universal newborn screening for congenital hip disease using ultrasound is being done in a number of European centres, but the incidence of infants judged to be in need of treatment differs considerably in different centers, suggesting that the diagnostic methods and criteria need further study.[2] In another study, ultrasound was used only for those newborns whose hips were "doubtful" after clinical assessment; the authors report good results with this approach.[3] Until there is good evidence that routine ultrasound leads to better long-term outcome than physical exam of the hips, the latter approach continues to be recommended.

Effectiveness of Prevention and Treatment

In 1977 Dershewitz and Williamson[7] reported the results of a randomized controlled trial of the prevention of childhood household injuries through an educational program. They found no differences in the total household hazard scores between the experimental and control groups. However, the two groups were of above average socioeconomic status. Thus, a reasonably high level of safety may have existed in both groups prior to the intervention. More recent randomized controlled trials involving lower socioeconomic groups have shown that safety education during visits for well-baby care can lower the risk of injury.[8] However, very large samples are required to show significant differences in the actual rates of injury, and these studies did not have significant power to do so. Educational programs designed to enhance infant protection in cars do not appear to be effective in jurisdictions where such protection has not been

Safety education during visits for well-baby care can lower the risk of injury

legislated. This subject is reviewed in detail in Chapter 44 on Prevention of Motor Vehicle Accident Injuries.

In a randomized controlled trial involving low-income families prenatal and postnatal counselling with anticipatory guidance in 19 visits of 1 hour each during the first 3 years of life were compared with routine well-baby care in the control group. The intervention was associated with less anemia, better infant nutrition and fewer behavioral problems at 5 and 6 years of age. In current clinical practice, whether the schedule recommended by the Canadian Pediatric Society (eight visits in the first 2 years) or that of the American Academy of Pediatrics (nine visits) is followed, the amount of time spent in counselling and anticipatory guidance (usually a few minutes) is far less than was provided in the aforementioned study.[9] As a result of iron supplementation of food in Canada iron deficiency anemia is rare. The issue of iron deficiency is discussed in detail in Chapter 23 on prevention of Iron Deficiency Anemia in Infants.

Night-time crying, a particularly vexing problem, frequently arises as an issue during visits for well-baby care. There is now level I evidence (from a randomized controlled trial) that counselling significantly reduces the prevalence of this problem.[5]

The early detection of certain physical problems, such as deafness, strabismus and congenital hip dislocation, can lead to effective interventions that prevent important physical and emotional difficulties. Although there have been no randomized controlled trials of the effectiveness of combined screening and intervention programs for such problems, the natural histories of undetected congenital deafness, strabismus and hip dislocation indicate considerable suffering and disability.

A study involving children with profound hearing loss (at least 70 dB in the speech frequencies) compared intervention with hearing aids and special training begun before and after 3 years of age. Sentence construction of those exposed to early (as opposed to late) intervention more closely matched that of control subjects with normal hearing. Unfortunately, confounding variables such as parent education were not assessed.

Although there is some controversy surrounding the exact age at which correction of congenital esotropia is essential to prevent amblyopia or failure of binocular vision,[10] current ophthalmological practice has been influenced by a cohort study in which infants whose eyes were aligned before 24 months of age had significantly fewer problems with binocularity.[11]

In a study of congenital hip dislocation the amount of open surgery required was much less and the long-term results much better among infants whose condition has been diagnosed at birth and treated with abduction splints before 1 month of age than among those diagnosed later in the first year.[6]

Other than the specific instances of phenylketonuria and hypothyroidism (usually diagnosed in the neonatal period) few measures to prevent mental retardation are available. For environmentally deprived infants an enriched environment may enhance mental development.

Frequency of Visits for Well-baby Care

A recent randomized controlled trial in Canada, involving healthy term neonates in intact families from all social classes, showed that the goals of well-baby care were achieved as well in a group randomly allocated to 5 or 6 visits coinciding with immunizations, as compared with a group allocated to 10 visits during the first 2 years. There were no differences in 1) physical status (assessed by a pediatrician blinded to group assignments); 2) developmental status at 2 years of age (assessed by the Mental Development Index of the Bayley scales of infant development; 3) maternal knowledge of child-rearing or maternal anxiety (as measured by the Hulka Infancy Questionnaire); 4) safety and infant stimulation in the home (determined by the Home Observation for Measurement of the Environment test); and 5) parent-initiated visits as a result of illness. The sample size provided adequate statistical power to detect any clinically significant differences.

Recommendations of Others

In 1990 the College of Family Physicians of Canada, concurred with the recommendations of the Task Force for an additional visit within the first month for infants of primiparous women. The Canadian Pediatric Society also recommended a visit within the first month as well as an additional visit at nine months for all well babies.

In 1989, the U.S. Preventive Services Task Force recommended that clinical prudence should be used to provide counselling on measures to reduce the risk of unintentional household or environmental injuries from falls, drownings, fires or burns, poisoning, and firearms. They also recommended that clinicians should be alert for signs of ocular misalignment when examining infants and that the height and weight of children should be measured regularly and plotted on a growth chart throughout infancy and childhood.[12] Their recommendation on screening for hearing impairment is currently under review.

Conclusions and Recommendations

There is good evidence for counselling about risk factors for accidental injury in the home during all well-baby visits. (A Recommendation) Anticipatory guidance particularly with regard to night-time crying beyond the expected age is also recommended

(A Recommendation). Although repeated examination of hips and hearing is recommended, (A Recommendation) there is insufficient evidence at this time to recommend that routine use of ABR or OCE for hearing screening of healthy babies should replace regular assessment of hearing during well-baby visits using parental questioning and the clap test. Additionally, there is insufficient evidence at this time to recommend that routine ultrasound examination of the hips should replace clinical assessment of the hips in the nursery and during well-baby visits. Repeat examination of the eyes for strabismus is recommended during well-baby visits, especially during the first six months (A Recommendation). There is fair evidence to assess developmental milestones at each visit, since, for infants with developmental delay due to lack of stimulation, an enriched environment may be effective (B Recommendation). There is fair evidence for serial measurements of height, weight and head circumference (B Recommendation).

Unanswered Questions (Research Agenda)

1. Is routine hearing screening of healthy babies using ABR or OCE more effective than traditional means during well-baby visits, in terms of the long-term outcome of oral language development?

2. Is routine hip screening using ultrasound more effective than clinical assessment in terms of long-term outcome?

3. The optimum frequency and timing of well baby visits needs to established.

Evidence

A MEDLINE search from 1990 to May 1993 was conducted for the mesh headings hip dislocation, congenital, heart defects, congenital, mass screening, ocular motility disorders, hearing disorders, counselling, accident, child abuse, crying, sleep disorders, child development disorders, and child behavior. This review was undertaken in May 1993 and updates a report published in 1990. Recommendations were finalized by the Task Force in March 1994.

Selected References

1. Canadian Task Force on the Periodic Health Examination: The periodic health examination, 1990 update: 4. Well-baby care in the first 2 years of life. *Can Med Assoc J* 1990; 143(9); 867-872

2. Rosendahl K, Markestad T, Lie RT: Ultrasound in the early diagnosis of congenital dislocation of the hip: the significance of hip stability versus acetabular morphology. *Pediatr Radiol* 1992; 22: 430-433

3. Krikler SJ, Dwyer NS: Comparison of results of two approaches to hip screening in infants. *J Bone Joint Surg Br* 1992; 74(5): 701-703

4. Early identification of hearing impairment in infants and young children. *NIH Consens Statement* 1993; 11(1): 1-24

5. Rickert VI, Johnson CM: Reducing nocturnal awakening and crying in infants and young children: a comparison between scheduled awakenings and systematic ignoring. *Pediatrics* 1988; 81: 203-212

6. Dunn PM, Evans RE, Thearle MJ, *et al*: Congenital dislocation of the hip: early and late diagnosis and management compared. *Arch Dis Child* 1985; 60: 407-414

7. Dershewitz RA, Williamson JW: Prevention of childhood injuries: a controlled clinical trial. *Am J Public Health* 1977; 67: 1148-1153

8. Kelly B, Sein C, McCarthy PL: Safety education in a pediatric primary care setting. *Pediatrics* 1987; 79: 818-824

9. Reisinger KS, Bires JA: Anticipatory guidance in pediatric practice. *Pediatrics* 1980; 66: 889-892

10. Lang J: The optimum time for surgical alignment in congenital esotropia. *J Pediatr Ophthalmol Strabismus* 1984; 21: 74-75

11. Schweinhart LJ, Wikart DP: What do we know so far? A review of the Head Start Synthesis Project. *Young Children* 1986; 41: 45-55

12. U.S. Preventive Services Task Force: *Guide to Clinical Preventive Services: an Assessment of the Effectiveness of 169 Interventions*. Williams & Wilkins, Baltimore, Md, 1989: 315-320

Well-Baby Care in the First 2 Years of Life

MANEUVER	EFFECTIVENESS	LEVEL OF EVIDENCE	RECOMMENDATION
Counselling to reduce risk factors in the home	Families counselled about risk factors for accidental injury in the home have fewer risk factors at follow-up visits than those not counselled.	Randomized controlled trial<7> (I)	Good evidence to include in periodic health examination (A)
Anticipatory guidance for night-time crying	Families complying with appropriate counselling have fewer problems with night-time crying than those not counselled.	Randomized controlled trial<5> (I)	Good evidence to include in periodic health examination (A)
Repeated examination of hips, eyes and hearing, especially in the first year of life	Outcome better with early than with late detection and treatment of congenital hip dislocation, amblyopia and hearing impairment.	Cohort studies<2,3,6-8> (II-2); expert opinion<4> (III)	Good evidence to include in periodic health examination on basis of good detection maneuvers, effective treatment and alleviation of burden of suffering (A)
Enquiries about the achievement of milestones at each visit	Other than the prevention of phenylketonuria and hypothyroidism (usually diagnosed by screening in the neonatal period) few preventive measures are available for mental retardation; for environmentally deprived infants an enriched environment may enhance normal mental development.	Cohort study<11> (II-2)	Fair evidence to include in periodic health examination (B)
Serial measurements of height, weight and head circumference	Treatment effective and efficacious for short stature due to hypothyroidism, hypopitutitarism, and congenital adrenal hyperplasia.	Cohort<2> (II-2)	There is fair evidence to include in the periodic health examination (B)
	The appropriate frequency of measurement is unclear.	Expert opinion<2,12> (III)	

Note: For recommendations on other pediatric issues see section on Pediatric Preventive Care and Immunizations of Children and Adults

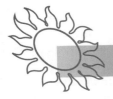

CHAPTER 25

Screening Children for Lead Exposure in Canada

By William Feldman and Patricia Randel

Screening Children for Lead Exposure in Canada

Adapted to the Canadian context by **William Feldman, MD, FRCPC**[1] and **Patricia Randel, MSc**[2] drawing freely from the manuscript prepared for the U.S. Preventive Services Task Force[3]

Lead is a heavy metal that can affect virtually every organ system in the body, particularly the nervous, hematologic and gastrointestinal systems. It is widely distributed throughout the environment because of contamination from energy production, metallurgy and associated processes.

In 1991, the U.S. Centers for Disease Control and Prevention (CDC) revised their intervention level for lead toxicity from blood lead (BPb) levels of 25 µg/dL to 15 µg/dL.<1> The CDC now recommends I) screening virtually all children for lead exposure at 12 and 24 months; 2) screening children at high risk every 6 months beginning at 6 months of age; and 3) using direct measurement of BPb rather than erythrocyte protoporphyrin (EP) to screen.

A recommendation for universal screening with BPb assumes that many children have mild (10-24 µg/dL) or moderate (25-44 µg/dL) lead exposure, that this condition can be accurately and reliably detected by available screening tests, that the condition is harmful to children, that detection results in meaningful health benefits, and that such benefits outweigh the risks associated with intervention. (Note: The units µg/dL will be used throughout this chapter. To convert to umol/L, divide by 20.72.)

In adapting these criteria to the Canadian context the Canadian Task Force finds fair evidence to support targeted screening by blood lead (BPb) determination in high-risk infants and children (B Recommendation) but insufficient evidence to recommend for or against universal screening in Canada. (C Recommendation).

---

[1] Professor of Pediatrics, Preventive Medicine and Biostatistics, University of Toronto, Toronto, Ontario
[2] Research Associate for the Canadian Task Force on the Periodic Health Examination, Department of Pediatrics, Dalhousie University, Halifax, Nova Scotia
[3] By Carolyn DiGuiseppi, Science Advisor, U.S. Preventive Services Task Force, Washington, D.C.

This review examines published evidence regarding mild and moderate lead exposure in order to determine whether a recommendation for universal screening to detect these levels is supportable in Canada. Studies of adults occupationally exposed to lead were excluded from consideration.

Burden of Suffering

Short-term acute exposure to high levels of lead can cause a metallic taste, abdominal pain, vomiting, diarrhea, convulsions, coma or even death. Long-term exposure may lead to anemia, learning disabilities and hyperactivity, problems with memory and attention span, as well as lack of appetite, abdominal pain, irritability and impaired kidney function.

Prevalence

The prevalence of neurotoxic lead levels in asymptomatic children in Canada is unknown. Surveys which have been conducted in Canada in the last fifteen years revealed that most Canadian children have blood lead levels below 10µg/dL and that the levels of lead exposure have declined. However variations in the reported prevalence of lead exposure in different communities and populations suggest that important local differences may exist. Clinically recognized lead poisoning is a rare event among Canadian children, and chelation therapy is rarely used. Lead poisoning is insignificant when compared to poisoning by other drugs.

Clinically recognized lead exposure is a rare event among Canadian children, and chelation therapy is rarely used

In 1978, *The Canada Health Survey*, the only national survey of blood lead levels in children, reported that 90.3% of boys and 100% of girls aged 3 to 4 years had blood lead levels below 10 µg/dL. In 1986, the Royal Commission on Lead in the Canadian Environment concluded that the blood lead levels for children and adults above the action level of 25 µg/dL were substantially less prevalent in Canada than in the large urban areas of other countries and were the lowest reported for all countries from which comparable data were available. These findings also applied to "hot spots", such as downtown areas, near lead smelters, lead-using industries, mines, concentrators, or other metallurgical industries.

A recent summary of blood lead surveys in Canada from 1979 to 1989 also found that the mean blood lead level in preschool children was less than 10 µg/dL, except in areas where the soil was contaminated.

The Ontario Ministry of Public Health, Public Health Branch have conducted surveys of blood lead levels from 1984 to 1992 in 4-6 year olds in downtown Toronto and estimated that under 4% of Ontario 4-6 year olds were in the 11-14 µg/dL range. They also reported that the mean blood lead levels in this age group had fallen from 12 µg/dL in 1984 to 3.5 µg/dL in 1992. Two recent Canadian studies comparing blood lead levels of pre-school children in smelting towns (Trail B.C., and Rouyn-Noranda, P.Q.) from the mid-1970s to the late 1980s have also reported similar findings, reporting declines of about 45%.

Cross-sectional studies of blood lead levels in urban, suburban and rural Quebec and Ontario children found geometric means of ≤10 µg/dL.[2,3] In a 1989 study in Vancouver about 7% of preschool children had a blood lead level of 9.94 µg/dL and mean blood lead level was 5.39 µg/dL.

A 1991 cross-sectional study in Saint John, New Brunswick revealed that among 23 children and 68 adults tested, 53% had blood lead levels above 25 µg/dL. A second survey of 205 individuals found that 50 were above 25 µg/dL. In a third study of 97 city children aged 1-3 years, 11.3% of participants had levels above 25 µg/dL. Mean blood lead levels were 4.77 µg/dL (range 1.2 µg/dL-18 µg/dL) in males and 5.6 µg/dL (range 1.4- 17.6 µg/dL) in females.[4]

Studies conducted on neonates in urban Toronto and urban, suburban and rural Quebec reported a geometric mean of <2 µg/dL.[5] Ninety-nine percent of the Toronto infants studied had cord blood lead levels below 7.04 µg/dL as compared to 34% in a similar study conducted in Boston and in Port Pirie, Australia, a high-risk area.

In the U.S., a national survey of BPb levels conducted as part of the National Health and Nutrition Examination Survey II (NHANES II) in 1976-1980 found that average blood lead levels, adjusted for race, sex, age, urbanization, etc., had decreased approximately 37% between 1976 and 1980. This decline correlated significantly with the concurrent decline in the use of leaded gasoline. Wide variations between communities suggested that community rather than national prevalence surveys were required to determine the need for screening and intervention.

Periodic population-based samples of BPb levels from Europe also have shown continuing declines in blood lead levels associated with reductions in the use of leaded gasoline over the past decade.[6,7]

Sources of Lead in the Environment

Sources of environmental lead exposure include: lead-based paint; soil and dust from paint, gasoline, and industrial sources; drinking water; certain occupations and hobbies; airborne lead from point sources such as lead smelters; and lead-contaminated food (from sources such as lead-soldered cans, the rain and soil in which food plants were grown, storage and serving vessels, and dust in the home).<1> Certain traditional ethnic remedies have also been associated with lead exposure.<8>

The individual contributions of each of these lead sources to the overall body burden of lead is not well-defined, primarily because of the lack of large population-based representative samples of concurrent measures of BPb levels and environmental lead exposures.

In Canada, the *Hazardous Product Act* has imposed strict federal legislation which has reduced lead levels in food, interior paint, furniture, and coatings of children's toys. Lead pipes and solder are prohibited but may still contribute to increased levels of lead in drinking water in areas with highly acidic water.

Paint

In the United States, lead-based paint is thought to be the most common high-dose source of lead exposure for children, and is an important source of household dust lead.<1> By contrast, in Canada, elevated blood lead levels due to lead dust from paint and pica are less commonly reported at levels higher than 10µg/dL, although cases may go undetected and/or unreported. Lead-based paint was in widespread use until the 1950s when the use of lead-based paint and its lead concentration began to decline. The manufacture of leaded paint was banned in Canada in 1972 and in the United States in 1978 although it is still available for industrial, military and marine use.

Although most Canadian experts feel that paint as a source of lead exposure is dramatically less significant in Canada than in the United States, a recent article cautions that "sound scientific data supporting this position are lacking".<2>

Lead paint exposure from housing has been associated with lead toxicity as measured by BPb levels.<4,9,10> Houses built prior to 1950 are the most likely to contain paint with high concentrations of lead. The risks of exposure from leaded paint and household dust are greatest when the paint is in deteriorated condition, as when chipped or peeling. In a recent cross-sectional study, peeling paint was found to be a significant factor associated with elevated blood lead levels in children living in the city of Saint John, New Brunswick.<4>

Remodelling and renovations of older houses can also produce increased levels of lead in the environment, increasing children's risk of toxicity.

In its 1986 report, the Royal Commission on Lead in the Canadian Environment was unable to identify any case where lead paint was definitely implicated in raised blood lead levels among groups of children. Since then isolated cases of acute lead poisoning with profound sequelae from chronic ingestion of lead-based paint have been reported in London, Ontario, Winnipeg, Manitoba and Halifax,

Nova Scotia. Other cases may have occurred but are not easily identified or are asymptomatic.

Air

Blood lead levels of Canadians have shown a consistent decline over the past fifteen years, attributed largely to the removal of lead from gasoline.

Blood lead levels of Canadians have shown a consistent decline over the past fifteen years

Soil

Lead in soil and dust are also important sources of exposure, despite recent declines in its use in paint, gasoline, and industry. Soil lead levels near roadways and adjacent to lead smelters are typically thousands of times higher than natural levels.

Water

Water lead concentration has also been found to correlate with BPb concentrations.<2,11> In the city of Saint John, New Brunswick, it was reported in 1990 that 13% of homes surveyed had lead levels of 50 parts per million (ppm). The acceptable level according to the Canadian Guideline is 0.01 ppm. Blood lead levels have been found to be significantly associated ($p<0.05$) with living in certain areas of the city, lead pipes from the main water line leading into the home or lead pipes in the home and using hot water directly from the tap in preparing food.<4>

Risk Factors for Increased BPb Levels

Risk factors for elevated BPb levels relate either directly or indirectly to the sources of lead exposure described above. The most important demographic risk factor is probably age. Blood levels tend to rise after birth, peak between 18 months and 2 years of age, and decline gradually through adolescence.<12,13> Possible contributors to this age effect include ingestion of lead in food at a greater quantity relative to body weight compared to adults, increased efficiency of gastrointestinal lead absorption, and normal hand-to-mouth activity in young children that results in their frequently placing their dirty hands and other objects into their mouths.

Several recent cohort studies have attempted to clarify the contributions of various sociodemographic risk factors to BPb levels with conflicting results.<4,14> Given the correlational nature of sociodemographic risk factors, however, it is possible that both lead indices and social factors may be associated with other unmeasured factors related to environment lead exposure. This is particularly important because of their potential role as confounders in evaluating the effects of lead on childhood growth and development, since sociodemographic factors have important independent effects on these outcomes.

Household members may also be exposed to high lead levels from clothing or waste material brought home by workers in lead-based industries or hobbies.[1]

Neurobehavioural Effects of Lead

Exposure to very high levels of inorganic lead associated with blood lead levels >70 µg/dL can cause convulsions and coma, sometimes resulting in death or long-term sequelae.[1] Neurotoxic effects may occur at BPb levels much lower than 80 µg/dL; the threshold (if any) for such effects in humans, particularly children, is unknown. The principal concern of recent research has been the risk of neurodevelopmental dysfunction in children, related to the effects of lead on the immature, rapidly developing nervous system.

Evidence that reductions of moderate BPb levels (25-55 µg/dL) may benefit children's cognitive function comes from a recent prospective cohort study evaluating chelation therapy and iron supplementation (for iron deficient or depleted children) in 154 children aged 13-87 months, all of whom received "largely successful" household lead abatement.[15] At 6-months follow-up, changes in cognitive function were significantly associated with reductions in BPb level after controlling for confounding variables. The cognitive index increased 1 point for every 3 µg/dL decrease in BPb level over the 6 month period.

No prospective studies evaluating associations between reductions in mildly elevated BPb and improvements in cognition have been identified. There is currently fair evidence that low level lead exposure as measured by BPb has a statistically significant effect on IQ or related measures of cognitive function but the clinical significance is unknown. In the past two decades, many studies[12-39] have evaluated lead exposure (as measured by BPb) and cognitive function in children, but few have found a significant effect of mild to moderate exposure on neurobehavioural function in children. Results from different studies have been inconsistent, effect sizes have been small, and few associations have been statistically significant. Many studies included children with moderate rather than low (10-24 µg/dL) BPb levels. The effects, if any, of low BPb levels on cognition are likely to be even smaller.

It is possible, however that these studies were unable to demonstrate a major effect because 1) intelligence may not be the best measure of neurologic damage due to lead; 2) sample sizes were too small to detect an effect; or 3) BPb may be an inadequate measure of exposure.

BPb levels primarily reflect recent exposure (i.e. over the last 3-5 weeks) and correlate poorly with lead levels in shed deciduous teeth,[17] which may better represent chronic or cumulative exposure. Mean dentine lead levels increase with duration of exposure to high levels of domestic water lead, and with age. Tooth (or dentine) lead may therefore represent cumulative lead exposure, in which case the causal linkage between cognitive function and high tooth lead levels would be clearer than between cognitive function and high BPb levels. Studies of tooth lead therefore may raise fewer methodologic questions than those of BPb, and a number of such studies have recently been conducted. Studies using dentine lead concentrations have shown consistent associations between increased lead and decreased IQ, although effect sizes have been quite small and not always statistically significant,[16,17,40-46] and some of these studies have suffered from methodologic errors.

There is fair evidence that lead exposure as measured by tooth lead is associated with (perhaps not causally) a small reduction in IQ test scores. There is limited evidence that tooth lead is associated with inferior long-term scholastic achievement.[40,41] Studies of the effects of mild lead exposure, as reflected by tooth lead levels, on long-term scholastic achievement need to be replicated. Continued research on the effect of lead on neurobehavioural function, with attention to improved measurement of lead burden and to adequate control of potential confounding, is essential.

One problem with evaluating the neurobehavioral effects of lead exposure using IQ tests is that they may not be the best measure of neurologic dysfunction. Significant, associations between concurrent BPb and visual-motor integration and delayed reaction times at low to moderate levels have been reported.[17,18,20,21] The clinical significance of this finding is unclear and may reflect attentional deficits.

While large cross-sectional studies have suggested an association between current BPb levels and stature, the study designs limit their ability to establish a causal relationship. There is fair evidence that prenatal mild and moderate lead exposure does not affect growth, and insufficient evidence to support or refute an adverse effect of postnatal lead exposure on growth. Continued research appears warranted.

Lead and Anemia

Lead exposure also affects red blood cells, typically causing anemia. There have been few reports of anemia due to lead exposure at BPb levels ≤25 μg/dL.

Maneuver

Most studies of lead effects have used blood lead concentrations as the indicator of lead toxicity, in part because it is a relatively simple and inexpensive test to perform. A single blood lead level cannot distinguish between recent exposure to a high level of lead and chronic exposure resulting in a steady state level.

The precision and reliability of BPb measurements at low and moderate levels may be affected by environmental lead contamination during blood collection and by laboratory analytic variation. Skin lead contamination may also be a problem, particularly with capillary blood sampling. However, studies have demonstrated that adequate attention to methods that minimize the risk of contamination using either capillary or venous sampling results in similar BPb levels.<47-49> Regarding analytic variation, current proficiency testing program criteria for blood lead require that reported results are within ±4 μg/dL of target values for values ≤40 μg/dL.<50> At BPb levels as low as 10-25 μg/dL, analytic variability of ±4 μg/dL and small errors caused by environmental contamination could lead to inappropriate decisions regarding intervention. Sending a repeat specimen to a different laboratory could increase analytic variation, since between-method variability tends to exceed within-laboratory variability.<1,50,51> Methods for determining BPb have good precision and accuracy but tend to be expensive, cumbersome and relatively slow.<50-52> Among Canadian laboratories specializing in blood lead analysis one would expect at least 10% of the samples to be misclassified if the cutoff point were 10 μg/dL. Changes in BPb levels up to ±8 μg/dL may be due to error and variability.

Erythrocyte Protoporphyrin (EP) measurement is inexpensive, unaffected by environmental lead contamination, is easily performed on capillary blood specimens, and is a better indicator of chronic lead exposure than BPb measurement. However, it appears to lack sensitivity and specificity for lead exposure in the low to moderate range, using BPb as the reference standard.

Inexpensive, non-invasive methods for assessing total body lead burden are clearly needed, particularly for low levels. Until such methods are available, measuring BPb appears to be the best alternative for screening for lead exposure.

Effectiveness of Prevention and Treatment

There have been no controlled trials to demonstrate that routine screening for BPb results in better clinical outcomes than either targeted screening or case-finding, but uncontrolled time series have suggested that screening high-risk populations may be effective in improving clinical outcome when compared to case-finding.<53,54> No controlled trials of targeted screening, and no studies of any kind evaluating universal screening or the health benefits of screening to detect mild or moderate lead exposure, were found in our literature review.

There have been no controlled trials to demonstrate that routine screening for BPb results in better clinical outcomes than either targeted screening or case finding

The rationale behind detecting BPb >10 µg/dL is that identification of such levels allows initiation of interventions that will prevent complications of lead toxicity or will prevent subsequent increases in BPb to toxic levels. Controlled trials demonstrating that interventions for persons who have mild to moderate lead exposure produce better outcomes than no intervention have not been reported. Without intervention, mean BPb levels are known to decrease as children age (after a peak at about age 2 years).[12,13] To evaluate adequately the effects of interventions on BPb levels, studies must take into account changes over time, preferably by using untreated controls.

Environmental Lead Abatement

There is good evidence against the use of soil-abatement to reduce BPb levels in children with mild lead exposure, and no evidence concerning clinical benefits of this intervention.[55] There is fair evidence that residential deleading results in significant BPb reductions in children with BPb levels $\geq$25 µg/dL.[56] Data of a beneficial effect on cognitive function of residential deleading with children who have moderately elevated lead levels are limited to a single cohort study.[12] Most studies of residential deleading suffer from important design flaws, particularly the absence of adequate controls and limited follow-up. One-time dust abatement has little effect on BPb in children with mild exposure,[55] but frequent, careful cleaning to reduce lead dust levels appears to cause modest, long-term reductions in BPb levels in children with moderate lead exposure,[57] and is likely to cost substantially less than deleading.

Pharmacologic Intervention

In children with symptomatic, severe lead exposure, treatment with dimercaprol (BAL) plus $CaNa_2$-EDTA appears to reduce morbidity and mortality (Comparisons of times and places, Grade II-3) evidence.[58-64] Treatment of children with severe ($\geq$ 55 µg/dL), asymptomatic lead exposure with EDTA or succimer reduces BPb levels to the range where the risk of encephalopathy or death is low, and these effects (at least for EDTA) may be long-lasting (Grade II-3) evidence).[61,65-69]

A large cohort study of EDTA chelation therapy in children aged 13-87 months with BPb levels between 25 and 55 µg/dL[15,70] found no association between chelation and reductions in BPb, bone lead or EP concentration, or improvements in cognitive function. Chelating agents have been associated with short-term reduction in BPb levels in before-after studies,[71-73] but these effects have not been sustained in the absence of other interventions.

Succimer, an oral chelating agent, was approved by the U.S. Food and Drug Administration in 1991 for use in children with BPb levels >45 µg/dL, and appears to have fewer adverse effects than BAL or EDTA. Neither has been evaluated in placebo-controlled trials in children with asymptomatic exposure at levels below 55µg/dl.

Penicillamine has been evaluated in two recent retrospective cohort studies of patients with BPb levels 25 to 40 µg/dL[72,73] with encouraging results. However, neither study describes results of long-term follow-up.

No controlled trials evaluating the efficacy or effectiveness of nutritional intervention (such as caloric, calcium or iron supplementation) for children with mild or moderate lead exposure were found.

Adverse Effects of Screening

The adverse effects of venipuncture for initial screening for lead toxicity are minimal, including rare complications of infection or bleeding. Problems may be associated with follow-up findings including financial costs and the inconvenience and anxiety associated with EDTA lead mobilization tests (LMT), although none of these effects have been evaluated in controlled studies. The LMT requires intramuscular or intravenous infusion, a stay at the clinical center for at least 8 hours, and for young children, application of urine collection bags, which are clearly not minor inconveniences. The potential risks associated with EDTA mobilization tests include those of EDTA therapy (see Adverse Effects of Intervention below), which primarily affects renal function. The use of EDTA alone in patients with very high BPb levels has been reported to aggravate neurologic symptoms.[1] However, no evidence of adverse neurologic effects from the current dosage used for the LMT in patients with moderate lead exposure has been reported. A recent study of low income California children revealed that only 0.12% had BPb >25 µg/dl and with a calculated cost of $19,139 to detect each of these children. The 6 children so identified were asymptomatic. Public health resources used to identify these children might have been used more effectively elsewhere.[74]

Adverse Effects of Intervention

For patients identified with lead exposure, interventions in the form of lead abatement or chelation therapy may also produce adverse effects. Residential deleading may result in significant increase in BPb levels during or immediately after the abatement process among resident children and lead abatement workers.[56,75-77]

Both EDTA and BAL treatment have substantial toxicity, are invasive (requiring intravenous or intramuscular injection) and generally require hospitalization.[1] Side effects, including mild fever, transient elevations of hepatic transaminase, lacrimation, paresthesias, tachycardia and increases in blood pressure have been reported in 30 to 50% of patients although most side effects are transient.

Early case reports of EDTA use at high doses have described acute renal failure and death in a number of patients.[78] Therapeutic EDTA at the lower doses currently used has been reported to cause transient increases in serum creatinine in 13% and reversible oliguric acute renal failure in 3% of 130 children.[79] However, in a series of 608 children treated with EDTA (± penicillamine) over a two year period, only one patient developed proteinuria and edema.[53] EDTA is a non-specific chelator, and has been associated with a 17-fold increase in the daily rate of zinc loss in urine.[80]

The principal adverse effects of d-penicillamine are penicillin-sensitivity-like reactions, such as rashes, leukopenia, and eosinophilia.[53,69,72]

Adverse effects reported in studies of succimer have been uncommon and mild, although clinical experience with this drug is limited compared to other chelators.

Recommendations of Other Groups

The Federal/Provincial Committee on Environmental and Occupational Health is currently finalizing recommendations which will be published in the fall of 1994. *The Final Report of The Royal Society of Canada*, had the following recommendations: 1) surveys of blood lead levels for the identification of "hot spots"; 2) annual screening during periods of clean-up; and 3) that wherever possible, such surveys be included in surveys undertaken for other purposes. The U.S. Preventive Services Task Force recommendation is currently under review. The U.S. Centers for Disease Control and Prevention (CDC)[1] recommend: 1) universal screening for all children ages 6 months to 6 years, except in communities where it has been demonstrated in large numbers of children (number not specified) that no lead exposure exists; 2) BPb levels beginning at 6 months for children defined as high-risk for high-dose lead exposure based on a brief questionnaire, and at 12-15 months for all other children, with follow-up screening schedules based on risk assessment and previous BPb levels; and 3) that pediatric health-care providers teach parents how to prevent lead exposure, tailoring guidance to likely hazards in the community.

Conclusions and Recommendations

Recent studies suggest that in populations presumed to be at high risk (based on sociodemographics or housing characteristics), the prevalence of mild, moderate, and severe lead exposure is highly variable, with 10-fold differences among different communities. These data suggest a need for each community to conduct its own surveys to determine actual risk. The need for screening is dictated in part by the likelihood of detecting substantial numbers of cases.

A questionnaire developed by the CDC appears to have a sensitivity of 64-87% (based on published studies) for detecting PBb ≤10 µg/dL, but its sensitivity for detecting moderate or severe lead exposure is unknown and it was not designed as a screening tool. No studies evaluating the CDC or any other questionnaire in a Canadian setting have been reported. Although specificity is poor, use of a validated questionnaire of known and acceptable sensitivity could reduce substantially the number of children requiring screening with BPb to detect those with increased levels.

While there is fair evidence that modest neurobehavioral dysfunction in children is associated with mild to moderate lead exposure as measured by tooth lead levels, the same association with low BPb levels is not clearly established. Since high BPb levels are clearly associated with neurotoxic effects, it is possible that the small effects likely to be seen with mild to moderate BPb exposure are not detectable with current psychometric tests, or that BPb is not a sufficiently accurate measure of lead exposure to detect these effects. Since lead is known to have many toxic effects, it may have effects at low levels, although the clinical importance of such effect sizes for the individual is questionable. On a population basis however, the cumulative effects of small reductions in IQ might be substantial.

For moderate lead exposure (25-49 µg/dL), no association was found between chelation with EDTA and improvements in IQ, and other interventions have not been evaluated with regard to morbidity. Scientific studies of adequate quality evaluating the ability of chelation or residential deleading to produce sustained reductions in moderately elevated BPb levels appear to have given equivocal results. In the experimental setting, twice monthly dust abatement by a research assistant has shown modest long-term reductions of moderately elevated (30-50 µg/dL) BPb levels, although the effectiveness of counselling families to provide this intervention in their homes has not been evaluated.

We found no studies that evaluated the effectiveness of early detection of mild lead exposure in improving clinical outcomes. Good evidence from a randomized controlled trial showed little effect on low BPb levels from either soil abatement or one-time interior dust abatement. Adequate studies evaluating chelation, residential deleading or other interventions, such as nutrition counselling, for mild lead exposure have not been reported.

One might argue that results from studies at high levels should be extrapolated to lower levels. However, the available evidence shows little or no benefit from intervention at low to moderate levels. In addition, there are important risks associated with such interventions, including substantial increases in BPb levels with residential deleading, and the potential for adverse effects from chelation therapy.

Given the low prevalence of elevated BPb levels in the general Canadian population, the relatively small burden of suffering from low to moderate lead exposure, and the limited data demonstrating the effectiveness of intervention, there is currently insufficient evidence to recommend for or against universal BPb screening of children to detect mild or moderate lead exposure (C Recommendation).

On the other hand, there are children who are at high risk for severe lead exposure either because of individual risk factors or because the prevalence in their community is high. These children may already be at increased risk for neurobehavioral dysfunction because of poverty, malnutrition, etc., and are more likely to have BPb levels in the range for which intervention has shown some effectiveness. They are therefore more likely to benefit from screening for lead toxicity (B Recommendation). In communities known to have very high prevalences of lead exposure (e.g., in certain inner cities, or near lead smelters), targeted screening may be more efficient and is most sensitive.

Clinical Intervention

Children found to have BPb ≥50 µg/dL should be treated according to current standards for chelation and/or environmental deleading. There is currently insufficient evidence to recommend for or against chelation therapy or residential deleading as a preventive maneuver for children with blood lead levels 10-49 µg/dL. Soil abatement and one-time household dust abatement are not recommended for the households of children with BPb levels ≤20 µg/dL.

For primary prevention of lead exposure, clinicians should consider informing families living in homes built before 1950, especially those in deteriorated condition, of the potential benefits of regular cleaning to reduce lead dust, including twice monthly wet-mopping with a high-phosphate detergent cleanser of all surfaces containing (or presumed to contain) high lead levels.

Unanswered Questions (Research Agenda)

The following have been identified as research priorities:

1. Evaluation of the many other contributors to neurologic dysfunction that may interact with lead, such as nutritional factors, genetic susceptibilities, and other toxins (including cigarettes and alcohol).

2. Evaluation of the ability of residential abatement, oral chelation therapy, nutritional interventions, and physician counselling to reduce low to moderate BPb levels, especially on a long-term basis.

3. Determination of the long-term effects on neurobehavioral dysfunction of reducing low to moderate lead levels.

4. Validation of questionnaires to screen for children at increased risk of lead exposure, particularly in rural and minority populations.

Evidence

The literature was identified using a MEDLINE search in the English language using the key words: Lead or lead Poisoning or plumbism with subheadings for potential lead sources such as dust and paint, screening methods, neurobehavioral testing and dysfunction in children, reproductive outcomes, environmental abatement and chelating agents for the years 1989 through October 1993. The review was initiated by the Task Force in March 1993 and the Recommendations finalized in January 1994.

Acknowledgements

The Task Force thanks Sarah Shea, MD, FRCP, Assistant Professor, Department of Pediatrics, Dalhousie University, Halifax, NS, for reviewing the draft report.

Selected References

1. Centers for Disease Control: *Preventing lead poisoning in young children. A statement by the Centers for Disease Control – October 1991*. Atlanta: U.S. Department of Health and Human Services, 1991

2. Levallois P, Weber JP, Gingras D, *et al*: Lead exposure of children living in the Quebec city area. *Environ Geochem Hlth* 1990; 13: 308-314

3. Poon HC, Carson R, Peter F, *et al*: The lead program at CPRI. *Clin Biochem* 1989; 22: 213-219

4. Balram C: *Study of blood lead levels in children living in Saint John, New Brunswick*. Health and Community Services, New Brunswick, June 1993

5. Rhainds M, Levallois P, Bernard PM, *et al*: 8th International conference in heavy metals in the environment, Edinburgh, 16-20 Sept. 1991

6. Ducoffre G, Claeys F, Bruaux P: Lowering time trend of blood lead levels in Belgium since 1978. *Environ Res* 1990; 51: 25-34

7. Schutz A, Attewell R, Skerfving S: Decreasing blood lead in Swedish children, 1978-1988. *Arch Environ Health* 1989; 44: 391-394

8. Centers for Disease Control and Prevention: Lead poisoning associated with use of traditional ethnic remedies – California, 1991-1992. *MMWR Morb Mortal Wkly Rep* 1993; 42: 521-524

9. Agency for Toxic Substances and Disease Registry: The nature and extent of lead poisoning in children in the United States: a report to Congress. Atlanta: U.S. Department of Health and Human Services, Public Health Service, 1988; DHHS document no. 99-2966

10. Schwartz J, Levin R: The risk of lead toxicity in homes with lead paint hazard. *Environ Res* 1991; 54: 1-7

11. Davies DJA, Thornton I, Watt JM, *et al*: Lead intake and blood lead in two-year-old U.K. urban children. *Sci Total Environ* 1990; 90: 13-29

12. Cooney GH, Bell A, McBride W, *et al*: Low-level exposures to lead: the Sydney Lead Study. *Devel Med Child Neurol* 1989; 31: 640-649

13. Dietrich KN, Succop PA, Bornschein RL, *et al*: Lead exposure and neurobehavioural development in later infancy. *Environ Health Perspect* 1990; 89: 13-19

14. Baghurst PA, Tong SL, McMichael AJ, *et al*: Determinants of blood lead concentrations to age 5 years in a birth cohort study of children living in the lead smelting city of Port Pirie and surrounding areas. *Arch Environ Health* 1992; 47: 203-210

15. Ruff HA, Bijur PE, Markowitz M, *et al*: Declining blood lead levels and cognitive changes in moderately lead-poisoned children. *JAMA* 1993; 269: 1641-1646

16. Needleman HL, Gatsonis CA: Low-level lead exposure and the IQ of children. A meta-analysis of modern studies. *JAMA* 1990; 263: 673-678

17. Bergomi M, Borella P, Fantuzzi G, *et al*: Relationship between lead exposure indicators and neuropsychological performance in children. *Devel Med Child Neurol* 1989; 31: 181-190

18. Winneke G, Brockhaus A, Ewers U, *et al*: Results from the European multicenter study on lead neurotoxicity in children: implications for risk assessment. *Neurotoxicol Teratol* 1990; 12: 553-559

19. Ernhart CB, Wolf AW, Sokol RJ, *et al*: Fetal lead exposure: antenatal factors. *Environ Res* 1985; 38: 54-66

20. Winneke G, Beginn U, Ewert T, *et al*: Comparing the effects of perinatal and later childhood lead exposure on neuropsychological outcome. *Environ Res* 1985; 38: 155-167

21. Winneke G, Brockhaus A, Collet W, *et al*: Modulation of lead-induced performance deficit in children by varying signal rate in a serial choice reaction task. *Neurotoxicol Teratol* 1989; 11: 587-592

22. Wigg NR, Vimpani GV, McMichael AJ, *et al*: Port Pirie Cohort Study: childhood blood lead and neuropsychological development at age two years. *J Epidemiol Community Health* 1988; 42: 213-219

23. McMichael AJ, Baghurst PA, Wigg NR, *et al*: Port Pirie Cohort Study: environmental exposure to lead and children's abilities at the age of four years. *N Engl J Med* 1988; 319: 468-475

24. Baghurst PA, McMichael AJ, Wigg NR, *et al*: Environmental exposure to lead and children's intelligence at the age of seven years. The Port Pirie Cohort Study. *N Engl J Med* 1992; 327: 1279-1284

25. Cooney GH, Bell A, McBride W, *et al*: Neurobehavioural consequences of prenatal low level exposures to lead. *Neurotoxicol Teratol* 1989; 11: 95-104

26. Bellinger DC, Needleman HL, Leviton A, *et al*: Early sensory-motor development and prenatal exposure to lead. *Neurobehav Toxicol Teratol* 1984; 6: 387-402

27. Bellinger D, Leviton A, Needleman HL, *et al*: Low-level lead exposure and infant development in the first year. *Neurobehav Toxicol Teratol* 1986; 8: 151-161

28. Bellinger D, Leviton A, Waternaux C, *et al*: Longitudinal analyses of prenatal and postnatal lead exposure and early cognitive development. *N Engl J Med* 1987; 316: 1037-1043

29. Bellinger D, Sloman J, Leviton A, *et al*: Low-level lead exposure and children's cognitive function in the preschool years. *Pediatrics* 1991; 87: 219-227

30. Bellinger D, Leviton A, Sloman J: Antecedants and correlates of improved cognitive performance in children exposed in utero to low levels of lead. *Environ Health Perspect* 1990; 89: 5-11

31. Bellinger DC, Stiles KM, Needleman HL: Low level lead exposure, intelligence and academic achievement: a long-term follow-up study. *Pediatrics* 1992; 90: 855-861

32. Dietrich KN, Krafft KM, Bornschein RL, *et al*: Low-level fetal lead exposure effect on neurobehavioural development in early infancy. *Pediatrics* 1987; 80: 721-730

33. Dietrich KN, Krafft KM, Bier M, *et al*: Early effects of fetal lead exposure: neurobehavioural findings at 6 months. *Int J Biosocial Res* 1986; 8: 151-168

34. Dietrich KN, Succop PA, Berger OG, *et al*: Lead exposure and the cognitive development of urban preschool children: the Cincinnati Lead Study Cohort at age 4 years. *Neurotoxicol Teratol* 1991; 13: 203-211

35. Dietrich KN, Succop PA, Berger OG, *et al*: Lead exposure and the central auditory processing abilities and cognitive development of urban children: the Cincinnati Lead Study cohort at age 5 years. *Neurotoxicol Teratol* 1992; 14: 51-56

36. Ernhart CB, Wolf AW, Kennard MJ, *et al*: Intrauterine exposure to low levels of lead: the status of the neonate. *Arch Environ Health* 1986; 41: 287-291

37. Ernhart CB, Morrow-Tlucak M, Marler MR, *et al*: Low level lead exposure in the prenatal and early preschool periods: early preschool development. *Neurotoxicol Teratol* 1987; 9: 259-270

38. Ernhart CB, Morrow-Tlucak M, Wolf AW, *et al*: Low level lead exposure in the prenatal and early preschool periods: intelligence prior to school entry. *Neurotoxicol Teratol* 1989; 11: 161-170

39. Ernhart CB, Greene T: Low level lead exposure in the prenatal and early preschool periods: language development. *Arch Environ Health* 1990; 45: 342-354

40. Needleman HL, Gunnoe C, Leviton A, *et al*: Deficits in psychologic and classroom performance of children with elevated dentine lead levels. *N Engl J Med* 1979; 300: 689-695

41. Needleman HL, Schell A, Bellinger D, *et al*: The long-term effects of exposure to low doses of lead in childhood. An 11-year follow-up report. *N Engl J Med* 1990; 322: 83-88

42. Hansen ON, Trillingsgaard A, Beese I, *et al*: A neuropsychological study of children with elevated dentine lead level: assessment of the effect of lead in different socio-economic groups. *Neurotoxicol Teratol* 1989; 11: 205-213

43. Lyngbye T, Hansen ON, Grandjean P: Bias from non-particiaption: a study of low-level lead exposure in children. *Scand J Soc Med* 1988; 16: 209-215

44. Smith M, Delves T, Lansdown R, *et al*: The effects of lead exposure on urban children: the Institute of Child Health/Southampton Study. *Dev Med Child Neurol* Suppl 1987; 47: 1-54

45. Rabinowitz MB, Wang JD, Soong WT: Dentine lead and child intelligence in Taiwan. *Arch Environ Health* 1991; 46: 351-360

46. Rabinowitz MB, Wang JD, Soong WT: Children's classroom behavior and lead in Taiwan. *Bull Environ Contam Toxicol* 1992; 48: 282-288

47. Lyngbye T, Jorgensen PJ, Grandjean P, *et al*: Validity and interpretation of blood levels: a study of Danish school children. *Scand J Clin Lab Invest* 1990; 50: 441-449

48. Jacobson BE, Lockitch G, Quigley G: Improved sample preparation for accurate determination of low concentrations of lead in whole blood by graphite furnace analysis. *Clin Chem* 1991; 37: 515-519

49. Calder IC, Roder DM, Esterman AJ, *et al*: Blood lead levels in children in the north-west of Adelaide. *Med J Aust* 1986; 144: 509-512

50. Parsons PJ: Monitoring human exposure to lead: an assessment of current laboratory performance for the determination of blood lead. *Environ Res* 1992; 57: 149-162

51. Osterloh JD, Sharp DS, Hata B: Quality control data for low blood lead concentrations by three methods used in clinical studies. *J Anal Toxicol* 1990; 14: 8-11

52. Subramanian KS: Determination of lead in blood by graphite furnace atomic absorption spectrometry – a critique. *Sci Total Environ* 1989; 89: 237-250

53. Sachs HK, Blanksma LA, Murray EF, *et al*: Ambulatory treatment of lead poisoning: report of 1,155 cases. *Pediatrics* 1970; 46: 389-396

54. Browder A, Joselow M, Louria DB, *et al*: Evaluation of screening programs for childhood lead poisoning by analysis of hospital admissions. *Amer J Public Health* 1974; 64: 914-915

55. Weitzman M, Aschengrau A, Bellinger D, *et al*: Lead-contaminated soil abatement and urban children's blood lead levels. *JAMA* 1993; 269: 1647-1654

56. Farfel MR, Chisolm JJ Jr: Health and environmental outcomes of traditional and modified practices for abatement of residential lead-based paint. *Am J Public Health* 1990; 80: 1240-1245

57. Charney E, Kessler B, Farfel M, *et al*: Childhood lead poisoning. A controlled trial of the effect of dust-control measures on blood lead levels. *N Engl J Med* 1983; 309: 1089-1093

58. Ennis JM, Harrison HE: Treatment of lead encephalopathy with BAL (2,3-dimercaptopropanol). *Pediatrics* 1950; 5: 853-867

59. Coffin R, Phillips JL, Staples WI, *et al*: Treatment of lead encephalopathy in children. *J Pediatr* 1966; 69: 198-206

60. Chisholm JJ Jr, Harrison HE: The treatment of acute lead encephalopathy in children. *Pediatrics* 1957; 19: 2-20

61. Chisholm JJ Jr.: The use of chelating agents in the treatment of acute and chronic lead intoxication in childhood. *J Pediatr* 1968; 73: 1-38

62. Graziano JH, Siris ES, Lolacono N, *et al*: 2,3-Dimercaptosuccinic acid as an antidote for lead intoxication. *Clin Pharmacol Ther* 1985; 37: 431-438

63. Friedheim E, Graziano JH, Popovac D, *et al*: Treatment of lead poisoning by 2,3-dimercaptosuccinic acid. *Lancet* 1978; 1234-1236

64. Selander S, Cramer K, Hallberg L: Studies in lead poisoning. Oral therapy with penicillamine: relationship between lead in blood and other laboratory tests. *Brit J Industr Med* 1966; 23: 282-291

65. Moel DI, Sachs HK, Drayton MA: Slow, natural reduction in blood lead level after chelation therapy for lead poisoning in childhood. *Am J Dis Child* 1986; 140: 905-908

66. Chisolm JJ Jr: Chelation therapy in children with subclinical plumbism. *Pediatrics* 1974; 53: 441-443

67. Vitale LF, Rosalinas-Bailon A, Folland D, *et al*: Oral penicillamine therapy for chronic lead poisoning in children. *J Pediatr* 1973; 83: 1041-1045

68. Graziano JH, Lolacono NJ, Moulton T, *et al*: Controlled study of meso-2,3-dimercaptsuccinic acid for the management of childhood lead intoxication. *J Pediatr* 1992; 120: 133-139

69. Marcus SM: Experience with d-Penicillamine in treating lead poisoning. *Vet Hum Toxicol* 1982; 24: 18-20

70. Markowitz ME, Bijur PE, Ruff H, *et al*: Effects of calcium disodium versenate (CaNa$_2$EDTA) chelation in moderate childhood lead poisoning. *Pediatrics* 1993; 92: 265-271

71. Graziano JH, Lolacono NJ, Meyer P: Dose-response study of oral 2,3-dimercaptosuccinic acid in children with elevated blood lead concentrations. *J Pediatr* 1988; 113: 751-7

72. Shannon M, Graef J, Lovejoy FH Jr: Efficacy and toxicity of D-penicillamine in low-level lead poisoning. *J Pediatr* 1988; 112: 799-804

73. Shannon M, Grace A, Graef JW: Use of penicillamine in children with small lead burdens. [letter] *N Engl J Med* 1989; 321: 979-980

74. Gellert GA, Wagner GA, Maxwell RM, *et al*: Lead poisoning among low-income children in Orange County, California: A need for regionally differentiated policy. *JAMA* 1993; 270: 69-71

75. Amitai Y, Brown MJ, Graef JW, *et al*: Residential deleading: effects on the blood lead levels of lead-poisoned children. *Pediatrics* 1991; 88: 893-897

76. Rey-Alvarez S, Menke-Hargrave T: Deleading dilemma: pitfall in the management of childhood lead poisoning. *Pediatrics* 1987; 79: 214-217

77. Feldman RG: Urban lead mining: lead intoxication among deleaders. *N Engl J Med* 1978; 298: 1143-1145

78. Wedeen RP, Batuman V, Landy E: The safety of the EDTA lead-mobilization test. *Environ Res* 1983; 30: 58-62

79. Moel DI, Kumar K: Reversible nephrotoxic reactions to a combined 2,3-dimercapto-1-propanol and calcium disodium ethylenediaminetetraacetic acid regimin in asymptomatic children with elevated blood lead levels. *Pediatrics* 1982; 70: 259-262

80. Thomas DJ, Chisolm JJ Jr: Lead, zinc and copper decorporation during calcium disodium ethylenediamine tertaacetate treatment of lead-poisoned children. *J Pharmacol Exp Ther* 1986; 239: 829-835

Screening Children for Lead Exposure in Canada

MANEUVER	EFFECTIVENESS	LEVEL OF EVIDENCE <REF>	RECOMMENDATION
Blood lead (BPb) targeted to high- risk children*	Fair evidence of modest neurobehavioural dysfunction in children with mild to moderate lead exposure.	Cohort studies and case series with meta-analysis <12,13,16-46> (II-2)	There is fair evidence for targeted screening of high-risk children* (B)
	Screening tests can reliably and precisely detect lead exposure.	Cross-sectional and case-control studies <9,10,11,14> (II-2); comparison between times and places <6,7> (II-3)	
	Screening high-risk populations using blood lead appears to result in improved clinical outcome.	Cross-sectional studies<47-52> (II-2); comparison between times and places<53,54> (II-3)	
	There is good evidence in symptomatic and fair evidence in asymptomatic for beneficial treatment with severe lead exposure. For mild and moderate lead exposure there is little evidence of benefit and fair evidence for serious adverse effects from environmental or pharmacologic intervention.	Randomized controlled trial<55> (I); cohort studies<15,70,72> (II-2); comparison between times and places<15,53,56,58-70,72,73,75,79,80> (II-3)	
	Many postulated adverse effects have not been adequately evaluated.	Controlled trial without randomization<71,56> (II-1); case reports <76-78> (III)	

* Children at high-risk include: children who live in or regularly visit homes built before 1950 with deteriorated paint or recent, ongoing, or planned renovation or remodelling; who have a sibling, housemate or playmate known to have had lead poisoning; who live with an adult whose job or hobby involves exposure to lead; or who live near lead industries or busy highways.

(Continued on next page)

Screening Children for Lead Exposure in Canada (concl'd)

MANEUVER	EFFECTIVENESS	LEVEL OF EVIDENCE <REF>	RECOMMENDATION
Universal screening of children (BPb and/or questionnaire)	No studies evaluating universal screening were found and no questionnaires have been validated on the Canadian population. Prevalence is low, the burden of suffering from low to moderate lead exposure is small and there are limited data on the effectiveness of intervention <30 µg/dL.	Cross-sectional<2,4,5> (II-2); case series<3> and expert opinion<1> (III)	Insufficient evidence to recommend for or against universal screening to detect lead exposure in the general population (C)

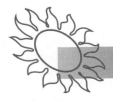

CHAPTER

26

Preschool Screening for Developmental Problems

By John W. Feightner

26
Preschool Screening for Developmental Problems

Prepared by John W. Feightner, MD, MSc, FCFP[1]

Preschool screening is directed at children 3 to 5 years of age and entails early detection of cognitive and behavioural problems that could jeopardize school performance. We evaluated primarily those screening tests that can be used in the primary care physician's office or in a relatively small system of care.<1> Remedial intervention for identified problems is usually carried out by professional educators, but often involves other health professionals such as speech and language therapists and occupational therapists. Early detection of developmental problems using the Denver Developmental Screening Test (DDST) has been shown not to improve school performance but to increase parental anxiety and is therefore not recommended. However, the benefits of other screening tools and remedial programs are controversial.

Burden of Suffering

A reasonable estimate of prevalence of school performance problems is 16-20%

Good data describing the prevalence of school performance problems are difficult to find. The reported prevalence has varied from 6% to 30%; an arguable estimate is 16% to 20%. The rates have depended on factors such as the socioeconomic status of the population studied (children in lower socioeconomic groups tend to have more difficulties), the definition of school problems and the stage in the educational process at which an outcome is measured.

The impact of poor school performance on the child and family can be wide-ranging and difficult to measure, but since society values education and school performance highly this problem has received much attention.

Maneuver

Measurement instruments have generally not been adequately evaluated for screening purposes

Measurement instruments have generally not been adequately evaluated for screening purposes. Sensitivity and specificity as well as predictive values for many instruments have been assessed through multiple analyses of one data set without testing the instrument on another population to confirm the findings.

The DDST is the most widely used test.<2> It is relatively easy to perform, takes little time and is inexpensive. It is effective among

---

[1] Professor of Family Medicine, McMaster University, Hamilton, Ontario

children with intelligence quotients (IQs) of less than 70, but its ability to identify less severe or specific developmental problems has been questioned. The reported sensitivity and specificity have varied considerably; in one study they were 29% and 89% respectively,<3> whereas in another they were 5% to 10% and 99%.<4> With an assumed prevalence rate of 20% the positive predictive value (proportion of true positive results) is 71% and the negative predictive value (proportion of true negative results) 81%; because of its low sensitivity, however, the DDST fails to identify 90% to 95% of children with developmental problems.

A revised version of the Denver Scale, the Denver-II, has added 20 new items primarily focusing on language expression and skills of articulation. There is, however, limited evidence to support its validity and indeed, work by Glascoe et al (1992),<5> raises serious concern regarding the sensitivity and specificity of the new version.

The Developmental Indicators for the Assessment of Learning<6> constitute a multi-dimensional instrument that reflects the school behaviour expected of children in a regular classroom setting. The instrument appears to have considerable potential (sensitivity 46% to 54% and specificity 93%<3>), but more research is required to establish its reliability and validity. Since a team of five to eight people and a moderate amount of equipment are required to administer the test its use is inappropriate for primary care physicians.<7>

The Early Screening Inventory<8> measures developmental abilities, is relatively easy to administer, takes 15 to 20 minutes to perform and has a high sensitivity (81% to 100%) although a lower specificity (67% to 72%).<9> Health care professionals could potentially administer the test, but the reliability of the results depends on the training of the examiner.<8>

The Minneapolis Preschool Screening Instrument<10> is educationally oriented, brief and economical to administer and has achieved a sensitivity of 60% to 63% and a specificity of 89% to 93%.<11> It shows promising reliability and validity.<10>

Other instruments such as the McCarthy Screening Test<12> and the Jansky Screening Index (JSI)<13> need further validation. A study using the JSI assessed teachers' ratings of overall reading skills in grade 1 against outcome in grade 2.<14> The teachers' ratings had both a sensitivity and a specificity of 93%, as compared with 50% and 90% to 92% respectively for the JSI. Furthermore, the teachers' assessments of children in grade 1 had a sensitivity of 61% and a specificity of 86% when compared with school performance in grade 6. The suggestion that the teacher is the best early identifier of future school problems has also been supported by other studies.<15>

Early grade teachers may be better predictors of future school performance problems than available detection tools

Effectiveness of Prevention and Treatment

Denver Developmental Screening Test

The only randomized controlled trial that examined the effectiveness of developmental screening and treatment encompassed three school districts and 4,761 children in the Niagara region of Ontario.[16] The control group comprised children who did not undergo the DDST (18% of the subjects). The remainder were randomly allocated to undergo the DDST with or without an intervention for those with positive results. The intervention consisted of referral to the child's physician for assessment, parent counselling, a review conference between the child's teacher and the school nurse, and monitoring of the child in school by the school nurse.

The children with positive results were assessed by various outcome measures such as the use of specialized educational services, academic achievement, cognitive and perceptual motor tests, and assessment of behavioural, social and emotional well-being. There were no statistically significant differences in outcome between the two screened groups; however, there was a statistically significant increase in worry about school work among the parents of the children in the intervention group. Since there was no benefit from the screening program and a potentially harmful labelling effect we caution against the widespread use of the DDST for screening purposes.

Intervention

Very few studies of specific interventions to improve problems such as reading performance were of sufficient methodologic quality to warrant consideration. However, some insight may be provided by a study of reading performance in older children (mean age 10.2 years) who had been referred by teachers because of poor academic performance.[17] Sixty-one children were randomly assigned to a control group or to a motivated remedial reading group in which each child received 54 sessions over 18 weeks. The intervention group obtained significantly higher scores in all reading tests than the control group did. However, the effect was transient, and the teachers did not rate the children in the intervention group as being significantly improved in general academic performance. Although these results are promising they do not provide sufficient evidence for a generalized adaptation of this strategy as an intervention, particularly among younger children.

Large-scale community programs aimed at high-risk or disadvantaged groups have resulted in mixed and controversial findings. These programs have often been characterized by early optimism followed by disappointment.

Information on the Head Start programs in the U.S. is extensive and open to multiple interpretations. Meta-analysis showed that significant and immediate gains in cognitive test scores, socio-emotional test scores and health status were achieved but the improvements were not long-lasting.[18] These findings have been disputed by others.[19]

In the Perry Preschool Program[20] disadvantaged children in Michigan received early intervention. Although conclusions about the effectiveness of the program remain controversial, at least one reviewer has argued that, in the long term, treated children had better school attendance, needed fewer special education services, were more likely to graduate and had lower rates of school drop-out, delinquency and teenage pregnancy than untreated children.[19] (Other evidence on disadvantaged children is reviewed in Chapter 32.)

Recommendations of Others

In 1986 the Committee on Children with Disabilities of the American Academy of Pediatrics (AAP) recommended that all children attending school be examined for developmental disabilities, preferably by their own pediatrician, before the time of registration or entrance to school. AAP includes elements of developmental screening in its recommended behavioural assessment at preschool visits.

Conclusions and Recommendations

There is fair evidence to recommend the exclusion of the Denver Developmental Screening Test (DDST) from the periodic health examination of asymptomatic preschool children (D Recommendation).

There is insufficient evidence to support either the inclusion or exclusion of other screening instruments (C Recommendation). Caution is advised, however, since problems exist with all current assessment tools, and no interventions have been conclusively proven to be effective. Large-scale community programs to prevent poor school performance in high-risk or disadvantaged groups have also given mixed and controversial results.

Unanswered Questions (Research Agenda)

The following have been identified as research priorities:

1. Assessment by teachers of children in kindergarten and grade 1 should be compared with preschool screening by health care professionals. The risk of teacher bias and the harmful effect of labelling students as having developmental problems should be studied.

2. Developmental screening instruments of acceptable quality need to be developed and evaluated.

3. Given the high costs associated with early education interventions, carefully designed and more focused studies should assess the effectiveness of remedial intervention once problems are identified.

Evidence

The literature was identified with a MEDLINE search to March, 1993 using the following MESH headings: child development; child development disorders; mass screening; reading or perceptual disorders; evaluation studies; longitudinal studies; randomized controlled trials.

This review was initiated in January 1993 and updates a report published in December 1989.[1] Recommendations were finalized by the Task Force in March 1993.

Selected References

1. Canadian Task Force on the Periodic Health Examination: The periodic health examination: 1989 update part 3, Preschool examination for developmental, visual and hearing problems. *Can Med Assoc J* 1989; 141: 1136-1140

2. Frankenburg WK, Dodds JB: The Denver Developmental Screening Test. *J Pediatr* 1967; 71: 181-191

3. Lichtenstein R: New instrument, old problem for early identification. *Exept Child* 1982; 49: 70-72

4. Cadman D, Chambers LW, Walter SD, *et al*: The usefulness of the Denver Developmental Screening Test to predict kindergarten problems in a general community population. *Am J Public Health* 1984; 74: 1093-1097

5. Glascoe FP, Byrne KE, Ashford LG, *et al*: Accuracy of the Denver-II in developmental screening. *Pediatrics* 1992; 89: 1221-1225

6. Mardell C, Goldenberg D: *Developmental Indicators for the Assessment of Learning (DIAL)*, Childcraft Education Corp, Edison, NJ, 1975

7. Lichtenstein R, Ireton H: *Preschool Screening: Identifying Young Children with Developmental and Educational Problems.* Grune, Orlando, Fla, 1984: 156-163

8. Meisels SJ, Wiske JS: *Early Screening Inventory*, Tchrs Coll, New York, 1983

9. Wiske MS, Meisels SJ, Tivan T: Development and validation of the Early Screening Inventory: a study of early childhood developmental screening. In Anastasiow NJ, Frankenburg WK, Fendal AW (eds): *Identifying the Developmentally Delayed Child*, Univ Park, Baltimore, 1982: 123-139

10. Lichtenstein R: *Minneapolis Preschool Screening Instrument*, Minneapolis Public Schools, Minneapolis, Minn, 1980

11. Ireton H, Thwig E: *Minnesota Pre-School Inventory*, Behavior Science Systems, Minneapolis, Minn, 1979

12. McCarthy D: *McCarthy Screening Test*, Psychological Corp, New York, 1978

13. Jansky JJ, de Hirsch K: *Preventing Reading Failure: Prediction, Diagnosis, Intervention*, Harper & Row, New York, 1972

14. Barnes KE: The Jansky Screening Index: a seven-year predictive evaluation and comparative study. In: Frankenburg WK (ed): *Early Identification of Children at Risk: an International Perspective*. Plenum Press, New York, 1985: 185-191

15. Cadman D, Walter SD, Chambers LW, *et al*: Predicting problems in school performance from preschool health, developmental and behavioural assessments. *Can Med Assoc J* 1988; 139: 31-36

16. Cadman D, Chambers LW, Walter SD, *et al*: Evaluation of public health preschool child developmental screening: the process and outcome of a community program. *Am J Public Health* 1987; 77: 45-51

17. Gittelmen R, Feingold I: Children with reading disorders – I. Efficacy of reading remediation. *J Child Psychol Psychiatry* 1983; 23: 167-191

18. Schweinhart LJ, Wikart DP: What do we know so far? A review of the Head Start Synthesis Project. *Young Children* 1986; 41: 45-55

19. Provence S: On the efficacy of early intervention programs. *J Dev Behav Pediatr* 1985; 6: 363-366

20. Schweinhart LD, Weikart DP: *Young Children Grow Up: the Effects of the Perry Preschool Program on Youths Through Age 15*. High/Scope Pr, Ypsilanti, Mich, 1980

Preschool Screening for Developmental Problems

MANEUVER	EFFECTIVENESS	LEVEL OF EVIDENCE <REF>	RECOMMENDATION
Denver Developmental Scale	Early detection of developmental problems followed by educational intervention did not improve school performance but increased parental anxiety.	Randomized controlled trial<15> (I)	Fair evidence to exclude from periodic health examination of children aged 3-5 years (D)
Other detection tools*	Other evidence regarding benefits of early detection and treatment of cognitive and behavioral problems remains controversial.	Nonrandomized controlled trial<16> (II-1) Before-after comparison<17,18> (II-3)	Insufficient evidence to include in or exclude from periodic health examination of children aged 3-5 years (C)

* Other detection tools include: the Developmental Indicators for the Assessment of Learning, the Early Screening Inventory, the Minneapolis Preschool Screening Instrument, the McCarthy Screening Test and the Jansky Screening Index.

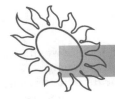

CHAPTER 27

Routine Preschool Screening for Visual and Hearing Problems

By John W. Feightner

Routine Preschool Screening for Visual and Hearing Problems

Prepared by John W. Feightner, MD, MSc, FCFP[1]

The 1979 Task Force report concluded that there was no justification for routine screening for visual deficits among asymptomatic individuals, although it did advocate that screening of children and adolescents be continued until better evidence became available. It stated that there was fair justification for physicians to actively identify people with a hearing impairment necessitating further diagnostic study. A subsequent review of the literature to 1988 resulted in changing the recommendation to include testing of visual acuity in the periodic health examination of preschool children based upon fair evidence.<1> The evidence, however, remained of insufficient quality to recommend the inclusion or exclusion of screening for hearing impairment among non-complainant preschool children.

Consistent with earlier evidence, a 1992 cohort study subsequently showed no benefit attributable to routine pre-school hearing assessment. Considering the resources required for hearing screening, the Task Force does not recommend routine hearing assessment of pre-schoolers although it remains in favour of visual acuity testing.

Visual Defects

Burden of Suffering

The prevalence of visual deficits in the preschool population is estimated to be 10-15%

On the basis of data from two Ontario communities, the prevalence rate of visual deficits in the preschool population is estimated to be 10% to 15%. The morbidity rate associated with such deficits depends on the degree of visual impairment and the acceptance of corrective lenses by the patient and by his or her family and peers. Estimates for amblyopia range from 1.2% to 5.6% with similar estimates for strabismus. The prevalence of combined amblyopia and strabismus is estimated to be in the region of 5%.

The identification of poor visual acuity by itself is accepted by many as being clinically important, however, firm evidence is lacking to link poor visual acuity to poor school performance.

---

[1] Professor of Family Medicine, McMaster University, Hamilton, Ontario

Maneuver

The use of simple visual charts to test visual acuity has been well developed and is widespread. Concerns have been raised about the need for further testing among preschool children, particularly for amblyopia.

Data on the sensitivity and specificity of the individual visual charts are limited, but instrument performance is far from perfect. Some insight into performance in the clinical setting is provided by evaluating the positive and negative predictive value of screening programs which have incorporated these instruments.

De Becker and co-authors[2] evaluated a program using visual inspection, assessment of visual acuity, and evaluation of stereoacuity. They found a negative predictive value of 98.7% for amblyopia, strabismus, and/or high refractive errors. MacPherson and colleagues[3] evaluated a similar program but with a limited gold standard assessment of outcome. Their findings suggested a positive predictive value of 72%. Kohler and colleagues,[4] in a Swedish population, evaluated a program assessing monocular visual acuity, stereoacuity, and the use of a "cover-test". They found a positive predictive value of 83.5% for all visual acuity problems, but only 43% for visual acuity problems requiring treatment.

Effectiveness of Early Detection and Treatment

No randomized controlled trials have evaluated the benefits of screening plus subsequent therapy. Once detected, simple refractive errors affecting visual acuity are readily treatable with eye glasses. However, evidence for the treatment of amblyopia is more controversial and inconclusive. It is widely held that for any potential benefit to be realized, amblyopia must be detected during the "sensitive" period, i.e. between birth and about the seventh year.

One well designed cohort study by Feldman and collaborators[5] examined the effects of preschool screening for visual and hearing problems on the prevalence of such problems six to twelve months later. Visual deficit was defined as an acuity of 20/40 or worse in one or both eyes. At follow-up six to twelve months later, the screened group had 50% fewer visual problems and 75% fewer severe visual deficits than the unscreened group. The impact on school performance, however, was not measured.

Six to twelve months later, screened children had 75% fewer severe visual deficits than an unscreened group.

Hearing Deficits

Burden of Suffering

Hearing problems in preschool children are best divided into short-term, transient problems that resolve and persistent problems. The latter category is composed primarily of persistent middle ear effusion and sensorineural deficits. The prevalence of short-term problems is approximately 15% while for persistent problems it is closer to 3%.

Maneuver

Tests available to evaluate hearing include clinical assessments such as the "whisper test" and pure tone audiometry. New instruments which evaluate the mobility of the tympanic membrane (tympanometry and acoustic reflexometry) have been used to screen for middle ear effusion, a common cause of transient hearing loss. While pure tone audiometry is often considered a gold standard, its appropriate application requires conditions and equipment which limit its use as a screening method.

The use of tympanometry is becoming more widespread. It requires some patient cooperation and a good seal within the ear canal. Karzon,[6] in a study of preschool children, generated two different sets of test characteristics depending on the criteria used. These test characteristics ranged from a sensitivity of 48% and specificity of 89% under one set of criteria to a sensitivity of 78% with a specificity of 68% using different criteria.

Studies evaluating acoustic reflexometry have indicated varying results. Again, the test characteristics generated depend on the criteria used in the specific studies. Myringotomy to establish the presence of middle ear effusion serves as the usual gold standard. While one study[7] indicated a sensitivity of 93% and the specificity of 83%, another study demonstrated a sensitivity of 88% with a specificity of only 44%.[8]

Effectiveness of Early Detection and Treatment

There have been no randomized controlled trials to evaluate the benefit of early detection of hearing problems and subsequent treatment.

However, Zielhuis and co-workers,[9] after screening preschool children with tympanometry for otitis media with effusion, randomized those with this condition to treatment with ventilation tubes or to no treatment. There was no difference between the groups in the main outcome measure of language development, but the authors acknowledge that the number of subjects (43) was quite small.

Two additional studies, one a cohort study and another a cohort analytic study, provide valuable data.

Feldman and associates,<5> in a well designed cohort study evaluated hearing in two groups of preschool children, one of which had been screened within the past year, another which had not. Hearing impairment was defined as the inability to hear sounds at 25 decibels in at least two of four speech frequencies. There was no statistically significant difference in the prevalence of hearing deficits between the two groups. The study did not evaluate the impact on school performance.

O'Mara and colleagues,<10> evaluated the outcome of screening 1,653 children aged 3 and 4 years using portable pure tone audiometry over a period of 18 months. 35 children failed the screening test and the results were reported to their parents. Of the 28 children reviewed in follow-up, two were already receiving treatment for hearing problems prior to the study. Eight of the remaining 26 were confirmed to have an underlying clinical problem but 3 of these had already been previously identified. All of the 5 "new problems" (0.3% of the original sample) were caused by middle ear effusion. The authors conclude that their results raise doubts about the potential benefit of such programs.

All "new hearing problems" (0.3% of 3-4 year-olds surveyed by audiometry) were caused by middle ear effusion

Recommendations of Others

The U.S. Preventive Services Task Force<11> and the American Academy of Family Physicians recommend that all children have testing for amblyopia and strabismus once before entering school, preferably at 3-4 years of age; routine visual acuity testing is not recommended for asymptomatic school-aged children. The American Academy of Ophthalmology, the American Academy of Pediatrics and the American Association for Pediatric Ophthalmology and Strabismus recommend that children have eye and vision screening performed as newborns and at approximately 6 months, 3 years and 5 years of age.

The American Academy of Family Physicians found there was insufficient evidence to recommend for or against universal hearing screening of children. The American Academy of Pediatrics recommends pure tone audiometry at 4 and 5 years of age and the American Speech-Language Hearing Association recommends annual pure tone audiometry for children 3-10 years of age. The recommendations of the U.S. Preventive Services Task Force on screening for hearing impairment are currently under review.

Conclusions and Recommendations

There is fair evidence to include testing of visual acuity in the periodic health examination of preschool children.

Two studies speak against including routine hearing assessment in the preschoolage periodic health examination. A cohort comparison study failed to demonstrate benefit of preschool screening. Second, the cohort analytic study of O'Mara and colleagues detected no new hearing problems of a sensorineural etiology after assessing 1,653 children. While hearing screening carries little or no risk to the individual child, it does detract resources (especially time) from other health maintenance maneuvers. This concern plus the lack of demonstrated benefit argue for excluding routine hearing assessment of pre-schoolers from the periodic health exam (D Recommendation).

Unanswered Questions (Research Agenda)

Studying the effect that correcting of visual or hearing deficits has on school performance.

Evidence

The literature was identified with a MEDLINE search to March 1993 using the following MESH headings or keywords: hearing disorders; vision disorders; child, preschool; mass screening, guideline or Canada. This review was initiated in March 1993 and the recommendation of the Task Force finalized in March 1994.

Selected References

1. Canadian Task Force on the Periodic Health Examination: The periodic health examination: 1989 update part 3, Preschool examination for developmental, visual and hearing problems. *Can Med Assoc J* 1989; 141: 1136-1140

2. De Becker I, MacPherson HJ, LaRoche GR, *et al*: Negative predictive value of a population-based preschool vision screening program. *Ophthalmology* 1992; 99(6): 998-1003

3. MacPherson H, Braunstein J, LaRoche GR: Utilizing basic screening principles in the design and evaluation of vision screening programs. *Am Orthopt J* 1991; 41: 110-121

4. Kohler L, Stigmar G: Vision screening of four-year-old children. *Acta Paediat Scand* 1973; 62: 17-27

5. Feldman W, Milner RA, Sackett B, *et al*: Effects of preschool screening for vision and hearing on prevalence of vision and hearing problems 6-12 months later. *Lancet* 1980; 2: 1014-1016

6. Karzon RG: Validity and reliability of tympanometric measures for pediatric patients. *J Speech Hear Res* 1991; 34: 386-390

7. Oyiborhoro JM, Olaniyan SO, Newman CW, *et al*: Efficacy of acoustic otoscope in detecting middle ear effusion in children. *Laryngoscope* 1987; 97(4): 495-498

8. Teele DW, Stewart IA, Teele JH, *et al*: Acoustic reflectometry for assessment of hearing loss in children with middle ear effusion. *Pediatr Infect Dis J* 1990; 9(12): 870-872

9. Zielhuis GA, Rach GH, van den Broek P: Screening for otitis media with effusion in preschool children. *Lancet* 1989; 1: 311-314

10. O'Mara LM, Isaacs S, Chambers LW: Follow-up of participants in a preschool hearing screening program in child care centres. *Can J Public Health* 1992; 83(5): 375-378

11. U.S. Preventive Services Task Force: *Guide to Clinical Preventive Services: an Assessment of the Effectiveness of 169 Interventions.* Williams & Wilkins, Baltimore, Md, 1989: 181-193, 193-200

Routine Preschool Screening for Visual and Hearing Problems

MANEUVER	EFFECTIVENESS	LEVEL OF EVIDENCE <REF>	RECOMMENDATION
Visual Acuity testing	Systematic screening for visual deficits has been found to decrease prevalence later.	Controlled trial without randomization<5> (II-1)	Fair evidence for inclusion in periodic health examination (B)
History-taking, clinical examination (pure-tone audiometry typanometry, acoustic reflexometry)	Detection of hearing impairment has not been found to significantly reduce prevalence later.	Controlled trial without randomization<5> (II-1); cohort analytic study<10> (II-2)	Fair evidence to exclude from periodic health examination (D)

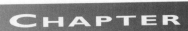
Prevention of Household and Recreational Injuries in Children (<15 years of age)

By R. Wayne Elford

Prevention of Household and Recreational Injuries in Children (<15 years of age)

Prepared by R. Wayne Elford, MD, CCFP, FCFP[1]

In the 1979 Canadian Task Force report,<1> home and recreational injuries were acknowledged to constitute an important proportion of accidents.[2] The report emphasized the particular risk for young children. At that time there was insufficient literature on the subject to justify a recommendation on scientific grounds. However, the maneuver of encouraging safety in the home and community in the context of periodic examinations scheduled for other purposes was made a "C" recommendation and included in the health protection packages for preschool to adolescent age groups. There is now considerable evidence describing the effectiveness of legislation and public health education in prevention of such injuries. There is, however, insufficient evidence to evaluate the effectiveness of physician counselling except as applied to poison treatment modalities (use of Ipecac and awareness of emergency poison control centre telephone numbers) and the identification of home hazards to prevent falls and burns. In these cases counselling is effective. Household and recreational injuries in adults (Chapter 45) and the elderly (Chapter 76) as well as motor vehicle accidents (Chapter 44) have been reviewed in other sections of the book.

Burden of Suffering

Injury is probably the most under-recognized major public health problem facing the nation today, and the study of injury presents unparalleled opportunities for reducing morbidity and mortality and for realizing significant savings in both financial and human terms – all in return for a relatively modest investment.<2>

Injuries are the leading killer of preschool children, school age children and adolescents in Canada

Injuries are the leading killer of our preschool and school-age children, and of adolescents. For Canadians aged 1 to 24, intentional and unintentional injury accounts for 63% of all deaths. In the developed world, injuries cause more than four times more childhood deaths than any other disease.<3> The leading cause of death in Canadian children is motor vehicle accidents, followed by drowning, burns, choking and falls.<4> Injury mortality rates for Canadian

---

[1] Professor and Director of Research and Faculty Development, Department of Family Medicine, University of Calgary, Calgary, Alberta
[2] "Unintentional injury" is more appropriate than "accident" in terms of terminology, however, many articles in the literature still use the term "accidental".

children aged 5 to 14 exceed those of children in Japan, Australia and most countries in Western Europe. These injury-related deaths are but the tip of the iceberg. For every fatal childhood injury, another 45 injuries will require hospital treatment; about 1,300 more will require a visit to an emergency department and an unknown number will result in a visit to a physician or clinic.[5] Disfigurement, disability, developmental delay and emotional problems are major sequelae of accidental injuries to children.[3] The Canadian Accident Injury Reporting and Evaluation (CAIRE) project identified the following top 10 circumstances involved in home accidents that resulted in visits to Children's Hospitals in 1989 – windows or window glass, bicycles, cribs, hot water (excluding other hot liquid), ladders, high chairs/child care, baseboard heaters/electric, glassware (excluding tempered), change tables/child care, and baby walkers.[6]

Table 1 summarizes the mortality and morbidity rates for the most common types of injury in children. A brief description of the predictable factors associated with each of the leading causes of accidental injury in children follows.

Falls

There were 2,100 deaths due to falls in 1988.[7] It is estimated that baby walkers are used in 80-90% of Canadian households with young infants; 300,000 Canadian infants would spend some time in them during the course of a year and 2,500 would require medical attention because of falls down stairs, tipping, jamming fingers or contact with a hot item.[8]

Drowning

429 Canadians drowned in 1987, 135 in boating accidents. It has been estimated that for each pediatric drowning fatality there are 3-4 hospital admissions and numerous children seen in emergency departments.[2] A review of Ontario coroners' reports for 1979-1981 showed that the young adolescent male was at particular risk of drowning, as were toddlers (aged 1-4) who may wander away from adult supervision. Approximately half of all accidental drownings took place in lakes or ponds; 75% of children who drowned in swimming pools were under 5 years of age.[9]

Burns, Scalds and Fire-Related Deaths

There were 402 deaths among Canadians caused by fire and flames in 1988 and 85% occurred in private dwellings.[10] More than one-third of childhood admissions to burn units are associated with scalding water (kettles and baths); boys are injured about twice as frequently as girls, and 74% are under 2 years old; 87% of accidents occur in the child's own home and about half of these take place in the kitchen.<11>

Poisoning

There were 424 fatal poisonings in Canada in 1987; however, only 2 of the deaths were among children under 15 years of age.<10> Data from poison control centres in Canada indicate that in 1986 there were 103,459 poisoning cases and 365 deaths (0.35% mortality rate).<12>

Suffocation

Of the 415 Canadian deaths by suffocation in 1987, 274 were related to ingestion of food and 102 to mechanical suffocation.<7> 36% were in children under 15 years of age.<10>

Bicycle and Other Sports-Related Injuries

There were 139 fatal pedal cycle injuries in Canada in 1987 and 86% of the casualties were male.<7> Deaths were most commonly associated with motor vehicles or trains; boys aged 10-14 years had the highest risk of death.<10> In 1988, 568 children were treated for bicycle-related injuries in an Ottawa study.<13> 70% were boys and the mean age was 9.4 years. Only 2% of the patients had been wearing a helmet at the time of the accident though 13% owned helmets. Over 60% of the accidents were attributed to carelessness or poor bicycle control. 97 children were admitted to hospital; 49% had head and skull injuries and 40% had skull fractures. Another observational study of 1,963 cyclists found 10.7% wore helmets; commuting and recreational cyclists had the highest level of helmet use (17.9% and 14.3% respectively) while helmet use among students (1.9%) was significantly lower.<14>

Firearm-Related

There were 60 deaths by firearms in Canada in 1988.<7> Most childhood deaths from firearms occur at a residence and defects in firearm performance were associated with 40%.<15>

Effectiveness of Intervention Maneuvers

The Haddon Matrix for generating countermeasures provides a multifactorial model for developing approaches to injury prevention.<16> Three widely adopted approaches to interventions for accidental injury based on this model are described in greater detail: public health education, environmental legislation, and individual counselling.

(i) *Public Health Education* – Numerous public health education campaigns have used combinations of leaflets, poster displays in public buildings and T.V. advertisements targeted towards high-risk populations. Several controlled studies have failed to demonstrate any resulting reduction in unintentional injuries.

(ii) *Legislative/Environmental* – Systematic identification and reduction of environmental hazards prevents accidents. Many studies have demonstrated a far greater impact on home and recreational safety through influencing legislators, who in turn modify the environment through building codes and safety legislation (see Table 2, Chapter 76 on Injuries in the Elderly).

Influencing legislators, who in turn can modify the environment through building codes and safety standards has the greatest impact

(iii) *Individual Counselling* – Several studies in the past decade have indicated that physicians can play a supportive role in preventing injuries through anticipatory guidance and counselling on safety measures. A recent publication[17] summarizing the impact of prevention counselling in primary care settings as determined by randomized controlled trials, supports the effectiveness of office counselling in improving parental knowledge and behaviours. Due to sample size and follow-up limitations these studies were unable to show an influence on morbidity or mortality.

Physicians can play a supportive role in preventing injuries through anticipatory guidance and counselling on safety measures

Falls

A 96% decrease in accidental falls from windows was reported following the "Children Can't Fly" program in New York City, in which owners of multiple dwellings were required to provide window guards in apartments where children 10 years or younger resided.[18] Safety features such as car restraints and window and stairway guards can reduce the incidence and severity of injury in infants.[19] To date, no studies of counselling parents about safety features in the home have demonstrated an impact on the rate of injuries even though intermediate outcomes such as "recognition of hazards" may have improved.

Drowning

Before there was legislation relevant to swimming pool design or water safety in Virginia (1982), Fairfax County had legislated comprehensive safety regulation; the death rate (per 100,000 population) for drowning was 1.6 for the 620,000 population, as compared with 17.3 for the remainder of Virginia.[20] The incidence of swimming pool submersions in public and semi-public pools regulated for fencing and self-closing gates by the Public Health Department decreased during 1974-1983 (from 13 in 1974-75 to 2 in 1982-83; p<0.03) while the incidence of unregulated private pool submersions remained unchanged.[21]

Children with pools on their own or neighbouring properties were 2.5 times more likely to be involved in accidents involving domestic pools. Expert opinion holds that toddler or early childhood swimming lessons not only provide a degree of improved survivability for the young child but also place the child in the swimmer category at an earlier age (the greatest proportion of drowning occurs in non-swimmers) and improve survival as an adult swimmer.[20]

An association between drowning and leaving young children alone in the bathtub has also been shown in a cohort study.[19]

Burns

Prior to 1953, flame burns were the leading cause of burn injury among children. The *Flammability Fabrics Act of 1967* substantially reduced this problem by improving safety standards in children's garments, especially sleep wear. Acquisition of safety features such as smoke detectors, non-inflammable sleepwear and lowering hot water thermostat settings reduces injury from scalds and burns.[21] In a controlled study, couples were randomly enrolled in one of two well-child care classes that did or did not include specific information on burn prevention (hot water heater settings and smoke detectors) in addition to information on nutrition, dental care, safety in the car and home, child development, child rearing, illness management and immunizations. Sixty-five percent of couples in the experimental group had their hot water temperature measured at 54°C or less and all but one had an operational smoke detector; all couples in the control group had hot water temperatures above 54°C (p=0.0001) but most had smoke detectors (p<0.12).[22]

Poisoning

The death rate due to poisonings of children under age 5 years declined from 2.0 per 100,000 in 1958 to 0.5 per 100,000 in 1978. Poison control centres in Canada reported a 50% decline in numbers of poisoning cases due to acetylsalicylic acid between 1982 and 1986. The decline in deaths from accidental poisoning in children was largely the result of increasing use of child-resistant packaging for chemicals and therapeutic drugs.[23]

Several demonstration projects have failed to document a major impact from educational programs on the prevention of poisoning.[24] In a controlled trial involving 403 families (with children 5 years old or younger) recruited from an emergency clinic, counselling on correct poison treatment methods (plus a written handout, telephone sticker and a bottle of ipecac) resulted in more self-reported ipecac storage (68% vs. 42%, p=0.005), familiarity with the use of ipecac (40% vs. 25%, p=0.04) and use of poison centre

phone number stickers at 6-month follow-up
(42% vs. 25%, p=.03).<25>

Bicycle and Sports-Related Injury

This topic is discussed in Chapter 45 on Injuries in Adults. However, a cohort analytic study has shown an association between the severity of head injury in cyclists and non-use of helmets.<26>

Recommendations of Others

In 1989, the U.S. Preventive Services Task Force recommended the following: "It may be clinically prudent to provide counselling on measures to reduce the risk of unintentional household or environmental injuries from falls, drowning, fires or burns, poisoning, and firearms."<27>

The American Academy of Pediatrics (AAP) has developed an Injury Prevention Program (TIPP) for use in office practice.<28> TIPP uses the Framingham safety survey to identify at-risk behaviour, safety sheets to reinforce information provided by the physician in discussion of questionnaire results and a model 12-session counselling schedule (from prenatal/newborn to 4 years). AAP's policy statement states that all physicians should advise parents to acquire the following items for their children's safety: 1) Currently approved child car restraints; 2) Smoke detectors in the home that would protect the child's sleeping area; 3) Safe hot water temperatures at the tap; 4) Window and stairway guards/gates to prevent falls; and 5) A 30-mL (1-oz) bottle of syrup of ipecac. No evaluation of the TIPP program has been published.

Conclusions and Recommendations

There is fair evidence (grade II-1) that window and stairway guards reduce the incidence and severity of injury in infants (B Recommendation). There is also fair evidence (grade I) to support counselling parents on the acquisition of such safety features in the periodic health examination of infants (B Recommendation).

There is fair evidence (grade II-2) that requiring conformity to water safety standards reduces deaths from drowning (B Recommendation) but insufficient evidence to support counselling parents of young children concerning early swimming class exposure and abiding by water safety guidelines (C Recommendation). A decision on such counselling may, however, be made on other grounds. There is fair evidence that parents of young children should never leave a child under 36 months of age alone in a bathtub (B Recommendation) but insufficient information about the ability of physicians to influence supervision of children in baths by counselling (C Recommendation).

There is fair evidence (grade II-2) that the acquisition of safety features such as smoke detectors, non-inflammable sleepwear, and hot water thermostat settings reduces injury from scalds and burns (B Recommendation). There is also fair evidence (grade I) concerning the effectiveness of counselling the parents of young children to acquire safety features such as smoke detectors, non-inflammable sleepwear, and hot water thermostat settings (B Recommendation).

There is good evidence (grade I) that parent awareness of poison control modalities reduces the incidence of poisoning in infants (A Recommendation). There is also fair evidence to support counselling on prevention of poisoning and the provision of ipecac and poison control centre phone number stickers to the parents of young children (B Recommendation).

There is fair evidence (grade II-2) that wearing helmets reduces the incidence and severity of head injuries in cyclists (B Recommendation). However, there is insufficient evidence that counselling will increase the rate of bicycle helmet use for those who ride the roadways (C Recommendation). Decision concerning such counselling may be made on other grounds.<29>

Unanswered Questions (Research Agenda)

Because of the multifactorial etiology of most injuries, a number of methodologic issues need further study. The problem of assessing or measuring exposure in the context of household and recreational injuries makes the design of analytic studies very difficult. There are persistent limitations in available data. For example, CHIRPP (Canadian Hospital Injury Reporting and Prevention Program) collects data in collaboration with all pediatric hospitals rather than from population-based sources.

Evidence

A MEDLINE search from 1981 to November 1991 was conducted using the following strategy: accidents as a major MESH heading with the subheadings diagnosis, economics, epidemiology, law and jurisprudence, mortality, prevention and control, standards and trends; and not aviation, occupational or traffic accidents. Other sources included Statistics Canada, Health and Welfare Canada, the Insurance Bureau of Canada, the Izaak Walton Killam Children's Hospital Poison Control Centre, supporting documents of other recommending bodies and references from identified literature.

This review was initiated in 1991 and the recommendations finalized by the Task Force in November 1992.

Selected References

1. Canadian Task Force on the Periodic Health Examination: The periodic health examination. *Can Med Assoc J* 1979; 121: 1193-1254

2. Division of Injury Control, Center for Environmental Health and Injury Control, Centers for Disease Control: Childhood injuries in the United States. *Am J Dis Child* 1990; 144: 627-646

3. Rivara FP, Thompson RS, Thompson DC, *et al*: Injuries to children and adolescents: Impact on physical health. *Pediatrics* 1991; 88: 783-788

4. Statistics Canada, Canadian Centre for Health Information: Hospital Morbidity 1985-86. Health Reports Supplement 1(2): Catalogue 82-003S. Minister of Supply and Services Canada. 1989; no paging; Tables 1 and 2.

5. Guyer B, Ellers B: Childhood injuries in the United States: Mortality, morbidity and cost. *Am J Dis Child* 1990; 144: 649-652

6. Stanwick RS: Prevention of Injuries in Canadian Children Aged 0-14 Years. Knowledge Development for Health Promotion: A Call for Action. Health Services and Promotion Branch Working Paper [HSPB 89-2]: March 1989: 51-59

7. Statistics Canada, Canadian Centre for Health Information: Causes of Death 1988. Catalogue No. 82-003S. Minister of Supply and Services Canada Health Reports 1990; 2(1 Suppl 11): 146-185

8. James W: Despite new regulations, caution a must when baby walkers are used. *Can Med Assoc J* 1988; 139: 73-74

9. MacLachlan J: Drownings, other aquatic injuries and young Canadians. *Can J Public Health* 1984; 75: 218-222

10. Canada Safety Council: Accident Fatalities, Canada 1987. Canada Safety Council 1988: 1-26

11. Herd AN, Widdowson P, Tanner NSB: Scalds in the very young: prevention or cure? *Burns Incl Therm Inj* 1986; 12: 246-249

12. Health and Welfare Canada: Poison Control Statistics. Minister of National Health and Welfare 1986: 9

13. Cushman R, Down J, MacMillan N, *et al*: Bicycle-related injuries: a survey in a pediatric emergency department. *Can Med Assoc J* 1990: 143: 108-112

14. Cushman R, Down J, MacMillan N, *et al*: Bicycle helmet use in Ottawa. *Can Fam Physician* 1990; 26: 697-700

15. Patterson PJ, Smith LR: Firearms in the home and child safety. *Am J Dis Child* 1987; 141: 221-223

16. Haddon W: Advances in the epidemiology of injuries as a basis for public policy. *Public Health Report* 1980; 95: 411-421

17. Bass J, Christoffel K, Widome M, *et al*: Childhood injury prevention counselling in primary care settings. *Pediatrics* 1993; 92: 544-553

18. Spiegal CN, Lindaman FC: Children can't fly: A program to prevent childhood morbidity and mortality from window falls. *Am J Public Health* 1977; 67: 1143-1145

19. Gallagher SS, Hunter P, Guyer B: A home injury prevention program for children. *Pediatr Clin North Am* 1985; 32: 95-112

20. Spyker DA: Submersion injury, epidemiology prevention and management. *Pediatr Clin North Am* 1983; 31(1): 113-125

21. Quan L, Gore EJ, Wantz K, *et al*: Ten-year study of pediatric drownings and near drownings: lessons in injury prevention. *Pediatrics* 1989; 83: 1035-1040

22. Thomas KA, Hassanein RS, Christophersen ER: Evaluation of group well child care for improving burn prevention practices in the home. *Pediatrics* 1984; 74(5): 879-882

23. Walton WW: An evaluation of the Poison Prevention Packaging Act. *Pediatrics* 1982; 69: 363-370

24. Fergusson DM, Horwood LJ, Beautrois AL, *et al*: A controlled trial of a poisoning prevention method. *Pediatrics* 1982; 69(5): 515-520

25. Woolf A, Lewander W, Filippone G, *et al*: Prevention of childhood poisoning: efficacy of an educational program carried out in an emergency clinic. *Pediatrics* 1987; 80: 359-363

26. Thompson RS, Rivara F, Thompson DC: A case-control study of the effectiveness of bicycle safety helmets. *N Engl J Med* 1989; 320: 1361-1367

27. U.S. Preventive Services Task Force: *Guide to Clinical Preventive Services: an Assessment of the Effectiveness of 169 Interventions*. Williams & Wilkins, Baltimore, Md, 1989: 321-329

28. Krassner L: TIPP usage. *Pediatrics* 1984; 74(Suppl): 976-980

29. Morris BA, Trimble NE: Promotion of bicycle helmet use among children. A randomized clinical trial. *Can J Public Health* 1991; 82: 92-94

Table 1: Canadian Mortality and Morbidity Rates for Unintentional Injury in 1989[1]
(per 100,000 – standardized to 1971 population)

| | Overall (0-85+ yr) | | | | Pediatric (0-14 yr) | | | |
| | Mortality | | Morbidity | | Mortality | | Morbidity | |
	M	F	M	F	M	F	M	F
Falls	6.77	4.16	425.0	384.0	.04	.24	420.5	283.5
Drownings	2.31	.63	2.78	1.38	1.86	.95	5.49	3.43
Burns/Fire related	2.11	.91	11.52	4.23	1.40	.91	11.01	4.88
Poisonings	1.88	.90	38.84	35.19	.13	.04	63.79	54.87
Suffocations	.72	.21	.39	.15	1.07	.48	.79	.37
Firearms	.57	.04	4.69	.52	.37	.11	3.32	.43

[1] Extracted from data, Bureau of Chronic Disease Epidemiology, Laboratory Centre for Disease Control, Health and Welfare Canada

Prevention of Household and Recreational Injuries in Children (<15 Years of Age)

MANEUVER	EFFECTIVENESS	LEVEL OF EVIDENCE <REF>	RECOMMENDATION
Use of window and stairway guards			
a) legislation	Association between falls in infants with hazardous environments (i.e. walkers and stairs).	Cohort analytic study<19> (II-1)	Fair evidence to implement (B)
b) individual counselling	Counselling can increase recognition of hazards in the home, but impact on injury unknown.	Randomized controlled trial<17> (I)	Fair evidence to include in periodic health examination (B)
Teach young children water safety and swimming skills			
a) Public Health Education/ Legislation	Requiring private and public pools to conform to safety standards reduces drownings.	Cohort study<21> (II-2)	Fair evidence to implement (B)
b) Individual counselling	Little information about ability of physician to influence teaching of water safety and swimming skills.	Expert opinion<20> (III)	Insufficient evidence to include or exclude in periodic health examination (C)
Never leave young children (<36 months) alone in bath tub			
a) Public Health Education	Association between drowning and unattended infants.	Cohort study<19> (II-2)	Fair evidence to implement (B)
b) Individual counselling	Little information about ability of physician to influence supervision of children in bath.	Expert opinion (III)	Insufficient evidence to include or exclude in periodic health examination (C)

(Continued on next page)

Prevention of Household and Recreational Injuries in Children (<15 Years of Age) (concl'd)

MANEUVER	EFFECTIVENESS	LEVEL OF EVIDENCE <REF>	RECOMMENDATION
Use safety devices such as smoke detectors, non-flammable sleepwear and hot water thermostat settings			
a) Public Health Education and legislation	Association between burns in young children with lack of safety features in their environment.	Non-randomized trial<22> (II-1)	Fair evidence to implement (B)
b) Individual counselling	Counselling can increase the number of safety features in the home but impact on injury is unknown.	Randomized controlled trial<17> (I)	Fair evidence to include in periodic health examination (B)
Use of Ipecac and Regional Poison Centre Awareness			
a) Public Health Education/ Legislation	Association between poisoning in young children and parental lack of awareness of poison treatment modalities.	Randomized controlled trial<24> (I)	Good evidence to implement (A)
b) Individual counselling	Counselling can generate a significant short-term improvement in the use of poison treatment modalities.	Comparison of times and places<25> (II-3)	Fair evidence to include in periodic health examination (B)
Use of helmets when riding bicycles			
a) Public Health Education/ Legislation	Association between severity of head injury in cyclists and non-use of helmets.	Case-control study<26> (II-2)	Fair evidence for implementing (B)
b) Individual counselling	Limited ability of physician to influence use of helmets.	Randomized controlled trial<29> (I)	Insufficient evidence to include or exclude in periodic health examination (C)

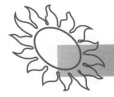

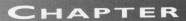

CHAPTER 29

Primary Prevention of Child Maltreatment

By Harriet L. MacMillan,
James H. MacMillan and David R. Offord

Primary Prevention of Child Maltreatment

Prepared by Harriet L. MacMillan, MD, FRCPC[1], James H. MacMillan, MSc[2] and David R. Offord, MD, FRCPC[3]

Child maltreatment includes the categories of physical abuse, neglect, sexual abuse and emotional abuse. In 1979, the Canadian Task Force on the Periodic Health Examination reported that there was fair justification for recommending that parenting problems, including child abuse and neglect, be included among those conditions considered in a periodic health examination. In evaluating the evidence since that time, this chapter considers the possibility of using screening to identify individuals at risk of maltreating children. It also examines programs for primary prevention of child maltreatment, such as perinatal and early childhood support programs (e.g. home visitation) and educational programs designed to teach children to recognize and respond to potentially abusive situations. The latter were included recognizing that parents may consult physicians regarding school-based programs. This chapter evaluates preventive programs based on the outcomes most closely related to maltreatment – for example, reports of verified or suspected abuse or neglect. Other more remote indices such as parenting attitudes were beyond the scope of the review.

Burden of Suffering

The term maltreatment includes all types of child victimization but is commonly divided into the subcategories of physical abuse, neglect, sexual abuse and emotional abuse. No national data are available in Canada regarding reports of child maltreatment. In the U.S., an estimated 45 reports of suspected child maltreatment per thousand children were received in 1992. However, many episodes of child maltreatment go unreported because of failure to detect, recognize or officially report the abuse. Deaths resulting from child maltreatment are also drastically underreported.

Estimates of both incidence and prevalence rates of child maltreatment have focused on two subcategories of child maltreatment: physical and sexual abuse. A U.S. national survey conducted in 1985 estimated the rate of severe physical violence against children by their caretakers as 11%. In the 1983 National Population Survey in Canada an estimated 15% of women and 8% of

[1] Assistant Professor of Pediatrics and of Psychiatry, McMaster University, Hamilton, Ontario
[2] Biostatistician, Glaxo Canada Inc., Mississauga, Ontario
[3] Professor of Psychiatry, McMaster University, Hamilton, Ontario

men reported that they had been victims of attempted or actual sexual intercourse before the age of 18 years. Other estimates of prevalence of childhood sexual abuse among girls 13 years or less vary from 10% to 12%.

Maltreated children are adversely affected in many ways. They may suffer from cognitive, emotional and social impairment in addition to physical disabilities. Many studies have pointed to an association between a history of childhood maltreatment and various psychiatric disorders including depression, personality disorders, anxiety, substance abuse, suicidal behaviour, conduct disorder and criminal behaviour. The human and fiscal costs associated with child maltreatment are clearly enormous.

Maneuver

Screening for Risk of Child Maltreatment

Most work in this area has focused on identifying people at increased risk for committing physical abuse or neglect. Methods of screening include three main approaches: a staff-administered checklist, a self-administered questionnaire and a standardized interview. The Family Stress Checklist[1] and the Dunedin Family Services Indicator[2,3] are examples of the first approach. Self-administered questionnaires include the Child Abuse Potential Inventory,[4] the Michigan Screening Profile of Parenting,[5] the Adult-Adolescent Parenting Inventory[6] and the Parent Opinion Questionnaire.[7] A standardized interview format has been used by Altemeier and collaborators.[8] Gray and colleagues[9] used a combination of approaches including interviews, questionnaire results and observations of parental behaviour. Leventhal, Garber and Brady[10] examined whether clinicians could correctly identify infants at high risk for abuse and neglect without the use of specific instruments.

Risk Indicators

A risk indicator is a factor associated with an increased likelihood of child maltreatment; it does not necessarily imply causation. Rates of physical abuse and neglect are similar among boys and girls. In contrast, girls are reported to be victims of sexual abuse 2.5 times more frequently than boys. Although children of all ages are at significant risk for physical abuse, those less than 5 years old and youths between 15 and 17 years old are at greater risk. Girls between 10 and 12 years are at increased risk of sexual abuse.

Risk indicators for committing physical abuse include low socioeconomic status, young maternal age, large family, single-parent family, parental childhood experience of physical maltreatment, spousal violence, lack of social support, and unplanned pregnancy or negative parental attitude toward pregnancy. The evidence regarding alcohol abuse and illicit drug use is unclear. Risk indicators of sexual abuse include: living in a family without a natural parent, growing up in a family with poor marital relations between the parents, presence of a stepfather, and poor child-parent relationships or unhappy family life.

Effectiveness of Screening

There is insufficient evidence to justify use of screening approaches to predict child maltreatment in the general population

      The main problem with the available approaches is the high false positive rate. For example, assuming a high prevalence rate for child maltreatment of 20%, screening 1,000 children with an instrument whose sensitivity is 80% and specificity 90% would result in 33% of the positive test results being false positive. With a lower prevalence rate of abuse, the number of false-positive results would be even higher. A sizeable number of individuals identified by such techniques as being "at risk for child maltreatment" would never go on to commit abuse. Such labelling may put people under increased stress and interfere with their ability to function as parents. Further, the validity of many of the screening approaches has not been adequately evaluated.

      Overall, screening may do more harm than good. Nevertheless, knowledge of risk indicators for child maltreatment can assist clinicians in making decisions regarding the provision of preventive interventions to individuals and families in high-risk populations. Although screening of individuals is not recommended, interventions can be targeted at all members of high-risk communities.

Maneuver

Preventive Interventions

      For the purpose of this review, primary prevention is defined as any intervention provided to stop maltreatment before it occurs. This includes interventions aimed at high-risk populations, sometimes referred to by others as secondary prevention. These interventions can be considered in two categories: 1) perinatal and early childhood hospital support, home visitation and parent training programs and; 2) education programs for children, parents and teachers. The former have generally focused on the prevention of physical abuse and neglect, whereas the education programs have primarily centred on the prevention of sexual abuse or abduction. Programs in both categories frequently used a spectrum of measures to evaluate effectiveness. This review includes the perinatal and early childhood programs that used official reports of verified or suspected abuse and neglect, in addition to the following proxy measures of maltreatment: rates of hospital admission, emergency visits and injuries. Effectiveness of education programs is frequently evaluated using measures of knowledge or behavioral responses under simulated conditions. Two systematic reviews provide a detailed description about the evaluation of these interventions.<11,12>

Effectiveness of Prevention

Perinatal and Early Childhood Programs

A randomized controlled trial (RCT) evaluated intensive pediatric contact plus home visitation by public health nurses (PHNs) and lay health visitors for 100 mothers identified as being at risk for abnormal parenting practices.<9> The number of verified reports of child maltreatment and accidents did not differ significantly between the intervention and control groups, however, the children of women in the control group were significantly more likely than those of women in the intervention group to require inpatient treatment for serious injuries. The number of central registry reports was greater in the intervention group, although the difference was not significant; one possible explanation for this result was increased surveillance among families in the intervention group.<9> This study suffered from inadequate follow-up; outcome was evaluated in only 50% of the families. Since this study examined a combined intervention of intensive pediatric contact plus home visitation, the lower number of seriously injured children in the intervention group cannot be attributed to intensive pediatric contact alone.

Several RCTs have evaluated home visitation as the primary preventive intervention. The two most rigorous studies demonstrated a reduction in the incidence of child maltreatment and outcomes related to physical abuse and neglect in the intervention groups. Olds and associates<13> evaluated home visits by nurses made to white primiparous women who were primarily young, single or of low socioeconomic status (85% of the 400 women met at least one of these criteria). Women in the control group received no services during pregnancy or free transportation for prenatal and well-child care; their infants underwent developmental screening. Of the two treatment groups, one was visited by a nurse during pregnancy (pregnancy-visited group) and the second during pregnancy and after birth until the child's second birthday (infancy-visited group). The babies in the latter group were taken to the emergency department significantly less often in the first (p=0.04) and second (p=0.01) years of life and were seen less frequently for accidents and poisonings in the second year (p=0.03) than babies in the comparison group. In a subgroup of mothers at highest risk for maltreatment (poor, unmarried teens), 19% of those in the comparison group and 4% of those in the infancy-visited group had instances of verified abuse and neglect (p=0.07). The incidence of outcomes in the pregnancy-visited group generally fell between the rates in the infancy-visited group and the comparison group.

Home visitation can prevent child physical abuse and neglect or outcomes associated with maltreatment among disadvantaged families

In a RCT, 290 black mothers of low socioeconomic status were assigned to receive either home visits beginning in the newborn period until the infant was 24 months of age or no such intervention.<14> Seventy-eight percent of the women were single and 23% primiparous. The home visitor was a woman from the community, with support provided through a health care program for children and youths. Children in the intervention group had significantly fewer admissions to hospital (p<0.01) and fewer episodes of suspected abuse or neglect (p<0.01) than those in the control group.[4] They also had fewer episodes of definite physical abuse and neglect (p<0.01).[4]

Siegel and colleagues<15> evaluated the effects of three types of intervention: 1) early and extended hospital contact after delivery between women and their newborns; 2) home visits by paraprofessionals during the first three months after birth; and 3) both. At one year follow-up, the three intervention groups did not differ from the control group in the number of reports of abuse and neglect, hospital admissions or visits to the emergency department. However, the visits continued only during the first three months of the infant's life.

O'Connor and associates<16> compared the effects of extended postpartum hospital contact (rooming-in) with routine care. Although the experimental group showed a reduction in parenting inadequacy, no significant differences were found in the number of hospital admissions, accidents, emergency department visits or reports of maltreatment to protective services. The outcome of parenting inadequacy was too broad to draw conclusions about prevention of child maltreatment. Evidence from the study was weakened because the study was not truly randomized.

A controlled trial without randomization and involving high-risk families evaluated contact by the project social worker after the mother's discharge from hospital and access to a drop-in-centre.<17> The proportion of children on the child abuse register, the rate of hospital admissions and rate of admissions because of trauma did not differ significantly between the intervention and control groups. Our statistical analysis of descriptive data provided by the authors revealed that the number of children seen in the emergency department was lower in the intervention group than in the control group (p<0.001). However, no statement was made about randomization or baseline comparison of groups. Given these problems, no conclusions can be drawn from the trial.

One RCT<18> and a non-randomized prospective controlled study<19> evaluated the effectiveness of parent training programs for mothers at risk of committing child abuse. Neither study evaluated reports of abuse or events (e.g. hospital admissions) related to child

---

[4] We conducted additional analyses using Fisher's exact test.

maltreatment, so once again no conclusions can be drawn about the prevention of child abuse and neglect.

Overall, the evidence regarding intensive pediatric contact,[9] home visitation over the short term (three months or less),[15] early and/or extended postpartum hospital contact,[15,16] use of a drop-in centre[17] and parent training programs[18,19] remains inconclusive. Several of the studies lacked sufficient statistical power to detect a difference between the groups in the outcomes evaluated in this review.[15-17] Two trials[13,14] provide evidence that home visitation can prevent child physical abuse and neglect or associated outcomes among disadvantaged families.

Specific recommendations about the intervention cannot be made based on the available evidence. Authors of the most rigorous trials of home visitation have emphasized three essential aspects: 1) the importance of building a supportive relationship between the home visitor and mother over time; 2) flexibility on the part of the home visitor; and 3) adequate backup support for the home visitor. Both programs extended until the newborn child reached two years of age. In the trial by Olds and colleagues[13] visits occurred every two weeks initially, gradually tapering to every six weeks by the time the infant was two years of age. In the second trial,[14] visits were scheduled initially every two months tapering to every three months. The duration of visits in the two trials ranged from 40 to 75 minutes. The visitor was free to tailor the curriculum to the specific needs of the parents.

Education Programs

The second group of interventions comprises primarily school-based programs aimed at identifying potentially abusive situations and teaching strategies to prevent sexual abuse or abduction.[20-28] The target group for most education programs has been children from 3 to 12 years of age. Other trials evaluating the effectiveness of preventive education for teachers and parents are beyond the scope of this review.

Identifying inappropriate touching or advances by an adult and saying "No" were common elements of the educational curricula.[20] Some programs also taught children to report advances of an adult or that a victim must report the abusive episode. Interventions used various modes of presentation including instruction (verbal and/or written material), film or videotape plus instruction, skits plus instruction, film plus instruction and printed material (e.g. a colouring book), behavioral rehearsal plus instruction, and a combination of instruction, film or videotape and behavioral rehearsal. The frequency and duration of the training sessions varied. The interveners also had a range of qualifications. Outcomes reported across trials fell into four main categories: 1) knowledge of prevention concepts; 2) assessment

Education programs improve knowledge but have not been shown to reduce the occurrence of child sexual victimization

of behavioral skills using responses to hypothetical vignettes; 3) behavioral responses under simulated conditions; and 4) disclosures of sexual abuse.

Numerous RCTs have demonstrated that education programs significantly increase knowledge about sexual abuse, enhance awareness of safety skills and modify children's behaviour in response to hypothetical vignettes.[20-25] In two studies[26,27] education programs were effective in modifying children's behaviour in response to a simulated abduction by a stranger. Disclosure of sexual abuse by children has been evaluated in a few trials. Due to methodologic problems (e.g. small control group), however, no conclusions could be drawn from these studies.[25,28] Participation in the trials has not been shown to be associated with negative effects but further assessment of both positive and negative long-term outcomes is necessary.[24]

The interpretation of outcome assessments remains a major dilemma. Researchers have assessed predominantly changes in knowledge assuming that increased knowledge leads to changes in behaviour. However, the appropriate response of a child in a research situation does not guarantee that the child will avoid abduction in real life. Although prevention of abduction and sexual abuse by strangers is a high priority, most sexual offenses are committed by people known to the child.

No study has produced evidence that the education of children about abduction and sexual abuse actually reduces the occurrence of such offenses. Without actual measures of abuse as outcome indicators, one cannot make firm recommendations about educational interventions for the prevention of sexual abuse and abduction.

Recommendations of Others

The second report of the U.S. Advisory Board on Child Abuse and Neglect released in September 1991, called upon the U.S. Federal Government to implement a universal voluntary neonatal home visitation system. The evidence reviewed in this chapter indicates that the effectiveness of home visitation programs in preventing child maltreatment has been demonstrated only in high-risk populations.

Conclusions and Recommendations

There is fair evidence not to recommend use of screening devices for identifying parents or families at risk for child maltreatment (D Recommendation) because of the high false positive rates and the harm associated with labelling parents as potential child abusers. However, physicians should know the risk indicators that characterize populations at increased risk for child maltreatment so that effective interventions for high-risk groups can be recommended (communities with high rates of poverty, and single and adolescent parenthood).

Two RCTs<13,14> provide evidence that home visitation can prevent child physical abuse and neglect or outcomes associated with maltreatment among disadvantaged families characterized by one or more of single parenthood, teenaged parenthood, and poverty. Thus, there is good evidence to recommend referral for home visitation during the perinatal period and through infancy to prevent child physical abuse and neglect for families of low socioeconomic status, single parenthood or teenaged parenthood (A Recommendation). There is inconclusive evidence regarding including or excluding a referral for intensive contact with a pediatrician, early and extended postpartum hospital contact or both, use of a drop-in centre, or parent training programs in the prevention of child maltreatment (C Recommendation). These interventions may be beneficial for other reasons and should be assessed on an individual basis; whether they reduce the incidence of abuse and neglect remains to be established.

Whether education programs for children reduce the incidence of sexual abuse and abduction remains to be established. Physicians making recommendations regarding such programs must do so on other grounds (C Recommendation).

Unanswered Questions (Research Agenda)

The following have been identified as research priorities:

1. Measuring the prevalence rates and distribution of child maltreatment and its subcategories in the general population including identifying populations at high-risk.

2. Investigating second-stage screening that would do more good than harm within high-risk populations.

3. Determining for different populations the optimal content, duration and frequency of visits, and qualifications of providers for home visitation program.

4. Further evaluation of interventions aimed at prevention of sexual abuse (effectiveness in reducing incidence of such episodes, in identifying children who have been sexually abused and any negative effects associated with the education programs).

Acknowledgements

The authors thank Drs. William R. Beardslee, Associate Professor of Psychiatry, Judge Baker Children's Center, Boston, Massachusetts, Leon Eisenberg, Professor Emeritus, Department of Social Medicine, Harvard Medical School, Boston, Massachusetts, USA, Kenneth M. McConnochie, Associate Professor of Pediatrics, University of Rochester, School of Medicine and Dentistry, Rochester,

New York, and David L. Olds, Professor of Pediatrics, University of Colorado Health Sciences Center, Denver, Colorado, for their helpful criticism of the background report.

Harriet MacMillan was supported by a New Faculty Research Fellowship from the Ontario Mental Health Foundation and the Chedoke-McMaster Hospitals Foundation. David Offord was supported by a National Health Scientist Award from Health Canada. Funding for this report was also provided by Health Canada under the Government of Canada's Family Violence Initiative.

Evidence

The medical literature was identified using the following search strategy for the years January 1979 to April 1993: 1) MEDLINE using the MESH headings child abuse, battered child syndrome, incest, and the textword prevent; 2) ERIC, PSYCINFO, CRIMINAL JUSTICE PERIODICAL INDEX and CHILD ABUSE AND NEGLECT using the descriptors child abuse, child neglect, incest, and prevention.

This review was initiated in 1992 and recommendations were finalized by the Task Force in January 1993. A report with a full reference list was published in January 1993.[29]

Selected References

1. Murphy S, Orkow B, Nicola RM: Prenatal prediction of child abuse and neglect: a prospective study. *Child Abuse Negl* 1985; 9: 225-235

2. Muir RC, Monaghan SM, Gilmore RJ, *et al*: Predicting child abuse and neglect in New Zealand. *Aust N Z J Psychiatry* 1989; 23: 255-260

3. Monaghan SM, Gilmore RJ, Muir RC, *et al*: Prenatal screening for risk of major parenting problems: further results from the Queen Mary Maternity Hospital Child Care Unit. *Child Abuse Negl* 1986; 10: 369-375

4. Milner JS, Gold RG, Ayoub C, *et al*: Predictive validity of the Child Abuse Potential Inventory. *J Consult Clin Psychol* 1984; 52: 879-884

5. Schneider CJ: The Michigan Screening Profile of Parenting. In Starr RH (ed): *Child Abuse Prediction: Policy Implications.* Ballinger, Cambridge, MA, 1982: 157-174

6. Bavolek SJ: Research and Validation Report of the Adult-Adolescent Parenting Inventory. Family Development Resources Inc., USA, 1989

7. Azar ST, Rohrbeck CA: Child abuse and unrealistic expectations: further validation of the Parent Opinion Questionnaire. *J Consult Clin Psychol* 1986; 54: 867-868

8. Altemeier WA, O'Connor S, Vietze P, *et al*: Prediction of child abuse: a prospective study of feasibility. *Child Abuse Negl* 1984; 8: 393-400

9. Gray JD, Cutler CA, Dean JG, *et al*: Prediction and prevention of child abuse. *Semin Perinatol* 1979; 3: 85-90

10. Leventhal JM, Garber RB, Brady CA: Identification during the postpartum period of infants who are at high risk of child maltreatment. *J Pediatr* 1989; 114: 481-487

11. MacMillan HL, MacMillan JH, Offord DR, *et al*: Primary prevention of child physical abuse and neglect: a critical review: Part I. *J Child Psychol Psychiatry* 1994; 35: 835-856

12. MacMillan HL, MacMillan JH, Offord DR, *et al*: Primary prevention of child sexual abuse: a critical review: Part II. *J Child Psychol Psychiatry* 1994; 35: 857-876

13. Olds DL, Henderson CR Jr, Chamberlin R, *et al*: Preventing child abuse and neglect: a randomized trial of nurse home visitation. *Pediatrics* 1986; 78: 65-78

14. Hardy JB, Streett R: Family support and parenting education in the home: an effective extension of clinic-based preventive health care services for poor children. *J Pediatr* 1989; 115: 927-931

15. Siegel E, Bauman KE, Schaefer ES, *et al*: Hospital and home support during infancy: impact on maternal attachment, child abuse and neglect, and health care utilization. *Pediatrics* 1980; 66: 183-190

16. O'Connor S, Vietze PM, Sherrod KB, *et al*: Reduced incidence of parenting inadequacy following rooming-in. *Pediatrics* 1980; 66: 176-182

17. Lealman GT, Haigh D, Phillips JM, *et al*: Prediction and prevention of child abuse – An empty hope? *Lancet* 1983; 1: 1423-1424

18. Wolfe DA, Edwards B, Manion I, *et al*: Early intervention for parents at risk of child abuse and neglect: a preliminary investigation. *J Consult Clin Psychol* 1988; 56: 40-47

19. Resnick G: Enhancing parental competencies for high risk mothers: an evaluation of prevention effects. *Child Abuse Negl* 1985; 9: 479-489

20. Wurtele SK: School-based sexual abuse prevention programs: a review. *Child Abuse Negl* 1987; 11: 483-495

21. Conte JR, Rosen C, Saperstein L, *et al*: An evaluation of a program to prevent the sexual victimization of young children. *Child Abuse Negl* 1985; 9: 319-328

22. Wurtele SK, Saslawsky DA, Miller CL, *et al*: Teaching personal safety skills for potential prevention of sexual abuse: a comparison of treatments. *J Consult Clin Psychol* 1986; 54: 688-692

23. Harvey P, Forehand R, Brown C, *et al*: The prevention of sexual abuse: examination of the effectiveness of a program with kindergarten-age children. *Behav Ther* 1988; 19: 429-435

24. Wurtele SK, Kast LC, Melzer AM: Sexual abuse prevention education for young children: a comparison of teachers and parents as instructors. *Child Abuse Negl* 1992; 16: 865-876

25. Hazzard A, Webb C, Kleemeier C, *et al*: Child sexual abuse prevention: evaluation and one-year follow-up. *Child Abuse Negl* 1991; 15: 123-138

26. Fryer Jr GE, Kraizer SK, Miyoshi T: Measuring actual reduction of risk to child abuse: a new approach. *Child Abuse Negl* 1987; 11: 173-179

27. Poche C, Yoder P, Miltenberger R: Teaching self-protection to children using television techniques. *J App Behav Anal* 1988; 21: 253-261

28. Kolko DJ, Moser JT, Hughes J: Classroom training in sexual victimization awareness and prevention skills: an extension of the red flag/green flag people program. *J Fam Violence* 1989; 4: 25-45

29. MacMillan HL, MacMillan JH, Offord DR with the Canadian Task Force on the Periodic Health Examination: Periodic health examination, 1993 update: 1. Primary prevention of child maltreatment. *Can Med Assoc J* 1993; 148: 151-163

Primary Prevention of Child Maltreatment

MANEUVER	EFFECTIVENESS	LEVEL OF EVIDENCE <REF>	RECOMMENDATION
Screening procedures (checklists, self-administered questionnaires, standardized interviews or clinical judgement) used to identify people at risk of maltreating children	High false positive rates, resulting in high risk of mislabelling people as potential child abusers.	Cohort studies <1-4,8-10> (II-2)	Fair evidence to exclude from the periodic health examination (D)
Home visitation during perinatal period through infancy for families of low socioeconomic status, single parenthood or teenaged parenthood	Decreased number of reports of abuse and neglect, emergency department (ED) visits, accidents and hospital admissions.	Randomized controlled trials<13,14> (I)	Good evidence to include referral for home visitation in periodic health examination (A)
Intensive contact with pediatrician plus home visitation	No significant reduction in number of reports of abuse and neglect or of accidents; children in intervention group were admitted to hospital because of serious injuries less often than those in control group.	Randomized controlled trial<9> (I)	Insufficient evidence to include in or exclude from periodic health examination; referral should be assessed on an individual basis (C)
Early or extended post-partum hospital contact or both	No significant reduction in number of reports of child abuse and neglect, ED visits, accidents, or hospital admissions in intervention group.	Randomized controlled trials<15,16> (I)	Insufficient evidence to include in periodic health examination but may be beneficial for other conditions (C)
Drop-in centre	Reduction in number of ED visits but not in number of reports of child abuse and neglect, hospital admissions or admissions because of trauma in intervention group.	Non-randomized controlled trial<17> (II-1)	Insufficient evidence to include referral in periodic health examination (C)

(Continued on next page)

Primary Prevention of Child Maltreatment (concl'd)

MANEUVER	EFFECTIVENESS	LEVEL OF EVIDENCE <REF>	RECOMMENDATION
Parent training program	Reports of child abuse and neglect as well as measures of events associated with child maltreatment not examined.	Randomized controlled trial<18> (I)	Insufficient evidence to include referral in periodic health examination but may be beneficial for other conditions (C)
Sexual abuse and abduction prevention programs for children	Improved knowledge of sexual abuse and enhanced awareness of safety skills; no studies have determined effectiveness of programs in reducing incidence of sexual abuse of abduction.	Randomized controlled trials<21-27> (I)	Insufficient evidence to include referral in periodic health examination; referral must be made on other grounds (C)

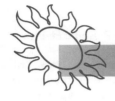

CHAPTER 30

Screening
for Childhood
Obesity

By William Feldman and Brenda L. Beagan

30

Screening for Childhood Obesity

Prepared by William Feldman, MD, FRCPC[1] and Brenda L. Beagen, MA[2]

In 1979, the Canadian Task Force on the Periodic Health Examination concluded that there was no satisfactory justification for including childhood obesity among conditions to be sought in a periodic health examination, based on the lack of an effective program directed to treatment and prevention of obesity in children. However, it was considered advisable to record height and weight on standard growth charts and identify any deviations from normal growth.

Since then, several studies have investigated the consequences of childhood obesity and several randomized controlled trials have been published on the effectiveness of treatment programs. In light of these developments, it was thought to be timely to reconsider our recommendations based on the new evidence. For more information on obesity on older age groups, consult Chapter 48.

Burden of Suffering

Estimates of Canadian prevalence rates for childhood obesity range from 7% to 43%, depending on whether the basis is self-reports or objective measures, and on what measure of obesity is used (e.g. body mass indices or skinfold thickness). The body mass index (BMI) or Quetelet's index, is weight divided by height squared (kg/m^2).

An inverse relationship has been shown between social class and prevalence of obesity in children aged 3-18 years, with rates ranging from 25% in low income families to 5% in high income families.

Recent adoption and twin studies suggest that family environment alone has no apparent effect on obesity but that genetic factors appear to predominate. The Swedish Adoption/Twin Study of Aging, combining the adoption and twin designs, showed that twins reared together were no more similar than twins reared apart, indicating that shared rearing environment had no effect on BMI. In a recent Canadian study of long-term overfeeding in 12 pairs of identical twins, the variance in weight gain and fatness gain between pairs was about six times greater than the variance within pairs. The authors

---

[1] Professor of Pediatrics and of Preventive Medicine and Biostatistics, University of Toronto, Toronto, Ontario
[2] Research Associate for the Task Force, 1990-92, Department of Pediatrics, Dalhousie University, Halifax, Nova Scotia

concluded that genetic factors influence the effect environmental factors have on weight status.

Fewer than 5% of obese children have an underlying disease producing obesity – the majority simply have an imbalance between energy expenditure and intake. However, several disease conditions can cause obesity, including endocrinopathies, central nervous system diseases, and specific congenital syndromes.

Infants and children who are obese are at somewhat increased risk of becoming obese adults.[1,2] That is, relative weight and skinfold thickness tend to "track" over time. However, the correlations are low, and the probability that an individual obese infant will be an obese adult is not high. Furthermore, the longer the age interval, the weaker the relation.

The probability that an individual obese infant will become an obese adult is not high

There are few known physical health risks to children who are obese. There is some indication of an association between obesity and hypertension in children, although false high blood pressure readings are not uncommon, a result of using cuffs that are too small for oversized arms.[3]

Obese children have been observed to have elevated levels of low-density lipoprotein cholesterol, and decreased levels of high-density lipoprotein.[4] Obesity in adults however, is not a strong independent contributor to heart disease risk in the absence of other coronary risk factors. Nevertheless, the same circumstances which produce the obesity may also increase other risk factors. It is unclear, then, whether obesity is a cause or a correlate.

In the Bogalusa Heart Study, 3,503 subjects of varying weights aged 5-24 showed marked and highly significant ($p<0.001$) clustering of three cardiovascular disease risk factors: systolic blood pressure, fasting insulin, and ratio of low- to high-density lipoprotein cholesterol.[5] When lipid risk factors were correlated to subscapular skinfold thickness, the relationship was not clear-cut; for example, it was not statistically significant for white or black males aged 5-9 and 20-24 years.

An earlier report from the Bogalusa Heart Study also indicated that there was an association between obesity and cardiovascular risk factors. However, the children who were studied were only those whose weight category "tracked" over the 6 year period under investigation (18% of the sample) and the children also tended to have other risk factors: high blood pressure, triglyceride levels and cholesterol levels.

Evidence from the Muscatine Ponderosity Family Study is also somewhat ambiguous[6] providing data on consistently heavy children and a "heavy gain group". Some but not all risk factor levels were high (considering total cholesterol, LDL cholesterol, apolipoprotein A-1, apolipoprotein B, and diastolic blood pressure). The above studies do not prove that obesity increases the risk of cardiovascular disease or that prevention or treatment of childhood obesity decreases adult coronary artery morbidity and mortality.

Abraham and colleagues conducted a retrospective cohort study examining the relationship between childhood weight status and adult morbidity.<7> They located 902 adult males for whom childhood weight and health records were available. Examination showed no association between weight status in childhood and adult cholesterol status, adult cardiovascular/renal disease, atherosclerosis or diabetes. The highest risk for hypertensive vascular and cardiovascular renal disease was found in those overweight adults who moved from a below average childhood weight category to an overweight adult group. Smoking status of adults was not assessed. It is possible that adult onset obesity is associated with more cigarette smoking and it is the smoking which is related to cardiovascular disease.

Studies have shown an association between infant or childhood obesity and increased incidence of acute respiratory infections, even when data is adjusted for factors such as social class, smoking, and overcrowding.<8,9>

Javier-Nieto et al<10> reviewed over 13,000 files on persons who were between 5-18 years old between 1933-1945. These were linked to census and death certificate records. The heaviest 20% during pre-puberty and adolescence had an adult mortality odds ratio adjusted for education and smoking status that was significantly greater than that of the lowest weight 20%. Must et al<11> did a follow-up of 508 people who were adolescents between 1922-1935. Overweight in adolescence (BMI top 25%) was associated with an increased risk of mortality from all causes and disease-specific mortality among men but not among women.

Severe obesity has been linked to increased mortality in adults, but there is no association between moderate childhood obesity and increased mortality, unless other risk factors are present.<4>

No association between moderate childhood obesity and increased mortality of adults exists, unless other risk factors are present

However, obese children may suffer significant social and psychological difficulties. In the Western world, there is strong cultural prejudice against obesity and a cultural obsession with thinness, which can lead to stigmatization and discrimination in academic and work environments, as well as in other social settings.<12> Obese children may be teased and harassed by their peers, may be socially ostracized, and may be treated as stupid and inferior by teachers and other adults.<13> Children share these negative cultural concepts about obesity, acquiring them very early, possibly as young as age 7.<14> Obese children therefore often have a very negative body image and generally low self-esteem.<4,13> One consequence of this poor self-image may be the development of eating disorders such as anorexia nervosa in adolescence.<13,14>

Maneuver

The assessment of obesity in children requires the use of reliable and valid measures of obesity. The use of body weight alone fails to allow for differences in height and stature. For adults there are acceptable tables of desirable weight for height based on the lowest mortality rates in an insured population e.g. the Metropolitan Life weight charts. However, there is no equivalent for children. There are some tables using average weight for age, height and sex, and several indices have been developed to attempt to standardize for height, such as the BMI.

The measurement of triceps or subscapular skinfold thickness to assess subcutaneous fat is a more direct measure of adiposity, and is better able than BMI to distinguish adiposity from muscularity and very large or very small stature. The correlation of multiple skinfold measures with total body fatness is in the range of 0.7-0.8.[3] However, the accuracy of skinfold measures decreases among very obese children. The Eid Index is the child's weight compared to the 50th percentile weight for the age at which the child's height is in the 50th percentile expressed as a percentage.

Effectiveness of Screening and Treatment

The benefits of early detection depend upon the availability of effective means to reduce body fat, and the feasibility of maintaining the loss and a resultant improvement in measures of mortality and/or morbidity.

The more drastic methods of fat reduction, such as surgery, pharmacotherapy, and gastric balloons are not appropriate for children, and very low calorie diets may impair their growth and development.

There is no evidence that traditional means of fat reduction – low calorie diets and/or increased exercise – produce successful results which are maintained on a long-term basis.[15] In one of the few intervention trials with adequate follow-up time, 21 children who were at least 30% overweight and as much as 144% overweight (n=21) lost an average of 33% on very low calorie diets.[16] On re-examination 4-10 years later, ten had maintained a reduced percentage overweight, by 3-61%; the other 11 children had gained back all the weight they had lost plus an additional 5-86% excess weight.

There is no evidence that low calorie diets and/or increased exercise produce long-term sustainable weight loss

Two types of exercise programs have been evaluated, life-style and aerobic. The evidence about whether diet plus exercise of either type improves results over diet alone (level II-2) is ambiguous.[16-19] In one study Epstein and his colleagues found it did,[19] but in an earlier study the same researchers found it did not.[20] However, the Task Force recommends the regular practice of moderate physical activity for the maintenance of a healthy body weight (Chapter 47).

Epstein and his colleagues have conducted a series of trials investigating the effectiveness of behavioral modification for weight reduction in children. Two of these studies were with children under the age of eight. In one trial in 5-8 year old girls (n=19), those in a family-based treatment program decreased their percentage overweight almost twice as much as control girls in a health education program.[21] In a later study, 17 children aged 1-6 years showed significant change in percentage overweight in a 12-month family-based treatment program.[22] At no point did the group mean go below obesity status (20% overweight).

There have also been several studies on preadolescents, children about eight to twelve years old. At least three of these have been controlled trials, where controls got no treatment. In all cases, the controls gained weight while children receiving treatment lost 6-20% excess weight.[20,23,24] The control group in each case was composed of children put on a waiting list to get into the treatment program – there is no way to know if that had any effect on the control children's weight status.

Some studies have examined the effect of including parents in treatment programs. There is some evidence that including parents in the program improves the success of both weight loss and maintenance of the loss. However, this is not unequivocal. In one trial, Epstein et al examined the importance of child self-control vs. parent control of the therapeutic process, randomly assigning 37 obese children to either of two groups (level I).[25] There was no significant difference in weight status after 5 years; all groups had returned to approximately baseline levels. In another small study, (n=30) Kirschenbaum et al found no evidence of superior results from including parents in the treatment programs.[24]

In a series of trials using behavioral modification therapy, with the "Traffic Light Diet" (green = low calories, yellow = moderate calories, red = high calories), Epstein et al found including parents does improve maintenance of weight loss.[26-28] They have recently published the results of a ten-year follow-up for this approach.[28] Children aged 6-12 years from intact, predominantly white, middle-class families (75 out of 185 applicant families met the study entrance requirements) were randomized to each of the three treatment groups (diet and exercise information plus behaviour modification for the child alone, for the parent and child, or information without behaviour modification). All groups attended 8 weekly meetings, and 6 additional meetings over the next 6 months.

Follow-up of 61 families was achieved at 10 years; six children had developed psychiatric problems and were excluded (final n=55). While initial amounts of weight lost were similar, after five years and after ten years members of the group in which both parents and children were targeted for behaviour modification were significantly less obese than members of the information only group. Not that obesity was completely prevented – even the parent-child information and behaviour modification group was about 35% overweight at the 10 year follow-up. This is the first evidence that the effects of treatment for obesity in childhood can persist into young adulthood. Moreover, the treatment does not appear to have had adverse effects, especially on ultimate height. Given the intensity of the intervention and the high motivation of these families caution in generalizing these results is indicated; they are nonetheless encouraging.[28]

There is little evidence regarding potential risks of treatment – it is generally assumed that weight control efforts are safe for children and infants. There is, however, some evidence that dietary restrictions at this age level may produce adverse effects. Mallick reviews several early studies which indicate that dietary restriction in infants and young children may result in retardation of growth and development, both physically and mentally, and these adverse effects may be permanent.[29] Other recent reviews also suggest that adolescents may not be safely subjected to calorie restriction at any point during their growth spurt.[30,31] Epstein[32] has argued that this previous research may have failed to consider the height of the children upon entry into weight loss programs.

Recommendations of Others

The American Academy of Pediatrics recommends that children's height and weight measurements be taken throughout infancy, annually from ages 1 to 6, and bi-annually thereafter. The U.S. Preventive Services Task Force recommends height and weight measurements be taken regularly and plotted on a growth chart throughout infancy and childhood;[33] this recommendation is currently being reviewed. Although the U.S. Task Force makes recommendations for nutrition and exercise counselling for adults, there are no specific recommendations for children.

Conclusions and Recommendations

It is understood that plotting the height and weight of infants and children during a periodic health examination will continue to be done, primarily to identify children who are failing to thrive. There is insufficient evidence that screening children for obesity is of value; nor is there evidence that screening for obesity is harmful (C Recommendation).[3]

There is insufficient evidence to include or exclude counselling about nutrition and exercise from the routine treatment of severely

---

[3] For highly motivated obese children and their families, there is good evidence that intensive diet, exercise, and family behaviour management counselling is successful in lowering the degree of obesity 10 years later, but these obese children were not identified by screening.

obese children (C Recommendation). However, the regular practice of moderate physical activity, taking into account current fitness levels, is recommended for all Canadians to maintain a healthy body weight (Chapter 47). There is fair evidence for excluding very low calorie diets from the routine treatment of pre-adolescent obese children (D Recommendation). Evidence is conflicting regarding the inclusion or exclusion of exercise from the routine treatment of obese children. (C Recommendation)

Unanswered Questions (Research Agenda)

1. Do family-based instruction and behaviour modification programs for childhood obesity improve the child's self-esteem?

2. If so, can these results be obtained in less advantaged, possibly less motivated groups?

3. Is there more eating disorders among adolescents who were previously involved in weight reduction programs?

4. If childhood obesity can be prevented or treated in childhood, what are the long-term benefits and risks?

Evidence

A MEDLINE search for January 1981, to February 1991, was undertaken using the key words, child and obesity. Additional references from articles retrieved were pursued. Current contents were retrieved and reviewed until December 1992. This review was initiated in February 1991 and the recommendations finalized by the Task Force in November 1992.

Selected References

1. Johnston FE: Health implications of childhood obesity. *Ann Intern Med* 1985; 103: 1068-1072

2. Garn SM: Continuities and changes in fatness from infancy through adulthood. *Curr Probl Pediatr* 1985; 15: 1-47

3. Merritt RJ: Obesity. *Curr Probl Pediatr* 1982; 12: 1-58

4. Leung AK, Robson WLM: Childhood obesity. *Postgrad Med* 1990; 87: 123-133

5. Smoak CG, Burke GL, Webber LS, *et al*: Relation of obesity to clustering of cardiovascular disease risk factors in children and young adults. *Am J Epidemiol* 1987; 125: 364-372

6. Burns TL, Moll PP, Lauer RM: The relation between ponderosity and coronary risk factors in children and their relatives: The Muscatine Ponderosity Family Study. *Am J Epidemiol* 1989; 129: 973-987

7. Abraham S, Collins G, Nordsieck M: Relationship of childhood weight status to morbidity in adults. *Public Health Rep* 1971; 86: 273-284

8. Tracey VV, De NC, Harper JR: Obesity and respiratory infection in infants and young children. *Br Med J* 1971; 1(739): 16-18

9. Somerville SM, Rona RJ, Chinn S: Obesity and respiratory symptoms in primary school. *Arch Dis Childhood* 1984; 59: 940-944

10. Javier-Nieto F, Szklo M, Comstock GW: Childhood weight and growth rate as predictors of adult mortality. *Am J Epidemiol* 1992; 136: 201-213

11. Must A, Jacques PF, Dallal GE, *et al*: Long-term morbidity and mortality of overweight adolescents: A follow-up of the Harvard Growth Study of 1922 to 1935. *N Engl J Med* 1992; 327: 1350-1355

12. Klesges RC, Klem ML, Hanson CL, *et al*: The effects of applicant's health status and qualifications on simulated hiring decisions. *Int J Obes* 1990; 14: 527-535

13. Wadden TA, Stunkard AJ: Social and psychological consequences of obesity. *Ann Intern Med* 1985; 103: 1062-1067

14. Feldman W, Feldman E, Goodman JT: Culture versus biology: children's attitudes toward thinness and fatness. *Pediatrics* 1988; 81: 190-194

15. Committee on Nutrition: Nutritional aspects of obesity in infancy and childhood. *Pediatrics* 1981; 68: 880-883

16. Ginsberg-Fellner F, Knittle JL: Weight reduction in young obese children. I. Effects on adipose tissue cellularity and metabolism. *Pediatr Res* 1981; 15: 1381-1389

17. Ballew C, Liu K, Levinson S, *et al*: Comparison of three weight-for-height indices in blood pressure studies in children. *Am J Epidemiol* 1990; 131: 532-537

18. Ward DS, Bar-Or O: Role of the physician and physical education teacher in the treatment of obesity at school. *Pediatrician* 1986; 13: 44-51

19. Epstein LH, Wing RR, Penner BC, *et al*: Effect of diet and controlled exercise on weight loss in obese children. *J Pediatr* 1985; 107: 358-361

20. Epstein LH, Wing RR, Koeske R, *et al*: Effects of diet plus exercise on weight change in parents and children. *J Consult Clin Psychol* 1984; 52: 429-437

21. Epstein LH, Wing RR, Woodall K, *et al*: Effects of family based behavioral treatment on obese 5-8 year old children. *Behaviour Therapy* 1985; 16: 205-212

22. Epstein LH, Valoski A, Koeske R, *et al*: Family-based behavioral weight control in obese young children. *J Am Diet Assoc* 1986; 86: 481-484

23. Israel AC, Stolmaker L, Sharp JP, *et al*: An evaluation of two methods of parental involvement in treating obese children. *Behaviour Therapy* 1984; 15: 266-272

24. Kirschenbaum DS, Harris ES, Tomarken AJ: Effects of parental involvement in behavioral weight loss therapy for preadolescents. *Behaviour Therapy* 1984; 15: 485-500

25. Epstein LH, Wing RR, Valoski A, *et al*: Long-term effects of parent weight loss on child weight loss. *Behaviour Therapy* 1987; 18: 219-226

26. Epstein LH, Wing RR, Koeske R, *et al*: Child and parent weight loss in family-based behavioral modification programs. *J Consult Clin Psychol* 1981; 49: 674-685

27. Epstein LH, Wing RR, Koeske R, *et al*: Long-term effects of family-based treatment of childhood obesity. *J Consult Clin Psychol* 1987; 55: 91-95

28. Epstein LH, Valoski, Wing RR, *et al*: Ten-year follow-up of behavioral, family-based treatment for obese children. *JAMA* 1990; 264: 2519-2523

29. Mallick MJ: Health hazards of obesity and weight control in children: a review of the literature. *Am J Public Health* 1983; 73: 78-82

30. Paige DM: Obesity in childhood and adolescence: special problems in diagnosis and treatment. *Postgrad Med* 1986; 79: 233-245

31. Kneebone GM: Childhood obesity – the diagnosis and management. *Aust Fam Physician* 1990; 19: 367-370

32. Epstein LH, McCurley J, Valoski A, *et al*: Growth in obese children treated for obesity. *Am J Dis Children* 1990; 144: 1360-1364

33. U.S. Preventive Services Task Force: *Guide to Clinical Preventive Services: an Assessment of the Effectiveness of 169 Interventions.* Williams & Wilkins, Baltimore, Md, 1989: 111-114

Screening for Childhood Obesity

MANEUVER	EFFECTIVENESS	LEVEL OF EVIDENCE <REF>	RECOMMENDATION
Detection 1) Measuring heights and weights of infants and children*	Insufficient evidence that screening for obesity leads to improved outcome. Effect of obesity on adult obesity and as a risk factor for morbidity and mortality (except psychological effect) is unclear.	Cohort studies <1,2,6-11> (II-2)	Insufficient evidence to include or exclude in health exam of children to prevent obesity (C)
2) Skin-fold thickness, body mass index (BMI) etc. for obesity	Insufficient evidence that screening for obesity leads to improved outcome. Effect of childhood obesity on subsequent obesity and as a risk factor for morbidity and mortality is unclear.	Cohort studies <1-3,5,11> (II-2)	Insufficient evidence to include or exclude in periodic health exam to prevent obesity (C)
Intervention 1) Very low calorie diets	Weight lost on very low calorie diets is poorly maintained.	Cohort studies <15,16> (II–2)	There is fair evidence for excluding very low calorie diets from the routine treatment of pre–adolescent obese children (D)
2) Exercise	Evidence is ambiguous regarding the role of exercise in initial weight loss or maintenance.	Cohort studies <16-19> (II–2)	There is insufficient evidence to include or exclude in the routine treatment of obese children (C)

*   Should continue to be done to screen for failure to thrive (see Chapter 24).

(Continued on next page)

Screening for Childhood Obesity (concl'd)

MANEUVER	EFFECTIVENESS	LEVEL OF EVIDENCE <REF>	RECOMMENDATION
3) Family-based nutrition and exercise education and behaviour modification	Weight loss has been maintained at 10-year follow-up in 6-12 year old obese children. Children were still about 35% overweight. High costs of these programs, lack of general availability and the extreme motivation of the families may limit generalizability. Other than weight, other outcome measures of interest (general health, self-esteem) were not measured. These programs are not readily applicable to primary care offices.	Randomized controlled trials<21-24,28,29> (I)	Insufficient evidence to include or exclude in the routine treatment of obese children (C)**

** There is evidence from a single study that moderate weight reduction can be achieved through intensive family-based instruction/behaviour modification program in intact, wealthy, well-motivated families. Whether this confers health benefits is unknown.

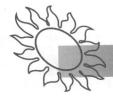

CHAPTER **31**

Screening for Idiopathic Adolescent Scoliosis

By Richard B. Goldbloom

Screening for Idiopathic Adolescent Scoliosis

Adapted by Richard B. Goldbloom, OC, MD, FRCPC[1] from the report prepared for the U.S. Preventive Services Task Force[2]

In 1979, the Canadian Task Force on the Periodic Health Examination reviewed the evidence then available and concluded that there was poor evidence to support the inclusion or exclusion of routine adolescent idiopathic scoliosis screening in the periodic health examination<1> (C Recommendation). A detailed review by one of the Task Force members was published subsequently.<2> A more recent, updated review of the evidence by the U.S. Preventive Services Task Force<3> using the same methodology, arrived at the same conclusion. The Canadian Task Force concurs with the U.S. Task Force analysis and conclusions.

Burden of Suffering

A study of over 29,000 children in a community health district of the province of Quebec demonstrated a prevalence of scoliosis of 42 per 1,000 in children aged 8-15 years. The Scoliosis Research Society defines scoliosis as a curve of 11° or greater. Such curves are reported to have a prevalence of 2-3% in adolescents at the end of their growth period. Curves which are greater than 40°-50° have a reported prevalence of 0.2% and cause disability and significant health problems later in life. Several investigators have reported the ratio of affected girls to boys as 1.5:1 and the prevalence of large and small curves is higher in girls. However, the prevalence of cases needing treatment in either sex is very low. Potential adverse effects include cosmetic deformity, back pain, social and psychological problems (e.g. poor self-image, social isolation), limited job opportunities, lower marriage rate and the financial costs of treatment.

Little firm epidemiological evidence suggests that persons with idiopathic scoliosis experience more back pain than the general population

There is little firm evidence from epidemiologic studies that persons with idiopathic scoliosis are at significantly greater risk of experiencing back pain than the general population. The incidence of back pain in the general population may be as high as 60-80% and it is unclear whether the incidence of pain is higher in persons with scoliosis. Pulmonary disease and other serious health effects attributable to idiopathic scoliosis occur in individuals with large curves that are easily detected without screening.

---

[1] Professor of Pediatrics, Dalhousie University, Halifax, Nova Scotia
[2] By Steven H. Woolf, MD, MPH, Science Advisor, U.S. Preventive Services Task Force, Washington, D.C. and Assistant Clinical Professor, Dept. of Family Practice, Medical College of Virginia, Richmond, Virginia

Maneuver

The principal screening test for scoliosis is physical examination including upright visual inspection of the back and the Adams forward bending test. The sensitivity and specificity of this examination in detecting curves greater than 10° have been reported as 73.9% and 77.8%, respectively.[4] In an Australian study, the positive predictive value (PPV) was 78% for curves greater than 5° in a population with an estimated prevalence for this degree of curvature of 3%.[5] A Canadian study involving specially trained school nurses reported a PPV of 18% in detecting curves greater than 20°.[6]

Based on an extensive prevalence study, Morais et al[6] estimated the PPV of the forward bending test as 42.8% for scoliotic curves of 5° or more, and only 6.4% when curves of 15° or more were considered. In typical screening settings where the prevalence and PPV are relatively low, for every curve >10° detected, there are 1-5 false positives; and for every curve >20° detected there are 3-24 false positives.[3] There is little evidence about the incremental value of repeat screening in individuals with previously normal results. There is insufficient evidence to evaluate the role of other tests, e.g. inclinometry or Moiré topography, as screening instruments.[7-9]

For every curve >20° detected, there are 3-24 false positives

Effectiveness of Screening and Treatment

Any proposal to screen for adolescent idiopathic scoliosis requires that several conditions be met:

1. That the screening test is accurate and reliable detecting curves that are both clinically significant and unlikely to be detected otherwise.

2. That earlier detection leads to improved health outcomes.

3. That effective treatment is available for cases detected through screening.

4. That scoliosis causes important health problems.

5. That small curves detected by screening are likely to progress to degrees of clinical significance.

6. That the benefits of early detection through screening outweigh any adverse effects of screening and treatment.

There have been no controlled studies to demonstrate that adolescents who are screened routinely for scoliosis have better outcomes than those who are not screened. There are no studies demonstrating a decrease in spinal fusions by screening or brace treatment. In communities that have adopted aggressive screening programs, favourable trends in curve size and surgery rates have been reported but it is unclear whether such changes are attributable to screening or to other temporal factors.[10-12]

No controlled studies demonstrate that adolescents screened routinely for scoliosis have better outcomes than the unscreened

Brace Therapy

There is inadequate evidence to determine whether brace therapy limits the natural progression of scoliosis in a significant number of cases. Most evidence concerning its effectiveness comes from uncontrolled case series reports. Early reports with limited follow-up had suggested significant degrees of correction. However, long-term studies involving more than 5 years of follow-up have shown a gradual loss of correction, with mean overall improvement averaging 2-4% compared with pre-brace curves.<13,14> One retrospective, case-controlled study showed that braced patients had a somewhat reduced rate of curve progression as compared to matched controls, but the difference was not statistically significant.<15> There have been no controlled studies that provide information on health outcomes such as back pain, self-esteem or psychosocial impact. Finally, compliance with the wearing of a brace is frequently poor.<16,17> An ongoing multicentre trial of brace therapy should provide additional information on its effectiveness.

Lateral Electrical Surface Stimulation (LESS)

Available studies of effectiveness offer little evidence that LESS results in better clinical outcomes than braces or other forms of conservative treatment.<18-23>

Exercise

Although published studies are few, exercise alone has historically demonstrated poor effectiveness in controlling curve progression

Exercise has been suggested as a means of preventing the need for more extensive treatment or as an adjunct to the wearing of a brace.<24> Although published studies are few, exercise alone has historically demonstrated poor effectiveness in controlling curve progression.<24,25> A school-based program failed to show any difference in curve progression after one year between a group treated with exercise and matched controls.<25> By contrast, a small randomized, controlled trial of scoliotic adolescents wearing a cast showed that exercise was more effective than traction in improving curves on lateral bending.<26> An uncontrolled cohort study showed improved vital capacity in hospitalized scoliosis patients who received physiotherapy;<27> and a report of an uncontrolled case-series suggested that some braced patients who performed a thoracic flexion exercise had reduced vertebral rotation and thoracic curves after exercise.<28> However, this study lacked controls, follow-up and an assessment of clinical outcomes.

Surgery

Surgery is currently recommended only if a curve progresses to more than 40-50° or if the procedure is requested for cosmetic reasons. The goals of internal fixation are to reduce the rib hump, correct spinal rotation and to obtain solid fusion and stability. The most well-established procedure is Harrington instrumentation. Others include Cotrel-Dubousset instrumentation, the Zielke procedure and Luque sublaminar wiring.

Surgical techniques appear to be effective in reducing, but not eliminating, the lateral scoliotic curve.<29-33> Axial rotation is less effectively controlled surgically, and deformities in the sagittal plane can be exaggerated.<34> Few controlled studies of functional status following surgery have been reported. There is no evidence that early detection of severe instances of scoliosis through screening improves surgical outcomes.

Adverse Effects of Screening and Treatment

Although the initial screening examination has insignificant adverse effects problems may be associated with follow-up testing of presumed abnormal findings. Roentgenograms are not obtained routinely on all follow-up evaluations however, many physicians obtain them to rule out significant deformity and to provide a baseline for future comparisons. Further evaluation of the patient may generate anxiety and affect future health insurance and work eligibility. These are postulated adverse effects and have not been proven in controlled studies.

Conservative treatment such as braces and LESS may have adverse medical and psycho-social effects. An association between brace wear and diminished self-esteem and disturbed peer relationships has been documented. LESS can produce uncomfortable sensations from the electrical stimulus, sleep disturbance and skin irritation but reliable data on these adverse effects are not available. There are few significant adverse effects associated with exercise therapy.

The potential adverse effects of surgery can be more substantial. In addition to the general risk of surgery they include financial cost, lost productivity and external immobilization with casts or braces, which may be required for months after surgery. Potential long-term effects occur generally in adults and include chronic pain syndromes and other complications that may require further surgery.<30,35-37>

Costs

There have been few formal analyses of the cost effectiveness of screening for scoliosis. A Quebec study estimated a cost of $2.31 per child for screening and $59.60 per child for the clinical evaluation of positive cases; the total cost of case finding was $194.27 per case of confirmed scoliosis and $3,505.49 per case of scoliosis brought to treatment. No studies have fully evaluated the direct and indirect costs of screening.

Recommendations of Others

The Scoliosis Research Society has recommended annual screening of all children aged 10-14 years. The American Academy of Orthopedic Surgeons has recommended screening girls at ages 11 and 13 years, and boys once at age 13 or 14 years. The American Academy of Pediatrics has recommended scoliosis screening at routine health supervision visits at ages 10, 12, 14 and 16. Fifteen of the U.S. States require scoliosis screening by law, and 31 have voluntary programs. Only two of the 10 Canadian provinces (Alberta and Prince Edward Island) are officially engaged in scoliosis screening, in one instance for research projects only. By contrast, the British Orthopaedic Association and the British Scoliosis Society issued a statement in 1983 advising against a national policy of screening for scoliosis in the United Kingdom. Individual authors who have conducted extensive reviews of the evidence have reached similar conclusions.

Conclusions and Recommendations

There is insufficient evidence from published clinical research to indicate that screening for idiopathic scoliosis in adolescents is either effective or ineffective in improving the outcome (C Recommendation). It is reasonable for clinicians to include periodic visual inspection of the back in their examination of adolescents seen for other reasons. Clinicians and public health personnel should bear in mind the limited current evidence regarding the effectiveness of scoliosis screening and treatment and the uncertainties about the natural history of the condition.

Unanswered Questions (Research Agenda)

Well-designed clinical trials are needed to evaluate the effectiveness or ineffectiveness of routine screening for adolescent idiopathic scoliosis. The cost-effectiveness of scoliosis screening cannot be determined until its clinical effectiveness has been demonstrated.

Evidence

The literature was identified with a MEDLINE search for the English language in the years 1980 to 1992, using the following strategy: MESH term scoliosis and key words screening, Cobb, brace, exercise or physical and surgery supplemented by references cited in bibliographies and reviewer comments.

This review was initiated in January 1993 and the recommendations finalized by the Task Force in June 1993.

Selected References

1. Canadian Task Force on the Periodic Health Examination: The periodic health examination. *Can Med Assoc J* 1979; 121: 1193-1254

2. Mann KV: Screening for scoliosis: a review of the evidence. In: Goldbloom RB, Lawrence RS, (eds). *Preventing Disease: Beyond the Rhetoric.* Springer-Verlag, New York, NY, 1990: 197-203

3. U.S. Preventive Services Task Force: Screening for adolescent idiopathic scoliosis: policy statement and review article. *JAMA* 1993; 269: 1664-2666

4. Viviani GR, Budgell L, Dok C, *et al*: Assessment of accuracy of the scoliosis school screening examination. *Am J Public Health* 1984; 74: 497-498

5. Chan A, Moller J, Vimpani G, *et al*: The case for scoliosis screening in Australian adolescents. *Med J Aust* 1986; 145: 379-383

6. Morais T, Bernier M, Turcotte F: Age- and sex-specific prevalence of scoliosis and the value of school screening programs. *Am J Public Health* 1985; 75: 1377-1380

7. Bunnell WP: An objective criterion for scoliosis screening. *J Bone Joint Surg* Am 1984; 66: 1381-1387

8. Amendt LE, Ause-Ellias KL, Eybers JL, *et al*: Validity and reliability testing of the Scoliometer. *Phys Ther* 1990; 70: 108-117

9. Laulund T, Sojbjerg JO, Horlyck E: Moiré topography in school screening for structural scoliosis. *Acta Orthop Scand* 1982; 53: 765-768

10. Torell G, Nordwall A, Nachemson A: The changing pattern of scoliosis treatment due to effective screening. *J Bone Joint Surg* Am 1981; 63: 337-341

11. Lonstein JE, Bjorklund S, Wanninger MH, *et al*: Voluntary school screening for scoliosis in Minnesota. *J Bone Joint Surg* Am 1982; 64: 481-488

12. Ferris B, Edgar M, Leyshon A: Screening for scoliosis. *Acta Orthop Scand* 1988; 59: 417-418

13. Mellencamp DD, Blount WP, Anderson AJ: Milwaukee brace treatment of idiopathic scoliosis: late results. *Clin Orthop* 1977; 126: 47-57

14. Carr WA, Moe JH, Winter RB, *et al*: Treatment of idiopathic scoliosis in the Milwaukee brace. *J Bone Joint Surg Am* 1980; 62: 599-612

15. Miller, JA, Nachemson AL, Schultz AB: Effectiveness of braces in mild idiopathic scoliosis. *Spine* 1984; 9: 632-635

16. Wynne EJ: Scoliosis: to screen or not to screen. *Can J Public Health* 1984; 75: 277-280

17. DiRaimondo CV, Green NE: Brace-wear compliance in patients with adolescent idiopathic scoliosis. *J Pediatr Orthop* 1988; 8: 143-146

18. Axelgaard J, Brown JC: Lateral electrical surface stimulation for the treatment of progressive idiopathic scoliosis. *Spine* 1983; 8: 242-260

19. McCollough NC: Nonoperative treatment of idiopathic scoliosis using surface electrical stimulation. *Spine* 1986; 11: 802-804

20. Bradford DS, Tanguy A, Vanselow J: Surface electrical stimulation in the treatment of idiopathic scoliosis: preliminary results in 30 patients. *Spine* 1983; 8: 757-764

21. Sullivan JA, Davidson R, Renshaw TS, *et al*: Further evaluation of the Scolitron treatment of idiopathic adolescent scoliosis. *Spine* 1986; 11: 903-906

22. Farady JA: Current principles in the nonoperative management of structural adolescent idiopathic scoliosis. *Phys Ther* 1983; 63: 512-523

23. Stone B, Beekman C, Hall V, *et al*: The effect of an exercise program on change in curve in adolescents with minimal idiopathic scoliosis. *Phys Ther* 1979; 59: 759-763

24. Dickson RA, Leatherman KD: Cotrel traction, exercises, casting in the treatment of idiopathic scoliosis. A pilot study and prospective randomized controlled clinical trial. *Acta Orthop Scand* 1978; 49: 46-48

25. Weiss HR: The effect of an exercise program on vital capacity and rib mobility in patients with idiopathic scoliosis. *Spine* 1991; 16: 88-93

26. Miyasaki RA: Immediate influence of the thoracic flexion exercise on vertebral position in Milwaukee brace wearers. *Phys Ther* 1980; 60: 1005-1009

27. Akbarnia BA: Selection of methodology in surgical treatment of adolescent idiopathic scoliosis. *Orthop Clin North Am* 1988; 19: 319-329

28. Thompson JP, Transfeldt EE, Bradford DS, *et al*: Decompensation after Cotrel-Dubousset instrumentation of idiopathic scoliosis. *Spine* 1990; 15: 927-931

29. Dickson JH, Erwin WD, Rossi D: Harrington instrumentation and arthrodesis for idiopathic scoliosis. A twenty-one-year follow-up. *J Bone Joint Surg Am* 1990; 72: 678-683

30. Kahanovitz N, Weiser S: Lateral electrical surface stimulation (LESS) compliance in adolescent female scoliosis patients. *Spine* 1986; 11: 753-755

31. O'Donnell CS, Bunnell WP, Betz RR, *et al*: Electrical stimulation in the treatment of idiopathic scoliosis. *Clin Orthop* 1988; 229: 107-113

32. LaGrone MO: Loss of lumbar lordosis: a complication of spinal fusion for scoliosis. *Orthop Clin North Am* 1988; 19: 383-393

33. Winter RB, Lonstein JE, VandenBrink K, *et al*: The surgical treatment of thoracic adolescent idiopathic scoliosis with a Harrington rod and sublaminar wires. *Orthop Trans* 1987; 11: 89-92

34. Christodoulou AG, Prince HG, Webb JK, *et al*: Adolescent idiopathic thoracic scoliosis. *J Bone Joint Surg Br* 1987; 69: 13-16

35. Shufflebarger HL, Crawford AH: Is Cotrel-Dubousset Instrumentation the treatment of choice for idiopathic scoliosis in the adolescent who has an operative thoracic curve. *Orthopedics* 1988; 11: 1579-1588

36. Moskowitz A, Moe JH, Winter RB, *et al*: Long-term follow-up of scoliosis fusion. *J Bone Joint Surg Am* 1980; 62: 364-376

37. Edgar MA, Mehta MH: Long-term follow-up of fused and unfused idiopathic scoliosis. *J Bone J Surg* Br 1988; 70: 712-716

Screening for Idiopathic Adolescent Scoliosis

MANEUVER	EFFECTIVENESS	LEVEL OF EVIDENCE <REF>	RECOMMENDATION
Physical examination of back including Adams forward bending test to detect curves	**Detection** High rate of over-referral (e.g. 3-24 false positives for every curve >20° detected).	Cohort and case-control studies<4-9> (II-2)	Poor evidence to include or exclude from the periodic health examination (C)
	Early detection has not been shown to lead to better outcomes.	Case series and temporal studies <10-12> (III)	
	Intervention Loss of correction and non-compliance limit the reliability of brace therapy.	Case-control studies<15> (II-2); case series<13,14,16,17> (III)	
	Lateral Electrical Surface Stimulation (LESS) has poor evidence of better outcomes than using braces.	Cohort studies<22> (II-2); case series <18-21,23> (III)	
	Exercise therapy shows poor evidence of effectiveness in preventing curve progression.	Randomized controlled trial<25> (I); case series<24,26-28> (III)	
	Harrington or Cotrel-Dubousset instrumentation reduces curves >40-50° in the frontal plane but clinical outcomes have not been adequately evaluated.	Cohort and case-control studies <35-37> (II-2); case series<29,30-34> (III)	

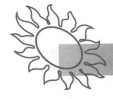
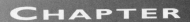

CHAPTER 32

Disadvantaged Children

By Ellen L. Lipman and David R. Offord

Disadvantaged Children

Prepared by Ellen L. Lipman, MD, FRCPC[1] and David R. Offord, MD, FRCPC[2]

Identification of disadvantaged children as an at-risk group for the Periodic Health Examination is very appropriate since there are currently over a million economically disadvantaged children in Canada. These children are at increased risk of morbidity and mortality, and may experience lifelong difficulties. Physician contact with disadvantaged children and their families is inevitable in most family practices, providing opportunities for health maintenance, detection of high-risk conditions, and appropriate interventions. Few studies have specifically examined primary care health maintenance among poor children. This chapter reviews the associations between socio-economic disadvantage and increased health risks and the evidence for effectiveness of selected interventions including public advocacy and multi-agency initiatives.

Burden of Suffering

The term disadvantage, as used here, refers principally to economic disadvantage or poverty. By definition, a child living in poverty in Canada lives in a family whose income is at or below the Statistics Canada low income cut-off.<1> In 1991, this definition identified those families spending greater than 58.5% of their income on food, shelter or clothing. The absolute value of the low income cutoff or poverty line varies with the size of the family and the place of residence. In addition to families below the low-income cutoff, there is a group of children living in families who are near poor, whose incomes fall only 10-20% above the Statistics Canada low income cut-off, and who differ little from those at the poverty line. Not all studies examining poor children use this poverty line, but instead may use more general measures such as level of income, area of residence, or eligibility for subsidies.

In Canada, the rates of child poverty have remained at the significant level of 16% over a 15-year span (1973-1988).<2> In 1988, this was estimated to represent over a million children under 18 years of age.<2> More recent figures suggest the current rate may be even higher.<3>

Children who grow up in economically disadvantaged circumstances are at increased risk for morbidity and mortality.<2,4-7> The mortality rate among children in the lowest

With over one million disadvantaged children in Canada, the burden of suffering is substantial for current and future morbidity

---

[1] Assistant Professor of Psychiatry, McMaster University, Hamilton, Ontario
[2] Professor of Psychiatry, McMaster University, Hamilton, Ontario

income quintile is twice that of those in the highest income quintile.<2> The increased morbidity among these economically disadvantaged children includes physical, emotional, social and educational health deficits.

Higher rates of chronic health problems have been found in children from poor families (i.e., whose income fell below the official Statistics Canada poverty line).<4> High morbidity and mortality rates have also been documented for treatable diseases such as asthma in children living in poor inner city areas.<5>

A significant association between economic disadvantage (measured by low income or parental welfare status) and child psychiatric disorders has also been demonstrated.<6,7> The risk of a poor boy, aged 6 to 11 years, having one or more psychiatric difficulties such as attention deficit hyperactivity disorder, conduct disorder or emotional disorder, was four times that of a non-poor boy (33 of 82 welfare boys with psychiatric difficulties vs. 187/1348 non-welfare boys).<6>

Similar associations have been demonstrated in the educational and social spheres,<7> including poor school readiness,<8> low math concept skills in the early grades<9> and later difficulties such as failing a grade or use of special education services.<7>

Disadvantaged children are clearly at increased risk for a wide range of health and psychosocial morbidities. A poor child may have difficulties in any of the physical, emotional, social or educational domains. Having any single deficit increases the likelihood of having other difficulties, so poor children tend to have multiple morbidities.

While the term "disadvantaged child" is being used interchangeably with "poor child" in this document, the actual disadvantage goes beyond a simple lack of money to include the context in which the child grows up. This includes such features as the characteristics of the family, neighbourhood and schools and the availability of preschool or recreational facilities. Characteristics of poor families include a family head with relatively little formal education, younger family heads, single parents, especially single mothers, and unemployed parents. Poor parents also have increased rates of physical or mental health problems. In terms of environmental circumstances, inadequate housing, unsafe neighbourhoods, neighbourhoods lacking in community resources or good schools, and homes lacking material resources or stimulation may be consequences of poverty. Each of these circumstances may have a negative impact on child growth and development. In turn, there is evidence that early interventions for children, such as an excellent preschool program, may have long-term beneficial effects that last into adulthood.<10>

The societal burden of suffering associated with child poverty in Canada is enormous, and continues to diminish opportunities for poor children as they grow. The mental and physical difficulties they experience do not necessarily resolve as they grow up. Instead, they may become adults with impairments in the physical, emotional, social, and occupational spheres. For example, approximately 40% of children with conduct disorder continue to experience serious psychosocial difficulties into adulthood.[11] This substantial lifelong impairment experienced by some poor children amounts to a large cost to society in areas such as physical and mental health costs, decreased occupational productivity, or use of social services.

Three maneuvers for assisting disadvantaged children will be discussed: contact in the family practitioners' office, referrals made by family physicians for child and parent assistance in the home and community, and advocacy by physicians and multi-agency initiatives.

Maneuver

Office Contact

Family physicians can provide disadvantaged children with preventive interventions known to be effective in the general population

Physician contact with disadvantaged children and their families is inevitable in most family practices. Office visits will likely be the most regular source of contact. Primary care contacts provide the opportunity for health maintenance, detection of high-risk conditions and intervention from infancy through the life span. Issues arising during office encounters discussed in this section are considered in terms of developmental stages of the child, and the context or environment in which the child lives.

Developmental Stages

There is no evidence that risk factors among poor children have different effects than they do among other children in the general population. However, exposure to multiple risk factors is more prevalent among poor children, thereby increasing associated detrimental outcomes. Maintaining an awareness of general risk factors as well as those with increased prevalence among disadvantaged populations will allow a family doctor to provide optimal care. Selected risk factors that are more prevalent among poor children are discussed below.

Prenatal Care

Adequate prenatal care for a poor mother is the first step in promoting the health of the disadvantaged child-to-be. Low-income mothers who have received inadequate prenatal care frequently give birth to low birth weight babies. Low birth weight is a major determinant of infant mortality, and can have major health consequences for babies who survive including serious illnesses, developmental disorders and lifelong handicapping conditions such as birth defects, mental retardation, cerebral palsy, and seizure disorders.<12> In addition to inadequate prenatal care, factors influencing low birth weight include poor nutrition, maternal prenatal stress, insufficient weight gain during pregnancy, drug and alcohol abuse, smoking, and obstetrical complications. Low birth weight is largely preventable, with an estimated 80% of women at risk identifiable at the first prenatal visit, allowing interventions to begin then to decrease the risks to the unborn child and mother.<12> Separate chapters on smoking during pregnancy (Chapter 3), prevention of low birth weight (Chapter 4) and preeclampsia (Chapter 13) are included in this volume but these reviews do not target the poor population specifically.

Childhood

Proper nutrition may be an issue in poor families due to such factors as inadequate funds for food, or poor knowledge of nutrition. Both types of growth disturbance, growth failure and obesity, have been documented among poor children.<13,14> Discussion of nutritional issues and monitoring of growth parameters is important, although mixed evidence has been presented regarding the association of poverty and retarded somatic growth.<13,14> In a case series of 82 children where anthropometric measures were found to be related to poor academic achievement, it was thought that environmental influences affected both the development of thought processes, and nutrient intake and therefore growth.<13> In 1979 the Canadian Task Force on the Periodic Health Examination found good evidence for prevention and treatment of malnutrition in high-risk populations, but poor children were not specifically studied as a high-risk population. The evidence for screening and treatment of another possible consequence of poor nutrition, iron-deficiency anemia, was fair in disadvantaged infants (also see Chapters 6 and 23).

Increased attention to preventable diseases should be maintained for low-income children and families. Increased morbidity from acute illnesses, such as asthma or infectious diseases, and maintenance of regular immunizations may be issues. There is good evidence from randomized control trials for effective prevention for immunizable infectious diseases by immunization (Chapter 33).<15> Prevention and treatment of hearing and vision problems (Chapter 27) should also be considered, although the general evidence for the effectiveness of prevention and treatment of these difficulties is less rigorous in general populations. Effectiveness specifically in poor populations has not been reviewed. Chronic medical illness has also been associated with poverty in children,<4> although this association has not been consistently demonstrated world-wide.<14>

Context (Environment)

Homelessness, or exposure to marginal or aged housing poses risks associated with inadequate shelter, or overcrowding. As well, specific health risks exist such as exposure to lead (e.g., through exposure to lead-based paint; see Chapter 25) with its hematologic and potential neurologic sequelae despite an asymptomatic clinical presentation.[16]

Evaluation of a poor child necessitates an understanding and appreciation of the context in which the child lives. Knowledge of the family and demographic history may alert the physician to possible problems. For example, chronic sociodemographic disadvantage, low maternal education, low family income, and poor family functioning have been shown to be associated with developmental delay, and psychosocial problems such as psychiatric, chronic health, social and educational difficulties.[7,17] Awareness that a family has these risk factors should increase vigilance for any of the above listed difficulties.

Careful attention to a poor child's family, and especially the primary caregiver, is needed. In a study of 155 children of single mothers recruited through social services and a local school in the U.S., economic hardship was found to be unrelated directly to child psychological functioning, but was related to mother's psychological functioning which was in turn related to their child's psychological functioning.[18] This highlights the need to assist poor mothers as well as their children since children are highly sensitive to their parents' emotional states. Other maternal difficulties which may influence the child, and also may necessitate maternal interventions include psychiatric disorders, tobacco and other drug and alcohol use. Current evidence for the effectiveness of prevention and treatment of psychiatric disorders and substance use as part of the Periodic Health Examination, with the exception of problem drinking (Chapter 42) and tobacco use (Chapter 43), is poor, and these areas are considered research priorities.

Three further points should be made. First, attention to language used, the nature of explanations given, reading material given, and attitude is important since all influence transmittal of information. Parents of disadvantaged children may themselves have low educational levels. Such parents require clear verbal explanations and literature written in easily understandable terms. There is evidence from the U.S. that poor families were more likely not to be completely satisfied with the primary care they received, and in particular, with the communication with the health care professional.[19] Second, consideration of drug costs, and whether medications are covered under drug plans such as those offered by welfare or family assistance, is important. Third, many poor parents do not feel comfortable in more formal or institutional settings such as a doctor's or a school principal's office. Primary practitioners can encourage parents to be advocates for their children and to feel empowered to seek optimal health and educational services for their children. There is evidence that by bridging the social and cultural gaps between home and school, a child's academic achievement can be enhanced.<20>

Child and Parental Assistance in the Home or Community

Studies in this area have focused on home- or community-based programs aimed at assisting families with children deemed to be at high risk for cognitive difficulties or developmental delay. Children have been identified as being at high risk based on disadvantaged intellectual, educational or social characteristics of the family.

Public Advocacy/Multi-Agency Initiatives

Public advocacy for disadvantaged children or involvement in multi-agency initiatives is beyond the scope of practice for many family physicians. However, as more municipalities focus on community initiatives for this (and other) disadvantaged populations, opportunities for multi-agency involvement will increase. As the awareness of the scope of morbidity, both immediate and long-term, for poor children increases, the importance of public advocacy on behalf of these children also increases.

Effectiveness of Treatment

Child and Parental Assistance in the Home or Community

The strongest evidence available to support a parental assistance program is found for community-based assistance to the parent and child. In one of only two randomized controlled trials available, 65 high-risk families were randomly allocated to one of three groups at the time of their child's birth.<21> Risk categorization was determined based on parental age and education, family income, maternal IQ, absence of father, poor school performance of siblings and other factors. One group were assigned to a Child Development Centre, a day care setting with a systematic developmental curriculum specialized in addressing cognitive and social difficulties, and family education, a home-based program to help parents foster appropriate cognitive and social development of their child. Notably the Child Development Centre also reserved spaced for non-high-risk children to have a socioeconomically diverse program. The Child Development program also had low teacher/child ratios, staff with considerable child-care experience, and provided staff training. An emphasis was put

There is good evidence to support recommending specialized day care or preschool programs for poor children

on intellectual/creative and social/emotional activities, and language stimulation. The second group of families received family education only, and the third acted as a control group. Follow-up of over 90% of enrolled families covered 54 months. Children in the group receiving combined educational day care and family education did significantly better (p<0.05) in cognitive performance than those with either of the other interventions (Bayley Scales of Infant Development at 12 and 18 months, Stanford-Binet Intelligence Test at 24, 36 and 48 months and the McCarthy Scales of Children's Abilities at 30, 42 and 54 months). Family education alone was not felt to be a sufficient intervention. The observed lack of effectiveness of family education alone is in contrast with results of other work, and the authors suggest that this difference may be related to factors such as intensity of training for home visitors and number of visits, or that short-term follow-up may not have detected potential later benefits. A weakness of this study is the lack of clarity about how families were recruited.

Martin and colleagues[22] estimated the effects of an experimental educational day-care program in the intellectual development of 86 preschoolers from high-risk families in a randomized controlled trial. High-risk status was determined by an index of risk factors for intellectual impairment. Children were allocated to the experimental or control groups between 6 and 12 weeks of age and remained in day care to 54 months (80% follow-up). The experimental program was designed to promote social and cognitive growth in an orderly, friendly environment. The IQs of experimental program children ranged from 8 to 20 points higher than those of control children and were higher on average (when maternal mental retardation and home environment were controlled p<0.0001). At 54 months, 93% of the experimental children and 69% of the control children had IQs within the normal range. There was an especially strong apparent effect on the IQs of children born to mentally retarded mothers, with none of the experimental children of retarded mothers having a subnormal IQ, but 6 of 7 control children of retarded mothers having subnormal IQ. Teenaged mothers in the experimental group were also found to be significantly more likely to have graduated from high school and to be self-supporting at the 54-month evaluation than were mothers in the control group.

Lee and co-workers[23] examined the longitudinal effects of an enriched preschool program aimed at disadvantaged black children (Head Start) vs. no preschool or other preschool programs for disadvantaged children using data from the National Longitudinal Study of Youth. Immediately after the program (one year follow-up), Head Start gains were favourable to both comparison groups. Beneficial effects were sustained into kindergarten and grade 1 for the Head Start program. These benefits were more pronounced when Head Start children were compared with children with no preschool experience, than when they were compared with children in other preschool programs. The authors suggest that this showed a beneficial effect of any preschool experience as compared to no preschool experience, rather than a benefit of Head Start per se.

Two other studies, including the only Canadian work identified from the MEDLINE search, provided descriptions of program development for home visiting or outreach programs for disadvantaged pregnant women[24] or low income mothers and infants.[25] Unfortunately, neither provided data evaluating outcomes. However, home visiting has been shown to prevent child maltreatment in American studies and is recommended by the Task Force during the perinatal period through infancy for families of low socioeconomic status, single parenthood or teenaged parenthood (A Recommendation – Chapter 29).

Halpern,[26] in a descriptive paper, outlined the need to address contextual factors impinging on parenting and child development, and warned not to expect parenting interventions to alter significantly the life chances of low income children. He noted, however, that there was evidence of a positive effect of parenting interventions. In some cases, increasingly positive parent-child relations were prompted through such programs.

Public Advocacy/Multi-Agency Initiatives

A series of descriptive and discussion papers supports the need for public advocacy and multi-agency initiatives. Recommendations for successful interventions include use of socioeconomic/cultural models vs. a purely medical model, assisting poor families to change their economic, and cultural beliefs and attitudes about health, linking educational and day care issues with access to preventive care, use of flexibility and collaborative spirit in these initiatives, providing programs for poor children and their families together, and changing government funding and policy around issues related to poor children and families. A strong plea has also gone out for increased funding of rigorous research to contribute to the solution of the medicosocial problems of these children.[27]

There is an increasing interest in public advocacy and multi-agency initiatives to assist disadvantaged children

Schorr[28] provides evidence of improved child outcome for children from programs that cut across traditional professional and bureaucratic boundaries, emphasize relationships of trust and respect, are deeply rooted in the community, are family focused, and that recognize the distinctive needs of those most at risk. In her discussion of the "cycle of disadvantage" she provides specific examples of successful U.S. programs that seem to meet these criteria. No systematic or scientific evaluation of similar Canadian programs was encountered in the literature reviewed. The Sparrow Lake Alliance in Ontario is working actively toward improving consultation and integration of children's services in the province. Its members include medical, community and government personnel. Initiatives promoted by the Alliance include an inner city outreach program which includes school, psychiatric and educational involvement, and a joining of personnel working in the adult addictions field and in the child care area to work with substance-using women and their children. No systematic evaluation of this program is available to date.

Recommendations of Others

Several advocacy groups have disadvantaged children as a specific focus. In Canada, these include the Child Poverty Action Group, and Campaign 2000, a nonpartisan national initiative to end child poverty in Canada by the year 2000. A number of other advocacy and research groups have an interest in this important area including, among others, the Canadian Academy of Child Psychiatry, the Canadian Pediatric Society, the Canadian Council on Children and Youth, the Canadian Council on Social Development, Canadian Child Welfare Association and the Centre for Studies of Children at Risk.

Most of the above agencies or groups have not made specific recommendations pertaining to the health and well-being of poor children. An exception is Campaign 2000, with its stated goal to eliminate child poverty. The only specific recommendations encountered came from the Society for Pediatric Research in the U.S. which outlined an 11-point plan to help solve health and other problems of poor children, and which included recognition of the importance of research, especially funding for long-term research initiatives.[27]

Conclusions and Recommendations

No specific studies have examined the effectiveness of preventive interventions during regular office contact between family physicians and disadvantaged children. Evidence from the general population exists to support efforts to prevent low birth weight, malnutrition in pregnant mothers and children, promote immunization, and identify hearing and vision problems. Awareness of other health risks such as homelessness, chronic medical problems and maternal difficulties should prompt efforts to prevent subsequent problems for children. These issues, however, have not been specifically studied among poor children (C Recommendation).

There is good evidence to support recommendations for specialized day care or preschool programs for disadvantaged children, particularly programs specially designed for this group (A Recommendation). There is insufficient evidence to recommend for or against home-based parenting programs for disadvantaged children and families (C Recommendation).

There is an increasing interest in public advocacy for disadvantaged children, and in developing multi-agency initiatives to assist these children. While individual family physicians may take an interest in such initiatives, these lie outside the context of the Periodic Health Examination.

Unanswered Questions (Research Agenda)

The following have been identified as research priorities:

1. Evaluating the effectiveness of specific screening interventions (e.g., for lead poisoning) in poor children.

2. Evaluating specific interventions for a disadvantaged child's mother (e.g., treatment of psychiatric disorder) in terms of its effect on the child.

3. Evaluating the effectiveness of other community-based interventions aimed at poor children (e.g., recreation programs or after-school programs).

4. Developing new and identifying pre-existing multi-agency collaborative programs involving physicians and government or educational personnel, and evaluating the effectiveness of these programs on the health and well-being of disadvantaged children.

Evidence

The literature was identified with a MEDLINE search from January 1984 to December 1992 using the following key words: unemployment, poverty, medical indigency, minority groups.

This review was initiated in January 1994 and the recommendations finalized by the Task Force in March 1994.

Acknowledgements

Ellen Lipman was supported by a Research Training Fellowship from the Ontario Mental Health Foundation. David Offord was supported by a National Health Scientist Award from Health Canada. The Task Force thanks Sarah Shea, MD, FRCPC, Assistant Professor, Department of Pediatrics, Dalhousie University, Halifax, NS, for reviewing the draft report.

Selected References

1. Statistics Canada low income cut-offs. Income distribution by size in Canada (Cat. No. 13-207), Statistics Canada, Ottawa, 1983: 32

2. Ross D, Shillington R: Children in poverty: toward a better future. Ottawa: Standing Senate Committee on Social Affairs, Science and Technology, 1991

3. Health and Welfare Canada: Countdown to the year 2000 Healthy Canada. Maclean's 1993; 106, Supplement: 8

4. Cadman D, Boyle MH, Offord DR, *et al*: Chronic illness and functional limitations in Ontario children: findings of the Ontario Child Health Study. *Can Med Assoc J* 1986; 135: 761-767

5. Weiss KB, Gergen PJ, Crain EF: Inner-city asthma. The epidemiology of an emerging US public health concern. *Chest* 1992; 101(6 Suppl): 3625-3675

6. Offord DR, Boyle MH, Jones BR: Psychiatric disorder and poor school performance among welfare children in Ontario. *Can J Psychiatry* 1987; 32: 518-525

7. Lipman EL, Offord DR, Boyle MH: Economic disadvantage and child psychosocial morbidity. *Can Med Assoc J* 1994; 151: 431-437

8. Hinshaw SP: Externalizing behaviour problems and academic underachievement in childhood and adolescence: causal relationships and underlying mechanisms. *Psychol Bull* 1992; 111: 127-155

9. Entwisle DR, Alexander KL: Beginning school math competence: minority and majority comparisons. *Child Dev* 1990; 61: 454-471

10. Schweinhart L, Weikart D, Lamer M: Consequences of three preschool curriculum models through age 15. *Early Childhood Res Quarterly* 1986; 1: 15-45

11. Offord DR, Bennet K: Prevention and treatment of conduct disorder: a critical review. *J Am Acad Child Adolesc Psychiatry* (In press)

12. Oberg CN: Medically uninsured children in the United States: a challenge to public policy. *J Sch Health* 1990; 60: 493-500

13. Karp R, Martin R, Sewell T, *et al*: Growth and academic achievement in inner-city kindergarten children. The relationship of height, weight, cognitive ability and neurodevelopmental level. *Clin Pediatr Phila* 1992; 31: 336-340

14. Carmichael A, Williams HE, Picot SG: Growth patterns, health and illness in preschool children from a multi-ethnic, poor socio-economic status municipality of Melbourne. *J Paediatr Child Health* 1990; 26: 136-141

15. Canadian Task Force on the Periodic Health Examination: The periodic health examination. *Can Med Assoc J* 1979; 121: 1193-1254

16. Landrigan PJ: Health effects of environmental toxins in deficient housing. *Bull NY Acad Med* 1990; 66: 491-499

17. Najman JM, Bor W, Morrison J, *et al*: Child developmental delay and socio-economic disadvantage in Australia: a longitudinal study. *Soc Sci Med* 1992; 34: 829-835

18. McLoyd VC, Wilson L: Maternal behaviour, social support and economic conditions as predictors of distress in children. *New Dir Child Dev* 1990; 16: 49-69

19. Wood DL, Corey C, Freeman HE, *et al*: Are poor families satisfied with the medical care their children receive? *Pediatrics* 1992; 90: 66-70

20. Comer JP: Educating poor minority children. *Scientific American* 1988; 259: 42-48

21. Wasik BH, Ramey CT, Bryant DM, *et al*: A longitudinal study of two early intervention strategies: Project CARE. *Child Dev* 1990; 61: 1682-1696

22. Martin SL, Ramey CT, Ramey S: The prevention of intellectual impairment in children of impoverished families: findings of a randomized trial of educational day care. *Am J Public Health* 1990; 80: 844-847

23. Lee VE, Brooks-Gunn J, Schnur E, *et al*: Are Head Start effects sustained? A longitudinal follow-up comparison of disadvantaged children attending Head Start, no preschool, and other preschool programs. *Child Dev* 1990; 61: 495-507

24. Woodard GRB, Edouard L: Reaching out: a community initiative for disadvantaged pregnant women. *Can J Public Health* 1992; 83: 188-190

25. Poland ML, Giblin PT, Waller JB, *et al*: Development of a paraprofessional home visiting program for low-income mothers and infants. *Am J Prev Med* 1991; 7: 204-207

26. Halpern R: Poverty and early childhood parenting: toward a framework for intervention. *Am J Orthopsychiatry* 1990; 60: 6-18

27. Kohl S: The challenge of care for the poor child: The research agenda. *Am J Dis Child* 1991; 145: 542-543

28. Schorr LB: Children, families and the cycle of disadvantage. *Can J Psychiatry* 1991; 36: 437-441

Disadvantaged Children

MANEUVER	EFFECTIVENESS	LEVEL OF EVIDENCE <REF>	RECOMMENDATION
Office contact with the primary care physician with a focus on risk factors for disadvantaged children	Routine primary care has not been evaluated. No studies with a specific focus on disadvantaged children.		Poor evidence to include or exclude specific maneuvers for poor children (C)*
Child and family assistance in the home or community	Enrolment in day care or preschool program helpful, particularly in specialized program for disadvantaged.	Randomized controlled trials<21,22> (I)	Good evidence to include recommendations for day care or preschool program for poor children in periodic health examination (A)
	Home-based parenting education program appears insufficient on its own, although long-term evaluation lacking.	Comparisons between places<21,23> (II-2)	Insufficient evidence to recommend for or against home-based parenting programs (C)

* Other Task Force recommendations on preventive health care for the general population should be followed (see Pediatric Preventive Care and Immunizations of Children and Adults). Also consider whether the children are at risk for iron deficiency anemia (Chapter 23), lead exposure (Chapter 25), or child maltreatment (Chapter 29).

Immunization of Children and Adults

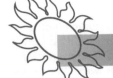

CHAPTER

33

Childhood Immunizations

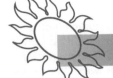

By Ronald Gold and Anne Martell

33

Childhood Immunizations

Prepared by Ronald Gold, MD, FRCPC, Peds, MPH[1] and Anne Martell, MA, CMC[2]

In 1979 the Canadian Task Force on the Periodic Health Examination strongly recommended that immunization be part of the care given at the time of the periodic health examination (A Recommendation).<1,2> In 1990, vaccination with diphtheria-pertussis-tetanus (DPT) and polio vaccines at 2, 4, 6 and 18 months (if oral polio vaccine (OPV) is used it should be given at 2, 4, and 18 months), measles-mumps-rubella (MMR) vaccine at 12 months and Hemophilus influenzae type b (Hib) vaccine at 18 months was reconfirmed regarding well-baby care in the first 2 years of life.<3>

The most effective way to reduce vaccine-preventable diseases is to have a high proportion of immune people. Universal immunization is therefore an important part of good health care and can be accomplished through routine and intensive programs carried out in physicians' offices and public health clinics. As the result of mass immunization, the incidence of diphtheria, Hib infection, measles, mumps, pertussis, poliomyelitis, rubella and tetanus has been greatly reduced in Canada except where there is poor access to health care.<4,5> A separate chapter has been prepared on hepatitis B immunization (Chapter 35).

Diphtheria-Tetanus-Pertussis

Burden of Suffering

Routine mass immunization with diphtheria toxoid has resulted in such significant declines in the incidence of diphtheria that it is now a very rare disease with <5 cases per year in Canada since 1987.<4,6> Diphtheria is mainly associated with poor socioeconomic conditions and occurs most frequently in unimmunized or partially immunized individuals.

Diphtheria toxoid is very effective in preventing disease, but does not prevent colonization and carriage of *C. diphtheriae*. Because the bacterium has not been eradicated, continued routine immunization is necessary to prevent diphtheria.

[1] Professor of Pediatrics and Microbiology, University of Toronto, Toronto, Ontario
[2] Martell Consulting Services Ltd., Halifax, Nova Scotia

Tetanus is an acute, often fatal disease caused by a potent neurotoxin produced by *Clostridium tetani*.<4,6> Routine mass immunization with tetanus toxoid has reduced reported deaths from approximately 60 a year in the pre-immunization period to virtually none today.

Pertussis is a highly contagious, acute infectious bacterial disease, caused by *Bordetella pertussis*. Pertussis was once a major cause of North American childhood morbidity and mortality.<4,6,7> While the incidence rates of pertussis in the 1980s have been about one tenth of those observed in the 1930s, well over 2,000 cases of pertussis are reported annually in Canada.<7> These statistics compare to the 1,000 to 3,000 cases reported annually in the United States.<6> The actual number of cases is 5-10 times greater in both countries because of significant under-reporting and under-diagnosis. Because of incomplete immunization coverage, the need for multiple doses of vaccine to achieve protection, the less than 100% efficacy of vaccine and continued circulation of the organism, cases and outbreaks of pertussis continue to occur in Canada.<7>

For various reasons, including less than 100% efficacy of vaccine, pertussis outbreaks continue to occur in Canada

Infants have suffered the highest attack rates in both epidemic and nonepidemic years and also have the highest hospitalization rates and the longest hospital stays. The case-fatality rate in the first year of life is 1 per 200.<7>

Maneuver

Whole-cell pertussis vaccines are prepared from suspensions of inactivated *B. pertussis* whole bacterial cells and are usually given combined with either adsorbed diphtheria and tetanus toxoids (DPT), or adsorbed diphtheria and tetanus toxoids plus inactivated polio vaccine (DPT-Polio). Pertussis vaccine is also available as a single non-adsorbed preparation.<4>

Effectiveness of Prevention

The current whole-cell vaccines have been shown to be 70% to 91% effective against pertussis following a primary course of at least three doses.<8> A recent U.S. study found that efficacy was 64%, 81% and 95% for case definitions of mild cough, paroxysmal cough, and severe clinical illness respectively.<9> The efficacy of the current Canadian pertussis vaccine is not well defined.

Whole-cell pertussis vaccines are associated with a variety of adverse events.<10> Local reactions (generally erythema and induration with or without tenderness) are common after the administration of vaccines containing diphtheria, tetanus or pertussis antigens. Mild systemic reactions such as fever, drowsiness, fretfulness, and anorexia occur frequently. Moderate to severe systemic events include high fever (temperature of ≥40.5 C); persistent, inconsolable crying lasting ≥3 hours; collapse (hypotonic-hyporesponsive episode); or short-lived convulsions. Other more severe neurologic events, such as a prolonged convulsion or encephalopathy, although rare, have been reported in temporal association with DTP administration.[10]

In August 1991, the Institute of Medicine released a report entitled *Adverse Effects of Pertussis and Rubella Vaccines* which examined 18 adverse events in relation to DTP vaccine.[10,11] The committee found that there is a causal relation between DTP vaccine and anaphylaxis and between the pertussis component of DTP vaccine and extended periods of inconsolable crying and screaming. The evidence was weaker but still consistent with a causal relation between DTP vaccine and two conditions — acute encephalopathy and hypotonic, hyporesponsive episodes. Evidence did not indicate a causal relation between the DTP vaccine and infantile spasms, hypsarrhythmia, Reye's syndrome, and sudden infant death syndrome. As well, there was insufficient evidence to indicate either the presence or absence of a causal relation between DTP vaccine and chronic brain damage and a variety of other rare events.[10,11]

Recommendations of Others

In its routine schedule for immunization against diphtheria, tetanus and pertussis, the National Advisory Committee on Immunization (NACI) recommends DTP vaccination at 2, 4, 6, 18 months and 4-6 years of age.[4] New NACI recommendations concerning cautions and contraindications for pertussis vaccine have been published.[12]

Conclusions and Recommendations

There is good evidence to recommend universal immunization at 2, 4, 6 and 18 months and 4-6 years of age (A Recommendation).

Unanswered Questions (Research Agenda)

In response to concerns relating adverse reactions to the whole-cell pertussis vaccines, acellular pertussis vaccines have been developed which contain purified components of *B. pertussis*. The safety and efficacy of these acellular vaccines in comparison to whole cell vaccine are currently under investigation in large-scale field trials.

Poliomyelitis

Burden of Suffering

Since August 1991, there have been no cases of paralytic poliomyelitis in the Western Hemisphere because of the success of the

Pan American Health Organization/World Health Organization (PAHO/WHO) polio eradication program using oral polio vaccine (OPV).<13> World-wide eradication by the year 2000 has been adopted as a major priority by the WHO.<14> Because of the persistence of poliomyelitis in many developing countries and the resurgence of paralytic polio in the parts of the former Soviet Union, the risk of importation of wild polio into Canada by immigrants, refugees, and travellers continues.

The risk of importation of wild polio virus into Canada by immigrants, refugees and travellers continues

Because both Canada and the United States have virtually eliminated disease due to indigenously acquired wild poliovirus by mass vaccination, vaccine-associated paralytic poliomyelitis (VAPP) has emerged as the predominant form of poliomyelitis.<15> The most current estimates of VAPP (U.S. data) for infant recipients are 1 case per 1.3 million infants; for household contacts <6 years old, 1 case per 22 million children; and for all others, 1 case per 29 million others.

Maneuver

Currently New Brunswick, Quebec, Manitoba, Alberta, British Columbia and the two Territories (57.9% of Canada's population) use OPV, while Newfoundland, Nova Scotia and Ontario (41.6% of the population) use inactivated polio vaccine (IPV). Prince Edward Island (0.5% of the population) uses a unique sequential IPV-OPV schedule.<16>

Effectiveness of Prevention

Both OPV and IPV are highly effective in preventing paralytic poliomyelitis in fully immunized persons. OPV is more effective in inducing mucosal immunity and in preventing spread of wild polio viruses.<4>

Although both oral polio vaccine and inactivated polio vaccine are highly immunogenic, OPV is more effective in preventing spread of wild virus

Recommendations of Others

The recommendations of the NACI concerning infant immunization for poliomyelitis remain unchanged. Either IPV or OPV can be used, depending on provincial preference. IPV is available as a combined DTP/IPV product. NACI does not recommend a sequential IPV/OPV schedule at this time because of the lack of data on which to base such a recommendation.

Conclusions and Recommendations

There is good evidence to recommend IPV or OPV, at 2, 4, 6 and 18 months and 4-6 years for IPV or at 2, 4 and 18 months and 4-6 years for OPV (A Recommendation).

Unanswered Questions (Research Agenda)

Determination of the optimal vaccination schedule, i.e. IPV alone versus sequential use of IPV and OPV.

Development of methods of improved surveillance, investigation and reporting of all cases of acute flaccid paralysis in order for Canada to be able to meet the WHO requirements for certification of eradication of polio.

Measles Immunization

Burden of Suffering

The introduction and use of measles vaccine beginning in 1963 led to a 95% decrease in incidence of measles. However, the number of reported cases in the U.S. and Canada increased in the past decade. While the U.S. outbreaks of measles have involved primarily unimmunized inner-city preschool children in the last 3-4 years, almost all of the Canadian outbreaks since 1988 have involved school-age children, with peak incidence in 10-19 year olds.<17>

Maneuver

Live measles virus vaccines are prepared from "further attenuated" Moraten or Schwarz strain viruses. They are available alone, or in combination with live mumps and rubella vaccines (MMR).<4>

Effectiveness of Prevention

Most measles vaccine failures are due to persistent maternal antibody or exposure of vaccine to excessive heat or light

Measles vaccine produces over 95% seroconversions, although the antibody titres achieved are lower than those that follow natural disease. Antibodies remain detectable for at least 17 years. In immunized individuals whose antibody titres had dropped below detectable levels, revaccination stimulates a rapid "booster-type" response.<4>

The primary failure rate after measles vaccination is about 5% among children immunized after 15 months of age.<18> The major reasons for primary vaccine failure are: 1) persisting maternal measles antibody; and 2) poor handling of vaccine resulting in death of the live vaccine by exposure to heat and/or light prior to use.

Indirect evidence for the effectiveness of a second dose in eliminating primary vaccine failures comes from several studies which show that attack rates during outbreaks are lower among persons who have had two doses of vaccine.<18,19> Additional evidence comes from experience with military recruits among whom measles has been virtually eliminated by revaccinating those whose screening sera suggest they are susceptible despite a history of vaccination.<20>

The current measles problem has resulted from failure to immunize and primary immunization failure. The rationale for recommending a second dose of vaccine appears to be strongest when considered as a strategy for eliminating primary vaccine failures. Current evidence suggests that most such individuals would become protected if given a second dose. Both experience in outbreaks where disease has spread over sustained periods even among groups with very high rates of previous immunization and mathematic modelling around estimated primary vaccine failure rates, suggest that protection rates achievable with a one-dose schedule of the current vaccine (seroconversion in 95% or more of recipients) are inadequate to prevent spread of the disease.<21>

The current measles problem has resulted from failure to immunize and primary immunization failure

At the level of expert opinion, the NACI recommended in 1990 that legislation requiring proof of measles immunity or valid exemption be enacted and enforced by all provinces and territories unless documented vaccination coverage of greater than 95% has been achieved by a voluntary program.<4,17>

Recommendations of Others

In 1989, both the Immunization Practices Advisory Committee, Centers for Disease Control and the Committee on Infectious Diseases of the American Academy of Pediatrics recommended the introduction of a routine two-dose schedule of measles vaccination.

The Canadian Measles Consensus Conference held in December 1992 targeted measles eradication in Canada for 2005 and established an immunization policy to include 100% MMR coverage of all infants by 15 months of age combined with a second dose of MMR at 4-6 years of age. These recommendations have been endorsed by NACI.<4,17>

Conclusions and Recommendations

All children should receive two doses of measles vaccine (A Recommendation). The first should be given as the combined measles-mumps-rubella (MMR) vaccine on, or as soon as possible after, the first birthday. A second dose of measles vaccine should be administered at 4 to 6 years of age. Ensuring that all children receive one dose of measles vaccine at the earliest appropriate age remains the priority.

There is also fair evidence to implement requirements for proof of measles immunization or valid exemption for children to attend school.

Mumps Vaccine

Burden of Suffering

Mumps is a common childhood disease caused by mumps virus. Mumps is more severe in older children and adults. Meningoencephalitis occurs commonly in mumps, and before vaccination became routine, was the commonest cause of aspetic meningitis. Epididymo-orchitis is the most common nonsalivary manifestation. Testicular involvement is generally unilateral but rarely may be bilateral. It may lead to atrophy of the involved testis, but rarely causes sterility.[4,22]

Maneuver

Live mumps virus vaccines are prepared from the Jeryl Lynn attenuated virus strain and are available in both monovalent form and in combination with live measles and rubella vaccines (MMR).[4]

Effectiveness of Prevention

In clinical trials an antibody response has been produced in over 95% of susceptible individuals through a single dose of the vaccine. The protective efficacy of the vaccine during outbreaks is 75 to 91%.[23]

Rubella Vaccine

Burden of Suffering

Rubella is one of the most benign of all infectious diseases in children. When contacted by pregnant women in the first 16 weeks of pregnancy, rubella frequently causes serious complications including miscarriage, abortion, stillbirth, and congenital rubella syndrome (CRS).[24]

The aim of universal immunization is to control CRS by interrupting transmission of rubella virus among young children through immunization of all children, male and female, on or after their first birthday, thereby decreasing the chances that a susceptible pregnant woman would be exposed to the virus. Screening and vaccinating adolescents and adults to prevent CRS are addressed in Chapter 12.

Maneuver

In both Canada and the United States a live attenuated virus, strain RA 27/3, is licensed as the rubella virus vaccine. The vaccine is administered as a single subcutaneous injection and is available either as a monovalent vaccine or in combination with mumps and measles vaccines (MMR).<4>

Effectiveness of Prevention

The current rubella vaccine is efficacious in preventing rubella infection and CRS when administered to children.<25> The recent increase in cases of rubella and CRS has been associated with outbreaks among unvaccinated persons rather than among persons with primary vaccine failure. It is expected that the incidence of CRS will continue to decline as the current cohort of highly immunized children and adolescents enters its child-bearing years.

The recent increase in cases of rubella and congenital rubella syndrome has been associated with outbreaks among unvaccinated persons

Conclusions and Recommendations

It is recommended that Canada establish a two-dose MMR vaccination schedule to produce enhanced immunity within the Canadian population, achieve eradication of indigenous transmission of measles and improve control of mumps and rubella.

Hemophilus Influenzae Type B

Burden of Suffering

Hemophilus influenzae Type b (Hib) has been a major cause of serious bacterial infections in young children from 3 months to 5 years of age, including meningitis, epiglottitis, facial cellulitis, pneumonia, pericarditis, septic arthritis, bacteremia, empyema and osteomyelitis.<26> Before the introduction of the newer Hib vaccines, it was estimated that Hib caused 2,000 cases of invasive infections annually in Canada, between 55% and 65% of which presented as meningitis.

Maneuver

Hib conjugate vaccines represent the second generation of vaccines against Hib disease, having replaced an earlier polysaccharide product (polyribose ribitol phosphate (PRP)). The conjugate vaccines include HbOC (oligosaccharide conjugate, HibTiter®), PRP-OMP (outer-membrane protein complex, PedVaxHIB®), PRP-T (tetanus toxoid, ActHIB®) and PRP-D (diphtheria toxoid, ProHIBit®).<26> The first 3 are approved for use in infants whereas the latter is used only in children 18 months and older.

Conjugate vaccines should be administered intramuscularly at 2, 4, 6, and 18 months of age and may be given simultaneously with DPT, polio and/or MMR vaccines. HbOC and PRP-OMP must be given in a separate syringe at a separate site. PRP-T is supplied as a lyophilized product which can be reconstituted with either saline or with DPT. DPT cannot be used to reconstitute other Hib vaccines.

Effectiveness of Prevention

Hemophilus influenzae type b vaccines show 95% efficacy after primary immunization and 100% protection following the booster dose

Results of efficacy trials of these Hib conjugate vaccines indicate >95% efficacy after completion of the primary series and 100% protection following the booster dose.<26–28> Surveillance at 10 pediatric tertiary care hospitals in Canada has demonstrated a 90% decline in the incidence of invasive Hib disease within 1 year of introduction of infant vaccine programs in Canada.<26>

Recommendations of Others

Recommendations on the use of the Hib vaccine have been updated recently by the NACI.<28> The Committee recommends that all infants receive conjugate Hib vaccine starting at 2 months of age. Although it is preferable to use the same product for all doses of the 2-3 dose primary series, when necessary HbOC, PRP-T, and PRP-OMP can be substituted for each other without restarting the primary series. A booster must then be given at 15-18 months of age. Previously unvaccinated children ≥15 months of age should be given a single dose of HbOC, PRP-OMP or PRP-T.

Conclusions and Recommendations

There is good evidence to recommend universal vaccination with Hib conjugate vaccine at 2, 4, 6, and 18 months (A recommendation).

Unanswered Questions (Research Agenda)

Development of combination vaccines containing DPT, IPV, and Hib conjugate vaccines.

Childhood Immunization Schedule

Recommendations of Others

Both the National Advisory Committee on Immunization and the Immunization Practices Advisory Committee recommend the establishment of programs aimed at ensuring that all children in all communities are immunized at the recommended ages.<4-6> The U.S. Preventive Services Task Force recommends childhood immunizations in accordance with the Immunization Practices Advisory Committee guidelines.<29>

Conclusions and Recommendations

The Canadian Task Force on the Periodic Health Examination finds that the evidence supports vaccination of all children with DPT, Polio vaccine, MMR, and Hib vaccine according to the schedules recommended by NACI.

Evidence

Review of evidence from 1988 to October 1993 has focused on determining the most effective and safe vaccines for the prevention of microbial diseases. The starting point for this review was the 4th edition of the *Canadian Immunization Guide*<4> and a draft report by the U.S. Preventive Services Task Force on measles immunization. Other literature was identified using a MEDLINE search with the following MESH headings: diphtheria-tetanus-pertussis vaccine; diphtheria; tetanus; whooping cough; meningitis, bacterial; hemophilus; mumps vaccine; rubella vaccine; measles vaccine; and poliovirus vaccine.

Acknowledgements

Funding for this report was provided by Health Canada under the Government of Canada's Brighter Futures Initiative. The Task Force thanks John C LeBlanc, Assistant Professor, Community Health and Epidemiology, Pediatrics, Dalhousie University, Halifax, Nova Scotia, for reviewing the draft report on measles.

Selected References

1. *Report of a Task Force to the Conference of Deputy Ministers of Health.* [cat no H39-3/1980E], Health Services and Promotion Branch, Department of National Health and Welfare, Ottawa, 1980

2. Canadian Task Force on the Periodic Health Examination: The periodic health examination. *Can Med Assoc J* 1979; 121: 1193-1254

3. Canadian Task Force on the Periodic Health Examination: The periodic health examination, 1990 update: 4. Well-baby care in the first 2 years of life. *Can Med Assoc J* 1990; 143: 867-872

4. Canadian Immunization Guide, Fourth Edition. Health and Welfare Canada, Ottawa, 1993, Minister of Supply and Services Canada (Cat. No. H41-8/1993E)

5. Advisory Committee on Immunization Practices: General recommendations on immunization. *Morbid Mortal Wkly Rep* 1994; 43(RR-1): 1-38

6. Immunization Practices Advisory Committee: Diphtheria, tetanus, and pertussis: guidelines for vaccine prophylaxis and other preventive measures. *MMWR Morb Mortal Wkly Rep* 1985; 34: 405-414,419-426

7. National Advisory Committee on Immunization, Advisory Committee on Epidemiology, Canadian Pediatric Society: Statement on management of persons exposed to pertussis and pertussis outbreak control. *Can Dis Wkly Rep* 1990; 16: 127-130

8. Fine PE, Clarkson JA, Miller E: The efficacy of pertussis vaccines under conditions of household exposure. Further analysis of the 1978-1980 PHLS/ERL study in 21 area health authorities in England. *Int J Epidemiol* 1988; 17: 635-642

9. Onorato IM, Wassilak SG, Meade B: Efficacy of whole-cell pertussis vaccine in preschool children in the United States. *JAMA* 1992; 267: 2745-2749

10. Howson CP, Fineberg HV: Adverse events following pertussis and rubella vaccines. Summary of a report of the Institute of Medicine. *JAMA* 1992; 267: 392-396

11. Howson CP, Howe CJ, Fineberg HV (eds): Adverse effects of pertussis and rubella vaccines. Washington, DC, National Academy Press, 1991

12. National Advisory Committee on Immunization: Statement on Pertussis Immunization. *Can Comm Dis Rep* 1993; 19: 41-45

13. Centres for Disease Control: Progress toward eradicating poliomyelitis from the Americas. *MMWR Morb Mortal Wkly Rep* 1989; 38: 532-535

14. Melnick JL: Poliomyelitis: eradication in sight. *Epidemiol Infect* 1992; 108: 1-18

15. Strebel PM, Sutter RW, Cochi SL, *et al*: Epidemiology of poliomyelitis in the United States one decade after the last reported case of indigenous wild virus – associated disease. *Clin Infect Dis* 1992; 14: 568-579

16. Varughese PV, Carter AO, Acres SE, *et al*: Eradication of indigenous poliomyelitis in Canada: impact of immunization strategies. *Can J Publ Hlth* 1989; 80: 363-368

17. Laboratory Centre for Disease Control: Consensus conference on measles. *Can Comm Dis Rep* 1993; 19: 72-79

18. Hutchins SS, Markowitz LE, Mead P *et al*: A school-based measles outbreak: the effect of a selective revaccination policy and risk factors for vaccine failure. *Am J Epidemiol* 1990; 132(1): 157-168

19. Nkowane BM, Bart SW, Orenstein WA, *et al*: Measles outbreak in a vaccinated school population: epidemiology, chains of transmission and the role of vaccine failures. *Am J Public Health* 1987; 77(4): 434-438

20. Crawford GE, Gremillion DH: Epidemic measles and rubella in air force recruits: impact of immunization. *J Infect Dis* 1981; 144(5): 403-410

21.   Markowitz LE, Preblud SR, Orenstein WA, *et al*: Patterns of transmission in measles outbreaks in the United States, 1985-1986. *N Engl J Med* 1989; 320: 75-81

22.   Bakshi SS, Cooper LZ: Rubella and mumps vaccines. *Pediatr Clin North Am* 1990; 37(3): 651-668

23.   Kim-Farley R, Barr S, Stetler H, *et al*: Clinical mumps vaccine efficacy. *Am J Epidemiol* 1985; 121: 593-597

24.   Cooper LZ: The history and medical consequences of rubella. *Rev Infect Dis* 1985; 7 (Suppl 1): S2-S0

25.   Herrmann KL: Rubella in the United States: toward a strategy for disease control and elimination. *Epidemiol Infect* 1991; 107(1): 55-61

26.   National Advisory Committee on Immunization: Statement on *Haemophilus influenzae* type b conjugate vaccines for use in infants and children. *Can Comm Dis Rep* 1992; 18: 169-176

27.   Scheifele D, Gold R, Law B, *et al*: Decline in *Haemophilus influenzae* type b invasive infections at five Canadian pediatric centers. *Can Comm Dis Rep* 1993; 19: 88-91

28.   National Advisory Committee on Immunization: Statement on Hemophilus influenzae type b conjugate vaccine for use in infants and children. *Can Med Assoc J* 1993; 148: 199-204

29.   U.S. Preventive Services Task Force: *Guide to Clinical Preventive Services: an Assessment of the Effectiveness of 169 Interventions*. Williams & Wilkins, Baltimore, Md, 1989: 359-362

Childhood Immunizations

MANEUVER	EFFECTIVENESS	LEVEL OF EVIDENCE <REF>	RECOMMENDATION
Vaccination with diphtheria-pertussis-tetanus (DPT) and polio vaccines at 2, 4, 6, 18 months and 4-6 years	Incidence of diphtheria, pertussis, tetanus and polio is greatly reduced in Canada compared to pre-vaccination era except where there is poor access to health care; no indigenous paralytic polio due to wild strains since 1979.	Dramatic differences between times and places, randomized controlled trials <4-7,13> (I)	Good evidence to include in periodic health examination (A)
Hemophilus influenzae type b (Hib) conjugate vaccine at 2, 4, 6 and 18 months	Incidence of invasive disease due to Hib decreased by >90% based on reported cases and pediatric hospital-based surveillance system.	Dramatic differences between times and places, randomized controlled trials <26-28> (I)	Good evidence to include in periodic health examination (A)
Measles-mumps-rubella (MMR) vaccine at 12 months and 4-6 years	Incidence of measles, mumps, rubella and congenital rubella syndrome is greatly reduced in Canada except where there is poor access to health care. Second dose of MMR is required for measles eradication and will improve immunity against mumps and rubella. Second dose of measles vaccine or MMR is not cost-effective but is essential for measles eradication.	Dramatic differences between times and places, randomized controlled trials<17,18,20,23,25> (I)	Good evidence to include in periodic health examination (A)

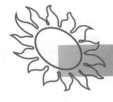

CHAPTER 34

Administration of Pneumococcal Vaccine

By Elaine E.L. Wang

Administration of Pneumococcal Vaccine

Prepared by Elaine E. L. Wang, MD, CM, FRCPC[1]

In its 1979 report the Canadian Task Force on the Periodic Health Examination recommended antipneumococcal vaccination for those with chronic debilitating illness, sickle cell anemia and anatomic or functional asplenia but not for the general population. In 1991 more detailed recommendations were made, based on the evidence for specific risk groups using a stringent measure of protective efficacy – the development of illness after exposure to the organism.

Burden of Suffering

The annual incidence of pneumococcal pneumonia in the United States has been estimated to be between one and five episodes per 1,000 subjects. One population-based study showed that pneumococcal bacteria were found in 18.7 subjects per 100,000 population, with an incidence of 53 per 100,000 among those 65 years or more. The incidence of pneumococcal pneumonia has been estimated to be three to five times this value. In Canada 7,069 people were admitted to hospital because of pneumococcal pneumonia during 1983-84; this represented 86,323 hospital days. The rate of death among such patients is approximately 15% to 20% despite appropriate antibiotic therapy.

S. pneumoniae is a major cause of otitis media, which has been estimated to occur in two-thirds of the general population by 3 years of age; about half will have had three or more episodes. It was responsible for 73 (37%) of the reported cases of bacterial meningitis in Canada in 1986.

Those at high risk for pneumococcal infections include: patients with anatomic or functional asplenia, those with Hodgkin's disease or nephrotic syndrome, and those receiving immunosuppressive therapy. Other groups in which such infections have been associated with increased rates of illness and death include those with chronic lung or cardiac disease or diabetes mellitus, those in institutions and over age 55. However, some authors conclude that there is no evidence to support an unusual frequency of pneumococcal infections in people with chronic cardiac, renal or hepatic disease or diabetes mellitus.

---

[1] Associate Professor of Pediatrics and of Preventive Medicine and Biostatics, University of Toronto, Toronto, Ontario

Maneuver

Pneumococcal vaccine, originally an octavalent vaccine, is now available as a 23-valent vaccine containing the strains of S. pneumoniae that have been isolated most often from patients with invasive disease. There have been no comparative studies of the old and new vaccines.

Effectiveness of Prevention and Treatment

Specific Patient Populations

The efficacy of pneumococcal vaccine was initially demonstrated in randomized controlled trials involving people working or living in close proximity to each other. Among South African miners[1,2] pneumococcal pneumonia or bacteremia developed in 17 of 1,493 vaccine recipients, as compared with 83 of 1,480 placebo recipients, for a vaccine efficacy rate of 78.5%.[1] Smit and collaborators[2] found an identical protective efficacy in a trial involving 983 recipients and 2,036 control subjects. Among 8,586 vaccine recipients in a study of U.S. military recruits[3] 4 had the pneumonia against which they were immunized, and 56 had other types of pneumonia; the corresponding numbers among the 8,449 saline recipients were 26 and 59.

Vaccine efficacy has also been confirmed in a cohort study involving patients with sickle cell disease and those who had undergone splenectomy.[4] Patients with Hodgkin's disease, on the other hand, have demonstrated poor antibody responses to the vaccine.[5]

General Pediatric Populations

In a randomized controlled trial in Australia involving 1,273 healthy children aged 6 to 54 months, there was no reduction in the number of respiratory and otic complaints among the vaccine recipients.[6] In addition, there were no differences in the rates of general hospital admission or admission because of respiratory tract infection. In a subgroup of patients, no difference was found between the recipients and the control subjects in nasal carriage rate of the S. pneumoniae serotypes included and not included in the vaccine.[7] In a multicentre study in Massachussetts 124 children aged 5 to 21 months were given the same vaccines.[8] The group that received the vaccine with the "target" serotypes had fewer infections than the other group but an equal number of ear infections.

For 179 infants in Alabama aged 6 to 21 months who had had at least one episode of otitis media before 10 months of age, no difference was observed in the overall infection rate between two

Pneumococcal vaccine has no role in preventing ear or respiratory infections in children

groups randomly assigned to receive vaccines containing "target" serotypes (those accounting for 75% of cases of otitis media) and "nontarget" serotypes.<9> The incidence of subsequent infections in black children 6 to 11 months of age was found to be decreased by half<10> but this may have been a chance occurrence resulting from multiple subgroup analyses. Makela and colleagues<11> examined the efficacy of vaccine in 827 Finnish children aged 3 months to 6 years. The subjects received either a 14-valent pneumococcal vaccine or *Hemophilus influenzae* type b vaccine in a double-blind manner. Although there was a significant reduction in the number of ear infections within the first 6 months after vaccination, the difference was lost with longer follow-up.

General Adult Populations

Shapiro and Clemens<12> conducted a case-control study of the efficacy of vaccine in patients at high risk for serious pneumococcal infections. In the 90 case-control pairs, 7% of the case subjects had received vaccine, as compared with 18% of the control subjects. The protective efficacy of the vaccine was estimated to be 67% (95% confidence interval (CI): 13% to 87%). This was mainly because of a reduction in the number of infections in the group at moderate risk; minimal efficacy was observed in the immunocompromised group. In an extension of this study, with 1,054 case-control pairs,<13> 13% of the case subjects and 20% of the control subjects had previously received vaccine, for a protective efficacy rate against vaccine serotypes of 56% (95% CI: 42% to 67%) for immunocompetent patients. The vaccine was not shown to be efficacious against infections caused by serotypes not represented in the vaccine (protective efficacy -73%; $p=0.15$) or for immunocompromised patients (protective efficacy 21%; $p=0.48$).

Using the same study design but excluding immunocompromised patients, Sims and co-workers<14> found that 8% of 122 infected patients had been vaccinated, as compared with 21% of 244 control subjects, for a vaccine efficacy rate of 70% (95% CI: 36% to 86%).

A case-control study involving 89 patients in hospital because of pneumococcal bacteremia showed no difference between the two groups in the vaccination rate or the distribution of responsible serotypes.<15> However, 30% of the subjects had hospital-acquired rather than community-acquired infection. The inclusion of people at high-risk who have previously been shown to respond poorly to vaccination and the small sample limit the significance of the findings.

In a two-year cohort study<16> involving elderly patients at two hospitals with long-term care facilities in Rochester, NY, the vaccine coverage was initially 84% (it was reduced to 65% by the end of the study). A small group of patients who refused to be vaccinated and a larger group of patients who were inadvertently not offered the vaccine acted as control subjects. The results of the first year revealed no significant difference between the two groups in the number of cases of pneumonia or deaths per 1,000 patient-years. This study is susceptible to volunteer bias and only a two-fold or greater difference in incidence would have been detected given the sample size. It has also been suggested that the etiologic serotypes in the elderly patients differed from the vaccine serotypes, which had been selected because they most frequently produced bacteremic disease in patients in general hospitals. However, there was no difference between the two groups when the vaccine serotypes were differentiated from nonvaccine serotypes.

In a cross-sectional analytic study[17] and among patients over 10 years of age, the proportions of isolates of vaccine serotypes (from blood and CSF samples) in vaccinated and nonvaccinated groups were 50% and 66% respectively, for an efficacy rate of 60%. The vaccine was not efficacious in a high-risk group with various immunologic or splenic disorders. In a subsequent study, involving more patients, efficacy was estimated to be 47%.[18] In addition, Bolan and associates[19] observed that the incidence of infection with pneumococcal serotypes found in the vaccine was higher among the nonvaccinated subjects (67%) than among the vaccinated subjects (49%). The efficacy rate was estimated to be 55% (95% CI: 2% to 82%) among patients with chronic cardiovascular disease, pulmonary disease or diabetes mellitus and 61% (95% CI: 3% to 99%) among those aged 61 years or more.

In several adult subpopulations, pneumococcal vaccine efficacy has been demonstrated in case-control studies, but not in randomized controlled trials

In a small randomized controlled trial of 1,300 mentally ill elderly patients randomly assigned to receive two hexavalent pneumococcal vaccines or saline placebo, there was no statistical difference in death rate or recovery rate of pneumococcal isolates (vaccine strains or all strains).[20]

A study involving 13,600 subjects aged 45 years or more who were not immunocompromised also demonstrated no difference in the incidence of radiologically diagnosed pneumonia or isolation of pneumococci from sputum samples.[20] This study had low statistical power because the incidence of pneumococcal pneumonia was low.

A trial involving 189 patients with severe chronic obstructive pulmonary disease[21] and the Veterans Administration Cooperative Study, involving 2,295 patients at high-risk,[22] also failed to detect differences in the rates of illness and death among vaccine recipients and control subjects. In the latter study the rate of death from lower respiratory tract infection was actually 15% greater among the recipients. The maximum achievable difference between the two groups would have been only 10%. The methodology of this study has been criticized regarding the lack of separation of colonization from infection, choice of endpoint, the possible failure of randomization and the high risk of ß error.

Kaufman and collaborators<23> conducted a 6-year study involving almost 11,000 inhospital patients over 40 years of age, about half of whom had received a divalent or trivalent vaccine. There were 99 cases of pneumonia in 5,750 vaccinated people, as compared with 227 cases in 5,153 control subjects (p<0.001). There were fewer deaths in the vaccinated group than in the control group (40 vs. 98, p<0.001).

In a randomized controlled trial, the vaccine was found to be efficacious in patients in geriatric hospitals and homes for the aged in France.<24> Patients with multisystem disease, and those who were immunocompromised were excluded. There were 1,234 patients aged 55 to 85 years without special risk factors, and 452 had diabetes or chronic cardiac, renal or pulmonary disease. Pneumonia occurred in 31 control subjects and 9 vaccine recipients, for a vaccine efficacy rate of 77% (95% CI: 51% to 89%). This study may be criticized because the cause of pneumonia was not confirmed and the pneumonia was not confirmed radiologically. It also differs from the U.S. studies because a higher frequency of pneumonia was observed in the control group.

Because of an absence of clinical studies controversy exists about recommendations for widespread vaccination in the general population. The efficacy of vaccine among people with chronic lung disease remains to be proven. Recent studies have shown that the proportion of people with serologic responses to the vaccine and the upper limit of the antibody concentration achieved were lower among elderly subjects with chronic lung disease than among young, healthy control subjects. These observations differ from those in previous studies in which some of the measured antibody was reactive to substances other than capsular polysaccharide.

Recommendations of Others

In 1989, the National Advisory Committee on Immunization recommended that a single dose of pneumococcal vaccine be given to all persons 65 or more years of age and to patients with chronic cardiorespiratory disease, cirrhosis, alcoholism, chronic renal disease, diabetes mellitus (adults), HIV infection, conditions associated with immunosuppression, asplenia, splenic disorders or sickle cell disease.

Conclusions and Recommendations

There is as yet no role for universal immunization with pneumococcal vaccine. Results of randomized trials have supported its use in studies of military recruits and South African miners under epidemic conditions but did not confirm a benefit among infants and young children. Therefore, there is good evidence to exclude pneumococcal vaccination from the periodic health examination of the

general population and of infants and young children
(E Recommendation).

The results of studies involving adults have been contradictory because of differences in study design, populations and end-points. In a cohort study the vaccine was effective in people with sickle cell disease and those who had undergone splenectomy. The efficacy rate of the vaccine in case-control studies has been from 60% to 70% among patients over 55 years of age, particularly if they have chronic pulmonary, cardiac or renal disease or are alcohol dependent. In cohort studies the rate has been 50% to 60%. Two randomized trials involving people in institutions have shown the vaccine to be efficacious. The data fit the model of increased exposure and incidence of infection observed among people living under crowded situations. Thus, there is good evidence to include vaccination in the periodic health examination of patients who have undergone splenectomy, those with sickle cell disease, immunocompetent elderly people living in institutions and adults living or working in crowded conditions (A Recommendation). Before the final decision to vaccinate is made, however, the physician must consider the overall condition of the person.

Immunocompromised patients do not seem to respond reliably to the vaccine, and the benefit in this group remains to be proven. There is fair evidence to exclude vaccination from the periodic health assessment of immunocompromised patients (D Recommendation).

Randomized trials in non-institutional settings have shown negative results, but all had limited power because of the low frequency of pneumonia as an outcome. If one assumes that 2.5 cases of pneumococcal pneumonia occur per 1,000 nonvaccinated people at high risk and a vaccine efficacy rate of 70% (the highest reported), then 571 subjects need to be vaccinated to prevent one case of pneumonia. The trend toward increased rates of death from lower respiratory tract infections among vaccine recipients in the Veterans Administration Cooperative Study prevents a stronger recommendation for vaccination considering its efficacy in the institutional setting. There is insufficient evidence to include vaccination in or exclude it from the periodic health examination of people over age 55 living independently (C Recommendation).

Unanswered Questions (Research Agenda)

1. Should pneumococcal vaccine be used in the ambulatory elderly population? We suggest conducting further trials, perhaps in countries where universal vaccination of those over 55 years of age has not been accepted, to replicate the Veterans Administration Cooperative Study.

2. Conjugate or other pneumococcal vaccines need to be developed that are more immunogenic in order to improve the efficacy rate among immunocompromised people.

Evidence

The literature was identified with a MEDLINE search to March 1993, using the following MESH headings: Bacterial vaccines, pneumococcal infections and human.

This review was initiated in March 1988 and the recommendations were finalized by the Task Force in September 1990. A report with a full reference list was published in March 1991.<25>

Selected References

1. Austrian R, Douglas RM, Schiffman G, *et al*: Prevention of pneumococcal pneumonia by vaccination. *Trans Assoc Am Physicians* 1976; 89: 184-194

2. Smit P, Oberholzer D, Hayden-Smith S, *et al*: Protective efficacy of pneumococcal polysaccharide vaccines. *JAMA* 1977; 238: 2613-2616

3. MacLeod CM, Hodges RG, Heidelberger M, *et al*: Prevention of pneumococcal pneumonia by immunization with specific capsular polysaccharides. *J Exp Med* 1945; 82: 445-465

4. Ammann AJ, Addiego J, Wara DW, *et al*: Polyvalent pneumococcal-polysaccharide immunization of patients with sickle-cell anemia and patients with splenectomy. *N Engl J Med* 1977; 297: 897-900

5. Addiego JE, Ammann AJ, Schiffman G, *et al*: Response to pneumococcal polysaccharide vaccine in patients with untreated Hodgkin's disease. *Lancet* 1980; 2: 450-453

6. Douglas RM, Miles HM: Vaccination against *Streptococcus pneumoniae* in childhood: lack of demonstrable benefit in young Australian children. *J Infect Dis* 1984; 149: 861-869

7. Douglas RM, Hansman D, Miles HB, *et al*: Pneumococcal carriage and type-specific antibody. Failure of a 14-valent vaccine to reduce carriage in healthy children. *Am J Dis Child* 1986; 140: 1183-1185

8. Teele DW, Klein JO, Bratton L, *et al*: Use of pneumococcal vaccine for prevention of recurrent acute otitis media in infants in Boston. The Greater Boston Collaborative Otitis Media Study Group. *Rev Infect Dis* 1981: 3 (Suppl): S113-S118

9. Sloyer JL, Ploussard J, Howie VM: Efficacy of pneumococcal polysaccharide vaccine in preventing acute otitis media in infants in Huntsville, Alabama. *Rev Infect Dis* 1981; 3 (Suppl): S119-S123

10. Howie VM, Ploussard J, Sloyer JL, *et al*: Use of pneumococcal polysaccharide vaccine in preventing otitis media in infants: different results between racial groups. *Pediatrics* 1984; 73: 79-81

11. Makela PH, Leinonen M, Pukander J, *et al*: A study of the pneumococcal vaccine in prevention of clinically acute attacks of recurrent otitis media. *Rev Infect Dis* 1981; 3 (Suppl): S124-S132

12. Shapiro ED, Clemens JD: A controlled evaluation of the protective efficacy of pneumococcal vaccine for patients at high risk of serious pneumococcal infections. *Ann Intern Med* 1984; 101: 325-330

13. Shapiro ED, Berg AT, Austrian R, *et al*: The protective efficacy of polyvalent pneumococcal polysaccharide vaccine. *N Engl J Med* 1991; 325(21): 1453-1460

14. Sims RV, Steinmann WC, McConville JH, *et al*: The clinical effectiveness of pneumococcal vaccine in the elderly. *Ann Intern Med* 1988; 108: 653-657

15. Forrester HL, Jahnigen DW, LaForce FM: Inefficacy of pneumococcal vaccine in a high-risk population. *Am J Med* 1987; 83: 425-430

16. Bentley DW, Ha K, Mamot K, *et al*: Pneumococcal vaccine in the institutionalized elderly: design of a nonrandomized trial and preliminary results. *Rev Infect Dis* 1981; 3 (Suppl): S71-S81

17. Broome CV, Facklam RR, Fraser DW: Pneumococcal disease after pneumococcal vaccination. An alternative method to estimate the efficacy of pneumococcal vaccine. *N Engl J Med* 1980; 303: 549-552

18. Broome CV: Efficacy of pneumococcal polysaccharide vaccines. *Rev Infect Dis* 1981; 3 (Suppl): S82-S88

19. Bolan G, Broome CV, Facklam RR, *et al*: Pneumococcal vaccine efficacy in selected populations in the United States. *Ann Intern Med* 1986; 104: 1-6

20. Austrian R: *Surveillance of Pneumococcal Infection for Field Trials of Polyvalent Pneumococcal Vaccines*. [rep DAB-VDR-12-84], National Institutes of Health, Bethesda, Md, 1980: 1-84

21. Leech JA, Gervais A, Ruben FL: Efficacy of pneumococcal vaccine in severe chronic obstructive pulmonary disease. *Can Med Assoc J* 1987; 136: 361-365

22. Simberkoff MS, Cross AP, Al-Ibrahim M, *et al*: Efficacy of pneumococcal vaccine in high-risk patients. Results of a Veterans Administration Cooperative Study. *N Engl J Med* 1986; 315: 1318-1327

23. Kaufman P: Pneumonia in old age. Active immunization against pneumonia with Pneumococcus polysaccharide: results of a six-year study. *Arch Intern Med* 1947; 79: 518-531

24. Gaillat J, Zmirou D, Mallaret MR, *et al*: Essai clinique du vaccin antipneumococcique chez des personnes âgées vivant en institution. *Rev Épidémiol Santé Publique* 1985; 33: 437-444

25. Canadian Task Force on the Periodic Health Examination: The periodic health examination, 1991 update: 2. Administration of pneumococcal vaccine. *Can Med Assoc J* 1991; 144: 665-671

Administration of Pneumococcal Vaccine

MANEUVER	EFFECTIVENESS	LEVEL OF EVIDENCE <REF>	RECOMMENDATION
Single dose of 23-valent pneumococcal vaccine	Vaccine is not beneficial in children. Vaccine does not prevent otitis media in infants and young children.	Randomized controlled trials<6-11> (I)	Good evidence to exclude from periodic health examination of infants and children (E)
	Vaccine is effective in patients with sickle cell disease and those having undergone splenectomy.	Cohort study<4> (II-2)	Good evidence to include in periodic health examination of people with sickle cell anemia and those having undergone splenectomy (A)
	Vaccine is ineffective in immunocompromised patients.	Case-control study<12> (II-2)	Fair evidence to exclude from periodic health examination of immunocompromised patients (D)
	Evidence of vaccine efficacy is contradictory for immunocompetent patients aged 55 years or more living independently.	Randomized controlled trials<20,22> (I); case control studies <12-14> (II-2); cross-sectional studies <17-19> (II-3)	Insufficient evidence to include or exclude from periodic health examination of immunocompetent individuals ≥age 55 years living independently (C)
	Vaccine has efficacy rate of 67% among immunocompetent patients aged 55 years or more in institutions.	Randomized controlled trials<23,24> (I)	Good evidence to include in periodic health examination of immunocompetent patients ≥age 55 years in institutions (A)

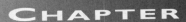

CHAPTER 35

Hepatitis B Immunization in Childhood

By Murray Krahn

35 Hepatitis B Immunization in Childhood

Adapted for the Canadian context by Murray Krahn, MD, MSc[1] from the report prepared for the U.S. Preventive Services Task Force[2]

Targeting high-risk groups for vaccination against hepatitis B infection has not had a major impact on the burden of disease. The incidence of both new hepatitis B infections and hepatitis B virus (HBV)-related deaths more than doubled between 1980 and 1989 in Canada.<1> Poor compliance and difficulties in reaching high-risk groups prior to infection have hindered efforts to control disease transmission. Also, 30-40% of new cases come from groups with no identifiable risk factors. A consensus has emerged among HBV experts and advisory groups in the United States and Canada that universal immunization is the key to controlling HBV infection.

Burden of Suffering

Current vaccination strategies have not been effective in controlling HBV infection

2,815 new cases of hepatitis B were reported in Canada in 1992 (Laboratory Centre for Disease Control, Ottawa, unpublished data). The true incidence rate is 5 to 10 fold higher, because HBV is under reported, and most infection is subclinical. Between 1980 and 1988, death certificate data indicated that 223 deaths were caused by hepatitis B.<1>

Most HBV infections in North America occur in adults, presumably through sexual transmission, intravenous drug use, or contact with contaminated blood products. However, acute infection was also reported in 253 children aged 0-19 years of age, accounting for 9% of cases. Most were in adolescents, but 41 cases occurred in children under age 10. Incidence in this age group may be much higher, because HBV infections in infants and young children are rarely symptomatic.

Most new hepatitis B infections in North America occur in adults, but childhood infection accounts for a large proportion of adult chronic liver disease

Illness related to hepatitis B may be acute or chronic. Acute hepatitis B infection is most frequently asymptomatic, but may cause illness characterized by jaundice, systemic symptoms, and even liver failure or death. Acute infection may be followed by a chronic carrier state. HBV transmitted from HBsAg-positive mothers to their newborns results in HBV carriage in up to 90% of infants. Children infected before 5 years of age become chronic carriers in 25-50% of cases, compared to 5-10% of those infected as adults. Thus, although

---

[1] Assistant Professor, Departments of Medicine and Clinical Biochemistry, University of Toronto, Toronto, Ontario
[2] By Carolyn DiGuiseppi, MD, MPH, Science Advisor, U.S. Preventive Services Task Force, Washington, D.C.

childhood infection is uncommon in North America, it accounts for a substantial proportion (40%, by one estimate<2>) of HBV-related chronic hepatitis, cirrhosis, and hepatocellular carcinoma in adults. One third of all carriers with a life expectancy of greater than 30 years will die from complications of HBV-related liver disease.

Children who are at substantially increased risk of HBV infection include immigrants and refugees (or those born to such persons) from HBV endemic areas, native Canadians, children living in homes for the developmentally disabled, household contacts of HBV carriers, and infants born to HBsAg-positive mothers. Among North American-born children of Southeast Asian refugees, the prevalence of horizontally acquired HBV infection is nearly 10%.

Maneuver

All hepatitis B vaccines contain purified HBsAg, and induce production of antibodies (HBsAb) which provide protection against acute infection. Two vaccines are licensed in Canada, Recombivax HB (Merck Sharp and Dohme) and Engerix-B (Smith Kline Beecham). Both vaccines are derived from yeast strains that have been genetically manipulated, and contain HBsAg adsorbed on aluminum hydroxide along with trace amounts of yeast-derived proteins, lipids, polysaccharides, and DNA. Plasma-derived hepatitis B vaccines are no longer available in Canada.

Effectiveness of Prevention and Treatment

Health Benefit

Controlled trials<3,4> and other studies have demonstrated that hepatitis B vaccine is 62-92% effective in preventing the development of the HBV chronic carrier state during the first 1-5 years of life when given to infants of HBsAg positive mothers soon after birth, again at 1 month, and then at either 6 months or 2 and 12 months of age. Efficacy in these studies has varied with dosage, vaccination interval, vaccine type, and hepatitis B e antigen status of the mother. The protective efficacy of vaccine when combined with hepatitis B immune globulin is higher (85-95%) than that of vaccine alone in these infants.

Controlled trials have shown that hepatitis B vaccine is effective in preventing new HBV infection and development of the carrier state

From controlled trials<5,6> and time series conducted in populations where horizontal HBV transmission is common, universal vaccination of infants and children with a 3 or 4 dose regimen has been estimated to be >87% effective in preventing HBV infection and >80% effective in preventing chronic HBV carriage. Mass vaccination of children in New Zealand and infants in Taiwan has also led to substantial reductions in the prevalence of acute HBV events and carrier status in the unvaccinated population.

The long term efficacy of the vaccine is less certain. In Gambian children vaccinated before 5 years of age, and in Senegalese vaccinated as infants, protective efficacy against HBV events (as evidenced by HBsAg or anti-HB core antigen positivity) declined somewhat over time. However, protection against chronic carriage persisted at least 5-6 years in Gambian children and in the vaccinated infants of carrier mothers. Time series from populations with high endemicity have reported loss of protective antibody levels in 11-17% of children (ranging in age from 0-19 years) at 3-7 year follow-up although the risk of infection remained low. Booster vaccinations in children result in anamnestic responses suggesting that immunologic memory is maintained despite the decline in antibody levels. It is unclear whether these studies are applicable to the North American population, since malnutrition and infectious diseases may contribute to the loss of antibody and continued exposure to HBV may contribute to the maintenance of immunity. The exact role of such factors is undefined.

Many of the studies cited above used the plasma-derived hepatitis B vaccine that is no longer available in Canada. However, the recombinant vaccines currently in use induce similar antibody responses and similar short term efficacy in children and adults. Information on long-term efficacy of recombinant vaccines is not yet available. Continued experience will determine whether booster doses are necessary to maintain long-term protection.

Adverse Effects

No serious adverse reactions have been reported with the use of HBV vaccine in children, though local soreness, irritability, and fever are not uncommon

Mild reactions to recombinant hepatitis B vaccine, including local soreness and induration, low grade fever, irritability and poor feeding, are reported by the parents of up to 13% of vaccinated children and 4-7% of vaccinated infants. No serious adverse effects have been reported in children, although an increased risk of Guillain-Barre syndrome associated with the plasma-derived vaccine has been suggested in adults. Neither the simultaneous administration of hepatitis B vaccine with diptheria-tetanus-pertussis and oral polio vaccines, nor modest alterations in timing to integrate the hepatitis B vaccine with other childhood vaccines, appears to interfere substantially with the immunogenic effect of the vaccine. Immunologic response to hepatitis B vaccine increases with increasing intervals between the first and third doses, suggesting some advantage to postponing the third dose to coincide with later visits (e.g., at 12 to 18 months of age) for those at low risk. A reduced response of preterm infants to hepatitis B vaccine has been described, with one study reporting an improved seroconversion rate when the first dose was delayed a mean of 31 days in preterm infants.

Costs

A recent cost effectiveness analysis<7> compared a policy of maternal screening and vaccination of high risk neonates (those born to HBsAg positive mothers) with HBIG and hepatitis B vaccine to a combined policy of maternal screening and universal infant vaccination. The combined strategy resulted in a cost of approximately $30,000 per additional year of life saved from a societal perspective, and $60,000 per year of life saved from a third-party payer perspective (costs and life years discounted). Results of the analysis were sensitive to assumptions about the duration of vaccine efficacy, and cost of the vaccine.

Another study<8> calculated that a universal vaccination strategy, when compared to no screening and no vaccination, resulted in a cost of approximately US$40,000 per year of life saved. Universal vaccination of adolescents, compared to no vaccination, resulted in a cost of US$100,000 per incremental life year (costs and life years discounted).

Recommendations of Others

The National Advisory Committee on Immunization (NACI) recommended that a universal immunization program during childhood be implemented, but stated that issues related to vaccine cost and optimal dose schedules should be resolved prior to implementation of a specific program.<9> NACI also recommended the vaccination of high-risk children: children living in communities of high HBV endemicity in Canada (e.g. some native populations in Labrador and the Northwest Territories), children of immigrants from areas of high HBV endemicity aged < 7 years, residents of institutions for the developmentally challenged, hemophiliacs, dialysis patients, and household contacts of HBV carriers.

The Canadian Pediatric Society has advised that initial steps be taken to develop a universal hepatitis B vaccination program for infants, and consideration be given to a "catch up" program targeted at adolescents.<10>

The American Academy of Pediatrics<11> and the Advisory Committee on Immunization Practices<12> advocate routine hepatitis B vaccination for all newborns, regardless of the HBsAg status of the mother. All groups recommend the addition of hepatitis B immune globulin (HBIG) to HBV vaccine for newborns of HBsAg-positive mothers, and vaccination of older children at high risk.

Conclusions and Recommendations

There is good evidence at this time to recommend that hepatitis B vaccination be incorporated in the childhood immunization schedule as a component of the periodic health examination (A Recommendation). Universal childhood immunization should be implemented to control HBV infection, but the appropriate target population (adolescents or newborns) and the optimal dose schedules have not yet been determined. Infants born to HBsAg positive mothers should receive HBIG and hepatitis B vaccine at birth, as well as two additional vaccine doses at 1 and 6 months. Vaccination of high risk groups (described above) according to recommended schedules<13> should continue to receive high priority. Booster doses in immunocompetent individuals are not recommended.

Unanswered Questions (Research Agenda)

The duration of vaccine efficacy in North American populations remains uncertain and requires further study. The optimal strategy for universal vaccination is unclear.

Evidence

The literature was identified with a MEDLINE search for the years 1988 to January 1994 using the following MESH headings: Hepatitis B, prevention and control, Canada, vaccination, and immunization. This review was initiated by the Task Force in January 1994 and recommendations finalized in March 1994.

Acknowledgements

The assistance of Sharon Smith in article retrieval and manuscript preparation is gratefully acknowledged.

Selected References

1. Ip HM, Wong VC, Lelie PN, *et al*: Hepatitis B infection in infants after neonatal immunization. *Acta Paediatr Jpn* 1989; 31: 654-658

2. Zhu QR, Duan SC, Xu HF: A six-year survey of immunogenicity and efficacy of hepatitis B vaccine in infants born to HBsAg carriers. *Chi Med J Engl* 1992; 105: 194-198

3. Coursaget P, Yvonnet B, Chotard J, *et al*: Seven-year study of hepatitis B vaccine efficacy in infants from an endemic area (Senegal). *Lancet* 1986; 2: 1143-1145

4. Sun Z, Zhu Y, Stjernsward J, *et al*: Design and compliance of HBV vaccination trial on newborns to prevent hepatocellular carcinoma and 5-year results of its pilot study. *Cancer Det Prev* 1991; 15: 313-318

5. Carter AO, Walsh, P: Hepatitis B in Canada: surveillance summary, 1980-1989. *Can Dis Wkly Rep* 1992; 17-31: 166-171

6.   West DJ, Margolis HS: Prevention of hepatitis B virus infection in the United States: a pediatric perspective. *Pediatr Infect Dis J* 1992; 11: 866-874

7.   Krahn M, Detsky AS: Should Canada and the United States universally vaccinate infants against hepatitis B? A cost effectiveness analysis. *Med Decis Making* 1993; 13: 4-20

8.   Bloom BS, Hillman AL, Fendrick AM, *et al*: A reappraisal of hepatitis B virus vaccination strategies using cost-effectiveness analysis. *Ann Intern Med* 1993; 118: 298-306

9.   National Advisory Committee on Immunization. Statement on hepatitis B vaccine. *Can Med Assoc J* 1993; 149: 1465-1471

10. Infectious Diseases and Immunization Committee Canadian Pediatric Society. Hepatitis B in Canada: the case for universal vaccination. *Can Med Assoc J* 1992; 146: 25-28

11. Committee on Infectious Diseases American Academy of Pediatrics. Universal hepatitis B immunization. *AAP News* 1992; 13-15: 22-22

12. Advisory Committee on Immunization Practices: Hepatitis B virus: a comprehensive strategy for eliminating transmission in the United States through universal childhood vaccination. *MMWR Morb Mortal Wkly Rep* 1991; 40 (RR-13):1-25

13. National Advisory Committee on Immunization: Statement on hepatitis B vaccine. *Can Commun Dis Rep* 1993; 19: 104-115

Hepatitis B Immunization in Childhood

MANEUVER	EFFECTIVENESS	LEVEL OF EVIDENCE <REF>	RECOMMENDATION
Immunization with hepatitis B vaccine and hepatitis B immune globulin (HBIG) in infants born to hepatitis B surface antigen (HBsAg) positive mothers	Effective in preventing hepatitis B virus (HBV) infection and development of the carrier state in infants born to carrier mothers.	Randomized controlled trials<1,2> (I)	Good evidence to include in periodic health examination (A)
Immunization with hepatitis B vaccine in infants born to HBsAg negative mothers	Effective in preventing new HBV events and development of the carrier state in areas of high endemicity.	Randomized controlled trials<3,4> (I)	Good evidence to include in periodic health examination (A)
Immunization of high-risk* children and adolescents	Effective in preventing new HBV events and development of the carrier state in areas of high endemicity.	Randomized controlled trials<3,4> (I)	Good evidence to include in periodic health examination (A)*
Universal vaccination of children and adolescents	Effective in preventing new HBV events and development of the carrier state in areas of high endemicity	Randomized controlled trials<3,4> (I)	Good evidence to include in periodic health examination (A)

* High-risk groups include: residents of institutions for the developmentally challenged, hemophiliacs, hemodialysis patients, household contacts of HBV carriers, residents in HBV endemic communities, children <age 7 in immigrant families from HBV endemic areas, travellers to HBV endemic areas for >6 months.

SECTION 4

Preventive Dental Care

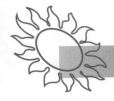

CHAPTER 36

Prevention of Dental Caries

By Donald W. Lewis and Amid I. Ismail

36 Prevention of Dental Caries

Prepared by Donald W. Lewis, DDS, DDPH, MScD, FRCDC[1] and
Amid I. Ismail, BDS, MPH, DrPH[2]

*In 1979, the Canadian Task Force on the Periodic Health
Examination using the evidence then available made
recommendations concerning the prevention of dental caries.[1]
Since then, significant reductions in the prevalence of dental
caries have occurred in Canada, and we have new understanding
of its epidemiology, diagnosis, risk factors and prevention.
Despite this improving picture and the accrued benefits of past,
largely fluoride-related preventive efforts, dental caries remains a
large problem for a significant proportion of the population, a
potentially increasing problem for an aging population retaining
more teeth and, surprisingly, in view of the overall decreased
caries prevalence, a growing major cost problem for Canadians
and those who insure their dental care.*

*In 1989 the U.S. Preventive Services Task Force published
guidelines for the prevention of dental caries[2] and a more
recent Canadian publication has provided more specific
preventive guidelines that are similar to those of the U.S. Task
Force.[3]*

Burden of Suffering

Dental caries results
from the interplay of:
dietary
carbohydrates,
cariogenic bacteria
within dental plaque
and susceptible
hardtooth surfaces

Dental caries (decay) is ubiquitous and is one of the most
prevalent infectious diseases of man. It is a localized, progressive
demineralization of the hard tissues of the crown (coronal enamel,
dentine) and root (cementum, dentine) surfaces of teeth. The
demineralization is caused by acids produced by bacteria, particularly
mutans Streptococci and possibly *lactobacilli*, that ferment dietary
carbohydrates. This occurs within a bacteria-laden gelatinous material
called dental plaque that adheres to tooth surfaces and becomes
colonized by bacteria. Thus, caries results from the interplay of three
main factors over time: dietary carbohydrates, cariogenic bacteria
within dental plaque, and susceptible hard tooth surfaces. Dental caries
is a dynamic process since periods of demineralization alternate with
periods of remineralization through the action of fluoride, calcium and
phosphorous contained in oral fluids.[4]

Dental caries is age-related. Prevalence begins soon after tooth
eruption in susceptible children and increases with age. Although

[1] Professor of Community Dentistry, University of Toronto, Toronto, Ontario
[2] Associate Professor and Chair, Department of Pediatric and Community Dentistry,
Dalhousie University, Halifax, Nova Scotia

current Canadian data are lacking, older data when dental caries were more prevalent suggest that caries incidence had three peaks: at about age 7 years for coronal decay of the primary dentition; at about age 14 years for coronal decay of the permanent dentition; and, for root surface decay, incidence began at about age 30-40 years with steady increases thereafter.

The different morphology of the pit-and-fissure surfaces of teeth makes them more susceptible to decay than the smooth surfaces. Thus, it is no surprise to find that the posterior molar and premolar teeth that have pit and fissure surfaces are more susceptible than the anterior teeth. Based on epidemiologic studies, the pit-and-fissure occlusal (biting) surfaces of molar teeth usually decay within three years of eruption or not at all.[5,6]

Although great international and regional intranational differences exist, the incidence and prevalence of coronal dental caries have declined in the industrialized countries over the past 20 years.[7] This change has been well documented for children and adolescents. Canadian children now have 33-50% lower dental caries prevalence and many children have experienced no decay or fillings at all.[6] In the U.S. in 1986-87, 50% of 5-17 year old children were completely free of decay and of restorations in their permanent teeth.[8] There has also been a shift in the types of surfaces displaying decay or fillings. Now an even greater proportion of childrens' decay (75-80%) occurs on pit-and-fissure surfaces.[6,7]

Coronal dental caries has declined dramatically over the past 20 years while root caries in adults has increased

In adults, there have been small reductions in the number of decayed, missing and filled teeth and in the rate of edentulism (total tooth loss).[7] In dentate adults, the decline in missing teeth has been more substantial.[9] While it is believed that the marked improvement in dental caries status and greater tooth retention experienced by children will eventually be evident in adults, a long transition period of about 40 years will be required before improvement is evident in all adult age groups. Longer tooth retention and aging of the population have combined to increase interest in root caries. Because of inconsistencies in studies, estimates of the incidence, prevalence and risk factors associated with root caries are problematic. A secular increase in root caries has, however, occurred. In the few studies completed, annual incidence rates of 1.6-1.8 surfaces per 1,000 surfaces at risk have been reported along with the observation that only a minority (30-40%) of the group studied bear the entire burden of root caries attack. Prevalence surveys have revealed wide variations in the percent displaying at least one decayed or filled root lesion (21-83%).

The extensive decline in dental caries has not benefited all children equally. U.S. data reveal that 20-25% of children still have high decay levels – the so-called high-risk children. Adults not yet benefiting from this decline still have decay and fillings characteristic of a previous era. Secondary decay around old fillings, replacement fillings and breakage of tooth cusps due to extensive fillings are commonplace in this age group and represent a large treatment backlog.

Children and adults with special medical problems are at higher risk for dental caries. These include bulimics, those with Sjögren's syndrome, and those receiving therapeutic head and neck radiation, chemotherapy, or prolonged treatment with drugs that reduce salivary flow.[10] Institutionalized and physically and mentally disabled persons are also at higher risk for dental caries.

The financial burden of diagnosing, preventing, treating and re-treating dental disease, particularly dental caries, is great. Canadian dental care costs in 1989 were estimated at $3.1 billion, higher than many medical conditions.[11] This represents a tripling of dental care costs since 1979.

Detailed reviews of the many risk factors and risk indicators for dental caries have been reported elsewhere.[10,12,13] Age, socioeconomic status and past dental caries are strongly linked with dental caries incidence; oral hygiene as practised by most people is not strongly related to dental caries occurrence. However, because of the impact on esthetics and gingival disease and, as a vehicle for self-application of fluoride dentifrice, regular oral hygiene practices are recommended. Although past research indicated that sugar was a definite risk factor, current research findings about the effect of contemporary dietary practices on dental caries have given equivocal results except possibly for those at high risk because of high sugar intake and poor oral hygiene.

Maneuver

Traditionally, the clinical detection of carious lesions on tooth crowns has involved the use of a sharp explorer, a viewing mirror, an artificial light source and air-drying of tooth surfaces to improve visibility. This visual and tactile approach is often supplemented by the use of selected radiographs to help in the diagnosis of small (incipient) lesions on the hidden surfaces between adjacent teeth. The early clinical detection of incipient carious lesions has attracted increased interest recently because of the possibility that primary preventive procedures (e.g. topical fluorides) used by patients or by dental personnel may enhance remineralization and even arrest dental decay.

The validity of visual detection of frank (more advanced) coronal decay using subsequent histological determination as the "gold standard", is represented by sensitivity and specificity values ranging between 0.78 and 0.84 and positive and negative predictive values of 0.63 to 0.92 (unadjusted for current prevalence).[3] Using radiographs for the diagnosis of caries between the teeth, sensitivities and specificities of 0.36 to 0.98 and (unadjusted) predictive values of 0.53 and 0.97 have been reported.[3]

Diagnosis of dental caries and treatment planning in clinical practice is idiosyncratic and plagued with considerable variation among dentists.<14,15> This has been demonstrated when the same group of patients and the same set of radiographs were examined.

Diagnosis of caries and treatment planning in clinical practice can be characterized as idiosyncratic and varies considerably among dentists

Effectiveness of Prevention and Treatment

Four types of primary prevention are reviewed: fluorides; fissure sealants; dietary counselling; and oral hygiene.

Systemic Fluorides

Despite the apparent reduction in effectiveness of water fluoridation due to declining caries levels (from about 50% reduction in decay to 20-40%), fluoridation of the water supply remains the single most effective, equitable and efficient means of preventing coronal and root dental caries.<16> The impact of water fluoridation on coronal decay in children, adolescents and adults has been studied in numerous community trials and economic evaluations and the impact on root caries has been evaluated in case-control studies. In areas having less than optimal F (0.7-1.2 ppm) in their water supplies, prescription of fluoride supplements is recommended, although compliance may be difficult.<17>

Because of the widespread availability of fluorides (in dentifrices, water, vitamin supplements, manufactured beverages and food), there is now concern about increases in the prevalence of (usually) very mild fluorosis in children's teeth. Although mild fluorosis is usually neither unsightly nor easily visible, it is, nevertheless, evidence of excess fluoride intake.

A principal reason for the observed increase in fluorosis appears to be inappropriate prescribing of systemic fluoride supplements by dentists and physicians<18> and/or overzealous use of these supplements by parents for their children. The currently recommended supplemental fluoride dose schedule, adjusted for the child's age and current fluoride content of water has been published elsewhere<3> as has a 1992 Canadian modification.<19> These modifications to avoid fluorosis suggest lower intakes of fluoride supplements because of increased use of fluoride toothpastes and ingestion of other food and beverage sources of systemic (and topical) fluoride that were not widely available when current guidelines were formulated.

Because of the caries decline and concerns regarding fluorosis, preventive interventions, although effective, must be selected carefully

Professionally-Applied Topical Fluorides

These agents, e.g., acidulated phosphate F gel in trays, have been proven efficacious in randomized clinical trials in children, though there have been few trials since 1980, the era of decline in caries incidence.[20] It has now been established that there is no need for a prophylaxis (cleaning) of the teeth prior to the application of a topical fluoride[20] but similar evidence for biannual rather than annual applications is lacking.

Today, costly professionally-applied topical fluoride cannot be recommended for use with most children in communities with water fluoridation[20] or, indeed, for most children generally because of the dental caries decline. However, this form of fluoride therapy is recommended for persons with active decay and at high risk, for those undergoing head and neck radiation therapy and for older adults experiencing root caries.[20]

Self-Applied Fluorides

These include the widely used fluoride dentifrices that are strongly recommended because of their ease of use, low cost and effectiveness on coronal and root caries prevention based on randomized clinical trials.[20,21] The primary reason for the caries decline in developed countries over the past 15-20 years is invariably ascribed to fluoride dentifrices. However, concerns about a possible increase in mild tooth fluorosis have prompted recommendations to use less dentifrice and supervise the toothbrushing of young children.[19]

Fluoride mouth rinses were recommended a few years ago for general use. However, because of the decline in caries and concerns about excess fluoride ingestion, they are now recommended only for those at high risk to dental caries and for those not regularly using a fluoride dentifrice.[22] None of these rinses are intended for use in children under age 5.

Fissure Sealants

These are resins applied by dental personnel to the pit-and-fissure surfaces of posterior teeth. They have been extensively tested since 1979 in randomized clinical trials and have proven to be effective in reducing this most common form of surface decay.[6,23] Because of their high cost, the general decline in decay and differential tendencies for certain fissures to decay, sealants should be applied selectively to high risk patients and to permanent molars only, within 2-3 years after tooth eruption.

Dietary Counselling

Encouragement to reduce sucrose intake and use dentally 'safe' substitutes may be less important now for the majority of persons. Two recent longitudinal (cohort) dietary studies revealed that dental caries incidence was low among study children despite their high sugar consumption.[24] In one study,[24] the only apparent etiologic role of sugar was related to decay of smooth surfaces between the teeth; however, this type of surface decay has rapidly declined in children recently. Thus, routine dietary counselling today may be misguided. As well, the effectiveness of dental counselling in inducing behaviour change is suspect.[25] Since sugars are one of the etiologic factors in the caries process,[4] selective counselling limited to high-risk children may still be indicated. Similarly, because of the high risk of severe decay to infants' teeth due to this practice, the majority of studies do not advise the nocturnal or other prolonged use of baby bottles containing liquids other than water.[26,27]

Oral Hygiene

Oral hygiene procedures consist of personal plaque removal by toothbrushing and/or flossing as well as the professional prophylaxis that often precedes a periodic dental examination. As ordinarily practised, in neither case is there evidence that these lead to caries reductions.[12,28] Daily personal oral hygiene (toothbrushing and flossing) is recommended in the interest of good hygiene and for the control of gingival disease. Toothbrushing is also required for the self-application of fluoride dentifrice, a proven caries preventive.

Recommendations of Others

The U.S. Preventive Services Task Force[2] has published recommendations for dental caries prevention (which are currently being reviewed), as have the Department of National Health and Welfare[6] (now Health Canada) and others.[16,20,22]

Conclusions and Recommendations

Lower dental caries prevalence and the need for efficiency in the provision of preventive and therapeutic dental services require selective use of dental caries preventives and targeting of services toward persons at greatest risk. The following recommendations are based on a review of the available evidence.

There is good evidence of effectiveness of the following measures in preventing dental caries (A Recommendation):

1. water fluoridation for preventing coronal and root caries;
2. fluoride supplements in low fluoride areas with careful adherence to low dosage schedules;
3. professional topical fluoride applications and self-administered fluoride mouth rinses for those with very active decay or at high future risk for dental caries;

4. fluoride dentifrices, with special supervision and the use of small amounts for young children;

5. professionally-applied fissure sealants for selective use on permanent molar teeth soon after their eruption.

There is poor evidence of effectiveness for the following measures in preventing dental caries (C Recommendation):

1. professional topical fluoride applications and self-administered fluoride mouth rinses for the majority of children and for adults who are not at high risk for dental caries;

2. toothbrushing (without a fluoride dentifrice) and flossing;

3. the traditional prophylaxis prior to a topical fluoride application or given at a dental recall visit;

4. dietary counselling to the general population about cariogenic foods.

Unanswered Questions (Research Agenda)

Methods of identifying early carious lesions accurately and of identifying individuals at high risk for dental caries are required; research aimed at defining appropriate restorative care and guidelines for restorative decision making is also indicated. Research is needed to confirm the relationship of vulnerability of occlusal surfaces to caries and time since tooth eruption. Prospective studies to examine all possible etiologic factors associated with nursing caries are needed. Since many different dental caries preventives have been proven effective, research into the most effective and efficient combinations of preventive interventions and the optimum frequency of use is important. Given the ubiquitous availability of fluorides and increased occurrence of mild fluorosis, the optimal use of systemic and topical fluorides to achieve maximum reduction of dental caries and minimum prevalence of dental fluorosis should be determined.

Evidence

Using the results of a literature search from 1980 to 1992 and significant review articles, relevant clinical findings were evaluated and categorized using the levels of evidence developed by the Task Force. This review was initiated in June 1992 and the recommendations finalized by the Task Force in September 1993. A more detailed review with a complete reference list is available.[3]

Acknowledgements

The authors are grateful to the following persons who reviewed the earlier publication[3] on which this chapter is based: D. Christopher Clark, BS, DDS, MPH, Associate Professor, University of British Columbia, Vancouver, BC; Dr David W. Banting, DDS, DDPH, MSc, PhD, FRCDC, Professor of Community Dentistry, University of Western Ontario, London, Ontario; Dr. David W. Johnston, BDS, MPH, Chair and Associate Professor, Department of Community Dentistry, University of Western Ontario, London, Ontario; Dr. James L. Leake, DDS, DDPH, MSc, FRCDC, Chair and Professor, Department of Community Dentistry, University of Toronto, Toronto, Ontario; and Dr. Wyatt R. Hume, BDS, PhD, DDSc, Professor and Chair, Department of Restorative Dentistry, University of California, San Francisco, San Francisco, CA, USA.

Selected References

1. Canadian Task Force on the Periodic Health Examination: Periodic Health Examination Monograph: *Report of the Task Force to the Conference of Deputy Ministers of Health* (cat H39-3/1980E), Health Services and Promotion Branch, Dept of National Health and Welfare, Ottawa, 1980

2. Greene JC, Louie R, Wycoff SJ: U.S. Preventive Services Task Force: Preventive dentistry 1. dental caries. *JAMA* 1989; 262: 3459-3463

3. Lewis DW, Ismail AI with the Canadian Task Force on the Periodic Health Examination: Periodic health examination, 1993 update: Dental caries, diagnosis, risk factors and prevention. *Can Med Assoc J*; (in press)

4. Dawes C: Fluorides: mechanisms of action and recommendations for use. *J Can Dent Assoc* 1989; 55: 721-723

5. Reid DBW, Grainger RM: Variations in the caries susceptibility of children's teeth. *Human Biol* 1955; 27: 1-11

6. Kandelman DP, Lewis DW: Pit and fissure sealants. In: Lewis DW (ed): *Preventive Dental Services second edition.* Ottawa: Minister of Supply and Services Canada. [Cat. No. H 39-4/1988E], 1988: 13-31

7. Graves RC, Stamm JW: Decline of dental caries. What occurred and will it continue? *J Can Dent Assoc* 1985; 51: 693-699

8. Brunelle JA, Carlos JP: Recent trends in dental caries in U.S. children and the effect of water fluoridation. *J Dent Res* 1990; 69(Spec): 723-727

9. Weintraub JA, Burt BA: Oral health status in the United States: tooth loss and edentulism. *J Dent Educ* 1985; 49: 368-378

10. Hunter PB: Risk factors in dental caries. *Int Dent J* 1988; 38: 211-217

11. Leake JL, Porter J, Lewis DW: A macroeconomic review of dentistry in the 1980's. *J Can Dent Assoc* 1993; 59: 281-284,287

12. Hunt RJ: Behavioral and sociodemographic risk factors for caries. In: Bader JD (ed): *Risk assessment in dentistry.* Chapel Hill: University of North Carolina Dental Ecology, 1990

13. Graves RC, Disney JA, Stamm JW, *et al*: Physical and environmental risk factors in dental caries. In: Bader JD (ed): *Risk assessment in dentistry.* Chapel Hill: University of North Carolina Dental Ecology, 1990

14. Klein SP, Bell RM, Bohannan HM, *et al*: The reliability of caries and radiographic examinations in the national preventive dentistry demonstration program. Santa Monica, *Rand Corp.* [Pub. R-313 8-WJ], 1984

15. Elderton RJ, Nuttall NM: Variation among dentists in planning treatment. *Br Dent J* 1983; 154: 201-206

16. Newbrun E: Effectiveness of water fluoridation. *J Public Health Dent* 1989; 49 (5 Spec No): 279-289

17. Driscoll WS: What we know and don't know about dietary fluoride supplements – the research basis. *ASDC J Dent Child* 1985; 52: 259-264

18. Woolfolk MW, Faja BW, Bagramian RA: Relation of sources of systemic fluoride to prevalence of dental fluorosis. *J Public Health Dent* 1989; 49: 78-82

19. Clark DC: Appropriate use of fluorides in the 1990s. *J Can Dent Assoc* 1993; 59: 272-279

20. Ripa LW: A critique of topical fluoride methods (dentifrices, mouthrinses, operator- and self-applied gels) in an era of decreased caries and increased fluorosis prevalence. *J Public Health Dent* 1991; 51: 23-41

21. Jensen ME, Kohout FJ: The effect of a fluoridated dentifrice on root and coronal caries in an older adult population. *J Am Dent Assoc* 1988; 117: 829-832

22. Leverett DH: Effectiveness of mouthrinsing with fluoride solutions in preventing coronal and root caries. *J Public Health Dent* 1989; 49(5 Spec No): 310-316

23. Weintraub JA: The effectiveness of pit and fissure sealants. *J Public Health Dent* 1989; 49(5 Spec No): 317-330

24. Burt BA, Eklund SA, Morgan KJ, *et al*: The effects of sugars intake and frequency of ingestion on dental caries increment in a three-year longitudinal study. *J Dent Res* 1988; 67: 1422-1429

25. Weinstein P, Milgrom P, Melnick S, *et al*: How effective is oral hygiene instruction? Results after 6 and 24 weeks. *J Pub Health Dent* 1989; 49: 32-38

26. Ripa LW: Nursing caries: a comprehensive review. *Pediatr Dent* 1988; 10: 268-282

27. Kroll RG, Stone JH: Nocturnal bottle-feeding as a contributory cause of rampant dental caries in the infant and young child. *J Dent Child* 1967; 34: 454-459

28. Andlaw RJ: Oral hygiene and dental caries – a review. *Int Dent J* 1978; 28: 1-6

Prevention of Dental Caries

MANEUVER	EFFECTIVENESS	LEVEL OF EVIDENCE <REF>	RECOMMENDATION
Water fluoridation	Even in era of caries decline caries reductions of 20-40% occur.	Controlled trials without randomization<16> (II-1)	Good evidence that water fluoridation is still effective, equitable and efficient (A)
Daily fluoride supplements (only where water fluoride levels are less than optimal)	Reductions in caries similar to water fluoridation, however, compliance is poor.	Controlled trials without randomization<17> (II-1)	Good evidence to recommend if proper dosage schedule is carefully followed (A)
Professionally applied topical fluorides	Effective if used selectively, otherwise expensive; prior teeth cleaning is not needed.	For coronal decay: randomized controlled trials<20> (I)	Good evidence to recommend for those at high risk (A)
Fluoride dentifrices	Daily use gives significant reductions in decay.	Numerous older and one recent randomized controlled trial for root caries<12,21> (I)	Good evidence to use daily as part of regular oral hygiene; concern about swallowing excess dentifrice requires supervision of young children (A)
Daily plaque removal by brushing and flossing	Without fluoride dentifrice not cariostatic.	Re: brushing and caries, expert opinion<12,28> (III) Re: flossing and teeth decay, controlled trial without randomization for very young children<28> (II-1)	Poor evidence to include strictly for caries prevention (C) BUT brushing essential for self-application of fluoride dentifrice (A) and prevention of gingivitis (B)
Fissure sealants	Statistically and clinically significant reductions in pit-and-fissure surface decay if sealants used selectively.	Numerous randomized controlled trials<6,23> (I)	Good evidence for selective use on recently erupted permanent molars of high-risk children (A)
Counselling: to reduce intake of cariogenic foods, and for infants to reduce nocturnal and long-term use of baby bottles containing liquids other than water as pacifiers	Despite early evidence recent data suggests less specific impact of dietary sugars on caries incidence in the general population.	Cohort studies<24,25> and case-control study for baby bottle caries<27> (II-2)	Poor evidence of dietary change as effective for population; (C) however for high-risk persons and regarding changes in infant feeding to prevent baby bottle caries may be clinically prudent

*   Because of space limitations details about dental fluoride mouth rinses and dental prophylaxis at periodic dental examinations have been omitted from this table.

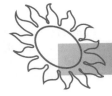

CHAPTER

37

Prevention of Periodontal Disease

By Amid I. Ismail, Donald W. Lewis
and Jennifer L. Dingle

37

Prevention of Periodontal Disease

Prepared by Amid I. Ismail, BDS, MPH, DrPH[1], Donald W. Lewis, DDS, DDPH, MScD, FRCDC[2] and Jennifer L. Dingle, MBA[3]

In 1979 the Canadian Task Force on the Periodic Health Examination found there was insufficient evidence to recommend for or against examination for periodontal diseases and encouragement of daily oral hygiene. Since that time, significant advances have occurred in the understanding of the histopathology, epidemiology, natural history, and effectiveness of prevention and management of multimicrobial infection leading to plaque-associated gingivitis and periodontitis.

Burden of Suffering

Periodontal diseases are the most prevalent chronic diseases affecting children, adolescents, adults, and the elderly. The periodontium is a complex, highly specialized, shock-absorbing and pressure-sensing system consisting of four interrelated tissues supporting the teeth: cementum, periodontal ligament, alveolar bone and junctional and sulcular epithelia (Figure 1).

Gingivitis is a necessary but not a sufficient prerequisite for initiation of periodontitis

The most common type of periodontal disease is gingivitis and its most common form is chronic plaque-associated inflammation – a polymicrobial infection with no single associated bacterial agent. Gingivitis is a necessary but not sufficient prerequisite for initiation of periodontitis. Loss of alveolar bone results in formation of a pocket around the tooth which then acts as a reservoir favouring the growth of anerobic bacteria.

In the most recent survey of American children and adolescents 60% of those examined had at least one tooth site with gingival bleeding; on average, less than 6% of the tooth sites per child had bleeding. The prevalence of gingival bleeding increases significantly until age 34 years when it reaches a plateau; overall, prevalence is 47-55%.

Periodontal diseases affect most adults but only 3-13% experience advanced periodontitis, usually involving only a few teeth

Periodontitis is highly prevalent, affecting 53% of 18-19 year-old American adults and 98% of individuals over 60 years of age. The prevalence of advanced periodontitis (defined by presence of a pocket depth of at least 6 mm) was 7.6% and 34% in adult and elderly Americans, respectively, and 12% for elderly Ontarians. In most people, advanced periodontitis affects relatively few teeth. Only 3-13% of the population is susceptible to rapid and advanced loss of

[1] Associate Professor and Chair, Department of Pediatric and Community Dentistry, Dalhousie University, Halifax, Nova Scotia
[2] Professor of Community Dentistry, University of Toronto, Toronto, Ontario
[3] Coordinator of the Canadian Task Force on the Periodic Health Examination, Department of Pediatrics, Dalhousie University, Halifax, Nova Scotia

periodontal attachment, while about 80% of adults experience low or moderate progression.

Dental plaque is the bacterial mass that adheres to and builds up on a tooth surface. There is good evidence that supragingival (above gingival line) plaque causes gingivitis.[1] Epidemiological studies have found a weak correlation between plaque mass and attachment loss but the presence of *Actinobacillus actinomycetemcomitans, Prevtella (Bacteroides) intermedia* and *orphyromonas (Bacteroides) gingivalis* in plaque has been associated with attachment loss.

Calculus or calcified dental plaque acts as a retention web for bacteria. It is associated with loss of attachment in patients with poor oral hygiene status who have limited access to professional dental care but not in those with excellent oral hygiene status. There is no evidence to support any direct causal role for calculus in the initiation of gingivitis or periodontitis but calculus is an important contributor to the chronicity of both.

A consistent association between cigarette smoking and periodontitis has been confirmed in both cross-sectional and longitudinal studies.[2-5] Use of smokeless tobacco has been associated with localized loss of periodontal attachment and oral leukoplakia but not with severe periodontal destruction.[6,7] Other risk factors are non-insulin dependent diabetes and possibly malocclusion and defective host defenses.

In 1981, the estimated treatment time required to manage all individuals with gingivitis and periodontitis in the U.S., over a 4-year period, was 120 to 133 million treatment hours, at a cost of U.S. $5 to $6 billion annually.

Maneuver

Gingival bleeding is a valid sign of inflammation in the gingiva regardless of the presence or absence of visual signs (redness and inflammation). Periodontal pocket depth provides a cross-sectional indicator of periodontitis but does not indicate whether the disease is active or not.

Specific bacterial identification methods such as DNA probes have recently been developed to identify periodontopathogens and aid dental practitioners in predicting when periodontal disease activity is occurring and may provide a promising tool in the future. As yet, the presence or absence of a certain bacterial species or specific antibody response are not reliable predictors of future periodontal destruction.

Effectiveness of Prevention

Prevention of gingivitis and periodontitis is based primarily on plaque and calculus control around the teeth. There have been no studies on the effectiveness of physician counselling (screening or referral) to prevent gingivitis and periodontitis.

Toothbrushing and Flossing (Personal Oral Hygiene)

Toothbrushing and flossing are effective in preventing gingivitis; frequency of professional care should depend upon periodontal disease status

Gingivitis develops in healthy adults after 10 to 21 days in the absence of personal plaque removal,[1] providing strong evidence for recommending at least daily toothbrushing.

Cross-sectional epidemiological studies have shown a negative correlation between periodontal disease and the frequency of toothbrushing. Cohort studies have shown an association between good oral hygiene and low prevalence of periodontitis.[8,9] A clinical trial[10] confirmed that effective plaque removal every 48 hours was associated with gingival health. However, the external validity of this study is limited because the participants cleaned their teeth under supervision.[11,12] The daily routine of the procedure was reported by the participants to be "very boring".[11]

In a unique longitudinal study (without a control group),[13] 375 participants received scaling and root planing (described below) to remove calculus every 2-3 months during the first 9 years of the study, and twice annually during the following 6 years. The participants were instructed on maintaining oral hygiene practices at home. After 15 years, the participants had no clinically detectable loss of periodontal attachment level. However, the costs and commitment required in such an intensive program may make this approach impractical.

A recent two-week clinical trial with adults found that while twice daily toothbrushing alone produced a 35% reduction in gingival bleeding, toothbrushing and flossing at home resulted in a 67% reduction.[14] No differences were found between waxed and unwaxed floss. This study again cannot be generalized to unsupervised flossing at home because the participants were checked daily. A recent clinical trial involving third grade schoolchildren found that toothbrushing was as effective as combined toothbrushing and flossing.[15] Nevertheless, flossing should be part of an oral hygiene program for children because of the need to build the skill and establish flossing as a habit.

There is no scientific evidence to support the superiority of any of the techniques (or styles) of toothbrushing. Physicians and dentists should advise their patients concerning the damaging effects of some toothbrushing techniques (for example, horizontal scrubbing can result in abrasion or systemic bacteremia and too frequent brushing leads to gingival recession).

There is no consistent evidence to support the long-term superiority of electric toothbrushes over manual brushes.[16-19]

While electric toothbrushes may help some patients to increase the frequency of toothbrushing and are very helpful in maintaining good oral hygiene in patients who cannot manage a manual toothbrush properly, the additional benefits should be judged relative to the higher cost.

Professional Care

The most common form of professional preventive care for gingivitis and periodontitis is scaling and polishing of teeth in a dental office. During scaling, specially designed sharp dental instruments are used to remove calculus and bacteria located either above the gingiva (supragingival) or inside the gingival crevice or pocket (subgingival). An abrasive is then applied to remove stains and plaque and to smooth the scaled areas. Another mechanical preventive procedure is root planing. Calculus is removed from the root surface using scalers. Root planing is performed either with or without surgical exposure of the root by opening a gingival flap.

The studies of Axelsson et al[13,20,21] have been used to support the contention that regular professional care is necessary for maintenance of periodontal health. However, these studies lack external validity and the frequency and techniques used for scaling are different from those used regularly in North America. Adults have also been shown to benefit from receiving 11 professional prophylaxes during a 3-year period.[22] Again the frequency of intervention was intensive. This does not mean that the conventional frequency of dental prophylaxis is harmful or not recommended, but rather that the scientific evidence supporting its effectiveness is weak.

For periodontally healthy adults, annual scaling has been shown to be as effective as scaling carried out more frequently in maintaining gingival health.[23-26] No recent clinical trial has been carried out to test the optimal frequency and efficiency of scaling for periodontally healthy individuals with excellent home maintenance vis-a-vis those who cannot personally maintain their periodontal health. The recall interval should be individualized based upon patient oral hygiene status and severity of gingivitis and periodontitis.

Antimicrobial Agents

An oral rinse with chlorhexidine (0.12% or 0.2%), an anti-bacterial agent, has been found to be effective in reducing supragingival plaque and gingivitis.[27-29] Unsupervised use of chlorhexidine for 6 months was more effective than sanguinarine and Listerine® (Warner-Lambert Canada Inc., Scarborough, Ontario) rinses in the reduction of plaque and gingival bleeding.[27] Side effects associated with chlorhexidine use include increased calculus formation, bad taste, and staining of teeth.[29]

For high-risk patients other effective measures include: smoking cessation, chlorhexidine or Listerine® rinse, and anticalculus toothpaste

There are also short-term studies (6 to 9 months) which have documented the effectiveness of Listerine® in the prevention of gingivitis when compared to a placebo.<30,31> Side effects of Listerine® are poor taste and a burning sensation in the mouth.

There are no long-term studies documenting the effectiveness of unsupervised use of over-the-counter mouthrinses such as Plax® (Pfizer Canada Inc., Kirkland, Quebec), Scope® (Procter and Gamble, Toronto, Ontario) and Cepacol® (Merrell Dow Pharmaceutical Inc., Richmond Hill, Ontario) in preventing gingivitis.

The use of antibiotics (tetracyclines) in the prevention of gingivitis and periodontitis in the population at large has not been tested because of possible side effects, and the potential development of resistant bacterial strains and patient hypersensitivity.

Anti-Calculus Toothpastes

"Anti-tartar" toothpastes contain soluble pyrophosphates which prevent calcification of plaque. The percentage reduction in supragingival (but not subgingival) calculus is between 32%<32> and 45%.<33> Cases of cheilitis and mucosal erythema have been reported<34> and the long-term value of these products in preventing gingivitis and periodontitis has not been established.

Recommendations of Others

In 1989, the U.S Preventive Services Task Force<35> recommended that all patients be encouraged to visit a dental care provider on a regular basis and that primary care providers should counsel patients regarding daily tooth brushing and dental flossing. Clinicians were advised to be alert for obvious signs of oral disease while examining the mouth and to counsel all patients regarding the use of tobacco products. These recommendations are currently under review.

Conclusions and Recommendations

Absence of gingival bleeding is a highly specific indicator of the lack of periodontal disease activity. While the presence of gingivitis cannot be used to predict periodontitis, assessment of gingivitis in a periodic dental examination is recommended. The presence of periodontal pockets and loss of periodontal attachment should also be recorded for all teeth. However, evidence for optimal frequency of professional care in preventing development or progression of periodontitis is not available for the population at large. The frequency of professional scaling should be based upon the patient's periodontal disease status and stability of periodontal health over time. The current practice of advising regular biannual or annual scaling for all patients is costly and cannot be supported for periodontally healthy patients.

There is evidence to recommend personal toothbrushing (B Recommendation) and flossing (A Recommendation) to prevent gingivitis in adults. In children there is fair evidence to support toothbrushing only (B Recommendation); however, flossing is recommended to develop the necessary skills and establish a habit (C Recommendation). Toothbrushing and flossing may prevent periodontitis; however, brushing and flossing are strongly recommended to prevent gingival inflammation and reduce the level of supra-gingival bacteria. Supervised toothbrushing and flossing is recommended for patients with malocclusion, diabetes or HIV infection based on poor evidence (C Recommendation). There is also fair evidence to recommend professional scaling and plaque removal in periodontally healthy individuals (B Recommendation).

There is also good evidence to recommend the use of chlorhexidine oral rinse as an adjunct to self-care in the prevention of gingivitis (A Recommendation) in special patients (mentally handicapped, cancer, or those who cannot clean their teeth because of a physical disability). Listerine is less effective than chlorhexidine (B Recommendation). There are no long-term studies of the effectiveness of other antimicrobial rinses marketed for home use (D Recommendation as effective alternatives available).

Anticalculus dentifrices are recommended for people with high levels of calculus formation to reduce the accumulation of supra-gingival calculus (B Recommendation) but for the general population the benefits are unclear (C Recommendation). Antibiotics are not recommended for the prevention of gingivitis or periodontitis (E Recommendation). There is fair evidence to recommend smoking cessation to reduce the risk of developing periodontitis (B Recommendation) (and good evidence overall, see Chapter 43 on Prevention on Tobacco-Caused Disease).

Physicians should ask patients during a periodic health examination whether they experience bleeding gingiva especially during chewing of foods or toothbrushing (C Recommendation). They should refer those patients who are diagnosed with any systemic condition (for example, diabetes or HIV infection) which may lead to a reduction of immune response or an increase of collagen tissue breakdown. Patients scheduled to receive chemotherapy or radiation therapy should also be seen by a dentist or periodontist.

Unanswered Questions (Research Agenda)

The identification of those at high risk for rapid progression of periodontitis is a major challenge for future research as is defining risk profiles for periodontal disease.

Evidence

A literature search was conducted for the period starting from 1980 to 1993 using MEDLINE with the keywords: periodontal diseases. Selected studies published prior to 1980 were also reviewed if there were no recent updates. This review was initiated in June, 1991 and recommendations were finalized by the Task Force in November, 1992. A report with a full reference list was published in 1993.<36>

Acknowledgements

Funding was provided by the Faculty of Dentistry, Dalhousie University, and the Faculty of Dentistry, University of Toronto.

Selected References

1. Loe H, Theilade E, Jensen SB: Experimental gingivitis in man. *J Periodontol* 1965; 36: 177-187

2. Bergstrom J, Eliasson S: Noxious effects of cigarette smoking on periodontal health. *J Periodont Res* 1987; 22: 513-517

3. Bergstrom J, Eliasson S: Cigarette smoking and alveolar bone height in subjects with a high standard of oral hygiene. *J Clin Periodontol* 1987; 14: 466-469

4. Rivera-Hidalgo F: Smoking and periodontal disease. A review of the literature. *J Periodontol* 1986; 57: 617-624

5. Ismail AI, Burt BA, Eklund SA: Epidemiologic patterns of smoking and periodontal disease in the United States. *J Am Dent Assoc* 1983; 106: 617-621

6. Ernster VL, Grady DG, Greene JC, *et al*: Smokeless tobacco use and health effects among baseball players. *JAMA* 1990; 264: 218-224

7. Robertson PB, Walsh M, Greene J, *et al*: Periodontal effects associated with the use of smokeless tobacco. *J Periodontol* 1990; 61: 438-443

8. Loe H, Anerud A, Boysen H, *et al*: The natural history of periodontal disease in man. The rate of periodontal destruction before 40 years of age. *J Periodontol* 1978; 49: 607-620

9. Loe H, Anerud A, Boysen H, *et al*: Natural history of periodontal disease in man. Rapid, moderate, and no loss of attachment in Sri Lankan laborers 14 to 46 years of age. *J Clin Periodontol* 1986; 13: 431-445

10. Lang NP, Cumming BR, Loe H: Toothbrushing frequency as it relates to plaque development and gingival health. *J Periodontal* 1973; 44: 396-405

11. Suomi JD, Peterson JK, Matthews BL, *et al*: Effects of supervised daily plaque removal by children after 3 years. *Comm Dent Oral Epidemiol* 1980; 8: 171-176

12. Lindhe J, Koch G: The effect of supervised oral hygiene on the gingivae of children. *J Periodontol Res* 1967; 2: 215-220

13. Axelsson P, Lindhe J, Nystrom B: On the prevention of caries and periodontal disease. Results of a 15-year longitudinal study in adults. *J Clin Periodontol* 1991; 18: 182-189

14. Graves RC, Disney JA, Stamm JW: Comparative effectiveness of flossing and brushing in reducing interproximal bleeding. *J Periodontol* 1989; 60: 243-247

15. Rich SK, Friedman JA, Schultz LA: Effects of flossing on plaque and gingivitis in third grade schoolchildren. *J Public Health Dent* 1989; 49: 73-77

16. Wilcoxon DB, Ackerman RJ Jr, Killoy WJ, *et al*: The effectiveness of a counterrotational-action power toothbrush on plaque control in orthodontic patients. *Am J Orthod Dentfacial Orthop* 1991; 99: 7-14

17. Walsh M, Heckman B, Leggott P, *et al*: Comparison of manual and power toothbrushing, with and without adjunctive oral irrigation, for controlling plaque and gingivitis. *J Clin Periodontol* 1989; 16: 419-427

18. Baab DA, Johnson RH: The effect of a new electric toothbrush on supragingival plaque and gingivitis. *J Periodontol* 1989; 60: 336-341

19. Glavind L, Zeuner E: The effectiveness of a rotary electric toothbrush on oral cleanliness in adults. *J Clin Periodontol* 1986; 13: 135-138

20. Axelsson P, Lindhe J: Effect of controlled oral hygiene procedures on caries and periodontal disease in adults. *J Clin Periodontol* 1978; 5: 133-151

21. Axelsson P, Lindhe J: Effect of controlled oral hygiene procedures on caries and periodontal disease in adults. Results after 6 years. *J Clin Periodontol* 1981; 8: 239-248

22. Suomi JD, Smith LW, Chang JJ, *et al*: Study of the effect of different prophylaxis frequencies on the periodontium of young adult males. *J Periodontol* 1973; 44: 406-410

23. Lightner LM, O'Leary JT, Drake RB, *et al*: Preventive periodontic treatment procedures: results over 46 months. *J Periodontol* 1971; 42: 555-561

24. Listgarten MA, Schifter CC, Laster L: 3-year longitudinal study of the periodontal status of an adult population with gingivitis. *J Clin Periodontol* 1985; 12: 225-238

25. McFall WT Jr: Supportive treatment. In: Nevins M, Becker W, Kornman K (eds): *Proceedings of the World Workshop in Clinical Periodontics*, American Academy of Periodontology, Princeton, NJ, 1989: IX-14

26. Suomi JD, Greene JC, Vermillion JR, *et al*: The effect of controlled oral hygiene procedures on the progression of periodontal disease in adults: results after third and final year. *J Periodontol* 1971; 42: 152-160

27. Grossman E, Meckel AH, Isaacs RL, *et al*: A clinical comparison of antibacterial mouthrinses: effects of chlorhexidine, phenolics, and sanguinarine on dental plaque and gingivitis. *J Periodontol* 1989; 60: 435-440

28. Banting D, Bosma M, Bollmer B: Clinical effectiveness of a 0.12% chlorhexidine mouthrinse over two years. *J Dent Res* 1989; 68 (Suppl): 1716-1718

29. Jolkovsky DL, Waki MY, Newman MG, *et al*: Clinical and microbiological effects of subgingival and gingival marginal irrigation with chlorhexidine gluconate. *J Periodontol* 1990; 61: 663-669

30. Gordon JM, Lamster IB, Seiger MC: Efficacy of Listerine antiseptic in inhibiting the development of plaque and gingivitis. *J Clin Periodontol* 1985; 12: 697-704

31. DePaola LG, Overholser CD, Meiller TF, *et al*: Chemotherapeutic inhibition of supragingival dental plaque and gingivitis development. *J Clin Periodontol* 1989; 16: 311-315

32. Lobene RR: A study to compare the effects of two dentifrices on adult dental calculus formation. *J Clin Dent* 1989; 1: 67-69

33. Rugg-Gunn AJ: A double-blind clinical trial of an anticalculus toothpaste containing pyrophosphate and sodium monofluorophosphate. *Br Dent J* 1988; 165: 133-136

34. Beacham BE, Kurgansky D, Gould WM: Circumoral dermatitis and cheilitis caused by tartar control dentifrices. *J Am Acad Dermatol* 1990; 22: 1029-1032

35. U.S. Preventive Services Task Force: *Guide to Clinical Preventive Services: an Assessment of the Effectiveness of 169 Interventions*. Williams & Wilkins, Baltimore, Md, 1989: 351-356

36. Ismail AI, Lewis DW with the Canadian Task Force on the Periodic Health Examination: The periodic health examination, 1993 update: 3. Periodontal disease: classification, diagnosis, risk factors and prevention. *Can Med Assoc J* 1993; 149: 1409-1422

Figure 1: A schematic longitudinal section through dento-gingival part of a healthy tooth and its periodontium

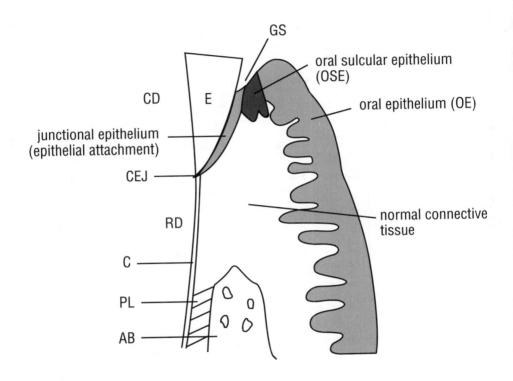

Caption:

E: enamel	CD: coronal dentin
RD: root dentin	PL: periodontal ligament
AB: alveolar bone	C: cementum
CEJ: cemento-enamel junction	GS: gingival sulcus

Source: Reprinted from Gillet IR, et al. J Clin Periodontology, 1990 with permission from © Munksgaard International Publishers Limited, Copenhagen, Denmark, April 14, 1992.

Prevention of Periodontal Disease

MANEUVER	EFFECTIVENESS	LEVEL OF EVIDENCE <REF>	RECOMMENDATION
Toothbrushing and flossing	Toothbrushing is effective in preventing gingivitis. Patients who are not motivated or dextrous may not comply.	Randomized controlled trial<10> (I); descriptive study<1> (III)	Fair evidence to recommend toothbrushing for prevention of gingivitis (B)
	Flossing is ineffective in preventing gingivitis in children.	Randomized controlled trials<11,12,15> (I)	Flossing is recommended to develop the skill and establish a habit but poor evidence to include or exclude (C)
	Flossing is effective in preventing gingivitis in adults.	Randomized controlled trial<14> (I)	Good evidence to recommend flossing in adults (A)
	Brushing and flossing may prevent periodontitis. **High risk groups:** There is no evidence that brushing or flossing is effective.	Cohort studies<8,9> (II-2)	Supervised toothbrushing and flossing is recommended for patients with malocclusion, diabetes or HIV infection based on poor evidence (C)
Use of electrically powered toothbrush	Electric toothbrushes are not superior to manual toothbrushes; the benefit to those with limited dexterity or motivation must be weighed against cost.	Randomized controlled trials<16-19> (I)	Fair evidence not to recommend (D) for general population but recommended for patients with limited dexterity based on poor evidence.
Professional scaling and prophylaxis	**In periodontally healthy patients:** Intensive professional oral hygiene and prophylaxis prevents chronic gingivitis and periodontitis. Annual scaling provides no additional benefit for those who maintain good oral hygiene.	Randomized controlled trials<13,20-26> (I)	Fair evidence to recommend professional scaling and prophylaxis depending on the periodontal disease status of the patient (B)

(Continued on next page)

Prevention of Periodontal Disease (concl'd)

MANEUVER	EFFECTIVENESS	LEVEL OF EVIDENCE <REF>	RECOMMENDATION
Use of chlorhexidine oral rinse as adjunct to toothcleaning	Effective in preventing gingivitis and as an antimicrobial. Reduces supragingival plaque but increases calculus formation. Rinse has bad taste and stains teeth.	Randomized controlled trials<27-29> (I)	Good evidence to recommend twice daily use of 0.12% chlorhexidine rinse (A) for those with difficulty cleaning teeth (e.g patients with disability, cancer)
Use of listerine® oral rinse	Less effective than chlorhexidine but effective in preventing gingivitis with over 6 months of use. Poor taste and burning sensation in mouth.	Randomized controlled trials<30,31> (I)	Fair evidence to recommend use by patients with severe gingivitis (B)
Use of other over-the-counter oral rinses	No long-term studies of effectiveness and alternatives available.		Fair evidence not to use (D)
Toothbrushing with anticalculus dentifrice	Effectiveness in preventing gingivitis not documented. Effectiveness in reducing supragingival calculus; no long-term evaluation.	Randomized controlled trials<32-34> (I)	No evidence to recommend for general population (C); fair evidence to recommend for patients at risk of calculus formation (B)
Antibiotic prophylaxis	No evidence of effectiveness in preventing gingivitis or periodontitis in the general population.		Good evidence not to recommend antibiotics for preventive use because of side effects (E)
Smoking cessation	Eliminates increased risk of periodontal disease due to smoking.	Cross-sectional and cohort studies<2-7> (II-2)	Fair evidence to recommend smoking cessation to prevent periodontal disease (B)
Screening for periodontal disease by physicians (reports of gingival bleeding during toothbrushing)	Not evaluated.		Insufficient evidence to evaluate but recommended in areas with no dental services (C)

Disorders of the Genitourinary Tract

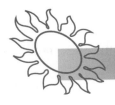

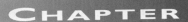

Dipstick Proteinuria Screening of Asymptomatic Adults to Prevent Progressive Renal Disease

By Ryuta Nagai, Elaine E. L. Wang and William Feldman

38

Dipstick Proteinuria Screening of Asymptomatic Adults to Prevent Progressive Renal Disease

Prepared by Ryuta Nagai MD, FRCPC[1], Elaine E. L. Wang MD, FRCPC[2] and William Feldman MD, FRCPC[3]

Dipstick urinalysis is a simple, noninvasive test for the detection of proteinuria, often a marker of unsuspected chronic renal disease. (Other analyses available on multiple dipstick urine tests are not considered in this review.) There is a strong correlation between urinary protein excretion and progression of renal failure. Ironically, patients with chronic renal failure and persistent proteinuria may remain minimally symptomatic until renal function is severely impaired, with the eventual need for endstage renal disease (ESRD) management (dialysis or transplantation). ESRD programs have a significant socioeconomic impact on our health care system. Unfortunately, effective, nontoxic therapy to arrest or slow disease progression is not available for most renal disorders, the exception being insulin dependent diabetes mellitus (IDDM) patients with proteinuria. Detection of microalbuminuria may be useful in patients with IDDM but this technique is not readily available in most primary care settings.

Although the cost of screening the general adult population would be equivalent to the cost of caring for 15 hemodialysis patients for one year, effective nontoxic therapy is not available for most renal diseases detected by dipstick urine testing. Thus, screening is not advocated except in those patients with IDDM.

Burden of Suffering

Over 13,000 patients are on ESRD programs (dialysis and transplantation) in Canada. An additional 2,000 patients enter dialysis programs every year, an annual increase of 7%.

The cost of health care incurred through dialysis and transplantation is enormous. The average cost of peritoneal or

---

[1] At time of writing, Research Associate, Department of Preventive Medicine and Biostatistics, University of Toronto, Toronto, Ontario

[2] Associate Professor of Pediatrics and of Preventive Medicine and Biostatistics, University of Toronto, Toronto, Ontario

[3] Professor of Pediatrics and of Preventive Medicine and Biostatistics, University of Toronto, Toronto, Ontario

hemodialysis is $50-58,000 per patient year with lower figures for long-term successful renal allografts. By comparison, the cost of a urine dipstick analysis is approximately 30 cents per test which translates to $7 million if all adults were to be screened in Canada. These fiscal calculations, however, do not take into consideration the diminished quality of life associated with long-term dialysis.

Maneuver

Most commercial dipstick urine tests for protein use a pH-dependent tetrabromphenol-blue indicator system. Sensitivity and specificity for proteinuria is between 95 and 99%, the latter reported in the laboratory setting.

Urine dipstick for protein is a noninvasive screening test with high sensitivity and specificity

False positives may occur in the presence of gross blood, very alkaline or decomposed urine. False negatives can occur with very dilute, acidic urine or with non-albumin proteinuria (e.g. tubular or light chain proteinuria). False negatives will mislabel patients as being normal with consequent failure to detect the renal disease and loss of the opportunity to treat comorbid disease that may accelerate progression to ESRD.

Eleven studies of both general and specialised adult populations were reviewed.<1-11> In all of these studies, not all patients who were found to have persistent proteinuria underwent the gold standard test (usually a renal biopsy). Thus, the positive predictive values (0-68%) likely represent an underestimate of the true prevalence of renal disease.

All patients who had persistent non-orthostatic proteinuria were designated as having "possibly significant renal disease" for the purpose of this review in order to give an overestimate of those with underlying renal disease at risk for developing ESRD. This gave an overall positive predictive value of 30% with a range of 6 to 70% depending upon the population under study.

A suggested algorithmic workup for those found to have dipstick positive proteinuria ($\geq$0.3 g/L) is presented in Figure 1. It should be noted that proteinuria itself may not actually represent a primary renal disorder. Proteinuria can be detected in patients with underlying cardiovascular diseases (e.g. chronic congestive heart failure) in the absence of an underlying primary renal disorder. Proteinuria in these clinical settings is likely not benign – a re-analysis of data from the Framingham study has demonstrated that dipstick positive proteinuria was associated with a higher mortality risk from cardiovascular disease. Although urine dipstick screening in the general adult population could provide another window of opportunity to screen for and modify cardiovascular risk factors in the general population, no study has yet addressed this issue.

Effectiveness of Prevention and Treatment

Specific therapy is not available for most diseases associated with chronic progressive renal disease

Those who are found to have significant disease are offered interventions to either arrest (in some cases, reverse) the disease process (designated forthwith as "specific" renal therapy) or slow the progression of the disease to ESRD ("nonspecific" renal therapy). Most studies to date have focused on nonspecific therapy to retard progression to ESRD. The paucity of specific therapy is largely due to the lack of understanding of the mechanisms for the initiation and progression of most renal diseases.

Specific therapy may be efficacious in the following disorders which can present with proteinuria (listed with their relative percentage contribution to ESRD in Canada): renovascular disease (6%); vasculitis and other treatable forms of glomerulonephritis (18%); tubulointerstitial disorders, including reflux nephropathy (8%); specific long-term infections of the urinary tract (tuberculosis, schistosomiasis) (<1%); and urinary tract tumors (<1%). Controlled clinical trials demonstrating the efficacy of treatment have been reported only for reflux nephropathy,[12] chronic urinary tract infections[13] and some forms of chronic glomerulopathies.[14,15] Consultation with a nephrologist or urologist is advised in specific cases as therapeutic measures vary depending upon disease severity and the presence of comorbid conditions.

Urine dipstick is indicated in IDDM patients as efficacious therapy is available for those found to have proteinuria

Diabetes accounts for approximately one quarter of the ESRD population in Canada. Specific therapy is not available to reverse established diabetic renal disease associated with persistent proteinuria. Antihypertensive agents, most notably angiotensin-converting enzyme inhibitors, have been shown to slow the progression to ESRD in patients with IDDM associated with proteinuria.[16-19] The recent Collaborative Study Group trial demonstrated that patient and renal mortality were significantly lower in those treated with captopril as compared to placebo over a 3.5 year follow-up period.[16] It should be noted that proteinuria can be detected earlier in the disease course (microalbuminuric stage) by more sensitive methods of protein excretion.[20] Early studies have shown benefit to treating IDDM patients at this stage with angiotensin-converting enzyme inhibitors.[21,22] Lack of wide availability of the detection method for microalbuminuria and lack of large long-term studies showing benefit of treatment makes this technique impractical for screening purposes.

A recent case-control study has suggested a benefit to the use of angiotensin-converting enzyme inhibitors in non-insulin dependant diabetes mellitus (NIDDM).[23] This has yet to be shown in a prospective blinded, controlled trial.

Small prospective trials have also shown a benefit of angiotensin-converting enzyme inhibitors in retarding progression to ESRD in various proteinuric disorders of non-diabetic etiology.[24,25] These studies have used surrogate outcome measures (rate of decline in kidney function). Moderate increases in serum potassium have been noted in some patients treated with the use of these agents.[24] They cannot be widely recommended for treatment at this time.

Systemic hypertension is prevalent among patients with chronic renal failure and has been suggested to accelerate the rate of progression to ESRD. Although several uncontrolled trials[26-28] suggest a benefit to blood pressure control in patients with mild to moderate hypertension associated with chronic renal failure, this has not been definitively demonstrated in a prospective controlled trial.[29] Data from large hypertension trials[30-38] looking at cardiovascular mortality as the primary outcome of interest, have suggested either no benefit or worse outcome for renal mortality in those with better blood pressure control. ESRD however, was not the outcome of interest. Although accelerated or malignant hypertension associated with renal failure has been shown to benefit from aggressive blood pressure control, this comprises a very small proportion of the hypertensive population in North America.[39]

Present nonspecific treatment in all forms of renal diseases to prevent progression to ESRD focuses on dietary protein restriction. There is good evidence to suggest that moderate protein restriction retards the rate of progression to ESRD[40] but its safety and long-term compliance have not been demonstrated (this question is the subject of the recently completed Modification of Diet in Renal Disease trial). Most trials have studied patients with moderate to advanced renal failure (glomerular filtration rate of 15-50 cc/minute) but a trend toward benefit has been observed in studies that included patients with mild renal failure.[41]

Recommendations of Others

A recommendation not to screen the general population is in keeping with previous Task Force recommendations, as well as those of Frame and Carlson[42] and the U.S. Preventive Services Task Force.[43]

Conclusions and Recommendations

A successful screening program is predicated on the principle that efficacious, nonharmful treatment is available early in the disease course. We thus do not recommend dipstick screening for proteinuria in the general adult population for the prevention of endstage renal disease (D Recommendation). Exceptions to this recommendation are IDDM patients as good recent evidence shows a benefit of therapy in early asymptomatic disease associated with proteinuria. (A Recommendation)

Unanswered Questions (Research Agenda)

Large clinical trials are needed to investigate the safety and effectiveness of angiotensin-converting enzyme inhibitors and other antihypertensive agents in non-diabetic progressive renal disease. Further basic science research is needed to elucidate mechanisms of initiation and progression of renal disease in order for new therapies to be developed.

Evidence

The literature was identified with a MEDLINE search for the years 1966 to December, 1992 using the following key words: evaluation studies, proteinuria, population studies, prospective studies, screening, protein restriction, hypertension, kidney disease, antihypertensive agents, diabetes mellitus and diabetic nephropathy.

This review was initiated in January, 1993 and the recommendations finalized by the Task Force in June, 1993. A draft technical report (1993) with a full reference list is available upon request.

Acknowledgements

Assistance was provided by Drs. David Churchill, FACP, ABIM (Nephrol), FRCPC, Professor, McMaster University, Hamilton, Ontario; and Stanley SA Fenton, MD, MB, BCh, BAO, FRCP(Ire), Associate Professor of Medicine, University of Toronto, Toronto, Ontario, in providing cost analyses of dialysis in Canada. The authors thank Lorraine Rosendall for the preparation of the manuscript and Patrick S. Parfrey, MD, FRCPC, FACP, Professor of Medicine, Memorial University of Newfoundland, St. John's, Newfoundland for reviewing the draft report.

Selected References

1. von Bonsdorff M, Koskenvuo K, Salmi HA: Prevalence and causes of proteinuria in 20-year-old Finnish men. *Scand J Urol Nephrol* 1981; 15: 285-290

2. Alwall N, Lohi A: A population study on renal and urinary tract diseases. *Acta Med Scand* 1973; 194: 541-547

3. Chen BT, Ooi B-S, Tan K-K, *et al*: Comparative studies of asymptomatic proteinuria and hematuria. *Arch Intern Med* 1974; 134: 901-905

4. Levitt JI: The prognostic significance of proteinuria in young college students. *Ann Intern Med* 1967; 66(4): 685-696

5. Haug K, Bakke A, Daae LN, *et al*: Screening for hematuria, glucosuria and proteinuria in people aged 55-64. *Scand J Prim Health Care* 1985; 3: 31-34

6. Muth RG: Asymptomatic mild intermittent proteinuria. *Arch Intern Med* 1965; 115: 569-574

7. Phillippi PJ, Reynolds J, Yamauchi H, *et al*: Persistent proteinuria in asymptomatic individuals: renal biopsy studies on 50 patients. *Mil Med* 1966; 131: 1311-1317

8. Turnbull JM, Buck C: The value of perioperative screening investigations in otherwise healthy individuals. *Arch Intern Med* 1987; 147: 1101-1105

9. Johnson H Jr, Knee-Ioli S, Butler TA, *et al*: Are routine perioperative laboratory screening tests necessary to evaluate ambulatory surgical patients? *Surgery* 1988; 104(4): 639-645

10. Akin BV, Hubbell FA, Frye EB, *et al*: Efficacy of the routine admission urinalysis. *Am J Med* 1987; 82: 719-722

11. Del Mar C, Badger P: The place of routine urine testing on admission to hospital. *Med J Aust* 1989; 151: 151-153

12. Weiss R, Duckett J, Spitzer A: Results of a randomized control trial of medical versus surgical management of infants and children with grades III and IV primary vesicoureteral reflux. *J Urol* 1992; 148 (5 Pt 2): 1667-1673

13. King CH, Mahmoud AA: Drugs five years later: praziquantel. *Ann Intern Med* 1989; 110(4): 290-296

14. Brodehl J: The treatment of minimal change nephrotic syndrome: lessons learned from multicentre co-operative studies. *Eur J Pediatr* 1991; 150(6): 380-387

15. Cameron JS: Membranous nephropathy and its treatment. *Nephrol Dial Transplant* 1992; 7: 72-79

16. Lewis EJ, Hunsicker LG, Bain RP, *et al*: The effect of angiotensin converting enzyme inhibition on diabetic nephropathy. *N Engl J Med* 1993; 329(20): 1456-1462

17. Bjorck S, Mulec H, Johnson SA, *et al*: Renal protective effect of enalapril in diabetic nephropathy. *BMJ* 1992; 304: 339-343

18. Parving H-H, Hommel E, Schmidt UM: Protection of kidney function and decrease in albuminuria by captopril in insulin dependent diabetics with nephropathy. *BMJ* 1988; 297: 1086-1091

19. Hommel E, Parving H-H, Mathiesen E, *et al*: Effect of captopril on kidney function in insulin dependent diabetic patients with nephropathy. *Br Med J Clin Res Ed* 1986; 293: 467-470

20. Tuttle KR, Stein JH, DeFronzo RA: The natural history of diabetic nephropathy. *Semin Nephrol* 1990; 10(3): 184-193

21. Marre M, Chatellier G, Leblanc H, *et al*: Prevention of diabetic nephropathy with enalapril in normotensive diabetics with microalbuminuria. *Br Med J* 1989; 299: 230-33

22. Mogensen CE: Prevention and treatment of renal disease in insulin-dependent diabetes mellitus. *Semin Nephrol* 1990; 10: 260-273

23. Gurwitz JH, Bohn RL, Glynn RJ, *et al*: Antihypertensive drug therapy and the initiation of treatment for diabetes mellitus. *Ann Intern Med* 1993; 118: 273-278

24. Apperloo AJ, de Zeeuw D, Sluiter HE, *et al*: Differential effects of enalapril and atenolol on proteinuria and renal haemodynamics in non-diabetic renal disease. *BMJ* 1991; 303(6806): 821-824

25. Rodicio JL, Praga M, Alcazar JM, *et al*: Effects of angiotensin converting enzyme inhibitors on the progression of renal failure and proteinuria in humans. *J Hypertens Suppl* 1989; 7(7): S43-S47

26. Brazy PC, Stead WW, Fitzwilliam JF: Progression of renal insufficiency: role of blood pressure. *Kidney Int* 1989; 35: 670-674

27. Rostand SG, Brown G, Kirk KA, *et al*: Renal insufficiency in treated essential hypertension. *N Engl J Med* 1989; 320: 684-688

28. Hartford M, Wendelhag I, Berglund G, *et al*: Cardiovascular and renal effects of long-term antihypertensive treatment. *JAMA* 1988; 259(17): 2553-2557

29. Weisstuch JM, Dworkin LD: Does essential hypertension cause end-stage renal disease? *Kidney Int Suppl* 1992; 36: S33-S37

30. Wolff FW, Lindeman RD: Effects of treatment in hypertension: Results of a controlled study. *J Chronic Dis* 1966; 19: 227-240

31. Veterans Administration Cooperative Study Group on Antihypertensive Agents: Effects of treatment on morbidity in hypertension. Results in patients with diastolic blood pressures averaging 115 through 129 mmHg. *JAMA* 1967; 202: 1028-1034

32. Veterans Administration Cooperative Study Group on Antihypertensive Agents: Effects of treatment on morbidity in hypertension II: Results in patients with diastolic blood pressure averaging 90 through 114 mmHg. *JAMA* 1970; 213: 1143-1155

33. United States Public Health Service Hospitals Cooperative Study Group: Treatment of mild hypertension: results of a ten-year intervention trial. *Circ Res* 1977; 40 (5 Suppl I): I98-I105

34. Report by the Management Committee: The Australian therapeutic trial in mild hypertension. *Lancet* 1980; 1: 1261-1267

35. Amery A, Birkenhager W, Brixko P, *et al*: Mortality and morbidity results from the European Working Party on High Blood Pressure in the Elderly Trial. *Lancet* 1985; 1: 1349-1354

36. Shulman NB, Ford CE, Hall WD, *et al*: Prognostic value of serum creatinine and effect of treatment of hypertension on renal function. *Hypertension* 1989; 13: I80-I93

37. Pettinger WA, Lee HC, Reisch J, *et al*: Long-term improvement in renal function after short-term strict blood pressure control in hypertensive nephrosclerosis. *Hypertension* 1989; 13: 766-772

38. Whelton PK, Klug MJ: Hypertension as a risk factor for renal disease. Review of clinical and epidemiological evidence. *Hypertension* 1989; 13: l19-l27

39. Whelton PK: Declining mortality from hypertension and stroke. *South Med J* 1982; 75(1): 33-38

40. Fouque D, Laville M, Boissel JP, *et al*: Controlled low protein diets in chronic renal insufficiency: meta-analysis. *BMJ* 1992; 304: 216-220

41. The Modification of Diet in Renal Disease Study Group: The modification of diet in renal disease study: design, methods and results from the feasibility study. *Am J Kidney Dis* 1992; 20(1): 18-33

42. Frame PS, Carlson SJ: A critical review of periodic health screening using scientific screening criteria. Part 3: Selected diseases of the genitourinary system. *J Fam Pract* 1975; 24: 189-194

43. U.S. Preventive Services Task Force: *Guide to Clinical Preventive Services: an Assessment of the Effectiveness of 169 Interventions*. Williams & Wilkins, Baltimore, Md, 1989: 155-161

Figure 1: Algorithm for dipstick positive proteinuria

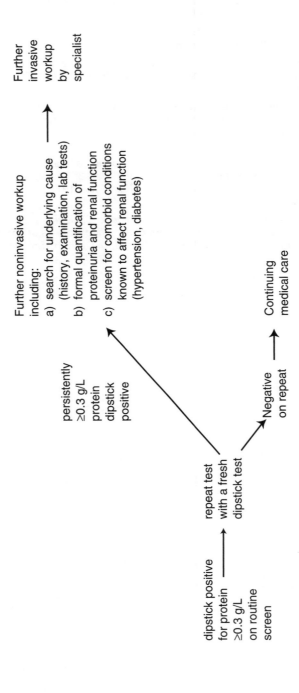

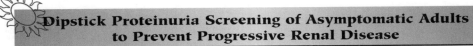

Dipstick Proteinuria Screening of Asymptomatic Adults to Prevent Progressive Renal Disease

MANEUVER	EFFECTIVENESS	LEVEL OF EVIDENCE <REF>	RECOMMENDATION
Urine dipstick for protein	Efficacious treatment not available in majority of patients with dipstick positive proteinuria.	Randomized controlled trials,<29-38,40,41> (I); cohort and case-control studies<27,28> (II-2)	Fair evidence to exclude dipstick screening for protein from the periodic health examination (PHE) of asymptomatic adults (D)
Urine dipstick for protein in adults with insulin dependent diabetes mellitus (IDDM)	Angiotensin converting enzyme inhibitors delay the onset of end-stage renal disease; test sensitivity and specificity over 95%.	Randomized controlled trial<16> (I)	Good evidence to include dipstick screening for protein in the PHE of adults with IDDM (A)

Prevention of Psychosocial Illness and Diseases of Lifestyle

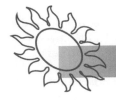

CHAPTER 39

Early
Detection
of
Depression

By John W. Feightner

Early Detection of Depression

Prepared by John W. Feightner, MD, MSc, FCFP[1]

Depression is a common problem that carries a high burden of suffering, which can include death from suicide. Effective treatment is available. However, in 1990 as in 1979 the Task Force recommended that routine screening for depression in asymptomatic individuals be excluded from periodic health assessments based on fair evidence that such screening by questionnaire did not improve detection rate or management.[1,2] However, physicians should be sensitive to the possibility of depression in their patients, particularly those at higher risk.

Burden of Suffering

Depressed individuals frequently present with physical symptoms, making diagnosis more difficult, particularly in the early stages of mild cases

Depression is frequently encountered in family practice and in ambulatory care settings. The lifetime prevalence of clinically significant depression is 15% to 30%; it is about twice as common among women as among men. The prevalence in the general population ranges between 3.5% and 27% depending on the definition used and the population studied; however, it is thought to have increased among children and adolescents. People who are single, divorced, separated, seriously ill, recently bereaved or those with a family history of depression have a greater incidence than others. Depressed individuals frequently present with physical symptoms, which may make diagnosis more difficult, particularly in the early stages and in mild cases. Important episodes of depression have been overlooked, so that instead of recognizing and treating the problem diagnostic testing or treatment for other illnesses is performed. Depression has a significant effect on the patient's quality of life and productivity, but psychiatric referral also has some negative implications regarding societal attitudes.

Spontaneous remission can occur over 6 to 12 months in up to 50% of affected people; however, about 50% of those who suffer from major depression become chronically depressed. Affected people are more likely than others to be suicidal: 30% to 70% of people who have committed suicide were previously identified as having major depression. In Canada, in 1986, suicide accounted for an estimated 97,600 potential years of life lost among men and another 25,300 years among women.

---

[1] Professor of Family Medicine, McMaster University, Hamilton, Ontario

Maneuver

The gold standard for diagnosing depression is careful application of standardized clinical criteria. In the primary care setting the problem must be recognized first and then properly evaluated. Several short (12-38 item), self-administered questionnaires have been proposed to assist with early recognition. When evaluated, these questionnaires have been generally sensitive to changes in clinical status but correlation with other tests or with clinical assessment has ranged from 0.40 to 0.89, with sensitivity 64-91% and specificity 56-82%. Hence, for many instruments, validity has not been fully established.

For many instruments, validity has not been fully established

Effectiveness of Early Detection and Treatment

Once identified, depression can be treated effectively with medication and psychotherapy; however, there is no conclusive evidence that treatment in the early stages of depression has greater long-term effects than intervention started later in the course of the illness.

Four randomized controlled trials have evaluated whether routine use of a screening questionnaire provided any benefit in terms of detection and management of depression. Shapiro and associates asked 1,242 patients attending an inner-city primary care teaching facility to complete the General Health Questionnaire (GHQ) before seeing a physician.[3] The provision of the GHQ information to the physician had no statistically significant effect on the detection of psychologic problems except among patients over 65 years of age. There was no ultimate effect on patient management, even in the group over 65 years of age.

Hoeper and collaborators found that physicians' knowledge of a "positive" GHQ result had no effect on the detection of psychologic distress among 1,469 patients in a Wisconsin primary care office.[4]

Using somewhat weaker methods in terms of identification of case and control subjects and choice of outcome measures, Johnstone and Goldberg used the GHQ to assess 1,093 patients.[5] New episodes of psychiatric illness were diagnosed and treated in 16% of the patients without data from the GHQ; an additional 11% were identified for treatment after the GHQ results were reviewed.

Zung and colleagues found that physicians informed of positive scores of the Zung Self-Rating Depression Scale detected depression in more patients (68% of 102) than when they were not informed of the results (15% of 41).[6] However, there were significant flaws in the design and execution of this study, particularly in terms of losses to follow-up.

In a well designed, randomized controlled trial, Magruder-Habib and coworkers used the Zung Self-Rating Depression Scale and a DSM-III screen to evaluate depression status in a group of subjects over age 45 attending a U.S. Veterans' Administration general medical clinic over a 12 month period.<7> Providing physicians with scores for patients whose depression was unrecognized in the clinical setting had an important impact on eventual recognition and management. However, in order to reduce the number of false positives, only patients scoring positive on both self-rating scale and a research assistant administered DSM-III checklist were identified to the attending physician. Hence, while the self-assessment instrument may be feasible in a primary care setting, the study does not evaluate the effectiveness or the impact of this instrument alone on the recognition and management of depression. The study did, however, provide valuable insight into the impact of informing physicians about unrecognized depression, and in conjunction with the Shapiro study indicates that further studies would be of value.

Recommendations of Others

The U.S. Preventive Services Task Force does not recommend routine screening but encourages physicians to have a high level of clinical suspicion.<8>

Conclusions and Recommendations

While routine screening isn't effective, physicians should be sensitive to the possibility of depression in their patients

Overall, these five trials fail to provide adequate evidence to support the use of routine screening tests for the early detection of depression. In fact, the current evidence supports not routinely using screening instruments but rather to maintain a high level of clinical sensitivity.

Unanswered Questions (Research Agenda)

The following have been identified as research priorities:

1. Conducting research into improved methods of identifying people at high risk for depression and developing a simple diagnostic test for use in this group by primary caregivers.

2. Evaluating the impact of questionnaires in the early detection of depression and subsequent management of patients over 65 years of age.

Evidence

The literature was identified with a MEDLINE search up to May 1993 using the following MESH headings: depression, mass screening.

This review was initiated in November 1992 and updates a report published in May 1990.<1> Recommendations were finalized in January 1994.

Acknowledgements

The original Task Force report was co-authored by Dr. Graham Worrall, MSc, DRCOG, MRCGP, CCFP, visiting lecturer, Community Medicine, Memorial University, St. John's, Newfoundland.

Selected References

1. Canadian Task Force on the Periodic Health Examination: The periodic health examination, 1990 update: 2. Early detection of depression and prevention of suicide. *Can Med Assoc J* 1990; 142: 1233-1238

2. Feightner JW, Worrall G: Early detection of depression by primary care physicians. *Can Med Assoc J* 1990; 142: 1215-1220

3. Shapiro S, German PS, Skinner EA, *et al*: An experiment to change detection and management of mental morbidity in primary care. *Med Care* 1987; 25: 327-339

4. Hoeper EW, Nycz GR, Kessler LG, *et al*: The usefulness of screening for mental illness. *Lancet* 1984; 1: 33-35

5. Johnstone A, Goldberg D: Psychiatric screening in general practice. *Lancet* 1976; 1: 605-608

6. Zung WW, Magill M, Moore JT, *et al*: Recognition and treatment of depression in a family medicine practice. *J Clin Psychiatry* 1983; 44: 3-6

7. Magruder-Habib K, Zung WW, Feussner JR: Improving physicians' recognition and treatment of depression in general medical care. *Med Care* 1990; 28(3): 239-250

8. U.S. Preventive Services Task Force: *Guide to Clinical Preventive Services: an Assessment of the Effectiveness of 169 Interventions*. Williams & Wilkins, Baltimore, Md, 1989: 261-263

Early Detection of Depression

MANEUVER	EFFECTIVENESS	LEVEL OF EVIDENCE <REF>	RECOMMENDATION
General Health Questionnaire and Zung Self-rating Depression Scale	Routine testing for depression by questionnaire did not improve detection rate or management.	Randomized controlled trials<3-6> (I)	Fair evidence to exclude testing from periodic health examination of asymptomatic people (D)

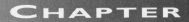

CHAPTER 40

Prevention
of
Suicide

By Jane E. McNamee and David R. Offord

Prevention of Suicide

Prepared by Jane E. McNamee, MA[1] and David R. Offord, MD, FRCPC[2]

In 1989 the Task Force recommended that primary care physicians routinely evaluate suicide risk among patients in high-risk groups. Available interventions include counselling, follow-up and, if necessary, referral to a psychiatrist.[1,2] Updated information shows changes in age-groups at increased risk for suicide.[3] Highest-risk groups in 1960 were men aged 70 years or more, and women aged 65 to 69 years. In 1991 highest-risk groups were men aged 20 to 24 years, and women aged 40 to 44 years. Other identified high-risk groups include people who have previously attempted suicide; those with a history of psychiatric illness; people with a history of drug and alcohol abuse especially those living in isolation; those with a chronic or terminal physical illness; Native people; people with a family history of suicide; and persons in custody. Additional groups identified recently are Aboriginal and Native youth in northern communities and new immigrants.

There is some evidence that physician education in treatment of affective disorders can reduce suicide rates. Studies evaluating suicide prevention in school-based intervention programs, community-based suicide prevention centres, or hospital-based intensive follow-up situations have shown that none reduced the incidence of suicide significantly. Studies evaluating medical treatment for reduction of suicidal ideation or depression have shown some reduction of depression. However there is insufficient evidence to recommend for or against the combination of routine evaluation of suicide risk with intervention programs.

Burden of Suffering

Suicide has accounted for about 2% of annual deaths in Canada since the late 1970s. (Unless otherwise stated, mortality rates cited here refer to deaths per 100,000 population). Between 1960 and 1991 the suicide rate in Canada increased from 7.8 to 12.8, peaking at 14.0 in 1986. In 1991, Alberta had the highest suicide rate (17.8), followed by Prince Edward Island (16.8) and Quebec (15.7). Between

---

[1] Research Associate, Department of Psychiatry, Chedoke McMaster Hospitals and Centre for Studies of Children at Risk, Chedoke McMaster Hospitals and McMaster University, Hamilton, Ontario

[2] Professor of Psychiatry, McMaster University, Hamilton, Ontario

1960 and 1991 the greatest increase in the provincial suicide rate was a three-fold increase in Quebec.

Eighty percent of all suicides reported in 1991 involved men. The male:female ratio for suicide risk was 3.8:1 (4.0:1 in 1960). In 1991 the highest suicide rate in males was in the group aged 20 to 24 years (33.3), followed by those aged 25 to 29 (29.7), and those aged 30 to 34 (29.2). The highest rate in females was in the group aged 40 to 44 years (8.3), followed by those aged 45 to 49 (7.7), and those aged 30 to 34 (7.3). Other groups, in decreasing order of risk, were males aged 35 to 39 (27.2), and 50 to 54 (26.7). Other at-risk groups among females were those aged 55 to 59 (7.2), 25 to 29 (7.1), and 65 to 70 (7.1). For both sexes the overall rates decreased with age, but began to increase again in later years.

Preferred methods of suicide remain unchanged. In 1991, males chose firearms (36%), hanging (30%) and by gas vapours (10%). Females chose to ingest solid or liquid substances (38%), hanging (24%) and drugs or medication (12%).<3>

In both males and females, the greatest increase between 1960 and 1991 occurred in the 15-to-19-year age group, with a four-and-a-half-fold increase for males, and a three-fold increase for females. Among males, other age groups at greater risk in 1991, compared with 1960, were those aged 10 to 14 (3.5:1), and 20 to 24 (2.7:1). Among females, other groups at greater risk in 1991, compared to 1961, were those aged 35 to 39 (2.2:1), and 40 to 44 (1.8:1). Despite the considerable increase in the suicide rate in young age groups, few reliable predictors of suicide in young people have been identified. One unexpected finding is that, since 1969, the rate of suicide in 15-19-year-old males has been higher in Canada than in the U.S., by as much as 50 percent, in many years.<4> The potential years of life lost (PYLL) to age 75 in 1986 due to suicide were 122,908 per 100,000 population, 97,613 among males and 25,295 among females in Canada.<5>

Despite the considerable increase in the suicide rate in young age groups, few reliable predictors of suicide in young people have been identified

Suggestions that Canadian suicide rates might be affected by under-reporting have recently been refuted. One study<6> found that under-reporting suicide in Canada did not substantially alter findings, suggesting that most conclusions based on official rates are essentially correct.

The public health impact of attempted suicide is substantial; the burden on casualty, general medical and psychiatric services is considerable. The risk of suicide after an attempt has been reported from 26.9:1 to 100:1. Among such individuals it is estimated that one-third have reported previous episodes of self harm and 15-20% will repeat within 3 months. The risk is highest within the first 3 years, especially during the first 6 months after an attempt.<7>

The mentally ill (those with affective disorder, schizophrenia, neurosis, personality disorder or organic brain syndrome) and people with drug and alcohol problems are at greater risk (by a factor of 2.4 to 23 times) than the general population.<8,9> Suicide is the chief cause of premature death among schizophrenics with a rate of 350-600 per 100,000 schizophrenic persons.<10> Depression and alcoholism are associated with suicide in elderly males living alone.<11> People with a chronic or terminal illness are at increased risk, from 4:1 among cancer patients to 66:1 among those with acquired immune deficiency syndrome (AIDS). In patients with symptomatic HIV infection the risk is thought to be even higher.<12>

Suicide rates for the Native population in Canada are more than twice the sex-specific rates, and three times the age-specific rates of non-Native Canadians

Suicide rates in the Canadian Native population are more than twice the sex-specific rates, and three times the age-specific rates of non-Native Canadians (56.3 for Native males and 11.8 for Native females). Among Aboriginal males, the rate for the 15-24 year age group was more than double that for all Aboriginal males (90.0:39.0).<13> Suicide among northern Native youth has reached epidemic proportions. In Alberta the rates in the northern region were 80.1, in the central region, 71.2, and in the southern area, 35.3.<14> An extremely high overall rate (180.2) has been found for 10-19 year-old Native males living on the northern coast of Labrador.<15> The 1991 Aboriginal Peoples Survey indicated that slightly more than two-fifths (41%) of Inuit, and 34.5% of Native Indians on reserves, report that suicide is a problem in their community.<16>

Suicide rates in federal and provincial prisons vary from 8 to 47 times rates in the general population. Suicide is the primary cause of death in Canadian penal institutions.<17> In addition to the high rate of completed suicide, the rate of nonfatal self-inflicted injuries among inmates is considerably higher than that for the general population (11.8:1 for males, and 45:1 for females). People with family member who committed suicide are nine times more likely than others to kill themselves.<18> Ethnicity has also been associated with suicide, with first generation immigrant females (2:1), particularly those of European and Asian origin being at higher risk.<19>

Maneuver

Out of every 10 persons who complete suicide, eight have previously signalled their intentions quite clearly

Physician involvement in suicide prevention is crucial. Out of every 10 persons who complete suicide, eight have previously signalled their intentions quite clearly. Distress signals about their suicidal impulses are often aimed at family physicians.<20> Studies show that many adolescents,<21> adults,<22> including physicians,<23> and elderly people<24> who commit suicide contact their family physician shortly before death. Successful intervention for suicide prevention depends on early detection, accurate assessment and diagnosis and appropriate treatment by the family physician. Physicians should routinely evaluate the risk of suicide among people in high-risk groups, particularly if there is evidence of psychiatric disorder. Assessment should include personal and sociodemographic risk factors, a thorough collection of clinical data, categorization of the problem and matching of the findings with well established risk factors.

Four maneuvers for treatment of suicidal patients have been identified: 1) medication (if indicated) targeted to the treatment of diagnosed mental illness. Prescriptions should be given for small amounts to reduce the risk of overdosage; 2) appropriate use of psychiatric consultations, referral and hospitalization where necessary; 3) psychosocial and psychotherapeutic interventions such as provision of social support, counselling and close follow-up visits, especially for depressed and isolated patients; and 4) environmental interventions, such as educating the patient and family members about the illness, identifying coping strategies and stress management, and development and utilization of a network of community social supports. Additionally, the physician may take a community leadership role among health care professionals, policy-makers, civic leaders and the general public to enhance support of suicide research and prevention programs, and development of "At-Risk-Clinics".

Effectiveness of Prevention and Treatment

Although there is only poor evidence (level III) supporting the effectiveness of intervention by the family physician in preventing suicide, there is fair evidence that family physicians may have a low rate of recognition of psychiatric disorders and suicide risk.[24] In one study of completed suicides, more than two-thirds of the victims had made previous attempts, but only 39% of their physicians were aware of their history.[24] Of the more than 30,000 people world-wide who have taken the suicide-prevention program at the Suicide Information and Education Centre (SIEC) in Calgary, physicians have constituted less than 1%.[25]

One recent study[26] has shown that physicians' knowledge of the risk and treatment of suicide patients improves after training in a suicide prevention program. Physicians' knowledge was compared, in pre-post situations, for three groups: those with no training, a group receiving written information only, and a group receiving the written information and seminar training. The last group showed significantly more knowledge about suicide prevention than the two other groups. However long-term follow-up of retention of knowledge, and its effect on the suicide rate, were not reported. Another pre-post study[27] reported decreased suicide rates after a systematic post-graduate training program for general practitioners. The program was directed at the diagnosis and treatment of patients with affective disorders. The study location was a geographically defined catchment area. Suicide rates were compared, pre- and post-program, with the area rates for previous years, and the Swedish national rate. A 50% reduction in the community suicide rate was found in the year following the program, which was attributed to the effects of the program. However no comparisons were made for subsequent years, and no long-term follow-up was conducted. Replication of this type of program in a controlled trial, with long-term follow-up is needed. Overall, there is fair evidence for both the benefit of physician education programs and reduction of suicide, after physician education, in selected groups.

The increase in attention given to adolescent suicide has led to a proliferation of school-based prevention programs. These programs have been described as ineffective, inefficient and even potentially deleterious in their attempts to reduce suicide risk. Program goals are to: 1) raise awareness of the problem of adolescent suicide; 2) train participants to identify adolescents at risk; and 3) educate participants about community mental health resources. The mean duration of U.S. programs is two hours. No evaluation of a Canadian curriculum-based suicide prevention programs exists. One descriptive survey[28] examined 115 U.S. school-based suicide prevention programs. It found that short-term educational interventions were not effective in the prevention of suicide among self-identified adolescent suicide attempters. It was suggested that such programs might actually facilitate suicide, or suicide behaviour, by not allowing adequate time to deal with issues raised by program content. A more recent study[29] which compared pre-post attitudes of curriculum-based suicide prevention programs for 758 teenagers with those of 680 control pupils also found little program impact. Both studies recommended caution in relation to prevention programs because of the possible stimulation of imitative behaviour in vulnerable youths. One recent study[30] advised physicians consulting to schools in the aftermath of a suicide, to resist the pressure to implement a curriculum-based prevention program that may have little or no impact. They suggested that physicians and other health care workers take a more active role in identifying children who may be at risk for suicidal behaviour, such as friends and relatives of the victim.

Suicide prevention centres differ from crisis centres and general help lines in the specificity of their focus on suicide. Evaluation of the effectiveness of the 97 Canadian suicide prevention and crisis intervention centres, listed in the 1993-1994 Handbook of the American Association of Suicidology, has not been carried out, due to non-comparability of data across centres. The consensus from evaluation studies in the United States suggests that suicide hotlines are minimally effective in reducing suicidal behaviour and community suicide rates. One descriptive survey[31] found that crisis centres do attract high-risk populations; centre clients were more likely to commit suicide than were members of the general population, and individuals who committed suicide were more likely to have been clients than were members of the general population. In another survey,[32] a slight reduction in risk in young white women, who were the most frequent users of such services, was found. Preliminary data from a descriptive evaluation survey of two suicide prevention centres in Quebec[33] showed that a significant number of callers feel less depressed at the end of a call, and that there was a reduction in suicidal urgency in a large number of callers. More work needs to be done in standardizing techniques used at different Canadian centres to achieve any meaningful evaluation of their reduction of suicide risk.

Medical treatment for the prevention of suicide involves mainly the treatment of depression and management of individuals who have attempted suicide previously. One early cohort study of hospitalized patients[34] admitted for self-inflicted injuries reported fewer subsequent suicide attempts in those who received psychiatric counselling, compared with controls who were discharged before seeing a psychiatrist. Another early survey of medical interventions[35] found that the risk of suicide among people with affective disorder was decreased when optimal pharmacotherapy was combined with routine psychiatric consultation. A more recent meta-analysis[36] which combined data from 17 double-blind clinical trials in patients with depressive disorder, showed that significantly fewer patients treated with fluoxetine suffered an increase in suicidal thoughts and actions, when compared to patients treated with placebo or a tricyclic antidepressant. Another descriptive survey of the use of antidepressants in the provocation or the prevention of suicide[37] concluded that antidepressants, with serotonin reuptake inhibitors, had a clear and consistent positive effect in reducing suicidal behaviour during treatment in depressed patients.

A review[38] of five British psychosocial intervention studies shows no statistically significant reduction in the risk of suicide, or episodes of deliberate self-harm in the active treatment groups. A study of parasuicides,[39] randomized to hospital admission or to discharge home, found no significant differences in psychological tests or further suicide attempts between the two groups at one week follow-up, but long term results were not evaluated. A more recent Canadian study,[40] which randomized suicide attempters to intensive follow-up or usual care, failed to reach its goal of halving the risk of repeat attempts in the intensive intervention group in the two years following the suicide attempt. Although not statistically significant, a 2% decrease of risk of a repeat suicide attempt was found in the intervention group. Of studies to date, none has shown a statistically significant benefit of psychosocial intervention on reducing suicide repetition rates. However, one limitation of these studies is that all except the Canadian study lacked sufficient power to assess whether an intervention reduced the risk of suicide repetition. That is, sample size was not adequate to detect clinically significant effects between groups. Also the results may not be generalizable to all persons attempting or completing suicide because of potential differences between persons attempting and persons completing suicide. Further evaluation of psychosocial interventions is required to assess their effectiveness.

Involuntary hospitalization may benefit persons with suspected suicidal intentions, and may be required for medical or legal reasons. However no data are available to assess the effectiveness of this intervention in reducing the risk of suicide.<41>

Recommendations of Others

In 1989, the U.S. Preventive Services Task Force recommended against routine screening for suicidal intent.<42> However, they also felt that clinicians should be alert to signs of suicidal ideation in persons with established risk factors; persons suspected of suicidal intent should be questioned regarding the extent of preparatory actions and referred for further evaluation if evidence of suicidal behaviour was detected.

Conclusions and Recommendations

There is poor evidence (based on expert opinion alone) to include or exclude routine evaluation of suicide risk in the periodic health examination (C Recommendation). Physicians should remain alert to the possibility of suicide in high-risk patients. They should routinely evaluate the risk of suicide, particularly if there is evidence of psychiatric disorder, especially psychosis, depression or substance abuse, or if the patient lives alone, recently attempted suicide, or a family member has committed suicide. Special attention should be paid to young Native and Aboriginal males. Physicians should be particularly alert when patients carry several known risk factors for suicide.

Physician education in the prevention of suicide, and the detection and management of depressed patients are promising approaches to the reduction of suicide risk. There is fair evidence to support physician education programs on suicide prevention (B Recommendation). There is insufficient evidence to evaluate school-based or community-based programs or interventions for those who have previously attempted suicide (C Recommendation). However, there is fair evidence to use medical therapy in the treatment of suicidal ideation (B Recommendation) and, where appropriate, for diagnosed depression (A Recommendation).

Unanswered Questions (Research Agenda)

The following have been identified as research priorities:

1. Evaluating the accuracy of family physicians in identifying psychiatric disorder and in determining suicide risk.

2. Obtaining better information on the factors that predict suicide among persons in high-risk groups, such as those who have a psychiatric disorder or have attempted suicide, particularly Northern Native and Aboriginal youth, or among those who abuse alcohol and other drugs.

3. Developing, monitoring and participation in education programs designed to increase physicians' effectiveness in identifying psychiatric disorder and people at high risk of suicide.

4. Evaluating the effectiveness of suicide prevention programs that combine identification of high-risk patients and subsequent intervention, with long-term follow-up.

5. Greater collaboration between physicians and school personnel in developing curriculum-based programs aimed at intervention/postvention or prevention, and the research of the reduction of adolescent suicide risk.

Evidence

The literature was identified with a MEDLINE search from January 1967 to November 1993 using the following key words: suicide, attempted suicide, parasuicide, epidemiology, at-risk populations, prevention, intervention, postvention.

Review of this topic was initiated in November 1993 and updates a report published in 1990.[1,2] Recommendations were finalized by the Task Force in March 1994.

Selected References

1. Canadian Task Force on the Periodic Health Examination: The periodic health examination, 1990 update: 2. Early detection of depression and prevention of suicide. *Can Med Assoc J* 1990; 142(11): 1233-1238

2. McNamee JE, Offord DR: Prevention of Suicide. *Can Med Assoc J* 1990; 142(11): 1223-1230

3. Statistics Canada: *Cause of Death 1991*. Minister of Industry, Science and Technology, [Cat. No. 84-208] Ottawa, 1993

4. Lyeenaars AA, Lester D: A comparison of rates and patterns of suicide in Canada and the United States, 1960-1988. *Death Studies* 1991; 16: 417-430

5. Mao Y, Hasselback P, Davies JW, *et al*: Suicide in Canada: an epidemiological assessment. *Can J Public Health* 1990; 81: 324-328

6. Speechley M, Stavraky KM: The adequacy of suicide statistics for use in epidemiology and public health. *Can J Public Health* 1991; 82: 38-42

7. Appleby L, Warner R: Parasuicide: Features of repetition, and the implications for intervention. *Psychol Med* 1993; 23: 13-16

8. Pokorny AD: Prediction of suicide in psychiatric patients. Report of a prospective study. *Arch Gen Psychiatry* 1983; 40: 249-257

9. Goldstein RB, Black DW, Nasrallah A, *et al*: The prediction of suicide. Sensitivity, specificity and predictive value of a multivariate model applied to suicide among 1906 patients with affective disorders. *Arch Gen Psychiatry* 1991; 48: 418-422

10. Caldwell CB, Gottesman II: Schizophrenia – a high-risk factor for suicide: clues to risk reduction. *Suicide Life Threat Behav* 1992; 22: 479-493

11. Lapierre S, Pronovost J, Dube M: Risk factors associated with suicide in elderly persons living in the community. *Canada's Mental Health* 1992; 40(Sept): 8-11

12. Marzuk PM, Tierney H, Tardiff K, *et al*: Increased risk of suicide in persons with AIDS. *JAMA* 1988; 259: 1333-1337

13. Grant C: Suicide and intervention and prevention among Northern Native Youth. *J Child Youth Care* 1991; 6: 11-17

14. Bagley C: Poverty and suicide among Native Canadians: A replication. *Psychol Rep* 1991; 69: 149-150

15. Aldridge D, St John K: Adolescent and pre-adolescent suicide in Newfoundland and Labrador. *Can J Psychiatry* 1991; 36: 432-436

16. Statistics Canada: *The Daily,* June 29 1993. [Cat No. 11-001E] Ottawa, 1993

17. Ramsay RF, Tanney BL, Searle CA: Suicide prevention in high-risk prison populations. *Can J Criminology* 1987; 29(3): 295-307

18. Giffin M, Felsenthal C: *A Cry for Help*. Doubleday, Garden City, NY, 1983

19. Strachan J, Johansen H, Nair C, *et al*: Canadian suicide mortality rates: First-generation immigrants versus Canadian-Born. *Heath Rep* 1990; 2: 327-341

20. Morrissette P: *Signalled Intention*: in Le Suicide de mystification, intervention, prevention, Quebec. Quebec City: Centre de prevention du suicide de Quebec, 1984

21. Hawton K, O'Grady J, Osborn M, *et al*: Adolescents who take overdoses: their characteristics, problems and contacts with helping agencies. *Br J Psychiatry* 1982; 140: 118-123

22. Barraclough B, Bunch J, Nelson B, *et al*: A hundred cases of suicide: clinical aspects. *Br J Psychiatry* 1974; 125: 355-373

23. Simon W: Suicide among physicians: prevention and postvention. *Crisis* 1986; 7: 1-13

24. Murphy GE: The physician's responsibility for suicide: 2. Errors of omission. *Ann Intern Med* 1975; 82: 305-309

25. Sutherland R: Alberta making major effort to overcome high suicide rate. *Can Med Assoc J* 1991; 144(8): 1050-1054

26. Michel K, Valach L: Suicide prevention: spreading the gospel to general practitioners. *Br J Psychiatry* 1992; 160: 757-760

27. Rutz W, von Knorring L, Walinder J: Frequency of suicide on Gotland after systematic postgraduate education of general practitioners. *Acta Psychiatr Scand* 1989; 80: 151-154

28. Garland A, Shaffer D, Whittle B: A national survey of school-based, adolescent suicide prevention programs. *J Am Acad Child Adolesc Psychiatry* 1989; 28: 931-934

29. Shaffer D, Gardland A, Vieland V, *et al*: The impact of curriculum-based suicide prevention programs for teenagers. *J Am Acad Child Adolesc Psychiatry* 1991; 30: 588-596

30. Adler RS, Jellinek MS: After teen suicide: issues for pediatricians who are asked to consult to schools. *Pediatrics* 1990; 86: 982-987

31. Dew MA, Bromet EJ, Brent D, *et al*: A quantitative literature review of the effectiveness of suicide prevention centers. *J Consult Clin Psychol* 1987; 55: 239-244

32. Miller HL, Coombs DW, Leeper JD, *et al*: An analysis of the effects of suicide prevention facilities on suicide rates in the United States. *Am J Public Health* 1984; 74: 340-343

33. Mishra BL, Daigle M: The effectiveness of telephone interventions by suicide prevention centres. *Canada's Mental Health* 1992; 40: 24-29

34. Greer S, Bagley C: Effect of psychiatric intervention in attempted suicide: a controlled study. *BMJ* 1971; 1: 310-312

35. Schou M, Weeke A: Did manic-depressive patients who committed suicide receive prophylactic or continuation treatment at the time? *Br J Psychiatry* 1988; 153: 324-327

36. Beasley CM, Dornseif BE, Bosomworth JC, *et al*: Fluoxetine and suicidality: a meta-analysis of controlled trials of treatment for depression. *BMJ* 1991; 303: 685-692

37. Montgomery SA, Bullock T, Daldwin D, *et al*: The provocation and prevention of suicide attempts. *Int Clin Psychopharmacol* 1992; 6 (Suppl 6): 28-34

38. House A, Owens D, Storer D: Psycho-social intervention following attempted suicide: is there a case for better services? *International Review Psychiatry* 1992; 4: 15-22

39. Waterhouse J, Platt S: General hospital admission in the management of parasuicide. A randomised controlled trial. *Br J Psychiatry* 1990; 156: 236-242

40. Allard R, Marshall M, Plante MC: Intensive follow-up does not decrease the risk of repeat suicide attempts. *Suicide Life Threat Behav* 1992; 22: 303-314

41. Wise TN, Berlin R: Involuntary hospitalization: an issue for the consultation-liaison psychiatrist. *Gen Hosp Psychiatry* 1987; 9: 40-44

42. U.S. Preventive Services Task Force: *Guide to Clinical Preventive Services: an Assessment of the Effectiveness of 169 Interventions*. Williams & Wilkins, Baltimore, Md, 1989: 265-269

Prevention of Suicide

MANEUVER	EFFECTIVENESS	LEVEL OF EVIDENCE \<REF\>	RECOMMENDATION
Routine evaluation of suicide risk if there is evidence of membership in one or more high-risk groups.*	Effectiveness of routine evaluation of suicide risk by primary caregivers has not been evaluated.	Expert opinion\<20,24,25\> (III)	Poor evidence to support either inclusion or exclusion from periodic health examination: evaluation recommended for people at high risk* because of burden of suffering (C)
Physician education in recognition and treatment of those at risk for suicide	Some evidence of increased knowledge and reduced suicide rate.	Pre-post comparison studies\<26,27\> (II-3)	Fair evidence for benefit of physician education programs on suicide prevention, and fair evidence for reduction of suicide rate in selected groups (B)
Curriculum or school-based intervention/ prevention and postvention programs	Few comparable programs or outcome measures; intervention described as ineffective, inefficient and potentially deleterious.	Matched cohort study\<29\> (II-2); descriptive survey\<28\> (III)	Insufficient evidence to recommend referral to this intervention (C)
Community-based suicide prevention programs, crisis centres and general help telephone lines	Few comparable programs or outcome measures.	Descriptive surveys\<31-33\> (III)	Insufficient evidence for or against referral to this service (C)
Medical treatment for reduction of 1) suicidal ideation 2) depression	Some evidence of reduced suicide risk, for those treated for suicidal ideation Good evidence of reduced suicide risk for those treated for depression.	Cohort study\<34\> (II-2); descriptive survey\<35\> (III) Meta-analysis of 17 randomized clinical trials\<36\> (I); descriptive survey\<37\> (III)	Fair evidence to use in the treatment of suicidal ideation, (B) and good evidence to use, where appropriate, for diagnosed depression (A)

* **High-risk groups include: those with a history of psychiatric illness, depression, drug & alcohol abuse especially those living in isolation, those with chronic terminal illness, Native & Aboriginal people especially young males, those with a family history of suicide, first generation immigrant women**

(Continued on next page)

Prevention of Suicide (concl'd)

MANEUVER	EFFECTIVENESS	LEVEL OF EVIDENCE <REF>	RECOMMENDATION
For those previously attempting suicide:			
Hospital admission or discharge home	No evidence of reduced risk between groups.	Randomized controlled trial<39> (I)	Insufficient evidence for or against referral to these interventions for those previously attempting suicide (C)
Intensive psycho-social follow-up using the Suicidal Risk Scale as an indicator of suicidal risk	No statistically significant evidence of reduced risk.	Randomized controlled trial<40> (I)	

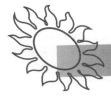

CHAPTER 41

Children
of
Alcoholics

By Jane E. McNamee and David R. Offord

Children of Alcoholics

Prepared by Jane E. McNamee MA,[1] and David R. Offord MD, FRCPC[2]

The topic, children of alcoholics (COA), has not been previously addressed by the Canadian Task Force on the Periodic Health Examination. However, related topics, such as fetal alcohol syndrome and problem drinking, have been covered elsewhere in this book. The focus of this report is children aged 0 to 18 years, who live with an alcoholic, or alcohol-abusing parent. Clinical and research evidence worldwide clearly shows that COA are an at-risk population for diminished intellectual capacity and development, increased emotional problems, and a wide range of psychological and behavioral disorders. As well as being at risk, these children are also likely to experience long-term adverse consequences. Increased risk status comes from three sources: 1) genetic influences; 2) teratogenic factors during pregnancy; 3) environmental conditions related to the upbringing of the child by addicted parents. Several screening tests have been derived to identify children of alcoholics of which the Children of Alcoholics Screening Test (CAST) is the most frequently used child self-completed questionnaire. Services to COA are nearly non-existent, being limited to referral of children to individual or group therapy in Al-Atot or Al-Ateen. Although physicians have a low recognition rate of alcohol abuse in parents of hospitalized children, there is no evidence to show that routine screening of non-complainant offspring of alcoholic parents would improve the detection rate of various morbidities, or management of these children. However, physicians should be sensitive to the possibility of alcohol-related stressors in offspring of alcoholic, or alcohol-abusing parents, particularly in high-risk groups, such as children hospitalized for injury. Additionally, physicians are encouraged to offer support to COA and to assist COA to recognise that they have a right to seek assistance (C Recommendation). A separate chapter has also been prepared dealing with problem drinking (Chapter 42).

Burden of Suffering

Although no large epidemiological studies have been conducted to identify the prevalence of children of alcoholics in Canada, there are indications that this is a sizable group. Russell and coworkers<1>

[1] Research Associate, Department of Psychiatry, Chedoke McMaster Hospitals and Centre for Studies of Children at Risk, Chedoke McMaster Hospitals & McMaster University, Hamilton, Ontario
[2] Professor of Psychiatry, McMaster University, Hamilton, Ontario

extrapolating data from the U.S. 1979 Drinking Practice Study[2] estimated that I out of 8 children in the United States lives in an alcoholic home. Using this ratio with 1991 Canadian population statistics[3] for children aged 0-19 years, it can be estimated that close to one million (approximately 945,150) children lived in an alcoholic home in Canada in 1991. This figure represents approximately 12% of children in any age group. Epidemiological evidence from other countries shows similar prevalence rates.[4]

Definitions of parental alcoholism have differed between studies and over time. Definitions ranged from self-reported family histories of heavy drinking or alcohol-dependency in the natural parent or grandparent in earlier studies[4,5] to parents who were described as "problem drinkers"[6,7] or "recovering alcoholics"[8,9] or "recovering-diagnosed-alcoholics",[10,11] or those who met the criteria systematically defining alcohol abuse or dependence in later studies. The strategy most commonly used to determine parental alcohol status was the DSM-III alcohol abuse or dependence criteria.[12,13,14] Questionnaires such as the Michigan Alcohol Screening Test,[15,16,17] or the four-question CAGE query[18,19,20] were also used to assess parental lifetime occurrence of impairments secondary to alcohol use, and alcohol dependence symptoms.

Systematic investigations of the transmission of alcoholism in family,[21] twin,[22] adoption[23] and half-sibling[24] studies have concluded that, compared with the general population, alcoholism in a biological parent is a consistent predictor of alcoholism in the offspring. A meta-analysis of the relationship between the sex-of-parent and sex-of-offspring on the transmission of alcoholism, indicates that across family studies, paternal alcoholism is associated with increased rates of alcoholism in both sons and daughters, whereas maternal alcoholism is solely associated with increased rates of alcoholism among daughters.[25] Biological sons and daughters of alcoholics are four times more likely than children of nonalcoholics to become alcoholics, and daughters of alcoholics are more likely to marry alcoholic men.[26]

The fetal effects of alcohol during pregnancy are well documented, particularly at the severe end of the syndrome in terms of the cluster of signs and symptoms known as the Fetal Alcohol Syndrome (FAS). There is also evidence that alcohol can result in more subtle changes such as mild forms of developmental delay and mental retardation.[27] More information on FAS is provided in Chapter 5.

In general, both cross-sectional and prospective longitudinal studies point toward a complex interaction between parental alcoholism and familial environment in increasing the vulnerability for psychopathology in the offspring. The home environments of COA with one alcoholic parent show there is diminished global functioning when compared with homes of children with neither parent alcoholic.<6> A comparison of the home environments of COA with one or more DSM-III diagnoses and those without psychiatric diagnoses shows that the homes of the "disturbed children" are characterised by greater exposure to the effects of parental drinking, more parent-child conflict and less parent-child interaction than the homes of the children who received no diagnoses.<6> The child-rearing practices of alcoholic fathers, compared to those of non-alcoholic fathers, are more likely to be rejecting, harsh and neglecting.<7> Living in a family with one active alcoholic parent seems to increase the risk of children being abused or neglected.<28> COA report a greater frequency of family violence than children from control families.<29> In a large U.S. survey,<12> children of mothers categorized as problem drinkers had a 2.1-fold relative risk (95% confidence interval (CI): 1.3-3.5) of serious injury (injuries resulting in hospitalization, surgical treatment, missed school, one-half day or more in bed) when compared with children of mothers who were non-drinkers. Children of two parents who were problem drinkers compared with children of nondrinkers had a 2.7-fold relative risk of serious injury (95% CI: 0.8-8.6).

Growing up in a household with alcoholic parents is more likely to produce lower self-esteem, greater dysphoria and more anxiety in adulthood.<30> Rates of emotional problems, especially anxiety, depression and nightmares are doubled in children of relapsed alcoholics as compared to children of non-alcoholics or to children of recovered alcoholics.<5> COA are more likely to describe their childhood as unhappy,<8> and to have a greater level of depressive affect, when compared to the general population.<31>

Parental alcoholism, in addition to creating an adverse family environment, increases the risk for maladjustments as measured by scores on the Child Behaviour Checklist (CBCL).<13> Children of alcoholic parents scored significantly higher on the total behaviour problem scale, as well as on both the internalizing and externalizing scales of the CBCL. They also scored significantly higher on the somatic complaints scale. In a comparison of COA and children of non-alcoholics,<16> the former reported more alcohol and drug problems, stronger expectancies for positive reinforcement from alcohol, higher levels of behavioral undercontrol, more neuroticism and more psychiatric distress. They also showed lower academic achievement and lower verbal ability than controls. Greater risk for overt child psychopathology was observed when both parental disorder and adverse family environment were present.

Preliminary studies have found significantly lower IQ scores in COA, when compared to children of non-alcoholic parents.<32> One longitudinal study on the island of Kauai, Hawaii,<33> followed 49 children of alcoholic parents. The children were reared in chronic poverty from birth to 18 years. Fifty-nine percent of the offspring of alcoholics appeared to cope well and had not developed serious

Growing up in an alcoholic family increases the child's risk of emotional disorders, health problems, sexual and physical abuse, and neglect

problems by the age of 18 years. However 41% of the children had coping problems, and scored significantly lower on verbal abilities as well as on reading and writing than the rest of the group.

A more recent study found no difference in cognitive functioning between children from alcoholic and non-alcoholic families.<34> Another study comparing children of male alcoholics with control children found that the former group was not compromised academically, and did not show more conduct problems. However, in this study daughters of alcoholics (but not the sons) showed more variability than controls in school attendance.<35>

Most research indicates a relationship between parental alcoholism and conduct problems in their children.<36> This appears to hold for both diagnosed conduct disorder as well as for specific conduct problems such as lying, stealing, fighting and truancy.<32> One recent prospective longitudinal study collected data from a consecutive sample of women from the general population visiting two mental health clinics in Sweden during the course of one year.<37> Of 497 liveborn children, 54 were born into families with an alcoholic parent. The study examined health, growth, mental development and psychopathology of children from before birth until school age. The childrens' physical health was tracked, and they were evaluated using the Griffiths Development Scales. By age 4 years, the children of alcoholic parents had a higher risk of pre- and post-natal death, poorer mental development and more symptoms of an overt psychiatric nature (DSM-III) than other children. However, delays in physical development observed during the infant years disappeared by age 4.

Not all children of alcoholics are equally vulnerable. Despite the risk to COA, at least 60% of COA do not themselves become alcoholic or psychiatrically ill. While it is true that this implies that not all COA are equally vulnerable, it may simply be that the unaffected subgroup has not inherited the genes conferring susceptibility from their parents. Present methods do not permit a distinction between biological and psychosocial vulnerabilities. One recent study<14> found that when factors such as low socioeconomic status and familial co-morbidity were controlled for, children from high-risk families with a multi-generational history of alcoholism or alcohol abuse, had similar rates of childhood disorders, when contrasted with low-risk children from community control families. However this study considered only childhood psychiatric disorders, and provided no information about the future risk of adult psychiatric disorders in these children. A longitudinal study<33> compared the characteristics of resilient children of alcoholics (59% of the sample) with the offspring who developed adjustment problems. Resilient children were found to have a responsible attitude, positive self-concept, adequate communication skills, at least average IQ, and more internalized locus of control. Another study examined the protective effects of positive family functioning in young adult children of alcoholic parents.<38> It found that a biological vulnerability, that is, being the offspring of an alcohol-dependent parent was not sufficient or necessary for children of alcoholics to develop alcohol dependency as young adults, although there was an increased risk. There appeared to be strong protective effects of positive family relationships on the potential negative effects of a family history of alcoholism.

Maneuver

Research on COA is of variable quality, but has mainly been criticized for missing pertinent information. Clear, consistent definitions of criteria to evaluate parental alcohol use are lacking and thus the strategies used to determine parental alcohol status varies among studies and are not necessarily comparable. Length of exposure of the child to the alcoholic parent and the differential impact of an alcoholic parent at various stages of the child's development are generally not considered. The role of gender needs further research; paternal alcoholism is associated with increased rates of alcoholism in both sons and daughters of alcoholics.[25] Often, confounding effects of factors other than parental alcoholism, such as parental divorce and subsequent family breakup, are not taken into account. Further, the focus of intervention programs has not been clearly defined and includes at least two conceptual approaches: 1) preventing COA from developing into alcoholics; and 2) prevention of the development of psychosocial problems in such children. Due to lack of comparability of programs, populations and outcome measures as well as the lack of control for confounding, in most cases there is insufficient evidence upon which to evaluate interventions for COAs.

Screening Tests

Although the family history method appears to be the most commonly used strategy for identifying COA, a number of instruments have been developed to assist in efficiently screening large numbers of subjects for a history of alcoholism in parents and other relatives. Some of these instruments represent adaptations of instruments originally developed for direct screening of alcoholism (eg. the MAST; see Chapter 42 on Problem Drinking) and are directed at adults. One test, the Children of Alcoholics Screening Test (CAST)[18] is directed at the impact of a parent's drinking on the child. The CAST is a 30-item inventory devised to identify children and adolescents who are living with at least one alcoholic parent. It measures children's feelings, attitudes, perceptions and experiences related to their parents' drinking behaviour. Positive responses to 6 or more of the questions have been found to significantly discriminate COA from a control group of children. It reliably identified 100% of the children of both clinically diagnosed and self-reported alcoholics.[18] However 23% of the children with no known history of parental alcoholism also scored above the cut-point. The drinking behaviour of the parents of children in the control group was not assessed, so there was no way to determine the true rate of alcoholism in parents of the control group. The reliability and validity of the CAST has been studied in adolescent,[19] adult[20] and psychiatric populations.[17] It has been found to discriminate between the offspring of alcoholic parents and the offspring of non-alcoholic parents. High CAST scores have been found to be significantly related to low family cohesion, and high family conflict, and low overall family support.[39] Children 8 years or younger need to have each CAST item read and interpreted. Children 9 years and older can usually complete the test with little difficulty.

Results from a study using the CAST with adolescent offspring of diagnosed alcoholic fathers,[19] show that CAST scores correlated positively with the Life Situations Check suggesting that the CAST is related to the occurrence of alcohol-related stressors within the family. Adult subjects who reported that one or more of their parents received treatment for alcoholism scored significantly higher on the CAST as compared to other subjects.[20] It has been suggested that a short form of the CAST (see Table 1) might be more appropriate as a screening instrument for clinical purposes.[17] Although the CAST appears to be a promising screening instrument, there is a need for more psychometric research and evaluation on both the full and the shortened CAST, especially since one study found that childrens' reports of parental drinking had little validity.[40]

The Children of Alcoholics Life-Events Schedule (COALES)[41] is another self-completed test directed at children. It is a stress scale for COA designed to determine the amount of parental drinking-related-stress which a child experiences. The rationale is that stress may be a factor that discriminates children who are most at risk from those who are resilient. A study[41] using this test showed that COA reported higher levels of negative events, and lower levels of positive events than did their peers from non-alcoholic homes. Scores on the positive and negative event subscales were significantly correlated with the children's scores on measures of anxiety and depression.

In contrast to using a multi-item self-report questionnaire for diagnosing a family history of alcoholism, several investigators have justified the use of single item measures to validly determine if an individual is a COA. Two such items are "Do you consider that either of your parents ever had a drinking problem?"[42], or "Do you consider that either of your parents may have, or may have had, an alcohol abuse problem?".[43] Although for research purposes such a subjective assessment is clearly inadequate, combined with a family history, these two assessment items provide a brief and cost-effective screening method for the general practitioner in an office setting.

Effectiveness of Prevention and Treatment

Physicians are in a unique position to identify and respond to substance abuse in the families of their patients

Physicians are in a unique position to identify and respond to substance abuse in their patients' families, but have been found to be slow to identify and respond to this problem. In a study of the detection of alcoholism in families of hospitalized children, physicians were found to have a low recognition rate of substance abuse in their patients' families.<44> It was suggested that alcohol problems are likely to go unnoticed in the absence of a conscious screening effort. In another study,<15> only 34% of physicians reported taking a family substance abuse history on their pediatric patients, compared with 62% who reported taking personal alcohol/drug use history from their adolescent patients. Physicians also reported little or no responsibility for substance abuse referrals of their patients' family members. However, when the identified patient was an adolescent, the number of referrals increased.

Physicians who treat both parents and children need to be aware of the potential role played by parental drinking. Data from a U.S. study of parental alcohol use, problem drinking and childrens' injuries,<12> suggest that the primary prevention of children's injuries might be enhanced if physicians included questions about parental alcohol use in the social history. It found that children of women who are problem drinkers have an elevated injury risk, and children with two parents who are problem drinkers are at even higher risk for injury. The association between parental drinking and child injuries might be used as motivation for behavioral change, as parents may respond more readily to a message concerning the effects of their behaviour on their children's health than to messages about the impact on their own health.<12>

With increased awareness of parental drinking problems, physicians need not make a diagnosis of alcoholism, but may recommend further exploration, leading to an expression of concern for parent and children, and promoting appropriate care for the alcoholic parent. (See Chapter 42 on Problem Drinking).

Intervention Programs

Consistent contact with the child by the health care provider may be the only continuous relationship the child has

Until recently most alcohol intervention programs were aimed at the alcoholic parent. Programs that exist for children are mainly for children of parents who are hospitalized for alcoholism. Interventions<45> for COA of Alcoholics are directed toward four main goals:

1. Establishing and maintaining a primary relationship with an adult; consistent contact with the child by the health care provider may be the only continuous relationship the child has;

2. Learning about alcoholism as a disease, and acknowledging that a parent is an alcoholic;

3. Learning about safety – knowing when and how to get help; and

4. Referral to a support group.

A brief review of the background literature on services available for the COA indicates that treatment is limited,[10] and that different types of agencies vary in the extent of family services provided. One U.S. study[46] found that despite the fact that a large number of COA have been identified, only 5% of children of alcoholics received the treatment they needed. A more recent study,[11] assessing the use of family services in 70 inpatient and 51 outpatient alcoholism treatment programs run by the Department of Veteran Affairs, found services for COA were nearly non-existent, being limited to the referral of teenage children to Al-Ateen. Nearly 90% of the programs did not offer services directed to the needs of the patients' family members, or to their children. Services investigated were individual therapy, group therapy or education groups.

Al-Ateen and Al-Atot (both offshoots of the Alcoholics Anonymous program) are anonymous support groups available to any adolescent or child who has an alcoholic parent. Groups exist in major towns across Canada. It is thought that identification and sharing experiences with other children who have similar problems may give a child a better understanding of their parent's problems and their own self-image. The success of these groups has not been well researched, due in part to the constraints of maintaining anonymity of the members. In an early non-replicated preliminary study of COA, those who attended Al-Ateen groups reported higher self-esteem and better school grades than those COA who did not attend meetings, but no behavioral changes were found.[9]

Although there is agreement that early intervention is needed to interrupt the development of problems, few school programs exist, and those that do have no comparable populations, programs, or outcome measures. A survey of school nurses reported that they have difficulty identifying COA, and lack the necessary knowledge and skills to intervene.[45] The efficacy of prevention programs for COA depends not only on the effectiveness of the intervention, but also on whether the target population is being reached. One study[47] has evaluated the effectiveness of a recruitment procedure to target COA in the general population. It used reports from all children in Grades 4 through 6 to determine the risk status of those responding to the recruitment process. Results showed that the level of concern about parental drinking was higher for children who showed interest in the program, than for those who showed no interest. Although the study showed that recruitment procedures attracted children at risk, this study was limited because childrens' reports[40] of parental drinking have been found to have little validity. Another study[48] attempted to evaluate the efficacy of a self-selection recruitment process, designed to attract fourth to sixth grade children into a school-based prevention program for COA. The recruitment process was not effective in recruiting children of alcohol abusing parents. A different study provided a possible reason for this.<49> It showed that any labelling of the children as COA may have detrimental consequences due to the negative stereotyping from peers that accompanies the label.

In summary, little work has been done to develop or evaluate treatment and prevention programs for COA in the general population, so the true efficacy of treatment has not yet been determined. At present available data are insufficient for drawing strong conclusions concerning the effectiveness of any of the treatment programs for COA.

Recommendations of Others

The U.S. Preventive Services Task Force<50>, the Institute of Medicine in the U.S., and the Alcohol Risk Assessment Intervention Project of the College of Family Physicians of Canada have recommended that all patients age 12 years or older be screened to assess their level of risk drinking. Thus the screening is directed at alcohol consumption and does not focus on COA or their emotional and behavioral problems. Additionally, the College of Family Physicians of Canada<51> suggests that physicians recognise that COA may feel isolated, depressed, inadequate, have deep-seated guilt feelings, and may tend to see their problems as minor when compared to their family's problems. The family physician is encouraged to offer help regularly and to assist COA to recognise that they have a right to seek assistance.<51>

Conclusions and Recommendations

There is poor evidence (based on expert opinion alone) to support the inclusion or exclusion of routine evaluation of asymptomatic offspring of alcoholic parents from the periodic health examination (C Recommendation). Physicians should be sensitive to the possibility of alcohol-related stressors in offspring of alcoholic, or alcohol-abusing parents, and in some high-risk groups, particularly children hospitalized for injury. Primary health care providers are in an excellent position to effect the primary prevention of some childrens' injuries by identifying, evaluating and assisting families in recovery from the effects of family alcoholism.

While there is fair evidence that the CAST can identify children at risk (B Recommendation) other screening questionnaires have not been evaluated (C Recommendation) and there is insufficient evidence of treatment efficacy to evaluate screening for management purposes

(C Recommendation). School and community-based programs have not been adequately evaluated (C Recommendations).

Unanswered Questions (Research Agenda)

While many basic research questions require further study and resolution before clinical questions can be addressed, the following questions have been raised:

1. Evaluating the accuracy of family physicians in identifying the prevalence of alcohol (and other drug) abuse and dependence in patients whether they be parents or children.

2. Further longitudinal studies aimed at identifying biological vulnerability and psychological risk factors in COA.

3. Evaluation of the methods of recruitment of populations to treatment, intervention and prevention programs.

4. Studies of the ethical issues involved in the potential harmful effects of labelling children as COA.

5. Rigorous evaluations of prevention, early intervention and treatment programs for COA.

6. Study of the protective factors which permit COA, despite known risk factors, to grow up and become successfully functioning adults.

7. Study of effects of societal change in family life of COA, especially the effects of single-parent families and sex roles on family alcohol problems.

Evidence

The literature was identified with a MEDLINE search from 1988 to October 1993, using the following key words: children of alcoholics. Review of this topic was initiated in October 1993 and recommendations were finalized by the Task Force in April 1994.

Acknowledgments

The Task Force thanks Michael Moffatt, MD, MSc, FRCPC, Associate Professor of Pediatrics and Child Health, Associate Head and Associate Professor of Community Health Services, University of Manitoba, Winnipeg, Manitoba, and Roberta Palmour, PhD, Associate Professor of Psychiatry and Human Genetics, McGill University, Montreal, Quebec, for reviewing the draft report.

Selected References

1. Russell M, Henderson C, Blume SB: Children of alcoholics: A Review of the Literature, New York: Children of Alcoholics Foundation, Inc., 1986

2. Clark WB, Midanik L: Alcohol use and alcohol problems among US adults: Results of the 1979 national survey. In: *Alcohol Consumption and Related Problems.* Alcohol and Health Monograph No.1, [DHHS Publication No. (ADM)82-119000]. Washington: Government Printing Office, 1982: 3-52

3. Statistics Canada: *Population Statistics 1991.* Minister of Industry, Science and Technology, [Cat. No. 93-310]. Ottawa, 1993

4. Macdonald DI, Blume SB: Children of alcoholics. *Am J Dis Child* 1986; 140: 750-754

5. Moos RA, Billings AG: Children of alcoholics during the recovery process: alcoholic and matched control families. *Addict Behav* 1982; 7: 155-163

6. Reich W, Earls F, Powell J: A comparison of the home and social environments of children of alcoholic and non-alcoholic parents. *Br J Addict* 1988; 83: 831-839

7. Udayakumar GS, Mohan A, Shariff IA, *et al*: Children of the alcoholic parent. *Child Psych Quart* 1984; 17: 9-14

8. Callan VJ, Jackson D: Children of alcoholic fathers and recovered alcoholic fathers: personal and family functioning. *J Stud Alcohol* 1986; 47: 180-182

9. Hughes JM: Adolescent children of alcoholic parents and the relationship of Alateen to these children. *J Cons Clin Psychol* 1977; 45: 946-947

10. Regan JM, Connors GJ, O'Farrell TJ, *et al*: Services for the families of alcoholics. A Survey of treatment agencies in Massachusetts. *J Stud Alcohol* 1983; 44: 1072-1982

11. Salinas RC, O'Farrell TJ, Jones WC, *et al*: Service for families of alcoholics: a national survey of Veterans Affairs Treatment Programs. *J Stud Alcohol* 1991; 52: 541-546

12. Bijur PE, Kurzon M, Overpeck MD, *et al*: Parental alcohol use, problem drinking and children's injuries. *JAMA* 1992; 267: 3166-3171

13. Rubio-Stipec M, Bird H, Canino G, *et al*: Children of alcoholic parents in the community. *J Stud Alcohol* 1991; 52: 78-88

14. Hill SY, Hruzka DR: Childhood psychopathology in Families with multigenerational alcoholism. *J Am Acad Child Adolesc Psychiatry* 1992; 31: 1024-1030

15. Duggan AK, Adger H Jr, McDonald EM, *et al*: Detection of alcoholism in hospitalized children and their families. *Am J Dis Child* 1991; 145: 613-617

16. Sher KJ, Walitzer KS, Wood PK, *et al*: Characteristics of children of alcoholics: putative risk factors, substance use and abuse and psychopathology. *J Abnorm Psychol* 1991; 100: 427-448

17. Staley D, el-Guebaly N: Psychometric Evaluation of the Children of Alcoholics Screening Test (CAST) in a psychiatric sample. *Int J Addict* 1991; 26: 657-668

18. Jones JW: *Children of Alcoholics Screening Test*, (CAST). Chicago, Ill. Camelot Unlimited, 1983

19. Dinning WD, Berk LA: The Children of Alcoholics Screening Test: Relationship to sex, family environment and social adjustment in adolescents. *J Clin Psychol* 1989; 45: 335-339

20. Pilat JM, Jones JW: Identification of children of alcoholics: Two empirical studies. *Alcohol Health Res World* 1985; 9: 27-36

21. Goodwin DW: *Is alcoholism hereditary?* 2nd Ed. New York; Ballentine Books, 1988

22. Kaprio J, Koskenvuo M, Langinvanio H, *et al*: Genetic influences on use and abuse of alcohol: a study of 5638 adult Finnish twin brothers. *Alcohol: Clin Exp Res* 1987; 11: 349-356

23. Cadoret RJ, Troughton E, O'Gorman TW: Genetic and environmental factors in alcohol abuse and antisocial personality. *J Stud Alcohol* 1987; 48: 1-8

24. Cloninger CR, Bohman M, Sigvardsson S: Inheritance of alcohol abuse: cross-fostering of adopted men. *Arch Gen Psychiatry* 1981; 38: 861-868

25. Pollock VE, Schneiders LS, Gabrielli WF Jr, *et al*: Sex of parent and offspring in the transmission of alcoholism: A meta-analysis. *J Nervous & Mental Dis* 1987; 173: 668-673

26. Schuckit MA: Biological vulnerability to alcoholism. *J Consult Clin Psychol* 1987; 55: 301-309

27. Steinhausen HC, Spohr HL: Fetal Alcohol Syndrome. In Lahey BB, Kazdin AE (eds): *Advances in Clinical Child Psychology.* New York, Plenum Press, 1986; 9: 217-243

28. Famularo R, Stone K, Barnum R, *et al*: Alcoholism and severe child maltreatment. *Am J Orthopsychiat* 1986; 56: 481-495

29. Black C, Bucky SF, Wilder-Padilla S: The interpersonal and emotional consequences of being an adult child of an alcoholic. *Int J Addict* 1986; 21: 213-231

30. Williams OB, Corrigan PW: The differential effects of parental alcoholism and mental illness on their adult children. *J Clin Psychol* 1992; 48: 406-414

31. Rolf JE, Johnson JL, Israel E, *et al*: Depressive affect in school-aged children of alcoholics. *B J Addict* 1988; 83: 841-848

32. West M, Prinz R: Parental alcoholism and childhood psychopathology. *Psych Bulletin* 1987; 102: 204-218

33. Werner EE: Resilient offspring of alcoholics: a longitudinal study from birth to age 18. *J Stud Alcohol* 1986; 47: 34-40

34. Johnson JL, Rolf JE: Cognitive functioning in children from alcoholic and non-alcoholic families. *Br J Addict* 1988; 83: 849-857

35. Murphy RT, O'Farrell TJ, Floyd FJ, *et al*: School adjustment of children of alcoholic fathers: comparison to normal controls. *Addictive Behaviours* 1991; 16: 275-287

36. Earls F, Reich W, Jung KG, *et al*: Psychopathology in children of alcoholic and antisocial parents. *Alcohol Clin Exp Res* 1988; 12: 481-487

37. Nordberg L, Rydelius PA, Zetterstrom R: Children of alcoholic parents: health, growth, mental development and psychopathology until school age. *Acta Paediatr* 1993; 82 (Suppl 387): 1-24

38. Hill EM, Nord JL, Blow FC: Young-adult children of alcoholic parents: protective effects of positive family functioning. *Br J Addic* 1992; 87: 1677-1690

39. Clair DJ, Genest M: The Children of Alcoholics Screening Test: reliability and relationship to family environment, adjustment and alcohol-related stressors of adolescent offspring of alcoholics. *J Clin Psychol* 1992; 48: 414-420

40. Roosa MW, Michaels ML, Groppenbacher N, *et al*: Validity of children's reports of parental alcohol abuse. *J Stud Alcohol* 1993; 54: 71-79,119-125

41. Roosa MW, Sandler IN, Gehring M, *et al*: The children of alcoholics, life-events schedule: A stress scale for children of alcohol-abusing parents. *J Stud Alcohol* 1988; 49: 422-429

42. Claydon C: Self Reported alcohol drug and eating disorder problems among male and female collegiate children of alcoholics. *Int J Group Psychother* 1987; 36: 111-116

43. Berkowitz A, Perkins HW: Personality characteristics of children of alcoholics: *J Consult Clin Psychol* 1988; 56: 206-209

44. Adger H Jr, McDonald EM, DeAngelis C: Substance abuse education in pediatrics. *Pediatrics* 1990; 86: 555-560

45. Scheitlin K: Identifying and helping children of alcoholics. *Nurse Practit* 1990; 15: 34-47

46. National Institute of Alcoholism and Alcohol Abuse (NIAA. Alcohol and Health. Fourth Special Report to the US Congress. Washington, DC: U.S. Department of Health and Human Services. (DHHS Pub. No. (ADM) 81-1080) US Government Printing Offices, 1981

47. Gensheimer LK, Roosa MW, Ayers TS: Children's self-selection into prevention programs: Evaluation of an innovative recruitment strategy for children of alcoholics. *Am J Community Psychol* 1990; 18: 707-723

48. Michaels ML, Roosa MW, Gensheimer LK: Family characteristics of children who self-select into a prevention program for children of alcoholics. *Am J Community Psychol* 1992; 20: 663-672

49. Burk JP, Sher KJ: Labeling the child of an alcoholic: negative stereotyping by mental health professionals and peers. *J Stud Alcohol* 1990; 51: 156-163

50. U.S. Preventive Services Task Force: *Guide to Clinical Preventive Services: an Assessment of the Effectiveness of 169 Interventions.* Williams & Wilkins, Baltimore, Md, 1989: 277-286

51. Steering Committee of The College of Family Physicians of Canada; Alcohol Risk Assessment and Intervention Project (ARAI). Mississauga, Ontario, 1994

Table 1: Children of Alcoholics Screening Test

Please check the answers below that best describe your feelings, behavior, and experiences related to a parent's alcohol use. Take your time and be as accurate as possible. Answer all 10 questions by checking either "yes" or "no".

YES	NO		
_____	_____	(1)	Have you ever thought that one of your parents had a drinking problem?
_____	_____	(2)	Have you every lost sleep because of a parent's drinking?
_____	_____	(3)	Did you ever encourage one of your parents to quit drinking?
_____	_____	(4)	Did you ever feel alone, scared, nervous, angry or frustrated because a parent was not able to stop drinking?
_____	_____	(5)	Did you ever argue or fight with a parent when he or she was drinking?
_____	_____	(6)	Did you ever threaten to run away from home because of a parent's drinking?
_____	_____	(7)	Has a parent ever yelled at or hit you or other family members when drinking?
_____	_____	(8)	Have you ever heard your parents fight when one of them was drunk?
_____	_____	(9)	Did you ever protect another family member from a parent who was drinking?
_____	_____	(10)	Did you ever feel like hiding or emptying a parent's bottle of liquor?

From Jones, J.W.: "Children of Alcoholics Screening Test", Chicago, Ill, Camelot Unlimited, 1983.

Children of Alcoholics

MANEUVER	EFFECTIVENESS	LEVEL OF EVIDENCE <REF>	RECOMMENDATION
Routine evaluation for evidence that one or more family members is alcoholic or abusing alcohol	Routine identification of risk by primary caregivers is not effective.	Descriptive survey<15,44> (III)	Insufficient evidence to support either inclusion or exclusion from periodic health examination: decision to examine should be made on other grounds. Evaluation and support recommended to children thought to be at high risk because of burden of suffering (C)
Screening procedures for detection of risk:			
1) The Children of Alcoholics Screening Test (CAST)	1) Effective in discriminating between children of alcoholic and non-alcoholic parents.	1) Cohort studies <17-19,35,39> (II-2)	1) Fair evidence for detection of risk (B)
2) Two screening questions	2) Has not been evaluated	2) Expert opinion<42,43> (III)	2) Insufficient evidence to include or exclude (C)
Screening procedure for management purposes	Insufficient data to evaluate treatment and prevention programs.		Insufficient evidence of treatment efficacy to include or exclude screening and subsequent intervention as a whole package for PHE (C)
Community based groups such as Al-Ateen, Al-Atot	Increased self-esteem and mood states, but behaviour not affected.	Cohort study<9> (II-2)	Insufficient evidence to include or exclude referral to these programs (C)
Curriculum-based or school-based intervention programs	Few comparable populations, programs or outcome measures adequately evaluated.	Cohort surveys <47-49> (II-2)	Insufficient evidence to include or exclude referral to these treatment programs (C)

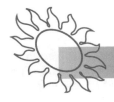

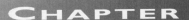

CHAPTER

42

Early Detection and Counselling of Problem Drinking

By Jean L. Haggerty

Early Detection and Counselling of Problem Drinking

Prepared by Jean L. Haggerty, MSc[1]

In 1989 the Canadian Task Force on the Periodic Health Examination concluded that there was fair evidence that routine case-finding for problem drinking, and that brief counselling intervention in patients identified thereby was effective in reducing alcohol consumption and related consequences.[1,2] The studies which yielded this evidence[3,4] have since been confirmed by seven new randomized controlled trials[5-11] in study populations that included both men and women aged 18-60 years. Standardized interviewing strategies and questionnaires are more sensitive than clinical judgement and can be used routinely with all adults to raise the index of clinical suspicion of problem drinking. When problem drinkers are identified, either simple advice or brief counselling is effective in reducing alcohol consumption and diminishing the negative consequences of drinking. The intervention of simple advice or brief counselling is appropriate for the patient with mild to moderate as opposed to severe alcohol dependency. Problem drinking or mild to moderate, rather than severe dependency is the focus of this report. There are separate chapters on Primary Prevention of Fetal Alcohol Syndrome (alcohol consumption among pregnant women – Chapter 5) and Children of Alcoholics (Chapter 41).

Burden of Suffering

Per capita consumption of alcohol in Canada has been steadily decreasing since 1981, and the decrease has been paralleled by a concomitant decrease in rates of mortality from alcoholic liver cirrhosis[12] and other possibly alcohol-related mortality such as suicide, upper gastrointestinal and respiratory cancers, duodenal and stomach ulcers, pneumonia, and accidents. Negative alcohol-related consequences have a dose-response relationship with individual alcohol consumption, and the risk of negative consequences increases dramatically after a threshold of regular consumption of 2-3 drinks/day in males and 1-2 drinks/day in females.

The nomenclature for alcohol-related problems can be confusing. In the literature, the terms alcoholism, alcohol abuse, and severe alcohol dependency are clinical diagnoses by DSM-IIIR criteria

---

[1] Coordinator, Canadian Task Force on the Periodic Health Examination, 1987-89, and Faculty Lecturer, McGill University, Montreal, Quebec

and correspond to an ICD-10 classification[2]. Alcohol consumption patterns (either excessive regular consumption or binge drinking) that put patients at high risk of physical, psychological or social consequences, are termed problem, hazardous, harmful, heavy, or excessive drinking, or mild to moderate alcohol dependency; no internationally-recognized criteria have been developed to classify problem drinking.

Severe alcohol dependency is present in 5-10% of the population, and problem drinking in 15-25%. In medical settings the rate of alcohol-related problems is even higher; routine screening with the instruments reviewed in this report have yielded prevalence rates of severe to mild dependency averaging 25% and as high as 36%.<13> Studies have repeatedly demonstrated that physicians fail to detect the majority of alcohol-related problems in their patients.

In medical settings, the prevalence of problem drinking is estimated to be between 15 and 35%

Maneuver

Case-finding

The traditional medical history-taking questions about average quantity and frequency of alcohol consumption underestimate problem drinking in patients, and the yield is highly dependent on the individual physician, patient, and clinical setting. For this reason, the use of standardized questionnaires or objective measures is generally favored. An exception may occur in patient populations where the prevalence of problem drinking is low, as shown in a screening study of pre-natal patients showing that quantity-frequency questions detected more problem drinkers than either the CAGE or the MAST questionnaires (see below).<14> Another suggested strategy to detect the problem drinker by history-taking is to use the two questions "Have you ever had a drinking problem?" and "Have you had a drink in the last 24 hours?". Positive responses to both yielded no false positives compared to the MAST when used to screen general medicine patients.<13>

The two most extensively validated and commonly used standardized questionnaires are the Michigan Alcoholism Screening Test (MAST) and the four-question CAGE query. The MAST is a 25-item questionnaire that takes 20 minutes to administer; borderline alcoholism is identified by positive responses to at least four of the alcohol-related problem behaviors. Shorter versions of the MAST are generally used, and the instrument has shown sensitivities of 59-100% and specificities of 54-95%.

Standardized questionnaires are currently the most practical, accurate and reliable instruments for screening

The CAGE is a mnemonic for the following questions: 1) ever felt the need to **cut** down on drinking? 2) ever felt **annoyed** by

---

[2] International Classification of Diseases

criticism of drinking? 3) ever had **guilty** feelings about drinking? 4) ever take a morning **eye-opener** drink? It can be easily incorporated into history-taking, and the presence of at least two positive responses in general medicine clinics has been shown to detect alcoholism with sensitivities ranging from 75%-89% and specificities from 68%-96%. Sensitivity and specificity are lower in populations where the prevalence of problem drinking is low,[14] or where problem drinking rather than severe alcohol dependency is the target.

Despite extensive validation, both the CAGE and the MAST have the limitations of being designed to detect severe alcohol dependency as opposed to problem drinking, and the questions are phrased in terms of lifetime occurrence, making it difficult to distinguish between current and previous problems. Neither instrument addresses "binge" drinking behavior, which has been found to be a more sensitive indicator of problem drinking in certain sub-groups such as women and inner-city populations.[15]

A promising screening questionnaire has recently been developed to address these issues. The Alcohol Use Disorders Identification Test (AUDIT, Table 1) is a 10-item questionnaire developed as part of a six-country World Health Organization (WHO) Collaborative Project on Identification and Management of Alcohol-Related Problems.[16] It is designed specifically to detect problem drinkers rather than alcoholics by placing emphasis on heavy drinking and frequency of intoxication rather than signs of dependency. The questions refer to lifetime alcohol experiences as well as those in the past year, thus distinguishing between current and previous problems. Its development in a broad range of cultures is thought to enhance cross-cultural validity, although further research is required to confirm this. In the WHO collaborative project, the sensitivity and specificity across the different countries were fairly consistent, averaging 80% and 98% respectively with a cut-off point of 10/40. It is currently being tested in various countries and sub-populations.

The reference criterion for problem drinking in the AUDIT is based on the expert judgement of the WHO Collaborative Project investigators, and this can reflect only the current knowledge and expert opinion since there are no internationally-recognized criteria to define hazardous drinking. Nonetheless, it appears to address criticisms of the CAGE and MAST effectively, and can be incorporated relatively easily into clinical practice. The yield of standardized instruments in clinical practice is still dependent on a neutral and sensitive approach by the clinician.

No biomarkers with adequate sensitivity or specificity for routine screening have yet emerged. Gamma-glutamyl transferase (GGT) continues to be used by researchers to identify excessive drinkers and to monitor the response to interventions; this, despite its poor sensitivity (40-52%) and specificity (78-89%). In a community sample of men one study found that the GGT was similar to the MAST for detecting problem drinkers, but the sensitivity of 50% is still inadequate for routine screening.<17> While not justified for detection, follow-up measures of GGT may be useful in patients attempting to reduce alcohol consumption. Researchers have also focused on the use of a combination of laboratory and clinical measurements to improve both sensitivity and specificity, but no consensus has emerged on what specific set of measures to use.

Counselling

The common elements in all eight studies of effective early interventions were: feedback to the patient about the results of the screening test, clarification of the association between excessive alcohol consumption and negative consequences, and advice to reduce alcohol consumption. This constitutes the maneuver of simple advice and should take about five minutes in the clinical encounter. Some of the interventions were more intensive and included problem clarification, goal setting, or discussion and/or guidance on how to reduce consumption; this maneuver is brief counselling and would a minimum of 15 minutes. Other components of successful interventions whose relative merit has not been investigated separately are: self-help pamphlets,<4-8> regular follow-up visits,<3,5,6,8,9> and objective laboratory biomarkers.<3,5,9,11>

There appears to be more acceptance in the alcohol treatment community of controlled drinking rather than abstinence as a treatment goal in problem drinkers.<18> Abstinence, however, continues to be the treatment goal in patients with severe alcohol dependency; these patients are generally not amenable to brief counselling interventions and should be referred for specialized treatment.

Effectiveness of Prevention and Treatment

Since the last report of the Task Force<1> several randomized controlled trials have confirmed that routine case-finding and counselling are effective in reducing alcohol consumption and alcohol-related problems in patients.<5-11> Five of the published trials are of good quality: two population-based screening trials which used elevated GGT levels to identify problem drinkers,<3,5> and three which used general health questionnaires and quantity-frequency measures of consumption in primary care populations in a variety of cultural contexts.<6-8>

In the Scandinavian population-based studies the intervention linked the elevated GGT to alcohol consumption; heavy drinkers were advised to reduce alcohol intake, and their progress was monitored regularly until the GGT levels normalized.<3,5> The Nilssen and

Problem drinking, as opposed to severe alcohol dependency, is amenable to a brief counselling intervention

colleagues study also evaluated the relative effectiveness of a second low-intensity intervention in which a more tenuous link was made between GGT levels and alcohol consumption, and subjects were given a pamphlet containing advice on GGT and alcohol consumption; no statistically significant differences were found between the two intervention groups at one-year follow-up. In the Kirstensen and coworkers study, the controls were informed by letter of their elevated GGT result and told to restrict alcohol, whereas no information was given to the controls in the Nilssen and colleagues study. This may account for the finding that in the Kirstensen and coworkers study, that GGT levels decreased significantly in both control and intervention groups, whereas in the Nilssen and colleagues study the statistically significant decrease in GGT levels and self-reported alcohol consumption was observed only in the intervention groups. The Kirstensen and coworkers study did, however, demonstrate a 61% reduction in hospital days and a 50% reduction in mortality in the intervention group after 5 years. The Kirstensen and coworkers study was limited to middle-aged males and a third of the subjects had symptoms of alcohol dependence. The Nilssen and colleagues study excluded alcoholics but included men and women aged 17-62 years; the effect by gender was stated to be homogenous. The limitation of both of these studies is the use of GGT as both a screening device and the principal outcome measure.

Two good quality primary care studies of adults aged 17-69 in the United Kingdom used comparable screening, intervention, and outcome measures.[6,7] Based on an independent two-stage screening procedure (self-administered health questionnaire, interviewer review of one-week drinking diary) patients were considered problem drinkers if males consumed more than 29 drinks per week or females more than 18 per week. Intervention subjects were referred to their general practitioner who gave the patient feedback about their consumption relative to national norms, advised them to reduce alcohol consumption to target levels of moderate drinking, and gave them a self-help pamphlet. Follow-up at one-year demonstrated that in the Wallace and associates study 45% of the intervention group reduced their drinking to target levels compared to 25% in the controls;[6] in the Anderson & Scott study the proportions were 18% and 5% respectively.[7] In the Wallace and associates study, intervention subjects were encouraged to return for at least one and up to 4 monitoring visits during the year and the study population included very heavy drinkers; these may account for the greater reductions in excessive drinking. The authors found that although the intervention was also effective in women, their reductions in reported consumption were not accompanied by reductions in mean GGT levels; the results for women were not reported in the Anderson & Scott study.

The early intervention study of the WHO Collaborative Project on Identification and Management of Alcohol-Related Problems did not use the AUDIT to identify problem drinkers because it was not completed by the initiation of the trial. Instead it used a general health and lifestyle questionnaire and a structures assessment interview to identify problem drinkers.<11> Based on the criteria of ≥ 2 intoxications/month or 29 drinks/week for men and 19 drinks/week for women, 1,559 problem drinkers aged 19-70 years in eight countries (Australia, the United Kingdom, Norway, Mexico, Kenya, the former Soviet Union, Zimbabwe, and the United States) were randomly assigned to either control, simple advice or brief counselling groups. After a 9-month average follow-up in 75% of the patients drinking behavior based on self-report was reduced in all groups, males in both intervention groups showed a significantly greater reduction in typical daily consumption and drinking intensity on the basis of self-report than did the controls. The intervention effect in the much smaller number of women was not statistically significant. There was no statistically significant difference between the simple advice and brief counselling intervention groups.

The results of these studies support the effectiveness of routine identification of problem drinkers and advice to reduce alcohol consumption, although in only one study<3> was the reduction corroborated by decreased morbidity and mortality over a longer period. None of the studies used the standardized screening instruments which have been reviewed in this report. Simple advice was found to be as effective as a brief counselling intervention.<5,11> Several authors suggested that the observed improvement in controls might be attributable to a therapeutic effect of the screening procedure itself. It is not clear whether the results can be generalized to the elderly. The effectiveness in these trials was less pronounced in women,<6,8,11> but a randomized trial of problem drinkers' responsiveness to different interventions showed that women were more likely to achieve problem-free moderate drinking than men.<19>

Recommendations of Others

The U.S. Preventive Services Task Force<20> recommends that all adolescents and adults be asked to describe their use of alcohol, but that routine measurement of biochemical markers not be the primary method of detecting alcohol abuse in asymptomatic persons. All persons who use alcohol, especially pregnant women, should be urged to limit their consumption.

The Alcohol Risk Assessment and Intervention (ARAI) Project of the College of Family Physicians of Canada recommends that all patients age 12 years or older be screened to assess their level of risk drinking, and that patients who drink at potentially problematic or problematic levels be counselled and followed-up to reduce their drinking; and that patients with severe problems be referred to appropriate specialized treatment with periodic follow-up by the primary care physician. The project provides aids for both physicians and patients.[3]

The Institute of Medicine in the United States recommends that all patients be screened for alcohol problems. If mild or moderate problems are detected, a brief counselling intervention should be provided and the patient be periodically monitored. If a severe problem is detected, the patient should be referred for specialized treatment.

Conclusions and Recommendations

Routine active case-finding of problem drinking by physicians is highly recommended on the basis of the high prevalence of this problem in medical practices, its association with adverse consequences before the stage of dependency is reached, and its amenability to a counselling intervention by physicians. Detection by biomarkers is not recommended, although these may be used to confirm clinical suspicions raised by use of the CAGE query, MAST or AUDIT questionnaires, and may be useful for monitoring the patient's progress. Either simple advice or the brief counselling intervention may be used with equal effectiveness in reducing alcohol consumption in problem drinkers. The counselling intervention is probably most effective in the context of an established and effective doctor-patient relationship.

Unanswered Questions (Research Agenda)

The most appropriate detection instruments and counselling interventions for women and the elderly still need to be addressed in well-designed trials. Further validation and use of the AUDIT is required. Broad consensus is required to establish internationally recognized criteria to define problem drinking.

Evidence

The literature was identified with a MEDLINE search for the years 1989 to October 1993 using the MESH headings, "alcoholism" and "alcohol drinking", with the sub-headings "epidemiology", "prevention & control", "therapy", and "rehabilitation". Only original studies reported in English or French were selected.

This review was initiated in August 1993 and the recommendations were approved by the Task force in March 1994.

---

[3] Alcohol Risk Assessment and Intervention Resource Manual for Family Physicians, 1994, College of Family Physicians of Canada, 2630 Skymark Avenue, Mississauga, Ontario, L42 5A4.

Acknowledgements

Assistance was provided by Douglas M.C. Wilson, MD, CCFP, FCFP, Professor, Department of Family Medicine, Faculty of Health Sciences, McMaster University, Hamilton, Ontario, and Martha Sanchez-Craig, PhD, Senior Scientist, Addiction Research Foundation of Ontario, Toronto, Ontario.

Selected References

1. Canadian Task Force on the Periodic Health Examination: The periodic health examination: 2. 1989 Update. *Can Med Assoc J* 1989; 414: 209-216

2. Carbonetto C, Battista RN, Haggerty JL: Early detection and counselling of problem drinkers. In: Goldbloom R, Lawrence RS (eds): *Preventing disease: Beyond the rhetoric*. Springer-Verlag, New York, 1990: 84-91

3. Kristenson H, Öhlin H, Hultén-Nosslin MB, *et al*: Identification and intervention of heavy drinking in middle-aged men: results and follow-up of 24-60 months of long-term study with randomized controls. *Alcohol Clin Exp Res* 1983; 7: 203-209

4. Chick J, Lloyd G, Crombie E: Outcome 1 year after a brief intervention among newly identified problem drinkers with social supports admitted to a general hospital – preliminary results of a controlled study. In: Chang NC, Chao HM (eds): Early identification of alcohol abuse. *National Institute on Alcohol Abuse and Alcoholism, Research Monograph* 1985; 17: 348-353

5. Nilssen O: The Tromso Study: identification of and a controlled intervention on a population of early-stage risk drinkers. *Prev Med* 1991; 20: 518-528

6. Wallace P, Cutler S, Haines A: Randomized controlled trial of general practitioner intervention in patients with excessive alcohol consumption. *Br Med J* 1988; 297: 663-668

7. Anderson P, Scott E: The effect of general practitioners' advice to heavy drinking men. *Br J Addict* 1992; 87: 891-900

8. Babor TF, Grant M (eds): *Project on Identification and Management of Alcohol Related Problems. Report on Phase II: A Randomized Clinical Trial of Brief Interventions in Primary Health Care*. World Health Organization, Geneva, Switzerland, 1992

9. Persson J: Early intervention in patients with excessive alcohol consumption: a controlled study. *Alcohol Alcohol Suppl* 1991; 1: 473-476

10. Elvy GA, Wells JE, Baird KA: Attempted referral as intervention for problem drinking in the general hospital. *Br J Addict* 1988; 83: 83-89

11. Maheswaran R, Beevers M, Beevers DG: Effectiveness of advice to reduce alcohol consumption in hypertensive patients. *Hypertension* 1992; 79-84

12. Mao Y, Morrison H, Johnson RJ, *et al*: Liver cirrhosis mortality and per capita alcohol consumption in Canada. *Can J Public Health* 1992; 83: 80-81

13. Goldberg HI, Mullen M, Ries RK, *et al*: Alcohol counselling in a general medicine clinic. A randomized controlled trial of strategies to improve referral and show rates. *Med Care* 1991; 29(7 Suppl): JS49-JS56

14. Waterson EJ, Murray-Lyon IM: Screening for alcohol-related problem in the antenatal clinic: an assessment of different methods. *Alcohol Alcohol* 1989; 24: 21-30

15. Barret TG, Vaughan-Williams CH: Use of a questionnaire to obtain an alcohol history from those attending an inner city accident and emergency department. *Arch Emerg Med* 1989; 6: 34-40

16. Saunders JB, Aasland OG, Babor TF, *et al*: Development of the Alcohol Use Disorders Identification Test (AUDIT): WHO Collabortive Project on Early Detection of Persons with Harmful Alcohol Consumption – II. *Addiction* 1993; 88: 791-804

17. Vanclay F, Raphael B, Dunne M, *et al*: A community screening test for high alcohol consumption using biochemical and hematological measures. *Alcohol Alcohol* 1991; 26: 337-346

18. Rosenberg H, Melville J, Levell D, *et al*: A 10-year follow-up survey of acceptability of controlled drinking in Britain. *J Stud Alcohol* 1992; 53: 441-446

19. Sanchez-Craig M, Spivak K, Davila R: Superior outcome of females over males after brief treatment for the reduction of heavy drinking: replication and report of therapist effects. *Br J Addict* 1991; 86: 867-876

20. U.S. Preventive Services Task Force: *Guide to Clinical Preventive Services: an Assessment of the Effectiveness of 169 Interventions*. Williams & Wilkins, Baltimore, Md, 1989: 277-286

Table 1:   Alcohol Use Disorders Identification Test (AUDIT)

Scoring[1]:				
0	1	2	3	4
1. How often do you have a drink containing alcohol?				
Never	Monthly or less	Two to four times a month	Two to three times a week	Four or more times a week
2. How many drinks containing alcohol do you have on a typical day when you are drinking?				
1 or 2	3 or 4	5 or 6	7 to 9	10 or more
3. How often do you have six or more drinks on one occasion?				
Never	Less than monthly	Monthly	Weekly	Daily or almost daily
4. How often during the last year have you found that you were not able to stop drinking once you had started?				
Never	Less than monthly	Monthly	Weekly	Daily or almost daily
5. How often during the last year have you failed to do what was normally expected from you because of drinking?				
Never	Less than monthly	Monthly	Weekly	Daily or almost daily
6. How often during the last year have you needed a first drink in the morning to get yourself going after a heavy drinking session?				
Never	Less than monthly	Monthly	Weekly	Daily or almost daily
7. How often during the last year have you had a feeling of guilt or remorse after drinking?				
Never	Less than monthly	Monthly	Weekly	Daily or almost daily
8. How often during the last year have you been unable to remember what happened the night before because you had been drinking?				
Never	Less than monthly	Monthly	Weekly	Daily or almost daily
9. Have you or someone else been injured as a result of your drinking?				
No		Yes, but not in the last year		Yes, during the last year
10. Has a relative or friend, or a doctor or other health worker been concerned about your drinking or suggested you cut down?				
No		Yes, but not in the last year		Yes, during the last year

[1]Cut-off point of 10/40 indicates problem drinking.

Early Detection and Counselling of Problem Drinking

MANEUVER	EFFECTIVENESS	LEVEL OF EVIDENCE <REF>	RECOMMENDATION
Case-finding: Standardized questionnaires and/or patient enquiry **Advice/Brief Counselling:** Clarification of association between alcohol consumption and alcohol-related consequences, advice to reduce consumption	Routine active case-finding followed by simple advice or brief counselling is effective in decreasing alcohol consumption and remediates adverse consequences.	Randomized controlled trials <3-11> (I)	Fair evidence to include routine detection and counselling in periodic health examination (B)

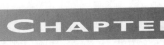

CHAPTER 43

Prevention of Tobacco-Caused Disease

By Mark C. Taylor and Jennifer L. Dingle

Prevention of Tobacco-Caused Disease

Prepared by Mark C. Taylor, MD, FRCSC[1] and Jennifer L. Dingle, MBA[2]

The reduction of tobacco-caused disease is a highly desirable goal for physicians. In 1986 the Canadian Task Force on the Periodic Health Examination recommended counselling for smoking cessation (A Recommendation). This chapter provides an update of evidence on strategies to achieve smoking reduction, again focusing on physician interventions. Smoking among pregnant women is addressed in a separate chapter (see Chapter 3).

Smoking cessation assistance (including nicotine replacement therapy) has been shown to be effective and is recommended. Reducing the number of young people who start smoking is critical but has been less intensively studied. Counselling to prevent smoking initiation is recommended (B Recommendation). There is also evidence to support referrals to other programs after giving cessation advice but insufficient evidence to evaluate counselling to reduce environmental tobacco smoke (ETS). Given the magnitude of the problem, educational programs, counselling and healthy public policies are all vital.

Burden of Suffering

Trends in Smoking

The use of tobacco in Canada has declined gradually since 1965. A November 1992 survey found that 28% of Canadians over the age of 18 were smokers.<1> It is estimated that roughly 6,700 Canadian adolescents start smoking every month.<2> The average age for starting to smoke has been reported to be 11-13 years. A 1986 survey found that 94% of smokers first tried smoking before age 17. The percentage of teenagers aged 15-19 years who smoke regularly (16%) has been cut to about a third of the rate that existed in the late 1970s (47% in 1979). In 1991, there were more regular female (20%) than male (12%) smokers in this age group.

The 1991 survey results from Statistics Canada<3> indicated for the first time that the number of regular female smokers was greater

---

[1] Clinical Fellow, The Toronto Hospital, Toronto, Ontario
[2] Coordinator, Canadian Task Force on the Periodic Health Examination, Department of Pediatrics, Dalhousie University, Halifax, Nova Scotia

than the number of males. The historically higher prevalence of smoking among men is no longer evident. Among women the overall decline in prevalence has been slight from 28% in 1966 to 26% in 1991.

Young women in Canada continue to start smoking at alarming rates

The 1986 Labour Force Survey found that smoking ranged from 18% among professional workers to over 40% among transportation workers and miners. Armed Forces personnel have also been identified as a high risk group; a 1992 study found 53% of junior navy personnel smoked.

By ethnic origin, the highest smoking rates in Canada are found among Canadian Native peoples (59% regular smokers in 1990). In addition to high smoking rates among Native children (51-71%), the high prevalence of use of smokeless tobacco has also been identified as a concern for Native children and other adolescents.

While data on exposure to environmental tobacco smoke (ETS) are limited, a 1991 survey found that 44% of the Canadian work force is exposed to second-hand smoke at work. Such exposure was inversely related to occupational status. Fifty-four percent of Canadian children live in households with at least one smoker, and they are twice as likely to be regular smokers as those who do not live with a smoker.[4]

Health Effects of Smoking

A large body of evidence has accumulated regarding the health effects of smoking. Tobacco use has been consistently linked with a variety of serious pulmonary, cardiovascular and neoplastic diseases. Evaluation of this evidence is beyond the scope of this chapter but detailed reviews[5-7] and estimates of relative risk for the many tobacco associated diseases[8] have been published elsewhere. Likewise, reviews of the evidence regarding the health consequences of ETS are published elsewhere.[9] In 1992 the U.S. Environmental Protection Agency (EPA) named ETS a Group A carcinogen (shown to cause cancer in humans) at typical environmental levels.[10]

Parental smoking is associated with smoking initiation by adolescents.[4] Exposure to smokers in the home may be the single most important factor in determining whether a teenager will smoke. Assistance which physicians provide for adult smokers to quit may have a powerful effect on children in the home.

It has been estimated that there were over 38,000 smoking-attributable deaths in 1989, or 20% of all the deaths in Canada.[8] This resulted in 271,497 potential years of life lost before 75 years of age. The decline in smoking prevalence has played a major role in the reduction of mortality from cardiovascular disease, as well as in projected declines in mortality from lung cancer and chronic obstructive pulmonary disease (COPD).

Health Effects of Smoking Cessation

In his 1990 report, *The Health Benefits of Smoking Cessation*,<11> the U.S. Surgeon General concluded that smoking cessation was highly beneficial. The health benefits of smoking cessation far exceeded any risks from the average 2.3 kg weight gain or any adverse psychological effects that followed quitting.

Tobacco is highly addictive.<12> Over 75% of adult smokers would like to stop and at least 60% have tried to quit at some time in their lives. Approximately one-third of smokers attempt to quit every year. About 20% reported quitting on the first attempt, while 50% succeeded after 6 tries.

In 1986, about 90% of successful quitters and 80% of unsuccessful quitters used individual methods of smoking cessation rather than organized programs; most of these smokers used a "cold turkey" approach. Research on self-help/minimal intervention strategies is ongoing.

Maneuver

Smoking Prevention Counselling

With adolescents, the most effective strategy to discourage smoking may be to concentrate on immediate issues, such as reduced athletic ability, cost, odours and poor appearance.<13> Teenagers can be shown that tobacco advertising falsely suggests that the majority smokes, and that smoking makes one sophisticated and attractive.<14>

Smoking Cessation Counselling and Community Action

The Canadian Consensus on Physician Intervention in Smoking Cessation<15> provides a guide on counselling strategies. While 85-94% of physicians have reported that they discuss smoking or tell most or all smoking patients to quit, U.S. surveys suggest that 43-50% of patients have never been advised to smoke less or to quit by a physician. A small study in Vermont found that only 40% of pediatricians routinely took a smoking history from parents. A 1989 study found that 91% of pediatricians in Maine advised parents who smoke to quit.

Physicians can also refer patients to smoking cessation programs; an inventory of self-help and group programs has recently been published.<16> Health care professionals can also promote non-smoking through a range of consulting and advocacy activities in health care settings as well as through communities, school boards, worksites, governmental agencies, legislatures and the media.

Effectiveness of Prevention

Prevention of Smoking Initiation

Since the 1960s, when tobacco was proven to be the cause of the majority of cases of lung cancer,[5] there have been formal educational programs in schools about the dangers of tobacco use. These programs have been effective in teaching children that tobacco use causes disease[17] but effectiveness in preventing smoking initiation has not been striking to date.[18] The 1994 Report of the U.S. Surgeon General found that in a variety of research studies (including several randomized trials and 4 meta-analyses) social influence programs for students decreased prevalence of smoking by 25 to 60%.[19] The difference persisted from 1 to 4 years. The report concluded that tobacco-use prevention programs that target the larger social environment of adolescents are both efficacious and warranted.

A 4-year cohort study[20] of Peer Assisted Learning (PAL) in Calgary grade 6 students found that the program prevented or delayed smoking initiation in 15% of males ($p<.05$). Its efficacy with females was negligible and the effect on prevention of regular as opposed to experimental smoking was unclear.

The educational programs which seem to show maximal effectiveness are those which emphasize the positive aspects of being smoke-free and promote self-esteem.[21] However, researchers have questioned whether educational programs on their own will ever lead to dramatic reductions in smoking initiation.[22]

When 12 to 17 year old smokers in Nova Scotia[23] were asked who should teach them about the effects of smoking on health, the option chosen by 23% was their family doctor. Also, 19% claimed that they would quit if their doctor so advised them. Several authors have suggested that the physician is strategically placed to advise young people effectively (expert opinion).[24]

The potential benefits in terms of prevention of addiction, the burden of morbidity and mortality for smokers and the effectiveness of counselling with regards to cessation (see below), provide further justification for counselling to prevent smoking initiation among children.

Smoking Cessation

In a 1988 meta-analysis of 39 smoking cessation trials, it was found that cessation rates for unselected patients who receive a clinical intervention average about 6% higher than for control patients after one year.[25] The most effective techniques were those involving more than one modality, that involved both physicians and

Counselling, with or without nicotine replacement therapy, can be effective in encouraging cessation

non-physicians, and that provided the greatest number of motivational messages for the longest period of time.

Nicotine replacement therapy has been found to be useful in many studies. The best results with nicotine chewing gum have been obtained with multi-component programs which have included some counselling and ongoing follow-up and support. In a 1987 meta-analysis by Lam and colleagues,[26] nicotine gum was superior to placebo gum in specialized cessation clinics (1-year abstinence rates of 23% versus 13%). Although nicotine gum was similar to placebo gum in general medical practice (11.4 versus 11.7%), nicotine gum was superior to the no gum control group (9% versus 5%).

Transdermal nicotine patches have been shown to improve 1-year cessation rates by 5-13%, in randomized controlled trials in comparison with placebo patches.[27-29] For the 24-hr patch, systemic side effects and/or withdrawal symptoms were reported in 32% of patch users as opposed to 24% of placebo patch users.[30] Local skin problems were reported by 14-50% of patch users and 0-13% of placebo patch users. Trials involving the 16-hour patch also suggest they may have fewer systemic side effects and local skin problems.[28] A 1994 meta-analysis of randomized controlled trials of nicotine replacement therapies including gum, patches, inhalers and nasal spray, found an overall odds ratio for abstinence with the use of nicotine adjuvants of 1.71 (95% confidence interval (CI): 1.56-1.87).[31] In a second meta-analysis of randomized trials of gum and patches,[32] nicotine 2 mg chewing gum had an overall efficacy of 6% (95% CI: 4%-8%), greater in self-referred subjects (responding to advertisements or attending anti-smoking clinics) than in invited (general practice or hospital patients) subjects (11% versus 3%). Efficacy was found to depend on the extent of dependence on nicotine as assessed by a simple questionnaire – the Fagerström test). It was 16% (7-25%) in "high dependence" smokers, but in "low dependence" smokers there was no significant effect. The 4 mg gum was effective in about 1/3 of "high dependence" smokers and appeared to be the most effective form of replacement therapy for this group. The efficacy of the nicotine patch (9% (6-13%) overall) was less strongly related to nicotine dependence, perhaps because the patch cannot deliver a bolus of nicotine to satisfy craving. While comparable in efficacy to other replacement therapies, the patch offers greater convenience and minimal need for instruction in its use. Other adjuncts to cessation therapy are available, but have undergone less thorough evaluation.

An intensive specific referral to a group smoking cessation program (counselling, videotape with testimonials and telephone call 1 week after referral) has also been shown to increase participation by patients in such programs (from 0.006% for those offered general advice to 11% for the intervention group in a study of 1380 smokers).[33] The authors recommend a brief office-based intervention preceding referral since most patients will not attend a group program.

Efforts to increase physician counselling have had some success. In randomized controlled trials, training, office systems and staff support have been shown to change physician behaviour<34> and doubling of quit rates among patients of physicians who had received training versus "control physicians" has been reported.<35> However, some trials have shown no statistically significant effect on quit rates although training may have had a small beneficial effect.<34,36> A randomized trial involving family physicians from the Hamilton, Ontario area found that 4 additional follow-up visits did not significantly improve cessation rates at 1 year (12.5% versus 10.2%).

While improving the cessation counselling offered by physicians has had mixed results, the evidence in support of counselling is clear. There is good evidence, based on multiple randomized controlled trials, to support cessation counselling and nicotine replacement therapy. Cessation interventions vary considerably in their effectiveness and many of the adjuncts to cessation counselling require further evaluation.

Counselling to Prevent ETS Exposure

A study<37> of a low-intensity physician's office-based strategy (telephone call and letter suggesting changes in household smoking behaviour not including cessation) aimed at reducing infant exposure to ETS was not effective in a study of 103 mother-infant pairs in which the mother smoked 10 or more cigarettes/day. However, the study sample size and drop-out rate was such that a small effect (less than 10% difference in cotinine measurements) could not be identified. Preschool education programs have been shown to create the intent to avoid second hand smoke in children,<38> but no other evidence evaluating the effect of such advice was identified. However, given the burden of suffering and the effectiveness of other counselling, it may be useful to combine counselling to avoid ETS exposure with cessation advice.

Community Action

Physicians have the potential to be highly influential community leaders on issues affecting health. An extensive review of smoking prevention programs concluded that adolescents will only change their behaviour if those changes are consistent with social norms.<39> Interventions must strive to make smoking widely perceived as "deviant behaviour".

Tobacco advertising and sponsorship make smoking appear acceptable and desirable. In countries where advertising has been banned or severely restricted, childhood smoking has declined.<40> In

Counselling and educational programs must be combined with healthy public policies to prevent smoking initiation

Canada, since the introduction of the Tobacco Products Control Act, overall consumption has declined by 17.1%. Smoking among youths aged 15-19 years has declined from 22.5% in 1986 to 16% in 1991.

There is strong evidence that the simplest approach to discouraging smoking initiation by adolescents is to keep the price out of reach. Investigators have found that price increases of the order of 10% lead to short-term reduction of teenage consumption by 14%.<41,42> Recent tobacco tax cuts, unfortunately may help to sustain the tobacco problem in Canada.

Other important strategies include reducing child access to tobacco through effective tobacco retailing restrictions,<43> and bans on smoking in public places. Physician activities as community leaders can have dramatic effects in this area.<44>

Recommendations of Others

The U.S. Preventive Services Task Force<45> recommends that tobacco cessation counselling be offered on a regular basis to all patients who use tobacco. The prescription of nicotine gum is thought of as an appropriate adjunct for some patients. They also recommend that adolescents and young adults who do not currently use tobacco products be advised not to start. Other medical organizations and agencies are consistent in their support of tobacco control measures.

Conclusions and Recommendations

There is good evidence to support counselling for smoking cessation in the periodic health examination of individuals who smoke (A Recommendation). Nicotine replacement therapy can be effective as an adjunct (A Recommendation).

There is fair evidence to support physicians also referring patients to other programs after offering cessation advice (B Recommendation).

There is fair evidence to support counselling to prevent smoking initiation for adolescents (B Recommendation). Educational programs have not been shown to significantly reduce tobacco initiation. Counselling by physicians has not been evaluated but given the burden of disease, the benefits of preventing addiction, the effectiveness of other smoking-related counselling and the support of expert opinion, all children and adolescents should be counselled on avoiding tobacco use.

There is insufficient evidence to evaluate counselling to reduce ETS exposure (C Recommendation) but it may be useful to combine such counselling with cessation advice, again based on the burden of suffering, the potential benefits of the intervention and the effectiveness of cessation advice.

Unanswered Questions (Research Agenda)

Research is needed into effective strategies to prevent teenage smoking initiation, specifically those which physicians can employ. The impact of tobacco industry sponsorship of sports and cultural events on tobacco initiation needs to be addressed.

Evidence

The evidence which forms the basis of this review was gathered from the collections of the authors and also identified using a MEDLINE search for 1988 to August 1993 using the key words: smoking and prevention, smoking cessation, tobacco, clinical trial or meta-analysis, Canada and physician.

This review was initiated in March 1993 and recommendations were finalized by the Task Force in January 1994.

Acknowledgements

The authors would like to thank Ms. Cathy Rudick, Executive Director of Physicians for a Smoke-free Canada, Ottawa, Ontario for reviewing the manuscript and providing research support. The Task Force also thanks Anthony F. Graham, MD, FACC, FACP, FRCPC Cardiology, Associate Professor of Medicine, University of Toronto and Past-President of the Heart and Stroke Foundation of Canada; Michael M. Rachlis, MD, MSc, FRCPC, Assistant Professor, Clinical Epidemiology and Biostatistics, McMaster University, Toronto, Ontario; and Douglas M.C. Wilson, MD, CCFP, FCFP, Professor of Family Medicine, McMaster University, Hamilton, Ontario for their review of the draft manuscript.

Selected References

1. Insight Canada Research: *Smoking in Canada: Warnings, Report on the findings of a nation-wide survey conducted on behalf of The Canadian Cancer Society, The Heart and Stroke Foundation of Canada, and the Canadian Council on Smoking and Health.* November 1992: 4-21

2. Sweanor DT: *The uptake of smoking among youth.* [unpublished] Non-Smokers Rights Association. Ottawa, October 1993

3. Statistics Canada: *General Social Survey, 1991* [Statistical Table 200W], Ottawa, 1993

4. Millar WJ, Hunter L: Household context and youth smoking behaviour: prevalence, frequency and tar yield. *Can J Public Health* 1991; 82: 83-85

5. U.S. Department of Health and Human Services: *Smoking and Health*. Washington, DC, Public Health Service, U.S. Department of Health, Education and Welfare, 1964, Public Health Service Publication No. 1103

6. U.S. Department of Health and Human Services: *Reducing the health consequences of smoking: 25 Years of progress. A report of the Surgeon General*. U.S. Department of Health and Human Services, Public Health Service, Centers for Disease Control, Center for Chronic Disease Prevention and Health Promotion, Office on Smoking and Health. DHHS Publication No.(CDC) 89-8411, 1989a, 703p

7. Stachenko SJ, Reeder BA, Lindsay E, *et al*: Smoking prevalence and associated risk factors in Canadian adults. *Can Med Assoc J* 1992; 146: 1989-1996

8. Collishaw NE, Leahy K: Mortality attributable to tobacco use in Canada, 1989. *Chr Dis Can* 1991; 12: 46-49

9. Spitzer WO, Lawrence V, Dales R, *et al*: Links between passive smoking and disease: a best evidence synthesis. A report of the Working Group on Passive Smoking. *Clin Invest Med* 1990; 13(1): 17-42

10. Office of Health and Environmental Assessment, Office of Research and Development, U.S. Environmental Protection Agency: *Respiratory Health Effects of Passive Smoking: Lung Cancer and Other Disorders*, Washington, DC, Dec 1992 EPA/600/6-90/006F

11. U.S. Department of Health and Human Services: *The health benefits of smoking cessation*. Public Health Service, Centers for Disease Control, Center for Chronic Disease Prevention and Health Promotion, Office on Smoking and Health, Rockville, MD, 1990, DHHS Publication No (CDC) 90-8416

12. Kozlowski LT, Wilkinson A, Skinner W, *et al*: Comparing tobacco cigarette dependence with other drug dependencies. Greater or equal 'difficulty quitting' and 'urges to use', but less 'pleasure' from cigarettes. *JAMA* 1989; 261: 898-901

13. Epps RP, Manley MW: The clinician's role in preventing smoking initiation. *Med Clin North Am* 1992; 76: 439-449

14. Cain JJ, Dudley TE, Wilkerson MK: Tar wars – a community-based tobacco education project. *J Fam Pract* 1992; 34: 267-268

15. *Guide your patients to a smoke free future, a program of The Canadian Council on Smoking and Health*. 1992

16. National Clearinghouse on Tobacco and Health: *Smoking Cessation Programs: An inventory of Self-Help and Group Programs*. Minister of Supply and Services, Canada, 1994 (Catalogue No. H39-296-1994)

17. Dooley DP: A look at the issue of adolescent smoking and prevention: What's happening in Canada. Masters Thesis, Department of Community Health Sciences, University of Calgary, 1990

18. Corbett S, Eaton F: Evaluation of the Peer-assisted Learning (PAL) Smoking Prevention Program – Summary Report. [unpublished] Prepared for Health and Welfare Canada, Ottawa, March, 1986

19. U.S. Department of Health and Human Services: *Preventing tobacco use among young people: a report of the Surgeon General*. U.S. Department of Health and Human Services, Public Health Service, Centers for Disease Control and Prevention, National Center for Chronic Disease prevention and Health Promotion, Office on Smoking and Health, Atlanta, Georgia, 1994

20. Abernathy TJ, Bertrand LD: Preventing cigarette smoking among children: results of a four-year evaluation of the PAL program. *Can J Public Health* 1992; 83(3): 226-229

21. Reid D: Prevention of children's smoking. Proceedings of the Fifth World Conference on Smoking & Health, Winnipeg, 1983; 2: 135-138, Canadian Council on Smoking and Health, Ottawa

22. Kozlowski LT, Coambs RB, Ferrence RG, *et al*: Preventing smoking and other drug use: let the buyers beware and the interventions be apt. *Can J Public Health* 1989; 80: 452-456

23. Freeman A, Mills T, Purcell J, *et al*: *Students and Tobacco: The 1990 Nova Scotia Council on Smoking and Health Student Survey*. NS Ministry of Health, Halifax, 1991

24. Fiore MC, Pierce JP, Remington PL, *et al*: Cigarette smoking: the clinician's role in cessation, prevention and public health. *Disease-a-Month* 1990; 36: 186-242

25. Kottke TE, Battista RN, DeFriese GH, *et al*: Attributes of successful smoking cessation interventions in medical practice: a meta-analysis of 39 controlled trials. *JAMA* 1988; 259: 2882-2889

26. Lam W, Sacks HS, Sze PC, *et al*: Meta-analysis of randomised controlled trials of nicotine chewing-gum. *Lancet* 1987; 2: 27-30

27. Transdermal Nicotine Study Group: Transdermal nicotine for smoking cessation. Six-month results from two multicenter controlled clinical trials. *JAMA* 1991; 266(22): 3133-3138

28. Tønnesen P, Nørregaard J, Simonsen K, *et al*: A double-blind trial of a 16-hour transdermal nicotine patch in smoking cessation. *N Engl J Med* 1991; 325: 311-315

29. Hurt RD, Dale LC, Fredrickson PA, *et al*: Nicotine patch therapy for smoking cessation combined with physician advice and nurse follow-up. One-year outcome and percentage of nicotine replacement. *JAMA* 1994; 271: 595-600

30. Müller P, Abelin T, Ehrsam R, *et al*: The use of transdermal nicotine in smoking cessation. *Lung* 1990; 168 Suppl: 445-453

31. Silagy C, Mant D, Fowler G, *et al*: Meta-analysis on efficacy of nicotine replacement therapies in smoking cessation. *Lancet* 1994; 343: 139-142

32. Tang JL, Law M, Wald N: How effective is nicotine replacement therapy in helping people to stop smoking? BMJ 1994; 308: 21-26

33. Lichtenstein E, Hollis J: Patient referral to a smoking cessation program: who follows through? *J Fam Pract* 1992; 34: 739-744

34. Cummings SR, Richard RJ, Duncan CL, *et al*: Training physicians about smoking cessation: A controlled trial in private practices. *J Gen Intern Med* 1989; 4: 482-489

35. Lindsay E, Wilson D, Best JA, *et al*: A randomized trial of physician training for smoking cessation. *Am J Health Promotion* 1989; 3(3): 11-18

36. Strecher VJ, O'Malley MS, Villagra VG, *et al*: Can residents be trained to counsel patients about quitting smoking? *J Gen Intern Med* 1991; 6: 9-17

37. Chilmonczyk BA, Palomaki GE, Knight GJ, *et al*: An unsuccessful cotinine-assisted intervention strategy to reduce environmental tobacco smoke exposure during infancy. *AJDC* 1992; 146: 357-360

38. Philips BU Jr, Longoria JM, Parcel GS, *et al*: Expectations of preschool children to protect themselves from cigarette smoke: results of a smoking prevention program for preschool children. *J Cancer Educ* 1990; 5: 27-31

39. Becker SL, Burke JA, Arbogast RA, et al: Community programs to enhance in-school anti-tobacco efforts. *Prev Med* 1989; 18: 220-228

40. Government tobacco promotion policies and consumption trends in 33 countries from 1970-1986. *World Smoking & Health* 1990; 15: 15-20

41. Ferrence RG, Garcia JM, Sykora K, *et al*: Effects of pricing on cigarette use among teenagers and adults in Canada 1980-1989. [unpublished] February 1991

42. Lewit EM: U.S. Tobacco Taxes: Behavioural Effects and Policy Implications. *Br J Addiction* 1989; 84: 1217-1234

43. Jason LA, Ji PY, Anes MD, *et al*: Active enforcement of cigarette control laws in the prevention of cigarette sales to minors. *JAMA* 1991; 266: 3159-3161

44. Traynor MP, Begay ME, Glantz SA: New Tobacco Industry Strategy to Prevent Local Tobacco Control. *JAMA* 1993; 270: 479-486

45. U.S. Preventive Services Task Force: *Guide to Clinical Preventive Services: an Assessment of the Effectiveness of 169 Interventions.* Williams & Wilkins, Baltimore, Md, 1989: 289-295

Prevention of Tobacco-Caused Disease

MANEUVER	EFFECTIVENESS	LEVEL OF EVIDENCE <REF>	RECOMMENDATION
Smoking cessation counselling and follow-up visits	Smoking cessation strategies by physicians are effective in reducing the proportion of smokers.	Meta-analysis of randomized controlled trials<25> (I)	Good evidence to support smoking cessation counselling (A); nicotine replacement therapy may be offered as an adjunct (A)
	Nicotine replacement therapy increases cessation rates.	Meta-analysis of randomized trials (gum);<26> randomized trials (patches);<27-29> meta-analysis randomized trials of nicotine replacement therapies<31> (I)	
Referral to smoking cessation programs	Referral by physician improves participation in group programs but majority do not attend.	Randomized controlled trial<32> (I)	Fair evidence to support referral to other validated programs after cessation advice (B)
Counselling to prevent smoking initiation	School-based social influence programs increase knowledge and decrease smoking prevalence by 25-60%; the difference persists 1-4 years.	Overview including meta-analyses of randomized trials and other evidence<19> (I)	Fair evidence to support counselling to prevent smoking initiation for children and adolescents (B)
	Counselling by physicians has not been evaluated but may have a valuable role in preventing addiction.	Expert opinion<19,24,45> (III)	
Counselling to prevent environmental tobacco smoke (ETS) exposure	Telephone and letter contact with mothers in a study with small sample size did not reduce ETS exposure.	Randomized controlled trial<36> (I)	Insufficient evidence to evaluate counselling to reduce ETS exposure (C) but may be useful to combine with cessation counselling
	Preschool education increases intent to avoid ETS.	Comparison of times and places<37> (II-3)	

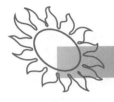

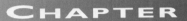

CHAPTER 44

Prevention of Motor Vehicle Accident Injuries

By R. Wayne Elford

Prevention of Motor Vehicle Accident Injuries

Adapted to the Canadian context by R. Wayne Elford, MD, CCFP, FCFP[1] from the 1989 report of the U.S. Preventive Services Task Force<1>

In 1979, the Canadian Task Force on the Periodic Health Examination recommended that physicians attempt to control underlying medical conditions, counsel the disabled, and encourage the use of seat belts by all drivers and passengers (C Recommendation). In 1989, the U.S. Preventive Services Task Force recommended that all individuals be urged to use occupant restraints (safety belts and child safety seats) for themselves and others, to wear safety helmets when riding motorcycles, and to refrain from driving while under the influence of alcohol or other drugs.<1> The Canadian Task Force concurs with these recommendations.

Burden of Suffering

Of the ten industrialized western countries Canada has the fourth highest injury mortality rate (37.5/100,000) and the sixth highest motor vehicle accident (MVA) fatality rate (15.8/100,000). In 1987, the crude fatality rate for males was 18.4/100,000 and 9.6/100,000 for females. Figure 1 displays the fatal injury rate from MVA according to the various age groups. Although the gender curves are of similar shape, the rate for males is consistently almost twice that of females. The risk of motor vehicle crashes is also increased for persons over age 60, but elderly motorists account for only 10% of fatal crashes, primarily because they drive less distance than younger persons.<2> Fatalities are but the tip of the iceberg; Figure 2 displays the nonfatal injury rate for the various age groups. The gender curves closely approximate each other except for the young adult group (19-34 yr). Motor vehicle injuries occur most commonly in males and in persons aged 15-24. This age group has the highest mortality rate and accounts for one-third of all deaths from motor vehicle crashes. Motor vehicle crashes are the leading cause of death in persons aged 5-24; in 1986 they accounted for 38% of all deaths in young persons aged 15-24.<3>

---

[1] Professor and Director of Research and Faculty Development, Department of Family Medicine, University of Calgary, Calgary, Alberta

High Risk Behaviours

The relationship between seatbelt use and the severity of injury is displayed in Figure 3. The rate of seat belt use among those persons fatally injured was considerably less than among those with nonfatal or no injuries from MVAs. The pattern of seatbelt use in Canada closely parallels the introduction of seatbelt legislation in the various provinces. For example, the rate in Alberta rose from 28% in 1986 to 83% in 1988 after the introduction of mandatory seatbelt legislation in July 1987 (Figure 4). About 40% of persons killed in motor vehicle crashes are intoxicated by alcohol.[4] Studies have consistently shown that fatally injured drivers are more likely to have a blood alcohol level of at least 0.10% than are drivers who are not killed. In addition to its role as a risk factor for causing motor vehicle crashes, alcohol intoxication increases the risk of death or serious injury during and after a crash, and can limit the ability of the victim to escape from the vehicle. Alcohol-intoxicated survivors with severe brain injuries appear to have longer hospitalizations and more persistent neurologic impairment than those who were not intoxicated. (For more information on problem drinking consult Chapter 42).

Motor vehicle crashes are the leading cause of death; about 40% of persons killed are intoxicated by alcohol

Medical Impairment

Impaired vision, impaired hearing, decreased flexibility and dexterity, and slowing of information processing capability result in abnormally high accident rates in the elderly when exposure is taken into account.[5] Less than 0.5% of all deaths of elderly people are the result of road accidents, but elderly drivers are over represented in low velocity, property-damage-only collisions. Whether drivers with concomitant medical conditions have excessive motor vehicle accidents is less clear. Most studies show that there is an excess of crashes among drivers whose medical condition is known to Departments of Motor Vehicles compared to drivers not reported to have medical problems.[6] An examination of the driving performance of drivers with selected medical impairments has resulted in the requirement for medically impaired drivers to obtain medical report forms from their physicians, and the development of tables of assigned weights for comorbid conditions. These tables are used by insurance companies and motor vehicle branches to designate different levels of restriction. Practitioners must comply with the obligation to report to the regional Department of Motor Vehicles patients who do not meet the criteria for maintaining a driver's license.

Off Road Vehicles

Most injuries associated with all-terrain vehicles (ATVs) occur when the driver loses control, the vehicle falls over, the driver is thrown from the vehicle, or the vehicle collides with fixed objects such as fences or trees. The 1987 data for numbers of vehicles in use and mortality, without reference to patterns of vehicle use, yielded annual death rates of 1.7/1000 for 3-wheeled and 1.2/1000 for 4-wheeled ATVs.[7] A review of data in 1986 identified 23 deaths and 572 hospitalizations in Quebec. Males accounted for 85% of hospitalizations. Canadian and U.S. studies have revealed the following risk factors: excessive speed, improper apparel and nonuse of helmets, inexperience, and alcohol abuse.[8]

Effectiveness of Prevention Maneuvers

Using occupant protection systems and avoiding driving after drinking significantly decreases the risk of injury or death

The effectiveness of occupant protection systems has been demonstrated in a variety of study designs that include laboratory experiments (using human volunteers, cadavers, and anthropomorphic crash dummies), postcrash comparisons of injuries sustained by restrained and unrestrained occupants, and postcrash judgements by crash analysts regarding the probable effects of restraints had they been used.[9] Based on such evidence it has been estimated that proper use of lap and shoulder belts can decrease the risk of moderate to serious injury to front seat occupants by 45-55% and can reduce crash mortality by 40-50%. When brought to the hospital, crash victims who were wearing safety belts at the time of the crash had less severe injuries, were less likely to require admission, and had lower hospital charges.[10] Airbags are in effect 100% of the time, whereas it is estimated that currently the 3-point seat belt is not worn by 25% of Canadians. Seat belts and airbags are not alternatives – they complement each other. The primary advantage of airbags is that they require no active participation by the occupants of the vehicle. High risk groups, in light-trucks and in rural areas are particularly vulnerable because of their lower rate of seat belt usage. The overall safety benefit of the combination of lap-shoulder belt and airbag system use has not yet been determined from field accident data, however, estimates based on the analysis of fatal crashes involving belted front seated occupants, a potential additional fatality prevention of 3-5% when a combination lap-shoulder belt and airbag system is used.[11] Child safety seats also appear to be effective. It has been reported that unrestrained children are over 10 times as likely to die in a motor vehicle crash than are restrained children,[12] although these data come from studies with important design limitations. Other studies suggest that child safety seats can reduce serious injury by 67% and mortality by 71%. Child restraints may also reduce noncrash injuries to child passengers by preventing falls both within and out of the vehicle. By wearing safety helmets, persons who operate or ride on motorcycles or ATVs can reduce their risk of injury or death from head trauma in the event of a crash. In regions where their use is required by law, such helmets have been shown to reduce mortality by about 30%. Head injury rates are reduced by about 75% among motorcyclists who wear safety helmets.[13] Regions that have repealed mandatory motorcycle helmet laws have experienced significant increases in motorcycle fatalities.

Effectiveness of Counselling

There is a paucity of information from clinical studies on the ability of physicians to influence patients to refrain from driving while intoxicated. Similarly, there have been few studies examining the effectiveness of physician counselling to use safety belts.<14> The strongest evidence that clinician counselling can be effective comes from programs that have encouraged parents to use infant safety seats before the practice became widely mandated by law. Results from such programs suggest that significant short-term improvements are possible immediately after newborns are discharged, but the effect is rarely maintained for more than a few months.<15> A controlled trial without randomization found that the combined intervention of pediatrician counselling, a prescription for an infant restraint, and a pamphlet on crash protection was associated with increased correct use of infant safety seats as assessed at the first two monthly well-baby visits. A small randomized study demonstrated that a "loaner seat" and instruction provided by a nurse resulted in increased use after two to four weeks. The same researchers in a subsequent trial found that a comprehensive hospital program combined with recent state legislation was effective in improving correct usage, but intensive counselling from pediatricians and nurses was of no additional benefit. Another controlled study found that personal discussion was of limited value; a subgroup receiving free infant restraints and literature demonstrated slightly higher correct usage at discharge, but there was no significant difference between the groups in two to four months. Finally, another study found that pediatrician counselling resulted in an immediate increase in safety belt use, but there was no difference in usage rates between the study group and controls at one-year follow-up.<16>

Recommendations of Others

The use of safety belts and child safety seats is widely recommended by organizations and agencies concerned with injury prevention. Child safety seats are required by law in all 50 states and all 10 Canadian provinces. Mandatory safety belt laws are in effect in most states and all the provinces of Canada. Recommendations specifically urging physicians to counsel patients to use occupant restraints have been issued by a number of organizations, including the Canadian Medical Association, the College of Family Physicians, and the National Highway Traffic Safety Administration. The Canadian Medical Association has made recommendations on a wide range of vehicle safety standards – restraint systems, running lights, motorcycle helmets, mopeds, all-terrain vehicles, minivans and light trucks; and supports legislation aimed at decreasing the incidence of drinking and driving. General Council resolutions have also been made regarding airbags and elimination of seat belt use exemptions for police officers and taxi drivers. The American Academy of Pediatrics also recommends counselling adolescents to abstain from intoxicants when driving; advising parents and children to discuss the proper use of alcohol at teen parties; and suggesting alternatives to driving while intoxicated or riding in a vehicle operated by an intoxicated driver.<17>

Conclusions and Recommendations

Counselling should be targeted towards high-risk groups: young adult males, persons who use alcohol or with medical impairments

There is good (grade I) evidence that persons who use occupant protection<9,10> and avoid driving while intoxicated<4,18> are at significantly decreased risk of injury or death from motor vehicle accidents. There is fair (grade II-2) evidence that wearing safety helmets when operating/riding motorcycles or all-terrain vehicles reduces the risk of accidental injury or death.<7,8> Expert opinion (grade III) suggests that many patients seen by clinicians could benefit from counselling to modify their behaviours as drivers and passengers in motorized vehicles.<15> Since motor vehicle crashes represent a leading cause of death and nonfatal injury, even modest successes through clinical interventions could have major public health value. In actual practice, however, it is not known how effectively clinicians can alter these behaviours. Counselling is most relevant for those at increased risk of motor vehicle injury, such as adolescents and young adults, persons who use alcohol or other drugs, and patients with medical conditions that may impair motor vehicle safety.<5> The optimal frequency for counselling patients about motor vehicle injury has not been determined and is left to clinical discretion.

Unanswered Questions (Research Agenda)

Ideally, the effectiveness of physician counselling concerning a number of efficacious practices related to the prevention of motor vehicle accident injuries should be evaluated. However, because many of the preventive maneuvers have become widely mandated by law, the evidence that clinician counselling can influence patient behaviour concerning these practices is unlikely to be defined.

Evidence

The Medline search strategy for this review identified articles for the years 1981-1991 using the following MESH headings:

1. Motor Vehicle,

2. Accident Prevention,

3. Primary Care Physician,

and produced 151 citations. The U.S. Preventive Services Task Force 1989 report[1] was used extensively and a number of their references were retained in the selected bibliography.

This review was initiated in June 1991 and recommendations were finalized in November 1992. A technical report with a full reference list dated February, 1993 is available upon request.

Selected References

1. U.S. Preventive Services Task Force: *Guide to Clinical Preventive Services: an Assessment of the Effectiveness of 169 Interventions.* Williams & Wilkins, Baltimore, Md, 1989: 315-320

2. *1987 Traffic Accident Injury Reporting (TRAID) System dataset.* Laboratory Centre for Disease Control, Health and Welfare Canada, Ottawa

3. Conn JM: Deaths from motor vehicle-related injuries, 1978-1984. *MMWR CDC Surveill Summ* 1988; 37: 5-12

4. Waller PF, Stewart JR, Hansen AR, *et al*: The potentiating effects of alcohol on driver injury. *JAMA* 1986; 256: 1461-1466

5. Evans L: Older driver involvement in fatal and severe traffic crashes. *J Gerontol* 1988; 43: S186-S193

6. Waller JA: Medical impairment and highway crashes. *JAMA* 1969; 208(12): 2293-2296

7. DeLisle A: Characteristics of three- and four-wheeled all-terrain vehicle accidents in Quebec. *Accid Anal Prev* 1988; 20: 357-366

8. Rodgers GB: The effectiveness of helmets in reducing all-terrain vehicle injuries and deaths. *Accid Anal Prev* 1990; 22(1): 47-58

9. Newman RJ: A prospective evaluation of the protective effect of car seatbelts. *J Trauma* 1986; 26(6): 561-564

10. Orsay EM, Turnbull TL, Dunne M, *et al*: Prospective study of the effect of safety belts on morbidity and health care costs in motor vehicle accidents. *JAMA* 1988; 260: 3598-3603

11. Viano DC: Limits and challenges of crash protection. *Accid Anal Prev* 1988; 20(6): 421-429

12. Margolis LH, Wagenaar AC, Liu W, *et al*: The effects of a mandatory child restraint law on injuries requiring hospitalization. *Am J Dis Child* 1988; 142: 1099-1103

13. Chenier TC, Evans L: Motorcyclist fatalities and the repeal of mandatory helmet wearing laws. *Accid Anal Prev* 1987; 19: 133-139

14. Kelly RB: Effect of a brief physician intervention on seat belt use. *J Fam Pract* 1987; 24: 630-632

15. Reisinger KS, Williams AF, Wells JK, *et al*: Effect of pediatricians' counselling on infant restraint use. *Pediatrics* 1981; 67: 201-206

16. Macknin ML, Gustafson C, Gassman J, *et al*: Office education by pediatricians to increase seat belt use. *Am J Dis Child* 1987; 141: 1305-1307

17. American Academy of Pediatrics, Committee on Adolescence: Alcohol use and abuse: a pediatric concern. *Pediatrics* 1987; 79: 450-453

18. McCarroll JR, Haddon W Jr: A controlled study of fatal automobile accidents in New York City. *J Chronic Dis* 1962; 15: 811-826

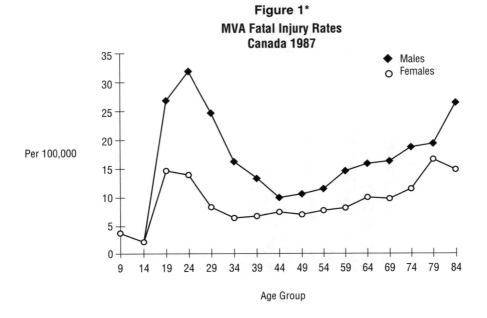

Figure 1*
MVA Fatal Injury Rates
Canada 1987

Per 100,000

Age Group

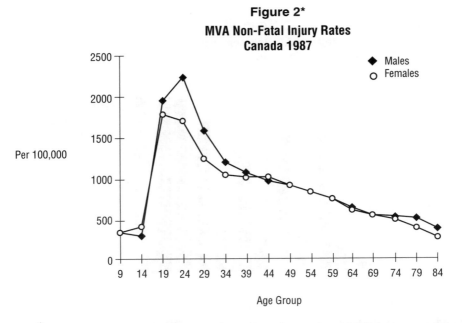

Figure 2*
MVA Non-Fatal Injury Rates
Canada 1987

Per 100,000

Age Group

*(Derived from: Traffic Accident Injury Reporting System (TRIAD) dataset. Laboratory Centre for Disease Control, Health and Welfare Canada; 1980's statistics, 1990 statistics not yet available at time of press.)

Figure 3*
Relationship Between Seatbelt use and Severity of Injury
Canada 1987

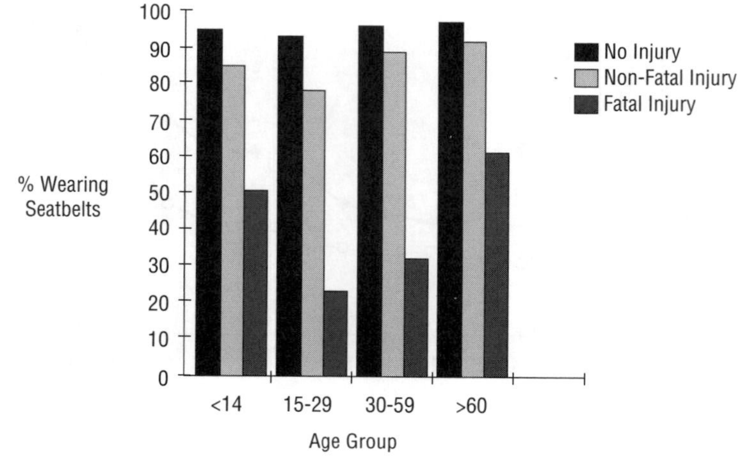

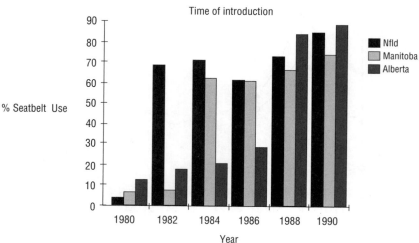

Figure 4*
Relationship Between Legislation and Seatbelt Use

* (Derived from: Traffic Accident Injury Reporting System (TRIAD) dataset. Laboratory Centre for Disease Control, Health and Welfare Canada; 1980's statistics, 1990 statistics not yet available at time of press.)

Prevention of Motor Vehicle Accident Injuries

MANEUVER	EFFECTIVENESS	LEVEL OF EVIDENCE <REF>	RECOMMENDATION
Use of seatbelt and/or child restraints			
a) legislation	Occupant protection systems reduce risk of motor vehicle accident (MVA) injury by 40-50%.	Controlled trials without randomization<9,10> (II-1)*	Good evidence to implement (A)
b) individual counselling	Physician can significantly influence short-term improvement in use of restraints among patients.	Comparisons between times and places<14,15> (II-3)	Fair evidence to include (B)
Use of helmet when riding motor-cycle or all-terrain vehicles			
a) legislation	Safety helmets reduce the risk of death or serious injury by more than 30%.	Cohort analytic studies<8,13> (II-2)	Fair evidence to implement (B)
b) individual counselling	Little information about ability of physician to influence patients to use helmets.	Expert opinion (III)	Insufficient evidence to include or exclude (C)
Do not drink and drive			
a) legislation	Alcohol intoxication increases risk of death and/or serious injury during and after a MVA.	Controlled trials without randomization<4,18> (II-1)	Good evidence to implement (A)**
b) individual counselling	Little information about ability of physicians to influence patients to refrain from drinking and driving.		Insufficient evidence to include or exclude (C)

* supplemented by randomized controlled trials (RCTs) using anthropomorphic crash dummies and/or simulations<9>

** an RCT can never be done and the existing evidence is compelling

(Continued on next page)

Prevention of Motor Vehicle Accident Injuries (concl'd)

MANEUVER	EFFECTIVENESS	LEVEL OF EVIDENCE <REF>	RECOMMENDATION
Monitor patient for medical impairment	Excess of crashes among persons with medical impairment.	Descriptive studies and expert opinion<5,11> (III)	Insufficient evidence to include or exclude (C)

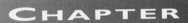

Prevention
of Household
and Recreational
Injuries in Adults

By R. Wayne Elford

Prevention of Household and Recreational Injuries in Adults

Prepared by R. Wayne Elford, MD, CCFP, FCFP[1]

In the 1979 Canadian Task Force report, home and recreational injuries<1> were acknowledged to constitute an important proportion of accidents.[2] At that time there was insufficient literature on the subject to justify a recommendation on scientific grounds. While there is currently fair evidence upon which to implement some legislative measures, there remains insufficient evidence to clarify the effectiveness of individual counselling by physicians (C Recommendations). Three other chapters deal with unintentional injuries in children (Chapter 28), the elderly (Chapter 76), and those due to motor vehicle accidents (Chapter 44).

Burden of Suffering

Injuries are the second highest cause of "potential years of life lost" before 65 years of age in Canada

Approximately 9,000 Canadians die annually of unintentional injuries, about 5% of all deaths. This review focuses on the seven leading causes of death from household and recreational injuries, namely, falls (21%), drownings (6.4%), burns and fire-related injuries (4.8%), suffocation (4.7%), poisonings (4.7%), bicycle/sports-related deaths (1.7%), and firearms (0.7%).<2> Because many of these injuries occur in the younger age groups the societal burden due to loss of productive years from prolonged dependency due to disabilities, and due to acute care (7.9% of all hospital days), is considerable. In 1989 injuries were the second highest cause of potential years of life lost (PYLL) before 65 years of age in Canada. The impact of these injuries is felt far beyond the injured person; family members, employers, health care systems and the community are affected. The individual and family burden of suffering is large in comparison to other types of unintentional injury because third party insurance is seldom in effect, and many of the financial obligations must be borne directly. Injury is probably the most under-recognized major public health problem facing the nation today, and the study of injury presents unparalleled opportunities for reducing morbidity and mortality and for realizing significant savings in both financial and human terms – all in return for a relatively modest investment.<3> Table 1 summarizes the mortality and morbidity rates for various types of adult injury. A brief

---

[1] Professor, Director of Research and Faculty Development, Department of Family Medicine, University of Calgary, Calgary, Alberta

[2] "Unintentional injury" is more appropriate than "accident" in terms of terminology, however, many articles in the literature still use the term "accidental".

description of the risk factors associated with each of the leading causes of unintentional injury in adults follows.

Falls

There were 2,100 deaths due to falls in 1988.<2> Falls were second only to motor vehicle traffic accidents among the leading causes of accidental death in Canada and were by far the leading cause of hospitalization for treatment of accidental injuries. Female exceeded male deaths, and falls resulting in serious injury or death were much more frequent among those aged 55 and over.<4>

Drowning

429 Canadians drowned in 1987, including 135 in boating accidents. Nearly one-quarter of drowning victims were youths 15-24 years of age. Drowning-site profiles varied by age and sex but also by climate and the accessibility of natural bodies of water and pools. Contributing factors were inability to swim, swimming outside patrolled areas, unfamiliarity with the beaches, pre-existing medical conditions and consumption of alcohol.<5> A review of Ontario coroners' reports showed that the young adolescent male was at particular risk of drowning. Among 263 deaths by drowning for young adults, males outnumbered females 3 to 1 and alcohol and/or drugs were detected in nearly 20% of victims.<6> For more information on problem drinking consult Chapter 42. In deaths involving boats, canoes and sail boats, only 25% of the drowning victims were wearing a personal flotation device or life-jacket. Diving, surfing and water skiing also account for a portion of spinal injuries.

Burns, Scalds and Fire-Related Deaths

There were 402 deaths among Canadians caused by fire and flames in 1988.<2> In 1987 there were 30,735 residential fires in Canada (including hotels), causing property damage of $382 million. Studies from the early 1980s indicated that cigarette smoking was associated with about half of residential fire deaths. The number of residential fires has declined continuously since 1980. This reduction in fires has been attributed to better education, more widespread use of smoke detectors, and fewer people smoking.<7>

Poisoning

Of the 424 fatal poisonings in Canada in 1987, most were by drugs and medications (58%); 23% were by solid and liquid substances, and 19% by gases and vapours.<4> Thirty-one percent were among persons aged 25-34;<4> the majority of these deaths (particularly where drugs and medication are involved) would be self-inflicted.

Canadian poison control centre data indicates that in 1986 there were 103,459 poisoning cases and 365 deaths (a 0.35% case fatality rate).<8>

Suffocation

Almost two-thirds of the 415 Canadian deaths by suffocation in 1987 resulted from inhalation and aspiration of food; 62% were in adults over 55 years of age.<4>

Bicycle and Other Sports-Related Injuries

There were 139 fatal pedal cycle injuries in Canada in 1987 and 86% of the casualties were male.<4> In a Calgary study, 67% of 107 patients hospitalized for bicycle-associated injuries had craniocerebral trauma; 20% overall involved a collision between bicycle and automobile.<9> Contusions, abrasions, open and crushing wounds and fractures were also common. Another study found that the most common sports and leisure activities resulting in death between 1982-88, were swimming (152 deaths), horse riding (117 deaths), motor sports (95 deaths), air sports (92 deaths among adults) and fishing (86 deaths). When the number of participants and hours of activity were taken into account, air sports, mountaineering, motor sports and horse riding were found to be the most hazardous activities – 10 to 100 times more hazardous than ball games or water sports.<10>

Firearms

There were 60 deaths by firearms in Canada each year in 1987 and 1988.<4> Elevated mortality rates for males aged 15-24 were documented in a study that found almost one-third of unintentional shooting deaths were hunting-related and that young hunters appeared to be at greatest risk of injury. There is some evidence (grade III) that keeping guns in the home unloaded and locked away reduces unintentional deaths among children.<11>

Alcohol and Drug Use in Association With Injury

Several studies from different countries have demonstrated that alcohol is an important contributing factor in many injury deaths, especially among adults. Higher proportions of positive alcohol readings occurred among home accident victims ($p<.001$) than among a comparison group of accident patients admitted to the same Boston hospital emergency service. Approximately half of several thousand deaths by drowning reviewed by autopsy in Auckland, Sacramento County, Baltimore, and Geelong, Australia showed evidence of alcohol consumption.<12>

Effectiveness of Prevention Maneuvers

During the past decade numerous descriptive studies concerning home and recreational injuries have been published. More important however, is the steady stream of experimental and quasi-experimental studies demonstrating that unintentional injury and death are not random, unpredictable events, but are predictable and preventable[13] and must be looked upon as being a disease whose prevention must be approached scientifically. One model for organizing preventive measures for unintentional injury and death is the Haddon Matrix,[14] named after a leading thinker in injury control. Three widely adopted approaches to interventions for accidental injury arising from this model are described in greater detail; namely, public health education, environmental legislation, and individual counselling.

Unintentional injury and death are not random, unpredictable events: they are predictable and preventable

(i) *Public Health Education* – Health professionals who wish to direct their efforts toward a major cause of death can give effective leadership to programs to prevent drowning by counselling patients that alcohol increases the hazard of water sports.[12] The well known dictum "do not drink and drive" also applies to water recreational activity in the modification, "do not drink and dive."

(ii) *Legislative/Environmental* – As influential as physicians may be with patients, they can have a far greater impact on promoting home safety by discussions with legislators, who in turn can modify the environment through building codes and safety legislation (see Table 2, Chapter 76 on Injuries in the Elderly). For example, barriers, bicycle paths and other design features that separate the cyclist from traffic and pedestrians or remove through-traffic are effective measures for reducing bicycle-related injuries.[15] In general, modifying the environment appears to be more effective than trying to change human behaviour.

(iii) *Individual Counselling* – While the evidence that physician counselling is effective in preventing injuries is inconclusive in some areas, minor reductions in injury rates would have major public health benefits. The evidence for these activities will be presented sequentially for each major type of home and recreational injury in adults.

Burns and Fire-Related Injuries

Smoke and carbon monoxide rather than heat or flame are generally responsible for fire-related deaths. Use of smoke detectors alone could reduce the residential fire fatality rate by about 50%. The relative risk of residential fire death rate in homes without a smoke detector relative to that in homes with one has been reported at 2.0–2.5.[16] Residential sprinklers are about 20 times more expensive but control the fire and concentration of combustion products so that those with poor mobility may not need to escape.

Suffocation

A review of before and after studies of programs teaching the Heimlich maneuver were reported to have resulted in 10-45% reductions in choking deaths.[17] The 1985 *Health Promotion Survey* in Canada found that only 34% of respondents indicated they knew how to administer CPR and/or the Heimlich maneuver.

Bicycle and Sports-Related Injury

A case-control study of injuries among bicycle riders experiencing crashes in greater Seattle showed that safety helmets reduced the risk of head injury by 85% (odds ratio 0.15; 95% confidence interval (CI): 0.07-0.29) and of brain injury by 88% (odds ratio 0.12; 95% CI: 0.04-0.40).[18] These results are confounded by the fact that those who choose to wear helmets would tend to have a different overall attitude toward safety; however, the physics of crashing suggest that helmet wearing is advisable.[19] In a survey of 894 South Australian bicycling enthusiasts, 197 had crashed and struck their head or helmet within the previous 5 years; a significant association was found between helmet use and reduced severity of head injury ($p<0.005$) which persisted ($p<0.05$) after adjustment for crash severity. Based on a cohort of 100 consecutive head injuries in Portsmouth, it was estimated that the wearing of safety helmets would prevent at least half of the minor head injuries and reduce the seriousness of major injuries sustained in cycle accidents.

Although bicycle helmets have been shown to reduce the rate of head and brain injuries from bicycle mishaps, the use of helmets is still uncommon. Educational programs promoting helmet use have shown no impact on the proportion of helmet wearers in a school age population.[20] Helmet design, peer pressure, lack of availability, and cost have been found to be reasons for non-use.

Alcohol and Substance Abuse Intervention for Prevention of Injuries

Alcohol testing and history taking in all cases of accidental injury has been suggested. When alcohol and/or other drugs are implicated in an injury, a number of expert groups have recommended that the connection should be authoritatively communicated to the patient with follow-up to self-help groups. This strategy is based on preliminary evidence that an appeal to fear fortifies adolescent intentions to eschew alcohol. The effectiveness of counselling regarding substance abuse to reduce recreational injury rates has not been evaluated.

Recommendations of Others

The "Year 2000 Injury Control Objectives for Canada" recommend that individual counselling be targeted particularly towards high-risk groups; namely, families with young children, the socio-economically disadvantaged, aboriginal people, situations where alcohol and/or substance abuse is suspected, and the elderly living alone.[21]

The American Academy of Pediatrics, based on expert opinion, makes the following recommendations concerning bicycle helmet use:[22]

1. Physicians should inform parents and patients of the importance of wearing bicycle helmets and the dangers of riding without a helmet.

2. Retail outlets should be urged to carry approved, inexpensive helmets that are available at the time of purchase of the bicycle.

3. The Consumer Product Safety Commission should develop mandatory, uniform safety standards for bicycle helmets.

4. Coalitions of physicians, parents, and community leaders should be encouraged to develop and support community-based programs to promote bicycle safety and helmet usage.

5. The popular media should be urged to depict the helmeted bicycle rider on television, in advertisements and in promotional materials.

The Technical Study Group on Fire Safety, in its report to the U.S. Congress (1987) advocated decreasing the number of cigarette smokers, flame retardant sleepwear and promotion of self-extinguishing cigarettes and matches as means to decreasing fire related injuries and deaths.

In 1989, the U.S. Preventive Services Task Force recommended the following: "Patients who use alcohol or other drugs should be warned against engaging in potentially dangerous activities while intoxicated. It may be clinically prudent to provide counselling on other measures to reduce the risk of unintentional household or environmental injuries from falls, drowning, fires or burns, poisoning, bicycle collisions, sports and firearms."[23]

Conclusion and Recommendations

There is fair evidence (grade II-2) that bicycle helmet use for those who ride the roadways reduces the rate of head injury and death[19] (B Recommendation). There is fair evidence

Counselling should be targeted towards high/risk groups: socio-economically disadvantaged, aboriginal people, where alcohol use is suspected, and elderly living alone

(grade II-2) that not drinking while being involved in water recreational activities reduces the rate of drowning among young adults<12> (B Recommendation). There is some evidence (grade III) that keeping guns in the home unloaded and locked away reduces unintentional deaths among children<11> (C Recommendation). There is some evidence (grade III) that adults learning the Heimlich maneuver can reduce deaths due to suffocation (C Recommendation). Expert opinion (grade III) evidence suggests that many patients seen by clinicians could potentially benefit from counselling to modify their accident prone behaviors. In actual practice, however, it is not known how effectively clinicians can alter these behaviors. Since unintentional injuries represent a leading cause of death and nonfatal injury, even modest successes through clinical interventions could have major public health value. Counselling is most relevant for those at increased risk of injury, such as adolescents and young adults, persons who use alcohol or other drugs. The optimal frequency for counselling patients about unintentional injury has not been determined and is left to clinical discretion.

Unanswered Questions (Research Agenda)

The Haddon Matrix for generating countermeasures provides a model for planning research. Most of the "energy vector" and "physical environment" aspects involve environmental design/engineering. Improving post-event performance is the domain of both formal and informal health care delivery systems. Provincial, regional, and local health care delivery effectiveness must constantly be assessed by quality assurance methods, and areas of poor performance must be addressed. An example of this process is the setting of the Year 2000 Injury Control Objectives.<15,21> The "social environment" sector is primarily the jurisdiction of the political/legislative institutions in our society but is greatly influenced by public pressure. The norms, values, and laws of our society must be constantly re-evaluated and revised as a better understanding of the balance between individual and corporate rights/privileges is derived. The "human" sector presents a major challenge for behavioral medicine (e.g., medication prescribing practices in the elderly). Much remains to be learned about lifestyle patterns and behaviour change strategies. It is in this last area that individual practitioners spend most of their time and energy. The "timing" of health education messages, the effectiveness of different motivational techniques, the counselling skills required by health care providers, and the most conducive atmosphere for anticipatory care, all require further elucidation.

Evidence

This review deals with household and recreational injuries without considering occupational or aviation related injuries. These limitations were incorporated in the MEDLINE search strategy: accidents as a major MESH heading under the subheadings diagnosis, economics, epidemiology, law and jurisprudence, mortality, prevention and control, standards and trends; and not aviation, occupational or traffic accidents. References were identified for the years 1981 – November 1992. Other sources included Statistics Canada, Health and Welfare Canada, the Insurance Bureau of Canada.

This review was initiated in January 1991 and recommendations were finalized by the Task Force in June 1993.

Selected References

1. Canadian Task Force on the Periodic Health Examination: The periodic health examination. *Can Med Assoc J* 1979; 121: 1193-1254

2. Statistics Canada, Canadian Centre for Health Information: Causes of death 1988. (Catalogue No. 82-003S). Minister of Supply and Services Canada. Health Reports 1990; 2(1 Suppl 11): 146-185

3. Division of Injury Control, Center for Environmental Health and Injury Control, Centers for Disease Control: Childhood injuries in the United States. *Am J Dis Child* 1990; 144: 627-646

4. *Canada Safety Council: Accident Fatalities, Canada 1987.* Canada Safety Council 1988: 1-26

5. Plueckhahn VD: Alcohol consumption and death by drowning in adults, a 24-year epidemiological analysis. *J Stud Alcohol* 1982; 43: 445-452

6. MacLachlan J: Drownings, other aquatic injuries and young Canadians. *Can J Public Health* 1984; 75: 218-222

7. *Insurance Bureau of Canada: Facts.* 17th Edition. December 1989: 14-17

8. Health and Welfare Canada: Poison Control Statistics, 1986, published by authority of the Minister of National Health and Welfare

9. Guichon DMP, Myles ST: Bicycle injuries: one-year sample in Calgary. *J Trauma* 1975; 15: 504-506

10. Avery JG, Harper P, Ackroyd S: Do we pay too dearly for our sport and leisure activities? An investigation into fatalities as a result of sporting and leisure activities in England and Wales, 1982-1988. *Public Health* 1990; 104: 417-23

11. Wintemute GJ, Kraus JF, Teret SP, *et al*: Unintentional firearm deaths in California. *J Trauma* 1989; 29: 457-461

12. Wintemute GJ, Kraus JF, Teret SP, *et al*: The epidemiology of drowning in adulthood: implications for prevention. *Am J Prev Med* 1988; 4: 343-348

13. Francescutti LH, Saunders LD, Hamilton SM: Why are there so many injuries? Why aren't we stopping them? *Can Med Assoc J* 1991; 144(1): 57-61

14. Haddon W Jr: Advances in the epidemiology of injuries as a basis for public policy. *Public Health Rep* 1980; 95: 411-421

15. Viano DC: A blueprint for injury control in the United States. *Public Health Rep* 1990; 105: 329-333

16. McLoughlin E, Marchone M, Hauger L, *et al*: Smoke detector legislation: it's effect on owner-occupied homes. *Am J Public Health* 1985; 75: 858-862

17. Day, R, Crelin, E, Dubois A: Choking: The Heimlich abdominal thrust vs backblows: an approach to measurement of inertial and aerodynamic forces. *Pediatrics* 1982; 70: 113-119

18. Thompson DC, Thompson RS, Rivara FP: Incidence of bicycle-related injuries in a defined population. *Am J Public Health* 1990; 80: 1388-1390

19. Thompson RS, Rivara F, Thompson DC: A case-control study of the effectiveness of bicycle safety helmets. *N Engl J Med* 1989; 320: 1361-1367

20. Morris BA, Trimble NE: Promotion of bicycle helmet use among schoolchildren: a randomized clinical trial. *Can J Public Health* 1991; 82: 92-94

21. Saunders LD (ed): Injury Control Objectives for Canada. Recommendations from National Working Group, May 1991 Proceedings

22. American Academy of Pediatrics Committee on Accident and Poison Prevention: Bicycle helmets. *Pediatrics* 1990; 85: 229-230

23. U.S. Preventive Services Task Force: *Guide to Clinical Preventive Services: an Assessment of the Effectiveness of 169 Interventions*. Williams & Wilkins, Baltimore, Md, 1989: 321-329

Table 1 :   Canadian Mortality and Morbidity Rates for Unintentional Injury in 1989[1]
(per 100,000 – standardized to 1971 population)

| | Overall (0-85+ yr) | | | | Adult (15-64 yr) | | | |
| | Mortality | | Morbidity | | Mortality | | Morbidity | |
	M	F	M	F	M	F	M	F
Falls	6.77	4.16	425.0	384.0	3.08	.74	296.2	204
Drownings	2.31	.63	2.78	1.38	2.46	.44	1.68	.51
Burns/Fire related	2.11	.91	11.52	4.23	2.03	.73	11.60	3.56
Poisonings	1.88	.90	38.84	35.19	2.68	1.24	22.84	21.98
Suffocations	.72	.21	.39	.15	.60	.09	.22	.04
Firearms	.57	.04	4.69	.52	.72	.01	5.79	.61

[1] Extracted from data, Bureau of Chronic Disease Epidemiology, Laboratory Centre for Disease Control, Health and Welfare Canada

Prevention of Household and Recreational Injuries in Adults

MANEUVER	EFFECTIVENESS	LEVEL OF EVIDENCE <REF>	RECOMMENDATION
Do not drink and dive (be involved in water sports)			
a) legislation	Association between use of alcohol/substance abuse and recreational drowning in adolescents.	Case control study<12> (II-2)	Fair evidence to implement (B)
b) individual counselling	Little information on ability of physician to influence adolescent behaviour.	Expert opinion<5> (III)	Insufficient evidence to include or exclude (C)
Use helmets when riding bicycles on roadways			
a) legislation	Association between severity of head injury in cyclists with non-use of helmets.	Case-control study<19> (II-2)	Fair evidence for implementing (B)
b) individual counselling	Limited ability of physician to influence helmet use.	Randomized controlled trial<20> (I)	Insufficient evidence to include or exclude (C)

(Continued on next page)

Prevention of Household and Recreational Injuries in Adults (concl'd)

MANEUVER	EFFECTIVENESS	LEVEL OF EVIDENCE <REF>	RECOMMENDATION
In the home make guns inaccessible; keep ammunition and gun separately			
a) legislation	Association between fire-arm related deaths and accessibility of loaded guns.	Expert opinion<11> (III)	Insufficient evidence to implement (C)
b) individual counselling	Little information on ability of physician to influence behaviour.		Insufficient evidence to include or exclude (C)
Use of Heimlich maneuver to treat choking on objects			
a) Public Health Education	Association between suffocation from choking on objects and lack of person to perform Heimlich maneuver.	Expert opinion<17> (III)	Insufficient evidence to implement (C)

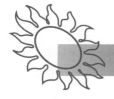

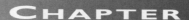

CHAPTER

46

Prevention of Unintended Pregnancy and Sexually Transmitted Diseases in Adolescents

By William Feldman, Anne Martell
and Jennifer L. Dingle

Prevention of Unintended Pregnancy and Sexually Transmitted Diseases in Adolescents

Prepared by William Feldman, MD, FRCPC,[1] Anne Martell, MA, CMC[2] and Jennifer L. Dingle MBA[3]

In 1987 the Canadian Task Force on the Periodic Health Examination recommended that physicians who see adolescents should advise those who are sexually active about the correct use of appropriate contraception (B Recommendation). Review of more recent evidence has not altered this recommendation, however oral contraceptives have been identified as the method of choice for adolescents in combination with a condom to protect against sexually transmitted diseases (STDs). Evidence from school-based clinics and community-based programs aimed at the reduction of adolescent pregnancy and STDs has also been evaluated, and supports the preventability of unintended teen pregnancy.

Burden of Suffering

In 1989, there were 39,600 teenage pregnancies in Canada. The teenage pregnancy rate for Canada (pregnancies per 1,000 women aged 15-19) was 44.1, down from 53.4 in 1975.

Teenage pregnancy levels are much lower in Canada than in the United States. In 1985, there were 37 pregnancies per 1,000 Canadian females aged 15-19 compared with 95 pregnancies per 1,000 females of the same age in the United States. In 1985, the fertility rate for Canadian teenagers (23 births per 1,000) was less than half that of the U.S. teenagers (52 per 1,000). The proportion of teenagers accepting abortion is comparable (38% in Canada and 44% in the U.S.) so that in 1985, the abortion rate for Canadian teenagers was 14 per 1,000, about one third of the U.S. rate (42 per 1,000).

The Risks/Effects of Teenage Pregnancy

The most serious physical risk to the teenage parent is death from pregnancy complications. For girls under 15 years the

---

[1] Professor of Pediatrics and of Preventive Medicine and Biostatistics, University of Toronto, Toronto, Ontario
[2] Martell Consulting Services Ltd., Halifax, Nova Scotia
[3] Co-ordinator of the Canadian Task Force on the Periodic Health Examination, Department of Pediatrics, Dalhousie University, Halifax, Nova Scotia

complication rate is 60% higher than the rate for all women and 2.5 times higher than the rate for mothers 20 to 24 years old. However, the increased risk of maternal complications may be associated more with socioeconomic factors than with age.

Teen mothers can expect to complete less education than those who do not bear children early. Teen mothers also reach lower levels of work success and of long-term income, and feel less satisfied with their vocational achievements. Satisfaction with career progress is also lower for married teenagers with children compared to married teenagers without children.

Adolescent mothers who marry subsequent to their child's birth are more likely than other adolescent couples to divorce or separate. Most teenage families with children are single-parent families.

Infants born to mothers less than 15 years of age are twice as likely as other infants to weigh less than 2,500 g (5 lb, 8 oz), a factor associated with increased infant mortality. 6.7% of live births in Canada during 1990 to women aged <20 years were of infants weighing <2,500 g, compared to 5.5% low birth weight babies born to mothers of all ages. Infants born to mothers less than 17 years of age are three times more likely to die in the first 28 days of life. However, cigarette smoking, poor gestational nutrition, low pre-pregnancy weight, primiparity and short stature are probably more important risk factors than maternal age.

Thus, adolescent pregnancy and childbearing may carry increased medical risk for mother and baby as well as lasting social, academic and economic disadvantages for mother, father and children. Except for academic and economic disadvantage, the evidence is weakened by lack of control for confounding variables.

Adolescent pregnancy may increase medical risk as well as social, academic and economic disadvantage

Sexually Transmitted Diseases

38,074 cases of genital chlamydia, 9,451 cases of gonococcal infection and 1,196 cases of syphilis were reported in Canada in 1992.

Given the prevalence of STDs in the adolescent population, the spread of HIV is particularly worrisome to health care providers. As of January 1, 1992, 22 cases of AIDS were reported in Canadians aged 15-19 years (<1% of all cases; 8 were reported in the 10-14 year age-group) and 1,092 cases (20%) were reported for those aged 20-29 years. Chapter 58 on HIV provides more extensive discussion of risk groups; there are several other related Chapters on STD prevention/screening.

Maneuver

Counselling for Contraception

All physicians who see adolescents should assess whether those who are sexually active are practising appropriate contraception. Although some physicians may be uncomfortable discussing these matters with young people, the third-person approach may be useful (e.g., "Some people your age are dating, some are having sexual intercourse. How about you?".)

Durant and colleagues[1] developed a model that can be used clinically to anticipate and recognize the multiple inter-relationships between factors that usually influence adolescent contraceptive behaviour. However, findings from empiric tests of the model indicate that among low socioeconomic black female adolescents, only a small part of the variation in frequency of intercourse or of engaging in unprotected coitus was explained. Clinical attempts to identify adolescent patients at risk of pregnancy using only one or two criteria will probably be unsuccessful. Thus, all adolescents should receive counselling.

Teenage Use of Contraception and Compliance

Eighty-five percent of adolescents saw their physician in the course of a year; only one-third of sexually active girls ever discussed contraception

Of all age groups, teens are the least likely to practice contraception. As one study noted "...the most notable feature of adolescent contraceptive behaviour is inconsistency." Although adolescents are thought not to visit a physician very often, a random sample of 1,000 teenagers in Ottawa (response rate 73%) revealed that 85% had seen their physician in the preceding year but only one-third of sexually active girls had ever discussed contraception with their physicians.

To eliminate the risk of pregnancy, an adolescent should understand that the only absolute method of contraception is abstinence. When this is not the adolescent's choice, however, appropriate contraceptive options should be offered.

Studies have shown that adolescent compliance is determined in part by the relationship established with health care providers. Accessible clinic hours, positive attitudes in the reception area, time spent waiting for the physician, care taken with the examination and assurances of confidentiality are all factors associated with adolescents' compliance. A further consideration may be financial as many adolescents have limited financial resources. Additionally, physicians should be open to some female adolescents' preference for a female examiner. Table 1 identifies actions a physician can take towards ensuring compliance. The effectiveness of these steps in ensuring compliance has not been systematically evaluated.

Contraceptive Options

Table 2 summarizes the available adolescent contraceptive methods with their advantages and disadvantages.<2> Table 3 provides additional information on estimates of contraceptive failure by type of contraception method over its first year of use.<3>

Oral Contraception

The oral contraceptive pill is highly effective in preventing pregnancy using reversible means. It has been reported to be the overwhelming favourite prescription method of contraception for adolescents (84% vs. 4% for IUD and 11% for diaphragm).<4> Additional advantages include its relative low cost and ease of use.

At the same time, however, clinicians are concerned that by relying solely on an oral contraceptive (OC), adolescents are leaving themselves open to STDs and particularly to HIV/AIDS. Experts recommend that adolescents who are sexually active should be advised to use condoms in combination with oral contraceptives.<5> This combination has not been evaluated.

Adolescents who are sexually active should be advised to use condoms in combination with oral contraceptions

Case-control studies have shown that OC's reduce the risk for endometrial cancer,<6> epithelial ovarian cancer,<2,7> pelvic inflammatory disease,<8> toxic shock syndrome<9> and ectopic pregnancy.<10> The potential association between OCs and cervical neoplasia is unsettled.<2> There is also some concern regarding a possible association between breast cancer and the use of OCs. However, many of the case-control studies evaluated in meta-analysis<11,12> were of low quality, without protection from bias or from the potentially confounding effects of duration of lactation, induced abortion, recent pregnancy or a history of diseases that are associated both with reduced use of OCs and reduced risk of breast cancer. One study<13> suggested that prognosis for breast cancer is worse for those who start oral contraceptives at an earlier age. Further evaluation is required.

While most epidemiologic studies have shown an association between oral contraceptive use and an increased risk of venous thrombosis and embolism, the risk for teenagers is very small. Finally, OCs can improve the quality of life by conferring protection against a number of common ailments that affect teenagers: primary dysmenorrhea, benign breast disease, ovarian cysts and iron deficiency anemia.

Expert opinion supports the use of OCs by teenagers as a safe method to avoid unwanted pregnancy since the overall risks of taking OCs are much less than the risks of pregnancy. Low-dose OCs have not been linked with either heart attack or stroke in contemporary U.S. studies and the evidence regarding breast cancer is contradictory. While the overall risk of thromboembolism in oral contraceptive users may be increased over that of the general population, the risk to teenagers, especially those who do not smoke, is minimal. As with all medical choices, the benefits of a treatment must be weighed against potential risks.

Benefits/Risks of Intrauterine Device (IUD)

While compliance is assured with intrauterine devices and effectiveness is comparable to that of OCs, they provide no protection from sexually transmitted diseases and the risk of adverse affects associated with IUDs appears to be higher for adolescents. Expert opinion supports their use mainly for older women in stable monogamous relationships.[14]

Barrier Methods and Spermicides

In their recent review,[15] Rosenberg and Gollub reported that observational studies show that condoms offer widely divergent degrees of protection against sexually transmitted diseases. Meta-analysis shows that for most outcomes, condoms decrease infection rates by approximately 50%. While protection seems to increase with more consistent use, condoms may not protect against organisms transmitted by external genital contact. The rate of condom use among 15-19-year old males in the United States was 58% in 1988, more than double the rate reported in 1979 (21%); 20% of sexually experienced females reported currently using condoms (47% at first intercourse), compared with 11% in 1982. Condoms are widely available but are less effective in preventing pregnancy than IUDs or OCs.

Foams, diaphragms and creams are unpopular with adolescents in North America.[2,16] Each of these options interferes with spontaneity, requires the adolescent to plan ahead, requires motivation and familiarity with technique, and is "messy". Diaphragms and cervical caps, which are assumed to be used in conjunction with spermicide, leave a portion of the vagina unprotected; observational studies indicate a reduction in sexually transmitted diseases of 50-100%.[15]

Long-Acting Contraceptives

The impact of new long-acting contraceptives such as the progestin implant (Norplant®) on the reduction of adolescent pregnancy is currently unknown and will likely depend on the cost and availability of the method and on teens' acceptance of these methods (including insertion discomfort and tolerance of menstrual irregularity). One observational study suggests Norplant is well accepted by adolescents.[17] Compliance is assured and effectiveness is high, but the methods again offer no protection from STDs.

Implant systems (for men) are under investigation as are vaginal rings releasing levonorgestrel and injectable hormone contraceptives. Birth control "vaccines" are also being developed, the most advanced being a vaccine inducing antibodies against human chorionic gonadotrophin (hCG).

The Morning-After Pill

Postcoital contraception (PCC) (the morning-after pill/ Ethinyl estradiol/dl-norgestrel in combination) has been shown to prevent pregnancy for most women when given after sexual intercourse. Termination of the pregnancy was not achieved for 1.1-2.0% of women treated, resulting in 15-30% of the expected number of pregnancies.[18-21] Side-effects include nausea (50%) and vomiting (20%). Women who rely on barriers, spermicide, withdrawal or periodic abstinence should be informed about the "morning-after pill".

Effectiveness of Prevention and Treatment

The Primary Care Physician

There have been no studies evaluating whether physicians identifying sexually active teenagers and counselling them on contraception will lead to more appropriate knowledge and behaviour. Most studies have evaluated interventions provided by non-physicians. However, the success of these interventions demonstrates that unintended pregnancy is preventable. There is no indication that physicians would be less successful.

A randomized controlled trial of 75 sexually active females in a clinic setting also showed that education programs increased knowledge of AIDS ($p < 0.001$).[22] No significant differences were noted regarding attitudes or condom acquisition and other changes in behaviour were not addressed. School-based AIDS-prevention curricula have had modest effects.

Community-based Programs

A recent report documented a successful community-based program to reduce adolescent pregnancy in counties of South Carolina characterized as rural, low income and undereducated. Their public health approach involved teenagers, parents, community leaders, ministers, schools, churches, and community groups. School sex education, use of mass media and training of adult leaders in the community were all included. The estimated pregnancy rate declined 35%, compared with pre-intervention levels (95% confidence interval (CI): -14% to -57%). Comparison communities (no intervention) had 5-16% increases in the rate of teenage pregnancy ($p < 0.002$). While the counties were comparable in terms of racial/ethnic composition, population density, income, and education, the comparison communities initially had lower estimated pregnancy rates (35-53% versus 61% in the target community).[23]

School-Based Programs

Most of the evidence regarding school-based programs (SBPs) comes from the United States. Most SBPs report a rate of use exceeding 75% of the school population once teens become aware of available services. An evaluation of the Baltimore SBPs' attendance suggests that their accessibility rather than any new or newly packaged information about sex, family planning or other new services was responsible for high student use.[24] St. Paul, Minnesota[25] and western Massachusetts[26] studies have shown that birth rates for teenagers can be reduced by more than 50% without major reliance on abortion, in a population which is not upper middle class, not college bound, and which has traditionally been viewed as very hard to reach.

Table 4 summarizes a number of examples of effective community-based and school-based programs operating in the United States.[23-29] This is grade II-3 evidence that comprehensive school-based efforts to lower the rates of teenage pregnancy can be effective.

Sex Education in the Schools

Education programs and computer games are effective in providing at least short-term knowledge and attitudinal change in adolescents but school sex education by itself appears to have little or no effect on adolescent sexual activity or pregnancy rates. However, a study of 536 low-income minority students in Atlanta showed that those who participated in a family planning outreach program for eighth graders led by older students, were less likely (p<0.01) to report initiation of sexual activity by the end of the 9th grade (24% versus 39% of students had not had sexual intercourse).[28]

Recommendations of Others

In 1989, the U.S. Preventive Services Task Force[30] recommended that clinicians should obtain a detailed sexual history from all adolescent patients. Empathy, confidentiality and a nonjudgemental supportive attitude were stressed. It was recommended that clinicians involve young pubertal patients and, where appropriate, their parents in early, open discussion of sexual development and effective methods to prevent unintended pregnancy and sexually transmitted diseases, and that sexually abstinent adolescents be encouraged to remain abstinent. Oral contraceptives and barrier methods (with spermicide) were recommended as the most effective means of reducing risk in sexually active persons, and complete sexual abstinence as the most effective method overall. The U.S. Task Force stated that sexual abstinence and the maintenance of a mutually faithful monogamous sexual relationship should be emphasized as two important measures to reduce the risk of sexually transmitted diseases. Patients who engage in sexual activity with multiple partners or with persons who may be infected with sexually transmitted organisms should be advised to use condoms and instructed in their proper use.

The American Ad Hoc Committee on Reproductive Health (Sub-committee of the Society for Adolescent Medicine)<5> and the Committee on Adolescence of the Council on Child and Adolescent Health<31> advocate more physician training regarding pregnancy counselling for adolescents. The Council also recommends that pediatricians who do not want to counsel their teenage patients about sexual matters, refer their patients to counselling facilities experienced and sensitive to the needs of adolescents.

Conclusions and Recommendations

Given prevention program successes in community- and school-based clinics, there is fair evidence that physicians can reduce the toll of unwanted pregnancy by provision of education and contraceptive services, by involving pubertal patients and, where appropriate, their parents in early, open discussion of sexual development, prevention of sexually transmitted diseases, and prevention of unwanted pregnancy. Physicians caring for sexually active adolescents should address their contraceptive practices and where indicated, should provide a combination of services: education, counselling, contraception and follow-up (this may include repeat D (Rh) blood group antibody screening before induced abortion or other obstetric procedures, see Chapter 11). Oral contraceptives combined with condoms are the first choice for adolescents who do not wish to be sexually abstinent.

Unanswered Questions (Research Agenda)

The following have been identified as research priorities:

1. Evaluating Canadian school-based clinics.

2. Evaluating the effectiveness of physicians in identifying sexually active and unprotected teenagers, counselling, prescribing contraceptives, and altering their behaviour.

3. Examining the effectiveness of a more widely available "morning-after pill" program because the majority of teenagers are unprotected during their first sexual encounter.

4. Further research into the reasons for noncompliance with oral contraception and the development of creative and effective solutions for non-compliance. Research into the effectiveness of counselling adolescents in the use of condoms in combination with oral contraceptives and with spermicide is also recommended.

Evidence

The MEDLINE search strategy undertaken for the years 1988 to November 1993 identified articles using the following key words: pregnancy, unwanted; adolescent; contraception; inject; contraceptive agents; contraceptive devices; human; contraception behaviour; and sex counselling.

This review was initiated in January 1993 and recommendations were finalized by the Task Force in October 1993.

Acknowledgements

Funding for this report was provided by Health Canada under the Government of Canada's Brighter Futures Initiative. The Task Force also thanks Dr. Steven Woolf, MD, MPH, Science Advisor, U.S. Preventive Services Task Force, Washington, DC and Assistant Clinical Professor, Department of Family Practice, Medical College of Virginia, Richmond, VA, USA for reviewing the draft report.

Selected References

1. Durant RH, Jay S, Seymore C: Contraceptive and sexual behaviour of black female adolescents. *J Adolesc Health Care* 1990; 11: 326-334

2. Sanfilippo JS: Adolescents and oral contraceptives. *Int J Fertil* 1991; 36 (Suppl 2): 65-79

3. Trussell J, Hatcher RA, Cates W Jr, *et al*: A guide to interpreting contraceptive efficacy studies. *Obstet Gynecol* 1990; 76(3 Pt 2): 558-567

4. Zelnik M, Koenig MA, Kim YJ: Sources of prescription contraceptives and subsequent pregnancy among young women. *Fam Plann Perspec* 1984; 16(1): 6-13

5. Society for Adolescent Medicine: Position Paper on Reproductive Health Care for Adolescents. *J Adol Hea* 1991; 12: 649-661

6. The Cancer and Steroid Hormone Study of the Centers for Disease Control and the National Institute of Child Health and Human Development: Combination oral contraceptive use and the risk of endometrial cancer. *JAMA* 1987; 257(6): 796-800

7. The Cancer and Steroid Hormone Study of the Centers for Disease Control and the National Institute of Child Health and Human Development: The reduction in risk of ovarian cancer associated with oral-contraceptive use. *N Engl J Med* 1987; 316: 650-655

8. Rubin GL, Ory HW, Layde PM: Oral contraceptives and pelvic inflammatory disease. *Am J Obstet Gynecol* 1982; 144: 630-635

9. Gray RH: Toxic shock syndrome and oral contraception. [letter] *Am J Obstet Gynecol* 1987; 156: 1038

10. Grady D, Rubin SM, Petitti DB, *et al*: Hormone therapy to prevent disease and prolong life in postmenopausal women. *Ann Int Med* 1992; 117: 1016-1037

11. Rushton L, Jones DR: Oral contraceptive use and breast cancer risk: a meta-analysis of variations with age at diagnosis, parity and total duration of oral contraceptive use. *Br J Obstet Gynaecol* 1992; 99(3): 239-246

12. Hawley W, Nuovo J, DeNeef CP, *et al*: Do oral contraceptive agents affect the risk of breast cancer? A meta-analysis of the case-control reports. *J Am Board Fam Pract* 1993; 6(2): 123-135

13. Ranstam J, Olsson H, Garne JP, *et al*: Survival in breast cancer and age at start of oral contraceptive usage. *Anticancer Res* 1991; 11(6): 2043-2046

14. Diagnostic and therapeutic technology assessment. Intrauterine devices. *JAMA* 1989; 261(14): 2127-2130

15. Rosenberg MJ, Gollub EL: Commentary: methods women can use that may prevent sexually transmitted disease, including HIV. *Am J Pub Health* 1992; 82(11): 1473-1478

16. McAnarney ER, Hendee WR: The prevention of adolescent pregnancy. *JAMA* 1989; 262(1): 78-82

17. Berenson AB, Wiemann CM: Patient satisfaction and side effects with levonorgestrel implant (Norplant) use in adolescents 18 years of age or younger. *Pediatrics* 1993; 92: 257-260

18. Percival-Smith RKL, Abercrombie B: Postcoital contraception with dl-norgestrel/ethinyl estradiol combination: six years experience in a medical clinic. *Contraception* 1987; 36(3): 287-293

19. Dixon GW, Schlesselman JJ, Ory HW, *et al*: Ethinyl estradiol and conjugated estrogens as postcoital contraceptives. *JAMA* 1980; 244: 1336-1339

20. Luerti M, Tonta A, Ferla P, *et al*: Post-coital contraception by estrogen/progestagen combination or IUD insertion. *Contraception* 1986; 33(1): 61-68

21. Van Santen MR, Haspels AA: Interception II: Postcoital low-dose estrogens and norgestrel combination in 633 women. *Contraception* 1985; 31(3): 275-293

22. Rickert VI, Gottlieb A, Jay MS: A comparison of three clinic-based AIDS education programs on female adolescents' knowledge, attitudes, and behavior. *J Adolesc Health Care* 1990; 11: 298-303

23. Vincent ML, Clearie AF, Schluchter MD: Reducing adolescent pregnancy through school and community-based education. *JAMA* 1987; 257(24): 3382-3386

24. Zabin LS, Hirsch MB, Smith EA, *et al*: Evaluation of a pregnancy prevention program for urban teenagers. *Fam Plann Perspect* 1986; 18(3): 119-126

25. Edwards EL, Steinman ME, Arnold KA, *et al*: Adolescent pregnancy prevention services in high school clinics. *Fam Plann Persp* 1980; 12(1): 6-14

26. Brann EA, Edwards L, Callicott T, et al: Strategies for the prevention of pregnancy in adolescents. *Adv Plan Parent* 1979; 14: 68-76

27. Kirby D, Waszak C, Ziegler J: Six school-based clinics: their reproductive health services and impact on sexual behaviour. *Fam Plann Perspect* 1991; 23(1): 6-16

28. Howard M, McCabe JB: Helping teenagers postpone sexual involvement. *Fam Plann Perspect* 1990; 22(1): 21-26

29. Orton MJ, Rosenblatt E: Adolescent pregnancy in Ontario: progress in prevention. Planned Parenthood Ontario, Report #2, February 1986: 149

30. U.S. Preventive Services Task Force: *Guide to Clinical Preventive Services: an Assessment of the Effectiveness of 169 Interventions*. Williams & Wilkins, Baltimore, Md, 1989: 341-349

31. American Academy of Pediatrics Committee on Adolescence: Counseling the adolescent about pregnancy options. *Pediatr* 1989; 83(1): 135-137

Table 1:   Steps to Encourage Compliance with Contraceptives

1. Discuss mechanism of action of contraceptive methods.	7. Provide close follow-up (every 8 to 12 weeks).
2. Discuss anticipated side effects.	8. Review instructions and the importance of compliance at each visit.
3. Assure patient confidentiality.	9. Provide a contact person.
4. Explain all tests.	10. Provide verbal rewards to patients who keep follow-up appointments and comply with instructions.
5. Give oral and written instructions.	11. Telephone patients who miss appointments.
6. Give samples at initial visit.	

Table 2:   Adolescent Contraceptive Methods[2]

Non-hormonal method	Advantages	Disadvantages	Cost[1]
Condom	Male shares responsibility; non-prescription; demonstrated protection against sexually transmitted diseases (STDs); highly effective when used with vaginal spermicide	Interferes with spontaneity and requires high degree of motivation.	12 @ $4.40-7.50; 12 @ $7-10 with spermicidal lubricant
Diaphragm	Some protection against STDs	Requires prescription (Rx) and fitting; "Messy" to use; increased risk of UTI; requires motivation, consistent compliance and forethought.	Physician visit; $30 and $4-5/tube of cream or jelly
Cervical cap	Some protection against STDs	Requires Rx and fitting; may not be able to fit; possible cervical abnormalities; associated with problems of odour, dislodgment, discomfort, difficulty inserting and removing, vaginal discharge, discomfort to partner, and bleeding.	Physician visit; caps not available (US$100); $4-5/tube of cream or jelly
Contraceptive sponge	Some protection against STDs; non-prescription	Need access to water prior to use; may be difficult to remove.	3 @ $8

[1] Cost at 1 Halifax location, January 26, 1993; U.S. prices 1991 publication[2]

Table 2: Adolescent Contraceptive Methods<2> – (Concl'd)

Non-hormonal method	Advantages	Disadvantages	Cost[1]
Vaginal spermicide	Some protection against STDs; non-prescription	Interferes with spontaneity; "Messy" to use; may need to wait for dissolution; less effective when used alone.	foam $17-20/container; $16-19/tube cream or jelly
Intrauterine device	Compliance assured; highly effective	Requires Rx and insertion; no protection against STDs; increased risk of pelvic infection; increased bleeding and cramping; high expulsion rate; inappropriate for use by adolescents, particularly nulligravidae.	Physician visit $50 lasts 1-4 years
Periodic abstinence	No chemicals or devices; reduces the risk of STDs	Fertile interval less predictable in adolescents; no protection against STDs; requires extensive education, high motivation, self-control; requires participation of partner.	Instructional visits; Thermometer and charts less than $10
Oral contra-ceptives	Highest degree of efficacy of reversible methods; long-term safety well documented; no complicated techniques to use; formulation can be tailored to individual needs	Requires Rx; compliance with schedule necessary for effectiveness; no protection against STDs.	Physician visit; $18-20/mo
Subdermal implantation (norplant)	Compliance assured; high degree of efficacy	Requires Rx; recently released in Canada; secondary effects may be unacceptable to adolescents; no protection against STDs.	Cost from the company $450; physician/ installation charges vary (US$750); lasts 5 years

[1] Cost at 1 Halifax location, January 26, 1993; U.S. prices 1991 publication<2>

Table 3: Lowest Expected and Typical Percentages of Accidental Pregnancy in the United States During the First Year of Use of a Method[3]

Method	Lowest Expected[1]	Typical[2]
Chance	85	85
Spermicides[3]	3	21
Periodic abstinence Calendar Ovulation method Sympto-thermal Post-ovulation	9 3 2 1	20
Withdrawal	4	18
Cap[4]	6	18
Sponge Parous women Nulliparous women	9 6	28 18
Diaphragm[5]	6	18
Condom[6]	2	12
Intrauterine device (IUD) Progestasert Copper T 380 A	2 0.8	3
Pill Combined Progestogen only	0.1 0.5	3
Injectable progestogen Depot Medroxyprogesteron acetate Norethisterone	0.3 0.4	0.3 0.4
Implants NORPLANT (6 capsules) NORPLANT (2 rods)	0.04 0.03	0.04 0.03
Female sterilization	0.2	0.4
Male sterilization	0.1	0.15

[1] Among couples who initiate use of a method (not necessarily for the first time) and who use it perfectly (both consistently and correctly), the author's best guess of the percentage during the first year if they do not stop use for any other reason.

[2] Among typical couples who initiate use of a method (not necessarily for the first time), the percentage who experience an accidental pregnancy during the first year if they do not stop use for any other reason.

[3] Foams and vaginal suppositories.

[4] Cervical mucous (ovulation) method supplemented by calendar in the preovulatory and basal body temperature in the postovulatory phases.

[5] With spermicidal cream or jelly.

[6] Without spermicides.

Table 4: Examples of Effective Community-Based and School-Based Programs

Study and Program	Services/Methodology	Results
Edwards Laura et al 1980<25> St. Paul Maternal & Infant Care Project	Operates a comprehensive clinic on the school premises. Screening, counselling and pelvic examinations are performed at school. Students requesting contraceptive services are referred to the same staff at a nearby clinic after school hours. Follow-up is performed at school. The clinic also provides prenatal and postpartum care, gynecologic exams, contraceptive education, counselling and referral and testing for STDs. Additional services include athletic and physical exams, weight-reduction program, well-child physical exams, immunizations and drug education and counselling.	Over the first three years of operation, the student birth rate was reduced by 56% from 70 per 1,000 (37 births out of approximately 470 female students) in the 1972-3 school year to 35 per 1,000 (13 births among 371 female students) in 1975-6. This decline was significant (p<.01) and was a more rapid decline than that which occurred in the nation as a whole. The percentage of mothers dropping out of school after delivery fell from 45% to less than 10%. The young mothers continuing their education have accepted contraception and have had no repeat pregnancies. The contraceptive continuation rate at 12 months was 86.4 per 100. By the end of the third year of the clinic, (1976) 50% of the entire student body had attended the clinic at least once and 92% of the pregnant students had obtained prenatal services.
Brann Edward A et al 1979<26> Family Planning Council of Western Massachusetts	Awareness Program at a vocational high school. Teachers in the schools' home economics department became concerned when they noted that approximately 40% of each class got pregnant before completing school. Together with the Family Planning Council they devised a special awareness program conducted twice yearly with the female students. The program consists of a film and group discussion.	Led to a decline in the pregnancy rate from 40% to approximately 4%. Over the 2.5 years the program was in place, there were only two pregnancies, one planned and carried to term and one intentionally aborted. The teachers also noted that the participants in the program were less eager to get married immediately upon graduation, a common event in the period before the program.

Table 4: Examples of Effective Community-Based and School-Based Programs – (Cont'd)

Study and Program	Services/Methodology	Results
Kirby Douglas et al 1991<27> Six diverse school-based clinics serving low-income populations. Five of the six serviced a predominantly black population.	Every clinic employed at least one part-time or full-time physician. They all provided primary health care, contraceptive counselling and pregnancy tests, but they differed in the emphasis placed on reproductive health, provision of sexuality education and family planning services.	Survey data collected indicated the clinics neither hastened the onset of sexual activity nor increased its frequency. At one school where pregnancy prevention was a high priority and staff issued vouchers for contraceptives, the use of condoms and pills were significantly higher than in the comparison school. Another school clinic which focused on high-risk youth, emphasized pregnancy prevention and dispensed birth control, recorded a significantly higher use of pills than its comparison school. Another clinic which focussed on AIDS education and prevention found condom use increased significantly over time but not pill use.
Brann Edward et al 1979<26> The Maryland State Department of Health and Mental Hygiene	Program in education and human sexuality for adolescents in two rural areas of the state. The program consisted of a combination of sex education in the schools taught by trained teachers, sensitization of county health departmental staff to the situation of teenagers, and access to contraception in distribution centres where teens were known to gather.	In Charles, Calvert and Worcester Counties, the combined fertility rate for 15- to 19-year-olds fell from 84 births per 1,000 females in 1972 to 56 per 1,000 in 1975, a 33% drop. In the 15 to 17 year old range, the rate fell from 66 per 1,000, to 42 per 1,000, a 36% drop.
Vincent Murray L et al 1987<23> The School/Community Program for Sexual Risk Reduction Among Teens in the western portion of a South Carolina county	The program consisted of the education of adults in the target community – parents, ministers, community leaders and the media. Sex education in the schools was only a small part of an overall effort to postpone the age of first coitus and to promote the consistent use of effective contraception. Central to the project was an educational program to help adults improve their skills as parents and as role models in the community.	In the pre-intervention years, the intervention and comparison portions of the county had similar average rates of 60.6 and 66.8 pregnancies per 1,000 females. In 1984 and 1985 (two and three years after implementation) the estimated pregnancy rate (EPR) declined in the intervention group to a level of 25.1 pregnancies per 1,000 females. This was significantly lower ($P<.01$) than the average EPR in the comparison counties.

Table 4: Examples of Effective Community-Based and School-Based Programs – (Concl'd)

Study and Program	Services/Methodology	Results
Zabin et al 1986<24> Baltimore	Pregnancy prevention program implemented in 1 inner-city junior and 1 senior high school with a predominantly black, low-income population. 2 schools serve as the control. Program provided students with sexuality and contraceptive education, individual and group counselling and medical and contraceptive services over a period of 3 years.	Decreases in pregnancy rate were reported in contrast to city-wide rate increases. Changes in sexual and contraceptive knowledge occurred; age at first intercourse was delayed (median 7 months); the percentage of students going to the clinic or doctor before first intercourse increased from 50 to 71% as did attendance during the first months of sexual activity; junior high boys used the clinic as freely as girls their same age. The authors conclude that access to free high-quality services was probably crucial to success.
Howard & McCabe 1990<28> Atlanta	Family-planning outreach program for eighth graders in a local school system. The program is led by older teenagers and focusses on helping students resist peer and social pressures to initiate sexual activity.	By the end of the eighth grade, students who had not participated in the program were as much as five times more likely to have begun having sex than were those who had had the program.
Orton & Rosenblatt 1986<29> Ontario	Combination program of school sexuality education and clinic contraception services.	A decline in teen births (-13%) plus the decline in the younger teen population (-10%) resulted in a 22% decline in the annual number of pregnancies to younger teens by 1981 – almost a thousand less than in 1976.

Prevention of Unintended Pregnancy and Sexually Transmitted Diseases in Adolescents

MANEUVER	EFFECTIVENESS	LEVEL OF EVIDENCE <REF>	RECOMMENDATION
Identification of sexually active adolescents; counselling on sexual activity and contraceptive methods; recommendation of appropriate contraception	Incidence of unwanted pregnancy decreases with appropriate use of contraception by compliant individuals. Intervention to enhance compliance is somewhat effective.	Comparison of times and places<2,3> (II-3) Comparisons of times and places <22,25,26> (II-3)	Fair evidence that sexually active adolescents be advised about correct use of oral contraceptives and condoms (B)

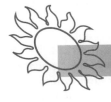

CHAPTER 47

Physical Activity Counselling

By Marie-Dominique Beaulieu

Physical Activity Counselling

Adapted by Marie-Dominique Beaulieu, MD, MSc, FCFP[1] from
materials prepared for the U.S. Preventive Services Task Force[2].

*There is fair evidence to support the effectiveness
of regular physical activity for the primary prevention of
cardiovascular heart disease and hypertension. Physical activity
can also contribute to the prevention of obesity, non-insulin
dependent diabetes and osteoporosis. There is insufficient direct
evidence to indicate whether physician counselling of patients to
incorporate regular physical activity into their daily routines will
have a positive effect on their behavior. However, qualifying
considerations suggest that such counselling may be clinically
prudent, especially for patients who are sedentary.*

Burden of Suffering

Research on the relationships between physical activity and
health are complex due to the variety of maneuvers and target
outcomes considered. It is important to distinguish between physical
activity and physical fitness. Physical activity or exercise are behaviors
and physical fitness is a set of attributes that represents the capacity
to perform the physical activities. Hence, physical activity, and its
opposite, sedentariness, are usually defined in terms of the amount of
time during the day devoted to certain types of physical activity or
exercise, either during work and/or leisure time. This review focuses
on the effects of physical activity levels on the primary prevention of
various health conditions, rather than on cardiorespiratory fitness or
specific training activities as primary or secondary prevention
measures.

The total burden of suffering attributable to a sedentary lifestyle
in Canada and the United States is difficult to ascertain. However,
sedentary lifestyle appears to be an independent risk factor for all-
cause mortality[1-3] and of developing certain chronic diseases,
particularly, coronary heart diseases (CHD)[4], hypertension[5,6]
and obesity.[7,8] Sedentariness has also been associated with
the risk of developing non-insulin dependent diabetes mellitus
(NIDDM)[9-11] and osteoporosis. Physical inactivity increases the
risk of CHD nearly twofold and is comparable to other major CHD

Physical inactivity
increases the risk of
CHD nearly two-fold
which is comparable
to other major CHD
risk factors

---

[1] Associate Professor, Department of Family Medicine, University of Montreal,
Montreal, Quebec

[2] By John Burress, MD, MPH, Research Fellow, Harvard School of Public Health,
Occupational and Environmental Medicine, Boston, MA; Donald M. Berwick, MD,
MPP, Associate Professor of Pediatrics, Harvard Medical School, and Vice Chair,
U.S. Preventive Services Task Force

risk factors.<4,12> In terms of attributable CHD risk, a sedentary lifestyle may carry a burden similar to that of smoking.<2,4>

In 1985, a review of eight national studies conducted in Canada and the United States showed that about 20% of the adult Canadian population exercised at a level recommended for cardiopulmonary fitness, 40% exercised at a level below that recommended for cardiopulmonary fitness but sufficient for other health benefits, and 40% were sedentary. The Canada Health Promotion Survey conducted in 1990 showed a slight decrease in the proportion of Canadians who qualified as regular exercisers, from 54% to 48%.

The relationship between the level of physical activity and socio-economic variables is unclear. Although individuals from higher socio-economic classes report performing vigorous physical activity during leisure time more frequently than those from lower classes, the level of daily physical activity is higher in lower socio-economic classes for both males and females. However, for most working people, physical activity on the job does not make up for sedentary leisure time. Women are as active as, or more active than, men between the ages of 25 and 64. However Canadians most likely to engage in daily exercise during their leisure time are men aged 65 and older.

Maneuver

The form of physical activity that is best suited to a given individual depends on that individual's needs, limitations, and goals. Current scientific knowledge suggests that the preferred general primary prevention maneuver is moderate-level physical activity performed consistently to accumulate 30 minutes or more over the course of most days of the week.<13> The following are considered moderate intensity physical activities (above 4.5 Mets): normal walking, golfing on foot, slow biking, raking leaves, cleaning windows, slow dancing, light restaurant work. Activities such as slow jogging, brisk walking, shovelling snow, heavy house repairing and gardening, racquet sports, to name a few, are considered vigorous activities. To improve cardiovascular fitness, exercise cannot be performed occasionally or seasonally, nor can one expect protection from CAD simply by having exercised regularly in the past.

Current knowledge suggests that the preferred prevention maneuver of moderate-level physical activity be performed consistently to accumulate 30 minutes or more over the course of most days of the week

Moderate physical activities have higher compliance rates than vigorous exercise activities, mesh better with daily lifestyles, and are well maintained over time.<3>

Potential Adverse Effects of Physical Activity

The benefits of exercise must be weighed against potential adverse effects, which include injury, osteoarthritis, myocardial infarction, and rarely, sudden death.

Data on the incidence of injury during non-competitive physical activity are scarce. One study randomly assigned 70-79 year-old men and women to strength training, walk/jog, or control groups. Injury rates were 8.7% for the strength training group during the full 26 weeks of the study, 4.8% for the walk group during weeks 1-13, and 57% for those who jogged during weeks 14-26 and had walked during their first 14 weeks. The risk of injury does not seem to be associated with age or sex. Most exercise-induced injuries are preventable. They often occur as a result of excessive levels of physical activity, and improper exercise techniques or equipment.

The concern that long-term physical activity may accelerate the development of osteoarthritis in major weight-bearing joints is not supported by case-control data. Reasonable recreational exercise performed within the limits of comfort while putting joints without underlying abnormality through normal motion does not inevitably lead to joint injury.

Adverse cardiovascular events are perhaps of greatest concern. Two recent large studies have confirmed that heavy physical activity increases the risk of acute myocardial infarction by a factor of 2.1 (95% confidence interval: 1.6-3.1)[14] to 5.9 (4.6-7.7)[15] However, a protective effect of regular physical activity was observed in both studies. As the weekly frequency of exercise increased, the relative risk of infarction during vigorous activity dropped consistently.[14,15] Studies suggest that sedentary individuals who engage in vigorous activity are at greater risk for sudden death than those who exercise regularly.[16]

Effectiveness of Prevention and Treatment

There is evidence that increasing the level of physical activity reduces morbidity and mortality for at least the following five chronic conditions: CHD, hypertension, obesity, NIDDM, and osteoporosis. Effectiveness of exercise counselling by primary care providers has not been studied as thoroughly and must be considered separately.

Primary Prevention of Coronary Artery Disease

Evidence from cohort studies has shown a consistent association between physical activity and reduced incidence of CHD.[3,4,12] Physical activity prevents the occurrence of major cardiovascular events, although there is no evidence that it reduces the severity of the events that do occur.[4] Similar benefits from exercise have been reported in older men (up to age 75). Although the physiological response to physical activity appears similar in men and women, epidemiologic data sufficient to confirm a primary preventive role of physical activity for CHD in women is not yet available.[3] The practice of regular exercise in men protects both from the risk of

CHD and the risk that strenuous physical activity triggers a myocardial infarction.<14,15>

All studies about the beneficial effects of exercise on all-cause and CHD mortality are subject to the "healthy volunteer" bias, even if care is taken in sampling and follow-up. In the above mentioned studies, the effects of exercise were independent of other CHD risk factors. In some studies, the cardiovascular benefits were augmented in the presence of other risk factors for CHD.<2,3> The observation that the protective effect of exercise disappears in individuals who discontinue the practice of regular physical activity supports the presence of a dose-effect relationship.

These data do not prove causal associations. Nonetheless, the consistency, strength, and suggestion of a graded response for the highest levels of fitness and physical activity being associated with decreased CHD is clear.<4>

Primary Prevention of Hypertension

Cohort studies suggest that physically inactive individuals have a 35-52% greater risk of developing hypertension than those who exercise. This effect appears to be independent of other risk factors for hypertension.<5,6> A graded inverse relationship between increasing fitness quartiles and blood pressure was noted in a large cohort.<17> However, randomized controlled trials of primary prevention have been either nonspecific or limited in sample size.

Primary Prevention of Obesity

Data from prospective population studies have shown an elevation in relative risk for the development of significant weight gain across leisure time physical activity categories.<7,8> Experimental data on secondary prevention of obesity show such a relationship. Although data confirms a significant effect of exercise alone on weight loss, the combination of regular exercise and balanced caloric consumption appears to be the most effective means of preventing obesity and maintaining ideal body weight.<18,19> Morbidity and mortality have been lower in overweight individuals who are physically active even if they remained overweight.<3>

Primary Prevention of Non-Insulin Dependent Diabetes Mellitus

Cohort data reveal an inverse relationship between the level of physical activity and the risk of developing NIDDM.<9-11> This effect is more pronounced among overweight men.<9> The age-adjusted risk of NIDDM is reduced by 6% for each 500-kcal increment in energy expenditure per week. The protective effect is especially pronounced in persons at highest risk for NIDDM (i.e., family history, obesity, hypertension).<11>

Primary Prevention of Osteoporosis

Recent non-randomized controlled trials have shown that postmenopausal women can retard bone loss through physical activity.<20-22> Cross-sectional studies suggest that physical activity can also reduce the rate of bone loss in pre-menopausal women.<23>

Direct evidence that physical activity reduces the incidence of hip fractures is limited to one case-control study and one cross-sectional study. The relationships between type and extent of physical activity and osteoporosis as well as postmenopausal fractures have recently been reviewed. Some studies have suggested that skeletal loads generating muscle pull, rather than gravity, may provide benefit.

However, the variation in bone mineral density attributable to differences in activity is thought to be modest (20%) compared to the genetic contribution. Experience in intervention trials suggests the following possible limitations of exercise as a prevention and treatment modality: 1) the training regimen is not feasible over the long-term even at moderate intensity, for many people; 2) the effect is not sustained upon detraining; 3) the amount gained is modest; 4) generic programs lacking individualization may result in high rates of musculoskeletal complications and noncompliance; and 5) optimal exercise prescription in terms of type, duration, intensity, and frequency is unclear at present. Screening for osteoporosis, hormone replacement therapy, and diet are addressed in Chapters 52 and 49.

Effectiveness of Counselling

The rationale and evidence for effectiveness of physical activity counselling was published in 1989 by the U.S. Preventive Services Task Force and is currently under review.<24> Studies that have demonstrated benefits from counselling provide little information about long-term compliance and are of limited generalizability, because they have not been representative of typical primary care physician counselling of healthy patients.

The latest version of *Canada's Health Promotion Survey* showed that of 42% of the adults who reported increasing their level of leisure time physical activity in the year prior to the survey, a majority (59%) did so because of increased knowledge of the risks of remaining sedentary. The example of others (46%), support from friends and family (43%), changes in social values (31%), and new life situations (30%) were also important factors in helping people become more active.

Recommendations of Others

Health Canada, Canada Fitness and most Canadian Provinces have developed community intervention programs to foster increased physical activity. The objectives of these initiatives are to encourage sedentary individuals to engage in moderately intense physical activities. The message of the federal government's "Green Plan" on "Active Living Environment Program" (ALEP) is "to encourage both individually and collectively, behavioral changes that support and encourage Canadians to engage in more responsible, active and healthier outdoor physical activities that are environmentally friendly".

In 1989, the U.S. Preventive Services Task Force recommended that clinicians should counsel all patients to engage in a program of regular physical activity, tailored to their health status and personal lifestyle.<24>

The American College of Sports Medicine (ACSM) has also issued guidelines for developing and maintaining cardiorespiratory fitness, body composition, and muscular strength and endurance, which are different objectives. A concise methodology for risk stratification prior to exercise testing based on age, coronary risk factors, signs and symptoms, and anticipated level of training has been published, along with guidelines for exercise prescription, including contraindications. Exercise stress testing to evaluate for CAD is not considered necessary, provided that the individual is contemplating initiation of low level physical activity and does not meet the criteria for high risk.

Conclusions and Recommendations

There is fair evidence that the regular practice of moderate intensity physical activity is an independent risk factor associated with a reduction in: all-cause and CHD mortality, incidence of CHD, hypertension and NIDDM, and the maintenance of a healthy body weight.<1-12> Considering the high prevalence of CHD, the benefits of regular physical activity in terms of decrease in CHD attributable risk is estimated to be comparable to that of smoking cessation. Recent data have also shown that individuals who practice moderate intensity physical activity regularly are less likely to be victims of myocardial infarction during strenuous exercise. The effectiveness of regular exercise on the primary prevention of osteoporosis is also supported by fair evidence. However, the attributable impact of exercising on the prevention of osteoporosis may be modest, considering the important contribution of genetic factors to bone mineral density.

High intensity physical activity by unfit people is associated with greater cardiovascular risk and increased risk of orthopedic injury.

The regular practice of moderate intensity physical activity is independently associated with a reduction in all-cause mortality

There is no scientific evidence that any general or specific counselling intervention by family physicians will influence sedentary individuals to practice regular physical activity. However, one must not forget that knowledge of the risk of sedentariness was the first reason to increase one's level of physical activity given by adults interviewed in *Canada's Health Promotion Survey*. Physicians, as part of the health care system, are a major source of health information and should be able to reinforce public health initiatives. They must also inform patients about the risks of excessively intensive physical activity under certain circumstances. Emphasis should be on encouraging a variety of self-directed, moderate-level physical activities (e.g., gardening, raking leaves, walking to work, taking the stairs) which can be more easily incorporated into an individual's daily routine. Sporadic exercise, especially if extremely vigorous in an otherwise sedentary individual, should be discouraged. If an individual requires additional direction or supervision, clinicians may wish to refer patients to an accredited fitness center or exercise specialist.

Unanswered Questions (Research Agenda)

The effectiveness of a short duration counselling intervention by the family physician in affecting long-term behavior patterns in sedentary individuals needs further investigation.

Evidence

The literature was identified by a MEDLINE search for the English language from 1988 to 1993 using the key words exertion, exercise, leisure activities, mortality, coronary disease, cardiovascular system, osteoarthritis, and obesity. This review was initiated in October 1993 and recommendations finalized by the Task Force in March 1994.

Selected References

1. Hahn RA, Teutsch SM, Rothenberg RB, *et al*: Excess deaths from nine chronic diseases in the United States, 1986. *JAMA* 1990; 264: 2654-2659

2. Paffenbarger RS Jr, Hyde RT, Wing AL, *et al*: The association of changes in physical-activity level and other lifestyle characteristics with mortality among men. *N Engl J Med* 1993; 328: 538-545

3. Blair SN, Kohl HW, Paffenbarger RS, *et al*: Physical fitness and all-cause mortality. A prospective study of healthy men and women. *JAMA* 1989; 262(17): 2395-2401

4. Berlin JA, Colditz GA: A meta-analysis of physical activity in the prevention of coronary heart disease. *Am J Epidemiol* 1990; 132(4): 612-628

5. Paffenbarger RS Jr, Jung DL, Leung RW, *et al*: Physical activity and hypertension: an epidemiological view. *Ann Med* 1991; 23: 319-327

6. Blair SN, Goodyear NN, Gibbens LW, *et al*: Physical fitness and incidence of hypertension in healthy normotensive men and women. *JAMA* 1984; 252: 487-490

7. Rissanen AM, Heliovaara M, Knekt P, *et al*: Determinants of weight gain and overweight in adult Finns. *Eur J Clin Nutr* 1991; 45: 419-430

8. Williamson DF, Madans J, Anda RF, *et al*: Recreational physical activity and ten-year weight change in a U.S. national cohort. *Int J Obes* 1993; 17: 279-286

9. Manson J, Nathan DM, Krolewski S, *et al*: A prospective study of exercise and incidence of diabetes among US male physicians. *JAMA* 1992; 268(1): 63-67

10. Manson JE, Rimm EB, Stampfer MJ, *et al*: Physical activity and incidence of non-insulin dependent diabetes mellitus in women. *Lancet* 1991; 338(8770): 774-778

11. Helmrich SP, Ragland DR, Leung RW, *et al*: Physical activity and reduced occurrence of non-insulin dependent diabetes mellitus. *N Eng J Med* 1991; 325: 147-152

12. Powell KE, Thompson PD, Caspersen CJ, *et al*: Physical activity and the incidence of coronary heart disease. *Annu Rev Public Health* 1987; 8: 253-287

13. Centers for Disease Control, American College of Sports Medicine: Summary Statement: Workshop on physical activity and public health. *Sports Med Bull* 1993; 28: 7

14. Willich SN, Lewis M, Lowel H, *et al*: Physical exertion as a trigger of acute myocardial infarction. *N Eng J Med* 1993; 329: 1684-1690

15. Mittleman MA, Maclure M, Tofler G, *et al*: Triggering of acute myocardial infarction by heavy physical exertion. *N Eng J Med* 1993; 329: 1677-1683

16. Kohl HW, Powell KE, Gordon NF, *et al*: Physical activity, physical fitness, and sudden cardiac death. *Epidemiolog Rev* 1992; 14: 37-58

17. Eklund LG, Haskell WL, Johnson JL, *et al*: Physical fitness as a predictor of cardiovascular mortality in asymptomatic North American men. The Lipid Research Clinics Mortality Follow-up Study. *N Eng J Med* 1988; 319: 1379-1384

18. Blair SN: Evidence for success of exercise in weight loss and control. *Ann Intern Med* 1993; 119: 702-706

19. Bouchard C, Tremblay A, Nadeau A, *et al*: Long-term exercise training with constant energy intake. 1: Effect on body composition and selected metabolic variables. *Int J Obesity* 1990; 14(1): 57-73

20. Smith EL, Gilligan C, McAdam M, *et al*: Deterring bone loss by exercise intervention in premenopausal and postmenopausal women. *Calcif Tissue Int* 1989; 44: 312-321

21. Dalsky GP, Stocke KS, Ehsani AA, *et al*: Weight bearing exercise training and lumbar bone mineral content in postmenopausal women. *Ann Int Med* 1988; 108: 824-828

22. Bloomfield SA, Williams NI, Lamb DR, *et al*: Non-weightbearing exercise may increase lumbar spine bone mineral density in healthy postmenopausal women. *Am J Phys Med Rehab* 1993; 72: 204-209

23. Harris SS, Casperson CJ, DeFriese GH, *et al*: Physical activity counselling for healthy adults as a primary preventive intervention in the clinical setting. *JAMA* 1989; 261: 3588-3598

24. U.S. Preventive Services Task Force: *Guide to Clinical Preventive Services: an Assessment of the Effectiveness of 169 Interventions*. Williams & Wilkins, Baltimore, Md, 1989: 297-303

Physical Activity Counselling

MANEUVER	EFFECTIVENESS	LEVEL OF EVIDENCE <REF>	RECOMMENDATION
Moderate-level physical activity* performed consistently to accumulate 30 minutes or more over the course of most days of the week	Regular practice of moderate intensity physical activity* has been associated with a reduction in all-cause mortality, incidence of coronary heart disease (CHD), high blood pressure (HBP) and non-insulin dependent diabetes mellitus (NIDDM) and protects against the risk that vigorous exercise triggers myocardial infarction.	Cohort studies: All-cause mortality<1,2>, CHD<3,4,12>, Risk of MI<14,15>, HBP<5,6,16>,Obesity <7,8,18,19>, NIDDM<9-11> (II-2)	There is fair evidence to recommend that individuals engage in the regular practice of moderate intensity physical activity (B)
Regular weight-bearing exercise by pre-menopausal and post-menopausal women	Weight-bearing exercise stimulates bone deposition. The specific type and duration of exercise necessary is still unknown.	Non-randomized trial<20-22> (II-1)	Evidence for or against a recommendation for women to engage in a specific type of exercise to reduce osteoporosis risk is lacking (C)
Inquiry on physical activity level and information on the health benefits of regular moderate activity and on the dangers of vigorous activity for unfit individuals	No studies on the effectiveness of counselling by physicians. Physicians are an important source of health advice. Important reduction of CHD risk attributable to physical activity.	Expert opinion<24> (III)	Evidence for or against a recommendation to include physical activity counselling in the periodic health exam is lacking (C)

* The following are considered moderate intensity physical activities (above 4.5 Mets): normal walking, golfing on foot, slow biking, raking leaves, cleaning windows, slow dancing, light restaurant work, etc.

Metabolic/ Nutritional Disorders

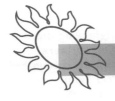

CHAPTER **48**

Prevention of Obesity in Adults

By James Douketis and William Feldman

Prevention of Obesity in Adults

Prepared by James Douketis, MD[1] and William Feldman, MD FRCPC[2]

The Canadian Guidelines for Healthy Weights and the Report of the Task Force on the Treatment of Obesity were published in 1988 and 1990 respectively. Both reports recognized that persons with a body mass index (BMI) of ≥ 27 kg/m^2, who were considered obese, were at increased risk of health problems.<1,2> The rationale for detecting the presence or absence of obesity is twofold: 1) To prevent the development of obesity in those with a normal BMI; and 2) To reduce weight in persons with obesity. It is hoped that detecting and treating obesity will decrease the incidence of coronary artery disease, diabetes, hypertension, hyperlipidemia and other diseases which have been linked to obesity. This, in turn, would reduce morbidity attributable to these diseases and lower overall mortality. This improvement in health status is predicated on sustained weight loss. At present there is insufficient evidence that these goals can be achieved based on the following conclusions: 1) Obesity prevention programs are ineffective in reducing the incidence of obesity; 2) Weight reduction is associated with a high rate of recidivism over the long term in the vast majority of persons, regardless of the weight loss method used; and 3) In obese persons there is no evidence that weight reduction will be longstanding and will translate into a reduction of morbidity (ie. reduced incidence of myocardial infarct, stroke, etc.) or lower mortality. However, one cannot exclude the possibility that weight reduction can have health benefits in a small minority of persons in whom long-term weight loss is successful. As well, in obese persons with coexistent diabetes, hypertension or hyperlipidemia, weight reduction can be recommended cautiously since this may improve the symptoms and management of these diseases. Obesity in children is discussed in a separate chapter (Chapter 30).

Obesity is very prevalent and has been linked to coronary artery disease, hypertension, hyperlipidemia, diabetes, and increased mortality

Burden of Suffering

In a cross-sectional study conducted between 1986-1990 in Canadians aged 18-74, the prevalence of obesity (BMI ≥ 27 kg/m^2) was 35% in men and 27% in women.<3> Three percent of men and 5% of women were found to be morbidly obese (BMI ≥ 35 kg/m^2). Factors

[1] Clinical Research Fellow in Thromboembolism, Department of Medicine, McMaster University, Hamilton, Ontario
[2] Professor of Pediatrics and of Preventive Medicine and Biostatistics, University of Toronto, Toronto, Ontario

associated with an increased prevalence of obesity include increased age, a low level of education, low physical activity, alcohol use in men and parity in women.<4> Obesity has been causally linked to several diseases including coronary artery disease, hypertension, hyperlipidemia and diabetes. The evidence supporting an independent association between obesity and these diseases is based on cross-sectional and longitudinal population-based cohort studies. These studies showed an increased prevalence of these diseases amongst obese persons as compared to non-obese persons, after controlling for potential confounding factors such as smoking and family history.<5-13> Recent data from several studies have suggested that the central form of obesity, as defined by an increased waist/hip ratio, correlates with the presence of the aforementioned diseases independent of the BMI.<11,12,14-18> Obesity has also been associated with other diseases including obstructive sleep apnea, cholelithiasis, venous thromboembolism, and certain neoplasms (breast, colon, endometrial, ovarian and prostate) although the evidence linking obesity to these conditions is not as extensive.<19> The psychological impact of obesity, although not as well studied, may be substantial, given the emphasis on a lean body image and the negative perception of an overweight state that currently exist in our society.

Obesity has also been independently associated with an increased mortality rate based on large prospective cohort studies.<5,7,19-21> These studies were of long duration, ranging from 10-26 years, were controlled for smoking behaviour, and eliminated early deaths during the follow-up period that may have been related to pre-existent sub-clinical disease unrelated to coexistent obesity.

Maneuver

The diagnosis of an obese state can be made using several methods (e.g. weight-height ratios, body circumference ratios, and skinfold thickness measurements). In Canada, the body mass index (BMI = weight/height^2) is the most widely accepted method of detecting the presence of obesity. This index is closely correlated with weight but largely independent of height. The BMI uses a statistical correction for height so that body weight will correlate maximally with adiposity. The BMI measurement is easily performed, reliable, and correlates well with body fat content.<22> In Canada, obesity is defined for both men and women as a BMI ≥ 27 kg/m^2. A BMI above this cut-off is associated with an increased health risk. Morbid obesity is defined as a BMI in men or women ≥ 35 kg/m^2.<1>

Effectiveness of Prevention and Treatment

At least two large community-based studies have assessed the effectiveness of educational programs aimed at encouraging weight reduction as part of an overall healthy lifestyle.<23,24> After five to ten years of intervention there was no significant difference in the average weight loss in the communities which received education as compared to control communities. Other educational interventions aimed at reducing cardiovascular risk factor prevalence have met with similarly disappointing results. (see Chapters 43 and 54)

The clinical approach to the management of obesity can be similar to the management of other chronic disorders such as diabetes, hyperlipidemia or most forms of hypertension. Lifelong dietary therapy and possibly long-term pharmacologic or behavioural treatment would be required to control obesity successfully. Given the high rate of recidivism following weight reduction, weight reduction targets should be realistic and modest weight loss or maintenance of a steady body weight may be appropriate therapeutic goals. The treatment of obesity should be individualized depending on each patient's age, BMI, and the coexistence of other diseases such as diabetes, hypertension or hyperlipidemia which have been linked to obesity.

Dietary Therapy

Two types of calorie restricted diets are currently used. Low calorie diets (LCD) provide 1,000-1,500 kcal of energy daily. Very low calorie diets (VLCD) provide <800 kcal per day and require physician supervision. Numerous cohort studies and randomized trials have demonstrated effective weight reduction over the short term but few randomized trials have assessed the effectiveness of weight reduction over a 3-5 year period. For both LCDs and VLCDs approximately 50-78% of participants who lost weight initially returned to their baseline weight within 1-3 years.<25,26> In studies with a longer follow-up of up to five years a similar pattern has occurred, with the vast majority of persons who lost weight eventually returning to their original pre-treatment weight.<27,28> Sustained weight loss may be achieved in a small number of persons.

Appetite-suppressant Drug Therapy

There have been many recent placebo-controlled clinical trials of various appetite-suppressant drugs as adjuncts to dietary therapy in the treatment of obesity. Drug therapies have been shown to be effective in reducing weight when combined with a diet but the effects have been limited to periods when the drug is taken or when a predetermined diet is maintained. In general, as with dietary restriction, drug therapy may be effective in the short-term but long-term (i.e. 3-5 year) benefits have not been demonstrated except in a small minority of persons.<29-31>

Behavioural Therapy

Behavioral therapy when used alone for the treatment of obesity will lead to only modest weight loss (i.e. 0.5-0.75 kg/week). Consequently, this form of treatment is usually used in concert with other weight reduction methods. It has been postulated that long-term behavioural therapy may reinforce the necessary lifestyle and cognitive changes required to maintain long-term weight loss. However, even in studies with long-term weight loss counselling, sustained weight loss has been difficult to achieve in all but a few subjects.<32,33>

Surgical Therapy

Surgical therapy for obesity is usually considered only for persons with morbid obesity in whom more conservative forms of treatment have been unsuccessful although it is combined with dietary, and often with behavioural therapy. Vertical band gastroplasty is currently considered to be the most effective and safest of all gastric lumen reducing procedures. A small cohort study has reported improved mortality benefit in selected patients.<34> The use of intragastric balloon insertion has been compared with dietary therapy in a placebo-controlled study; weight loss was not found to be significantly different in either group.<35,36>

Exercise and the Treatment of Obesity

When combined with dietary and behavioural weight reduction methods, there is little evidence that exercise augments weight loss unless there is significant change in the baseline exercise capacity.<37,38> Exercise has been recommended as an adjunct to any weight reduction program since it may help people maintain their diet through a sense of psychological well-being, and this in turn may prevent weight regain. However, the Task Force recommends the regular practice of moderate to intense physical activity for the maintenance of a healthy body weight (Chapter 47).

Benefits of Weight Reduction

There is substantial evidence that treatment of obesity can improve the management of many of the purported sequelae of obesity. Based on randomized trials and prospective cohort studies, weight reduction has been shown to reduce systolic and diastolic blood pressures amongst obese persons with hypertension, independent of sodium intake, thereby reducing their antihypertensive drug requirements.<39,40> In obese diabetics, weight loss can improve

Weight reduction can improve control of hypertension, diabetes and hyperlipidemia but other benefits may be limited by recidivism

glycemic control and reduce the need for or the dosage of oral hypoglycemics or insulin.<41> As well, weight loss can improve hyperlipidemic states and may significantly reduce symptoms in patients with obstructive sleep apnea.<42,43> The evidence that treating obesity will prevent major outcome events such as myocardial infarction, stroke or diabetes and will reduce mortality is sparse. This evidence is based on insurance company mortality data, retrospective analyses of prospective cohort studies and one retrospective study.<5,44,45> However, since weight reduction is usually short-lived this may attenuate or obscure any potential benefit that weight loss might achieve in terms of reduced major morbidity or mortality.

Risks Associated With the Treatment of Obesity

Weight reduction has been associated with several possible adverse effects, depending on the method of treatment. Diets of less than 1,000 kcal can cause orthostatic hypotension, fatigue, hair loss, transient menstrual irregularities and symptomatic cholelithiasis. Drug therapy can commonly cause drowsiness, fatigue and gastrointestinal discomfort. Gastroplasty and balloon insertion surgery can lead to gastric ulceration, perforation and bowel obstruction. Over the long term, weight reduction and fluctuations in weight (weight cycling) have been associated with increased cardiovascular morbidity and higher mortality.<46-48> These interesting results are based on observational studies that have certain methodologic limitations. Further prospective studies are required to address this important issue before definitive conclusions are made.

Recommendations of Others

In 1990 the Canadian Task Force on the Treatment of Obesity encouraged weight loss in obese persons with "coexistent health problems that can be ameliorated with weight loss and/or at risk of developing conditions associated with obesity (e.g., those with a family history of diabetes)". They advised weight loss in the presence of "upper body obesity" when the individual's BMI was ≥ 25 kg/m^2.<2> The U.S. National Institute of Health Technology Assessment Conference on obesity recommended treatment in persons with health problems that could be lessened by weight loss such as sleep apnea, hypertension or non-insulin-dependent diabetes mellitus, and that weight control might be appropriate in persons near the upper limit of the healthy weight range. The U.S. Preventive Services Task Force recommendation is currently under review.

Conclusions and Recommendations

There is insufficient evidence at this time to recommend the inclusion or exclusion in a routine physical examination of BMI measurement for persons aged 18-65, given the lack of long-term effectiveness of weight reduction therapy in the large majority of obese persons. Weight reduction can be cautiously recommended in obese persons with coexistent diseases who may benefit from weight loss, after taking into account the high recidivism rate and adverse effects of weight loss. For all persons, who are either obese or in the upper normal BMI range and in whom weight reduction is not indicated or has been unsuccessful, maintenance of a stable weight would be a reasonable alternative.<25> Moderate intensity physical activity, taking into account current fitness levels, is also recommended for all Canadians to maintain a healthy body weight (Chapter 47).

Unanswered Questions (Research Agenda)

The following are research priorities:

1. To develop a better understanding of the etiology and pathophysiology of obesity, and to clarify the clinical importance of central (android) obesity.

2. To design and execute long-term randomized trials or methodologically sound cohort studies so as to determine the effects of sustained weight reduction and weight cycling on well defined morbidity events and on mortality.

3. To develop effective obesity prevention strategies.

4. To develop effective weight reduction strategies in obese persons with coexistent diseases whose management may be improved by weight loss, and in other persons with obesity.

Evidence

The literature was identified with a MEDLINE search for the years 1966 to June 1993 using the following key words: Obesity, weight reduction. Further references were obtained from the bibliographies of review articles and recently published articles that had not yet appeared in the MEDLINE directory.

This review was initiated in March 1993 and the recommendations were finalized by the Task Force in January 1994.

Selected References

1. Health and Welfare Canada: *Canadian Guidelines for Healthy Weights*. Ministry of National Health and Welfare, Ottawa, October 1988

2. Levy AS, Heaton AW: Weight control practices of U.S. adults trying to lose weight. *Ann Intern Med* 1993; 119: 661-666

3. Reeder BA, Angel A, Ledoux M, *et al*: Obesity and its relation to cardiovascular disease risk factors in Canadian adults. *Can Med Assoc J* 1992; 146: 2009-2019

4. Evers S: Economic and social factors associated with obesity in adult Canadians. *Nutr Res* 1987; 7: 3-13

5. Hubert HB, Feinleib M, McNamara PM, *et al*: Obesity as an independent risk factor for cardiovascular disease: a 26-year follow up of participants in the Framingham Heart Study. *Circulation* 1983; 67: 968-977

6. Manson JE, Colditz GA, Stampfer MJ, *et al*: A prospective study of obesity and risk of coronary heart disease in women. *N Eng J Med* 1990; 322: 882-889

7. Rhoads GG, Kagan A: The relation of coronary disease, stroke and mortality to weight in youth and middle-age. *Lancet* 1983; 1: 492-495

8. Van Italie TB: Health implications of overweight and obesity in the United States. *Ann Intern Med* 1985; 103: 983-989

9. Stamler R, Stamler J, Reidlinger WF, *et al*: Weight and blood pressure. Findings in hypertension screening of 1 million Americans. *JAMA* 1978; 240: 1607-1610

10. Colditz GA, Willet WC, Stampfer MJ, *et al*: Weight as a risk factor for clinical diabetes in women. *Am J Epidemiol* 1990; 132: 501-513

11. Hartz AJ, Rupley DC Jr, Kalkhoff RD, *et al*: Relationship of obesity to diabetes: influences of obesity level and body fat distribution. *Prev Med* 1983; 12: 351-357

12. Freedman DS, Jacobsen SJ, Barboriak JJ, *et al*: Body fat distribution and male/female differences in lipids and lipoproteins. *Circulation* 1990; 81: 1498-1506

13. Larsson B, Bjorntorp P, Tibblin G: The health consequences of moderate obesity. *Int J Obes* 1981; 5: 97-116

14. Kannel WB, Cupples LA, Ramaswami R, *et al*: Regional obesity and risk of cardiovascular disease: The Framingham study. *J Clin Epidemiol* 1991; 44: 183-190

15. Ducimetiere P, Richard J, Cambien F: The pattern of subcutaneous fat distribution on middle-age men and the risk of coronary heart disease: The Paris Prospective study. *Int J Obes* 1986; 10: 229-240

16. Larsson B, Svadsudd K, Welin L, *et al*: Abdominal adipose tissue distribution, obesity, and risk of cardiovascular disease and death: 13 year follow-up of participants in the study of men born in 1913. *Br Med J Clin Res Ed* 1984; 288: 1401-1404

17. Lapidus L, Bengtsson C, Larson B, *et al*: Distribution of adipose tissue and risk of cardiovascular disease and death: a 12 year follow up of participants in the population study of women in Gothenburg, Sweden. *BMJ* 1984; 289: 1257-1261

18. Ohlson LO, Larson B, Svardsudd K, *et al*: The influence of body fat distribution on the incidence of diabetes mellitus. *Diabetes* 1985; 34: 1055-1058

19. Bray GA: Obesity: basic considerations and clinical approaches. *Dis Mon* 1989; 35: 449-537

20. Wilcosky T, Hyde J, Anderson JJ, *et al*: Obesity and mortality in the Lipid Research Clinics Program Follow-up Study. *J Clin Epidemiol* 1990; 43: 743-752

21. Keys A, Taylor HL, Blackburn H, *et al*: Mortality and coronary heart disease among men studied for 23 years. *Arch Intern Med* 1971; 128: 201-214

22. Stewart AW, Jackson RT, Ford MA, *et al*: Underestimation of relative weight by use of self-reported height and weight. *Am J Epidemiol* 1987; 125: 122-126

23. Taylor CB, Fourtmann SP, Flora J, *et al*: Effect of long-term community health education on body mass index. The Stanford Five City Project. *Am J Epidemiol* 1991; 134: 235-249

24. Jeffery RW: Minnesota studies on community-based approaches to weight loss and control. *Ann Intern Med* 1993; 119: 719-721

25. NIH Technology Assessment Conference Panel: Methods for voluntary weight loss and control. *Ann Intern Med* 1992; 116: 942-949

26. Wadden TA, Stunkard AJ, Brownell KD: Very low calorie diets: their efficacy, safety, and future. *Ann Intern Med* 1983; 99: 675-684

27. Holden J, Darga LL, Olson SM, *et al*: Long-term follow-up of patients attending a combination very-low calorie diet and behaviour therapy weight loss programme. *Int J Obes* 1992; 16: 605-613

28. Karvetti RL, Hakala P: A seven year follow up of a weight reduction programme in Finnish primary health care. *Eur J Clin Nutr* 1992; 46: 743-752

29. Guy-Grand B, Apfelbaum M, Crepaldi G, *et al*: International trial of long-term dexfenfluramine in obesity. *Lancet* 1989; 2: 1142-1145

30. Weintraub M: Long term weight control: The National Heart, Lung, and Blood Institute funded multimodal intervention study. *Clin Pharmacol Ther* 1992; 51: 581-646

31. Garrow J: Importance of obesity. *BMJ* 1991; 303: 704-706

32. Wing RR: Behavioural treatment of severe obesity. *Am J Clin Nutr* 1992; 55 (2 suppl): 545s-551s

33. Hakala P, Karvetti R-L, Ronnemaa T: Group vs. individual weight reduction programmes in the treatment of severe obesity – a five year follow-up study. *Int J Obes* 1993; 17: 97-102

34. Mason EE, *et al*: Impact of vertical banded gastroplasty on mortality from obesity. [abstract] *Obes Surg* 1991; 1: 115

35. Lindor KD, Hughes RW, Ilstrup DM, *et al*: Intragastric balloons in comparison with standard therapy for obesity – A randomized, double blind trial. *Mayo Clin Proc* 1987; 62: 992-996

36. Benjamin SB, Maher KA, Cattau EL Jr, *et al*: Double blind controlled trial of the Garren-Edwards gastric bubble: An adjunctive treatment for exogenous obesity. *Gastroenterology* 1988; 95: 581-588

37. Sweeney ME, Hill JO, Heller PA, *et al*: Severe vs. moderate energy restriction with and without exercise in the treatment of obesity: efficiency of weight loss. *Am J Clin Nutr* 1993; 57: 127-134

38. Troisi RJ, Heinold JW, Vokonas PS, *et al*: Cigarette smoking, dietary intake, and physical activity: effects on body fat distribution – the Normative Aging Study. *Am J Clin Nutr* 1991; 53: 1104-1111

39. Tuck ML, Sowers J, Dornfeld L, *et al*: The effect of weight reduction on blood pressure, plasma renin activity and plasma aldosterone levels in obese patients. *N Eng J Med* 1981; 304: 930-933

40. Stevens VJ, Corrigan SA, Obarzanek E, *et al*: Weight loss intervention in phase I of the Trials of Hypertension Prevention. *Arch Intern Med* 1993; 153: 849-858

41. Wing RR, Marcus MD, Salata R, *et al*: Effects of a very-low-calorie diet on long-term glycemic control in obese type 2 diabetic subjects. *Arch Intern Med* 1991; 151: 1334-1440

42. Wolf RN, Gundy SM: Influence of weight reduction on plasma lipoproteins in obese patients. *Arteriosclerosis* 1983; 3: 160-169

43. Wittels EH, Thompson S: Obstructive sleep apnea and obesity. *Otolaryngol Clin North Am* 1990; 23: 751-760

44. Borkan GA, Sparrow D, Wisniewski C, *et al*: Body weight and coronary disease risk: patterns of risk factor change associated with long-term weight change. *Am J Epidemiol* 1986; 124: 410-419

45. Lean MEJ, Powrie JK, Anderson AS, *et al*: Obesity, weight loss and prognosis in type 2 diabetes. *Diabet Med* 1990; 7: 228-233

46. Everhart JE: Contribution of obesity and weight loss to gallstone disease. *Ann Intern Med* 1993; 119: 1029-1035

47. Pamuk ER, Williamson DF, Serdula MK, *et al*: Weight loss and subsequent death in a cohort of U.S. adults. *Ann Intern Med* 1993; 119: 744-748

48. Jeffery RW, Wing RR, French SA: Weight cycling and cardiovascular risk factors in obese men. *Am J Clin Nutr* 1992; 55: 641-644

Prevention of Obesity in Adults

MANEUVER	EFFECTIVENESS	LEVEL OF EVIDENCE <REF>	RECOMMENDATION
Counselling to prevent obesity	Primary prevention programs are ineffective in reducing the incidence of obesity.	Prospective cohort studies<23,24> (II-2)	Insufficient evidence to recommend for or against primary prevention programs for obesity (C)
Measurement of height and weight, calculation of body mass index (BMI) (weight/ height²) and treatment of obesity	BMI is a reliable and valid method of determining body fat content and detecting obesity.	Prospective cohort study<22> (II-2)	Insufficient evidence to include or exclude from the periodic health examination (C); weight reduction can be cautiously recommended in persons with obesity and coexistent diabetes, hypertension or hyperlipidemia. In persons who are either obese or in the upper normal BMI range, in whom weight reduction is not being considered or has been unsuccessful, maintenance of a stable weight is a reasonable alternative
	In most obese persons weight reduction methods can be effective in the short term but over the long term weight loss is eventually regained. There is insufficient evidence that weight reduction will reduce morbidity and mortality but weight reduction may have health benefits for the small minority who achieve long-term weight loss.	Randomized trial<29, 30,35,36> (I); cohort studies<27, 28,33,34> (II-2)	
	Over the long term, weight reduction and weight cycling have been associated with increased cardiovascular morbidity and mortality.	Prospective cohort studies<46-48> (II-2)	

(Continued on next page)

Prevention of Obesity in Adults (concl'd)

MANEUVER	EFFECTIVENESS	LEVEL OF EVIDENCE <REF>	RECOMMENDATION
Measurement of height and weight, calculation of body mass index (BMI) (weight/ height^2) and treatment of obesity	**High-Risk Group*** Weight reduction can improve short-term control of coexisting diseases but there is insufficient evidence that weight reduction will reduce morbidity and mortality (e.g. myocardial infarct, stroke).	Randomized trial<40> (I); prospective cohort studies<41,42,44> and retrospective study<45> (II-2)	*(See previous page)*

* Persons with obesity and coexistent diabetes hypertension or hyperlipidemia.

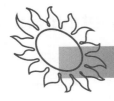

CHAPTER 49

Nutritional Counselling for Undesirable Dietary Patterns and Screening for Protein/Calorie Malnutrition Disorders in Adults

By Christopher Patterson

49

Nutritional Counselling for Undesirable Dietary Patterns and Screening for Protein/Calorie Malnutrition Disorders in Adults

Prepared by Christopher Patterson, MD, FRCPC[1] drawing from materials prepared for the U.S. Preventive Services Task Force[2]

The consumption or lack of consumption of certain nutrients has been associated with a wide variety of illnesses. This chapter focuses upon diseases induced by excessive consumption and selected deficiency states. There is a strong association between excessive consumption of saturated fats and coronary artery disease, and weaker associations between consumption of fats and malignancies of the breast, colon and prostate. (Also see chapters on childhood obesity (Chapter 30), obesity (Chapter 48), cholesterol screening (Chapter 54), and lung cancer (Chapter 64). Chapters making nutritional recommendations for pregnant women should also be consulted where possible: neural tube defects (Chapter 7), low birth weight (Chapter 4), iron supplementation (Chapter 6), breast feeding (Chapter 22), iron deficiency anemia (Chapter 23), and dental caries (Chapter 36)). There is good evidence for the efficacy of nutritional counselling by non-physicians. In 1979 the Canadian Task Force on the Periodic Health Examination concluded that there was insufficient justification to screen the general population for malnutrition, but recommended screening and/or case-finding for certain high risk groups.<1> High-risk groups included adolescent girls, pregnant women, women who breast feed for unusually long periods, the elderly (especially if living alone), Native peoples and food faddists.

[1] Professor and Head, Division of Geriatric Medicine, McMaster University, Hamilton, Ontario

[2] By Steven H. Woolf, MD, MPH, Science Advisor, U.S. Preventive Services Task Force, Paul S. Frame, MD, Clinical Associate Professor, Department of Family Medicine, and Department of Community and Preventive Medicine, University of Rochester School of Medicine and Dentistry, Rochester, NY, and Robert S. Lawrence, MD, Director, Health Sciences, The Rockefeller Foundation, New York, NY

Burden of Suffering

Dietary Excess

Diseases associated with dietary excess and imbalance rank among the leading causes of illness and death in the western world. Major diseases in which diet plays a role include coronary artery disease, some cancers and cerebrovascular disease. Coronary artery disease is the leading cause of death in Canada, accounting for about 46,600 deaths per year.<2> Cancer of the colorectum, breast and prostate are epidemiologically associated with nutritional risk factors and together cause 15,500 deaths annually.<3> Cerebrovascular disease is the third leading cause of death accounting for about 13,900 deaths per year.<2> Caloric intake exceeding energy expenditure can lead to obesity, which in turn is a risk factor for both hypertension and type II diabetes mellitus. Hypertension is also associated with excessive sodium intake. Sequelae of hypertension include stroke, cardiac and renal failure. Diabetes is a leading cause of neuropathy, peripheral vascular disease, renal failure and blindness.

Excessive dietary fat intake contributes to 75,000 deaths annually in Canada

Major disparities between recommended dietary practices and actual consumption are most notable in intakes of fat (30% vs. 38%) and complex carbohydrates (55% vs. 48%). There is also concern about excessive consumption of inappropriate vitamin and mineral supplements. Multivitamins are the most commonly consumed supplements, followed by vitamin C, calcium, vitamin E and vitamin A. Men and women over the age of 65 are the primary purchasers. While few individuals consume nutrient and vitamin preparations in amounts considered toxic, the need for these supplements for most people is questionable. Reasons cited for nutrient supplement use are often inappropriate (e.g. to improve general health, to prevent colds and other illnesses, to prolong youth, increase energy level, etc.). Most people receive advice on the use of supplements from unreliable sources. Large amounts of vitamin C can result in a rebound deficiency with clinical signs of scurvy when supplements are stopped abruptly. High doses of vitamin C may interfere with the absorption of vitamin B12, and lead to the formation of oxalate renal calculi. For fat-soluble vitamins, excess intake of Vitamin A may cause bone and joint pains, changes in the skin and hair, hepatomegaly and benign intracranial hypertension. Vitamin D excess may lead to hypercalcemia and excessive excretion of calcium with skeletal decalcification. Self administered calcium supplements from "natural sources" may be contaminated with toxic substances such as lead. Excessive doses of zinc may interfere with immune function.

Deficiency Disorders

Nutritional factor deficiencies have been linked to osteoporosis, diverticular disease, constipation, and iron deficiency anemia. Seventy-four to eighty percent of women do not meet the recommended requirement for calcium. Dietary deficiency of calcium has been implicated in the genesis of osteoporosis. Those who are less exposed to the sun, and hence less capable of dermal photosynthesis of cholecalciferol may be at particular risk; this includes many elderly living alone or in institutions. An estimated 40% of North American women will suffer from osteoporosis-related fractures by the time they reach age 70. Hip fractures are associated with significant pain, disability, decreased functional independence and high mortality. Deficiency of dietary fibre has been implicated in constipation and other gastrointestinal disorders such as diverticulosis. A large number of adults do not consume Recommended Nutrient Intakes (RNI) for dietary fibre. Constipation is a frequent complaint, and diverticular disease produces significant morbidity. Iron deficiency is common in menstruating women whose diet is deficient in foods containing available iron, especially meats. Pregnant women, and those who nurse for a prolonged period of time are also at risk for iron deficiency. Up to 63% of people over age 60 have been documented to have deficient iron intakes.

Chronic alcoholics are at high risk for deficiency disorders as they derive an excessive amount of energy from alcohol to the detriment of other nutrients, resulting in deficiency of water-soluble vitamins, particularly thiamine. Strict vegetarians are another vulnerable group for B group vitamin deficiency.

Five to six percent of males and 15-22% of females in Canada have a low body mass index (BMI less than 20) which may be associated with health problems. Malnutrition is associated with an increased prevalence of complications and high mortality among hospitalized patients. While those living alone are at risk, institutional care is associated with malnutrition in as many as 52-85%. Protein/calorie malnutrition (PCM) is characterized by inadequate intake of both energy and protein or a sufficient energy intake with a high carbohydrate, low protein diet. A weight loss of 10-20% from usual weight represents moderate PCM, and a loss greater than 20% indicates severe PCM. Due to the difficulty of defining PCM the true prevalence is unknown, but in a community study, Canada's Health Promotion Survey, 8% of younger women and 15% of women aged over 65 years had BMI values that placed them in the underweight category.<4> PCM has been reported in 17-44% of general medical and 30-65% of general surgical hospital in-patients.

RNI are based upon average intakes of healthy people, levels of intake that are known to be associated with deficiency, and a limited number of studies of nutrient supplementation. In one Canadian study,

10-28% of elderly were at risk for dietary deficiency of calcium, beta-carotene and vitamins A, D, and C.

Detection Maneuver

There are three principal methods to determine nutrient history: screening questionnaires, dietary records and dietary recall.

Self-administered questionnaires are believed to provide reasonable estimates of current nutritional intakes,[5] particularly for those nutrients that are highly concentrated in relatively few foods. The validity of food frequency questionnaires may be affected by gender, educational, cultural and other factors which influence recall. Alcohol is one of the most difficult items to quantify and underestimates are frequent. Other chapters address alcohol more directly: Chapter 5 on fetal alcohol syndrome, Chapter 41 on children of alcoholics, and Chapter 42 on early detection and counselling of problem drinking. Inaccuracies extend to other food items, and many people have difficulty reporting accurate portion size.[6]

The seven-day weighed dietary record has commonly been regarded as the gold standard for assessing habitual dietary intake. However, recent studies have found significant bias in reporting habitual energy intakes.[7-9] Dietary records are intrusive, which may interfere with compliance.

Recalled diet information more accurately characterizes former dietary intakes than does current diet information.[10] The Food Frequency Questionnaire is more reliable for the distant past than the recent past.[11] When individuals change food consumption during a four year period, their estimates of former consumption are biased towards their current consumption. Where food consumption remains stable, there is good agreement between recalled diet and original diet information.[12]

Determination of dietary intake for older people is problematic. Increased prevalence of memory disorders in old age may interfere with the accuracy of dietary recall. Twenty-four hour recall grossly underestimates actual intake. In young adults, recall is more likely to produce a reliable estimate of intake where a regular meal pattern is maintained, although snacking is often omitted from reports. In the case of dietary records and food weighing, the effort required to weigh food may result in unwillingness to participate, limiting the generalizability of results to those with greater compliance.

Physical Examination

Other than the finding of obesity, physical examination is unhelpful for determining whether appropriate quantities of nutrients are being consumed. In malnutrition, the early changes are not easily distinguished from changes of normal aging. Abnormally thin or sparse hair, changes to the tongue and angles of the mouth and lips may be seen, but require supporting dietary and biochemical evidence to establish a diagnosis of malnutrition. Anthropometric measures include height, weight and calculation of body mass index (BMI). As older people tend to become shorter, measurement may not reflect former adult height. Ulnar and fibular length appear to correlate well with former height in older people. Adiposity may be assessed by girth or skin fold measurements. Measuring triceps skinfold thickness (TSF) and arm muscle area (AMA) is simple, however interobserver variability is problematic with TSF and adequate norms have not been established for all age groups. Midarm muscle circumference (MAMC) and AMA do not correlate well with biochemical measures of protein status and are insensitive to early changes. In severe malnutrition, an AMA of less than 16 cm^2 correlates highly with 90 day mortality. Anthropometric measurements may be affected by the accuracy of location for each measurement, and the skill level of the observer.

Laboratory Measurement

Serum protein measurements are commonly used to assess nutritional status. Albumin levels change slowly, due to a long half-life (14 days) and a large pool. Reduced levels are not specific for protein deficiency, as concentrations tend to fall in advanced age and in the presence of chronic disease. Serum transferrin may be more responsive to rapid change due to a shorter half-life (8-10 days) and a smaller body pool of the protein. An absolute lymphocyte count of less than 1500/mm^3 indicates malnutrition if other causes of lymphopenia are excluded. Moderate to severe malnutrition is associated with more marked lymphopenia.

While measures of specific vitamins may be valuable to confirm deficiency, normal ranges for the elderly are not clearly established, and blood nutrient levels may not reflect whole body nutrient stores.

The Nutritional Risk Index (NRI) is a risk index based on data collected from personal interviews, anthropometric measurements, laboratory assay of nutritional perimeters, three day food records and medical records review. It is reported to be a valid measure of health status.<13>

Effectiveness of Prevention

Counselling

The media currently serve as the most popular source of nutrition information. Improper nutrition is often due to uninformed food selection, although lack of funds to purchase food is also a factor. The ability to change dietary habits of patients through nutritional counselling by non-physicians has been demonstrated in a number of

Numerous randomized trials establish the value of nutritional counselling to reduce dietary fat intake

clinical trials involving both specialized and community-wide programs.<14> The following randomized trials are representative of the available evidence: in each case the intervention has been carried out by non-physicians.

Comprehensive worksite nutritional intervention, consisting of classes and food demonstrations, labelling nutritional information in cafeterias and individual counselling, produces a small but significant decrease in mean dietary fat intake.<15> In a small study of hypercholesterolemic adults, an initial counselling session accompanied by the distribution of printed materials was effective in lowering dietary cholesterol levels and increasing dietary fibre intake. Follow-up counselling was effective in maintaining positive change.<16> A course of individual instruction, together with behavioral counselling in groups of 12 to 15, initially weekly, then biweekly and later monthly, was effective in reducing the percentage of energy derived from fat from 39% to 21% in middle-aged women; the control group who received no intervention showed no significant change in dietary fat intake.<17> In a study examining the effects of individual and group nutritional education in males recuperating from myocardial infarction, desirable changes in fat intake were seen only in those receiving education. Those receiving lectures did as well as those receiving food preparation demonstrations. Beneficial changes persisted up to 24 months.<18>

In a study designed to simulate the type of intervention possible within the primary care setting, five-minute interviews were conducted at which generic self-help educational materials were distributed by a registered nurse. Ten days later the treatment group received a follow-up telephone call. Three months later a telephone interview was carried out by individuals blind to subject assignment, to determine whether changes in dietary intake had occurred. Even with this brief intervention, small but significant reductions in fat intake and increases in fibre intake were evident, but only in those subjects who had some responsibility for meal preparation.<19> In the Women's Health Trial, groups of 8 to 15 women attended eight weekly sessions, eight bi-weekly sessions and subsequent monthly sessions. Substantial decreases in fat consumption occurred, from 38% of total calories to 21%. The husbands of women receiving the active intervention reported an average weight loss of 2.4 pounds and a reduction in saturated fat intake significantly different from the husbands of control group women.<20>

Although physicians may lack the time and skill to obtain a thorough dietary history, offer specific guidance on food selection, or address potential barriers to change eating habits, general guidelines can be provided, and referral made to others for further counselling.

Effectiveness of Dietary Changes

Reduced intake of dietary fat, especially saturated fat, can reduce the risk of developing coronary artery disease. A large body of epidemiologic evidence links serum cholesterol levels with the development of coronary atherosclerosis. Serum cholesterol levels can be modified by dietary measures. Controlled clinical trials in which diets low in saturated fat were given to asymptomatic middle-aged men with selected cardiac risk factors have reported a 10-15% reduction in serum cholesterol levels, and in most trials a decrease in the incidence of cardiac events such as myocardial infarction and sudden death.[21-26] All cause mortality was not reduced, however. Concern has been raised over studies which have shown that low-fat diets applied to outpatients with moderate hypercholesterolemia result in only a modest reduction of total serum cholesterol (about 5%) and a parallel reduction in HDL which might negate positive effects.[27] The association between dietary fat and various forms of cancer is currently under investigation. An epidemiologic correlation between dietary fat consumption and incidence of cancer of the breast, colon, prostate and lung is present in most case-control studies. There is as yet no evidence that modification of dietary fat intake in humans influences the incidence of these malignancies.

Increased intake of dietary fibre improves gastrointestinal motility. Certain types of fibre may also be useful in controlling carbohydrate intolerance, reducing weight and controlling lipid disorders. A high-fibre diet may be effective in reducing intracolonic pressure and preventing diverticular disease. The risk of developing colorectal cancer may also be influenced by dietary fibre intake. At least fifteen cross-cultural studies have shown an inverse relationship between dietary fibre intake and the incidence of colon cancer. Such studies do not provide direct evidence that high dietary fibre intake, rather than other population dietary characteristics (e.g. low fat intake) is directly responsible for lower cancer incidence rates. Although case-control studies have shown inconsistent results regarding the association between dietary fibre and colon cancer, meta-analyses of these studies suggest an overall benefit from dietary fibre.[28,29] Inappropriate supplementation with bran may impair the absorbtion of calcium, zinc and iron.

A diet emphasizing the consumption of foods high in complex carbohydrate and fibre (e.g. whole grain foods and cereal products, vegetables and fruits) is an important means of lowering dietary fat consumption. It is desirable to replace foods high in simple carbohydrates (table syrup, honey, corn sweeteners) with those containing starch and fibre. Foods high in complex carbohydrates and fibre have a lower caloric density, and are therefore preferred for maintaining caloric balance and healthful body weight.

Reduced intake of dietary sodium may be of clinical benefit to people who have hypertension, or who are likely to develop it in the future.<30> Cross-cultural studies have shown a correlation between the sodium intake of different populations and the incidence of hypertension. A multi-national study involving 52 sites also demonstrated an association between sodium excretion and the rate of change of blood pressure with age.<31> A number of clinical trials and recent meta-analyses have demonstrated the ability of dietary sodium restriction to lower blood pressure by at least several millimetres of mercury in some hypertensive and normotensive individuals.<32> Only prospective controlled trials can provide definitive evidence that normotensive persons who practice daily sodium restriction are at lower risk of developing hypertension and its complications than are those with more typical sodium consumption. Nonetheless there is at least suggestive evidence of potential benefit and no known harm associated with moderate sodium restriction.

Many North American women and adolescent girls consume less dietary calcium than the recommended nutritional intake (adults 800 mg per day, adolescent, pregnant or lactating women 1200 mg per day). Population cross-sectional studies suggest that reduced calcium intake among women may be an important risk factor for bone mineral loss and postmenopausal osteoporosis. Prospective studies in asymptomatic postmenopausal women have produced inconsistent results about the efficacy of increasing dietary calcium as a means of slowing bone loss. Although some studies have reported that a daily intake of 750-1040 mg per day can reduce significantly the rate of bone loss in asymptomatic postmenopausal women, other controlled studies have shown either no effect or an effect only on compact bone with doses as high as 1800-2000 mg per day. A meta-analysis of intervention and observational studies concluded that 1000 mg of calcium daily would prevent 1% of bone loss per year.<33> For more information on osteoporosis consult Chapter 52. While a high intake of calcium is seen as nutritionally desirable from the point of view of skeletal health, an association has been noted between a high intake of calcium and arterial calcification, and between consumption of milk and mortality from coronary artery disease.

In cases of clear cut specific nutritional deficiencies, supplementation with the deficient nutrient is appropriate. In those individuals who do not consume the RNI for specific nutrients, and who may have serum levels which fall below the accepted normal levels, but who do not have classic deficiency syndromes, controversy exists concerning any possible benefit from supplementation. For example, in a randomized trial of elderly long-term patients, vitamin C supplements reduced the incidence of purpuric spots and petechial hemorrhages, but produced no other beneficial change.<34> In a placebo-controlled trial involving 80 healthy elderly Irish women randomly selected from a population with marginal thiamine deficiency, 63% of those supplemented with thiamine reported increased appetite

Vitamin supplementation in asymptomatic individuals is not of established value

and enjoyment of meals, showed significantly higher energy intakes and weight gain. Fatigue lessened and well-being improved in 88% of treated subjects.<35> Ninety-six independently living healthy elderly individuals, mean age 74 years, were randomly assigned to receive an oral nutrient supplement containing standard doses of multiple vitamins, trace elements, minerals, or matching placebo. By 12 months those receiving active treatment showed improvements in various immunological parameters, and a decrease in the number of days of illness due to infection from 48 to 23.<36>

Recommendations of Others

Canada's Food Guide<37> suggests the following daily intakes for adults: 5-12 servings of grain products

5-10 servings of fruits and vegetables

2-4 servings of milk products and

2-3 servings of meat or alternates.

The guide recommends eating a variety of foods from each group every day, and choosing lower fat foods more often. The number of servings suggested depends on age, body size, activity level, gender, pregnancy or breast feeding.

The U.S. Preventive Services Task Force recommends a diet emphasizing consumption of foods high in complex carbohydrates and fibre (e.g. whole grain foods and cereal products, vegetables, and fruits) as an important means of lowering dietary fat and calorie consumption.<38> The Task Force also recommends that clinicians should provide periodic counselling regarding dietary intakes of calories, fat, (especially saturated) cholesterol complex carbohydrates (starches), fibre and sodium. Women should receive counselling on calcium and iron intake. Adults should be given guidance on how to reduce total fat intake to less than 30% of total calories and dietary cholesterol to less than 300 mg/day. Energy intake and expenditure should be balanced to maintain desirable weight. These recommendations are currently under review.

Specific recommendations for physicians to offer nutritional counselling to patients have been issued by the American Medical Association,<39> the American College of Physicians<40> and the American Heart Association.<41>

Conclusions and Recommendations

There is good evidence that reduction of the dietary intake of fat (especially saturated fat) and cholesterol leads to a reduced incidence of symptomatic coronary artery disease, although not of total mortality. There is no evidence at present that reduction of dietary fat intake has a beneficial effect on the incidence of cancers. Reduction in the proportion of calories derived from fat to 20-30% does not appear to have significant adverse effects. Avoidance of excessive body weight by reduction of total calories, replacement of refined carbohydrates by complex carbohydrates and increase in fibre intake is also supported by fair evidence. Restricting sodium intake may reduce the incidence of hypertension, and has no serious adverse effects.

While there is evidence that nutritional counselling is effective in changing diet, the role of the physician has not been adequately evaluated. Based on the effectiveness of dietary advice and the association between poor diet and disease, it is reasonable to provide general dietary advice (B Recommendation). For those at increased risk, it is prudent to consider referral to a clinical nutritionist or other professional with specialized nutritional expertise.

Although the prevalence of nutritional deficiency is high in certain groups such as alcoholics, and the elderly living alone and in institutions, there is insufficient evidence to recommend for or against a routine search for malnutrition (C Recommendation).

Evidence

MEDLINE search 1988-1992 identified articles using the following MESH headings: 1) Deficiency diseases or Malnutrition or Nutrition disorders or Nutrition assessment or Nutrition and 2) Adults or Aged.

This review was initiated in September 1992 and recommendations were finalized by the Task Force in January 1994.

Selected References

1. Canadian Task Force on the Periodic Health Examination: The periodic health examination. *Can Med Assoc J* 1979; 121: 1193-1254

2. Nair C, Colburn H, McLean D, *et al*: Cardiovascular disease in Canada. *Health Reports* 1989; 1: 1-22

3. National Cancer Institute of Canada: *Canadian Cancer Statistics 1993*. Toronto, Canada, 1993: 13

4. Health and Welfare Canada: Canada's Health Promotion Survey: Technical Report. Rothman I, Warren R, Stephens T, Peters L (eds): Ottawa: Minister of Supply and Services Canada, 1988 (Cat No H39-119/1988E ISBN 0-662-15981-0)

5. Willett WC, Sampson L, Browne ML, *et al*: The use of a self-administered questionnaire to assess diet four years in the past. *Am J Epidemiol* 1988; 127: 188-199

6. Flegal KM, Larkin FA: Partitioning macronutrient intake estimates from a food frequency questionnaire. *Am J Epidemiol* 1990; 131(6): 1046-1058

7. Nelson M, Black A, Morris J, *et al*: Between and within subject variation in nutrient intake from infancy to old age: estimating the number of days required to rank dietary intakes with desired precision. *Am J Clin Nutr* 1989; 50: 155-167

8. Livingstone MB, Prentice AM, Strain JJ, *et al*: Accuracy of weighed dietary records in studies of diet and health. *BMJ* 1990; 300: 708-712

9. Mertz W, Tsui JC, Judd JT, *et al*: What are people really eating? The relation between energy intake derived from estimated diet records and intake determined to maintain body weight. *Am J Clin Nutr* 1991; 54: 291-295

10. Wu ML, Whittemore AS, Jung DL: Errors in reported dietary intakes. II. Long-term recall. *Am J Epidemiol* 1988; 128: 1137-1145

11. Hislop TG, Lamb CW, Ng VTY: Differential misclassification bias and dietary recall for the distant past using a food frequency questionnaire. *Nutr Cancer* 1990; 13: 223-233

12. Persson P-G, Ahlbom A, Norell SE: Retrospective versus original information on diet: implications for epidemiological studies. *Int J Epidemiol* 1990; 19: 343-348

13. Prendergast JM, Coe RM, Chavez MN, *et al*: Clinical validation of a nutritional risk index. *J Comm Health* 1989; 14: 125-135

14. Glanz K: Nutrition education for risk factor reduction and patient education: a review. *Prev Med* 1985; 14: 721-752

15. Sorenson G, Morris D, Hunt M, *et al*: Work-site intervention and employees' dietary habits: the Treatwell program. *Am J Public Health* 1992; 82: 877-880

16. Milkereit J, Graves JS: Follow-up dietary counselling benefits attainment of intake goals for total fat, saturated fat, and fibre. *J Am Diet Assoc* 1992; 92: 603-605

17. Insull W Jr, Henderson MM, Prentice RL, *et al*: Results of a randomised feasibility study of a low-fat diet. *Arch Intern Med* 1990; 150: 421-427

18. Karvetti RL: Effects of nutrition education. *J Am Diet Assoc* 1981; 79: 660-667

19. Beresford SA, Farmer EM, Feingold L, *et al*: Evaluation of a self-help dietary intervention in a primary care setting. *Am J Publ Health* 1992; 82: 79-84

20. White E, Hurlich M, Thompson RS, *et al*: Dietary changes among husbands of participants in a low-fat dietary intervention. *Am J Prev Med* 1991; 7: 319-325

21. Dayton S, Pearce ML, Goldman H, *et al*: Controlled trial of a diet high in unsaturated fat for prevention of atherosclerotic complications. *Lancet* 1968; 2: 1060-1062

22. Hjermann I, Velve-Byre K, Holme I, *et al*: Effect of diet and smoking intervention on the incidence of coronary heart disease. Report from the Oslo Study Group of a randomised trial in healthy men. *Lancet* 1981; 2: 1303-1310

23. Rinzler S: Primary prevention of coronary heart disease by diet. *Bull NY Acad Med* 1968; 44: 936-949

24. Miettinen M, Turpeinen O, Karvonen MJ, *et al*: Effect of cholesterol-lowering diet on mortality from coronary heart disease and other causes. A twelve-year clinical trial in men and women. *Lancet* 1972; 2: 835-838

25. Turpeinen O, Karvonen MJ, Pekkarinen M, *et al*: Dietary prevention of coronary heart disease: the Finnish Mental Hospital Study. *Int J Epidemiol* 1979; 8: 99-118

26. Frantz ID, Dawson EA, Kuba K: The Minnesota Coronary Survey: effect of diet on cardiovascular events and deaths. *Circulation* 1975; 52(Suppl II): II-4

27. Hunninghake DB, Stein EA, Dujovne CA, *et al*: The efficacy of intensive dietary therapy alone or combined with lovastatin in outpatients with hypercholesterolemia. *N Engl J Med* 1993; 328: 1213-1219

28. Trock B, Lanza E, Greenwald P: Dietary fiber, vegetables, and colon cancer: critical review and meta-analyses of the epidemiologic evidence. *J Natl Cancer Inst* 1990; 82: 650-661

29. Howe GR, Benito E, Castelleto R, *et al*: Dietary intake of fiber and decreased risk of cancers of the colon and rectum: evidence from the combined analysis of 13 case-control studies. *J Natl Cancer Inst* 1992; 84: 1887-1896

30. Stamler J: Dietary salt and blood pressure. *Ann NY Acad Sci* 1993; 676: 122-156

31. Intersalt: an international study of electrolyte excretion and blood pressure. Results for 24 hour urinary sodium and potassium excretion. *BMJ* 1988; 297: 319-328

32. Cutler JA, Follman D, Elliott P, *et al*: An overview of randomized trials of sodium reduction and blood pressure. *Hypertension* 1991; 17 (Suppl I): I27-I33

33. Cumming RG: Calcium intake and bone mass: a quantitative review of the evidence. *Calcif Tissue Int* 1990; 47: 194-201

34. Schorah CJ, Tormey WP, Brooks GH, *et al*: The effect of vitamin C supplements on body weight, serum proteins, and general health of an elderly population. *Am J Clin Nutr* 1981; 34: 871-876

35. Smidt LJ, Cremin FM, Grivetti LE, *et al*: Influence of thiamin supplementation on the health and general well-being of an elderly Irish population with marginal thiamin deficiency. *J Gerontol* 1991; 46(1): M16-22

36. Chandra RK: Effect of vitamin and trace element supplementation on immune responses and infection in elderly subjects. *Lancet* 1992; 340: 1124-1127

37. Health and Welfare Canada: *Canada's Food Guide to Healthy Eating*. Minister of Supply and Services Canada, 1992 (Cat No H39-252/1992E ISBN 0-662-15981-2)

38. U.S. Preventive Services Task Force: *Guide to Clinical Preventive Services: an Assessment of the Effectiveness of 169 Interventions*. Williams & Wilkins, Baltimore, Md, 1989: 305-314

39. Council on Scientific Affairs: American Medical Association concepts of nutrition and health. *JAMA* 1979; 242: 2335-2338

40. American College of Physicians: *Nutrition: position paper*. Washington, D.C.: American College of Physicians, 1985

41. American Heart Association: Dietary guidelines for healthy American adults. A statement for physicians and health professionals by the Nutrition Committee. *Circulation* 1988; 77: 721A-724A

Nutritional Counselling for Undesirable Dietary Patterns and Screening for Protein/Calorie Malnutrition Disorders in Adults

MANEUVER	EFFECTIVENESS	LEVEL OF EVIDENCE <REF>	RECOMMENDATION
Nutritional Counselling	Effectively reduces intake of fat and increases intake of fibre.	Randomized controlled trials<16-19> (I)	Fair evidence to provide general dietary advice (B). For those at increased risk,* it is prudent to consider referral to a clinical nutritionist or other professional with specialized nutritional expertise
	Reduction of dietary fat intake reduces incidence of coronary artery disease but not all cause mortality.	Randomized controlled trials<21-26> (I)	
	Increase in dietary fibre improves gastrointestinal motility and may reduce colonic cancer; replacing fat foods with fibre reduces serum cholesterol.	Case-control studies<27,28> (II-2)	
Screening for protein/calorie malnutrition	Despite high prevalence in alcoholics, the elderly living alone and in institutions no evidence of benefit.	Expert opinion (III)	Insufficient evidence to recommend for or against a routine search for malnutrition (C)

*   High-risk group includes alcoholics and the elderly living alone and in institutions

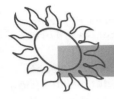

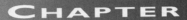

CHAPTER

50

Screening for Diabetes Mellitus in the Non-Pregnant Adult

By Marie-Dominique Beaulieu

Screening for Diabetes Mellitus in the Non-Pregnant Adult

Adapted by Marie-Dominique Beaulieu, MD, MSc, FCFP[1] from materials prepared for the U.S. Preventive Services Task Force[2]

In 1979 the Canadian Task Force on the Periodic Health Examination concluded that screening for diabetes mellitus (DM) in non-pregnant asymptomatic adults without risk factors was not part of the periodic health examination.<1> Review of further published evidence does not alter this conclusion. The screening test for DM in the absence of symptoms or risk factors has poor sensitivity and has never been associated with secondary prevention of diabetic complications (D Recommendation). Test characteristics are enhanced when applied to high risk populations, namely native Canadians, obese individuals and those with a strong family history of diabetes. Based on some evidence that treatment of overt diabetes may retard micro-vascular complications, a decision to screen in those populations could be considered. Screening pregnant women is discussed in Chapter 2 on Gestational diabetes.

Burden of Suffering

Diabetes Mellitus affects 3% of Canadians and is the leading cause of blindness and end-stage renal failure

The prevalence of DM in the general Canadian population is estimated to vary between 2% and 2.7%.<2> Prevalence increases with age. Estimates from the Manitoba data base yielded rates of 0.8% in adults less than 45 years, 3.5% among those between 45 and 64 years of age, and 7.6% among those 65 and or older.<3> Prevalence is higher in native Canadian populations. A study conducted in Northern Quebec revealed that 6.2% of the Cree population suffered from DM, with a prevalence rate of 20% in women over 50 years of age.<4> Other risk factors for diabetes include family history, obesity, impaired glucose tolerance, and a previous history of gestational diabetes.

Diabetes may cause life threatening metabolic complications and is an important risk factor for other leading causes of death such as coronary heart disease, congestive heart failure and cerebrovascular disease. Diabetes is the most common cause of polyneuropathy with approximately 50% of diabetics developing neuropathic disease within 25 years after diagnosis.<5> Diabetes is responsible for 40% of all

---

[1] Associate Professor, Department of Family Medicine, University of Montreal, Montreal, Quebec
[2] By M. Carrington Reid, MD, PhD, Fellow, Robert Wood Johnson Clinical Scholar, Yale School of Medicine, New Haven, CT and Harold C. Sox, Jr., MD, Joseph M. Huber Professor and Chairman, Department of Medicine, Dartmouth Hitchcock Medical Center, Lebanon, New Hampshire

nontraumatic amputations in Canada.<6> Diabetic nephropathy has now become the leading cause of end-stage renal disease.<7> Diabetes is also the leading cause of blindness in adults.<7> (Screening for diabetic retinopathy in the elderly is reviewed in Chapter 78, screening for pancreatic cancer in Chapter 71 and screening for end-stage renal disease in Chapter 28). Individuals with this disease have higher hospitalization rates, longer hospital stays and more ambulatory care visits than persons without diabetes.

Most of this burden of illness is due to type II, or non-insulin dependent DM (NIDDM), which comprises approximately 80-90% of all cases. Type II diabetes generally occurs after age 30. Type I, or insulin dependent DM (IDDM), generally begins before this age. This discussion of the efficacy of screening and detection of diabetes mellitus does not include type I DM. The low prevalence of this disease and the fact that it has a brief presymptomatic period are reasons against screening for type I DM.

Some authors have proposed to use immunopathologic markers, such as islet cell antibodies, to identify presymptomatic type I DM. These studies, which have been restricted to relatives of patients with type I DM, have shown asymptomatic periods ranging from months to years prior to the onset of clinical disease.<8> Many issues remain to be resolved before recommending screening for type I DM in the general population. The immunoassays for islet cell antibodies remain difficult to standardize.<8> Screening for these markers has largely been restricted to first degree relatives of patients with type I DM. Finally, firm evidence that treatment of individuals with immune markers prevents progression of disease or reduces complications is lacking.

Maneuver

There are two gold standard diagnostic criteria for DM depending on the presence or the absence of symptoms. In patients who have symptoms and signs of diabetes (polyuria, polydipsia, polyphagia, weight loss, fatigue, blurred vision etc.), the diagnosis of diabetes is made on the basis of either a random venous plasma glucose above 11.1 mmol/L (200 mg/dl) or at least two fasting venous plasma glucose levels over 7.8 mmol/L (140 mg/dl). The oral glucose tolerance test (OGTT) is unnecessary if the patient meets these criteria. In patients without symptoms, biochemical hyperglycemia must be confirmed by the 75 gr 2 hour OGTT.<7> The most commonly used diagnostic criterion for the OGTT is that of the National Diabetes Data Group (NDDG).<9> The test is considered abnormal when the 2-hour venous plasma glucose level is >11.1 mmol/L (200 mg/dl) and one glucose value before two hours is >11.1 mmol/L (200 mg/dl).

The National Diabetes Data Group recognizes an intermediate form of disordered glucose metabolism, i.e. impaired glucose tolerance (IGT). The diagnosis of IGT requires OGTT test results in which the 2-hour glucose value is between 7.8 mmol/L (140 mg/dl) and 11/1 mmpl/L (200 mg/dl), and one intervening value is greater than II.1 mmol/L (200 mg/dl). Thus, IGT is a point on a continuum between normal glucose tolerance and a diabetic state.

The OGTT must be positive on more than one occasion to establish a diagnosis of diabetes mellitus. Indeed, the OGTT is known for its test-retest variability. In an attempt to decrease some of the test-retest variability, the American Diabetes Association (ADA) recommends that the OGTT only be performed in patients who have had an unrestricted diet for three days preceding the test and that the test should be administered after an overnight fast.<10>

Several screening tests for DM have been proposed (fasting, random, or 2-hour post-prandial glucose). ADA states that the best screening test is the fasting plasma glucose, in which sampling occurs after the patient has refrained from any food or beverage for at least a 3 hour period.<7,10>.

The fasting plasma glucose has a wide range of reported diagnostic sensitivity varying between 21% and 73%.<11-13> The wide variability in test performance reflects the unimodal distribution of glucose levels in most populations. Test sensitivity and specificity will vary with the cutoff used to define a positive result on the index test and the gold standard test. Study populations that differ in disease prevalence and severity may also contribute.

A number of studies have evaluated measurement of glycosylated proteins, primarily HA1c and serum fructosamine, as screening tools for diabetes. Test characteristics compare with the fasting plasma glucose, with sensitivities ranging from 15-91% and specificities reported as 84-89%.<14>

Effectiveness of Screening and Treatment

Screening for diabetes mellitus in asymptomatic individuals can only be justified if treatment during the asymptomatic phase prevents complications more effectively than treatment instituted after symptoms have developed. Studies over the preceding 20 years have suggested an association between the degree of glycemic control, duration of disease and complication rates. However, there is no conclusive evidence supporting the increased effectiveness of early intervention.

Microvascular complications (e.g. diabetic nephropathy and retinopathy) are correlated with level of glucose control in longitudinal studies. Studies examining this question have utilized almost exclusively type I IDDM patients. The relevance of these findings to type II

NIDDM patients is unknown. The Diabetes Control and Complications Trial (DCCT), involving over 1,400 subjects, is the largest prospective randomized clinical trial to date and was designed to determine whether tight glycemic control in type I diabetic patients retarded the progression of preexisting diabetic complications (secondary prevention). The trial also evaluated whether tight glycemic control prevented long term sequelae in diabetic subjects without preexisting complications (primary prevention). Intensive therapy reduced progression of microvascular disease in both groups.[15] People randomized to intensive therapy had a three-fold increase in severe hypoglycemic events. The study findings provide supportive, but not conclusive, evidence that hyperglycemia mediates microvascular disease in diabetic subjects. Directly translating the DCCT results to the management of type II diabetic patients remains controversial at this time. While improved glycemic control may result in decreasing microvascular complications in the type II diabetic population, studies providing firm evidence for this have not been published yet. The U.K. Prospective Diabetes Study is designed to address this question and data is anticipated in the near future.

Patients with diabetes are also at significantly increased risk of developing atherosclerotic and peripheral vascular disease. There is evidence that disease duration and degree of glycemic control do not affect macrovascular complications in individuals treated for type II diabetes. The rate of increase in risk of CHD events in type II diabetic patients increases with disease duration but at the same rate as people without diabetes. A recent review of the World Health Organization (WHO) multinational study of vascular disease in diabetes found no increased risk of cardiovascular events in type II diabetic subjects after 8 years of follow-up.[16] There was no significant correlation between cerebrovascular and peripheral vascular events and diabetes duration. Difficulty in accurately ascertaining the time of disease onset has complicated the study of possible associations between macrovascular complications of type II diabetes mellitus and disease duration. However, the estimation of disease duration is quite unreliable, since some data suggest that in the United States, as many as 50% of diabetics ignore their condition. Some studies have shown that up to 21% of newly diagnosed diabetics have signs of retinopathy.[17]

The majority of individuals with disordered glucose metabolism are classified as having impaired glucose tolerance (IGT). There is little direct evidence that asymptomatic persons benefit from the detection and treatment of IGT[16,18] Most untreated asymptomatic persons with IGT do not develop diabetes. The rate of progression from IGT to diabetes ranges from 1% to 6% per year, with a higher rate found in some minority populations.[16] Thus, although IGT is an important risk factor for diabetes, it is not by itself an established indication for treatment.

Most asymptomatic adults with impaired glucose tolerance do not develop diabetes mellitus; however, up to 50% of individuals presenting overt diabetes ignore their condition

Recommendation of Others

In 1989, the U.S. Preventive Services Task Force recommended against routine screening for DM in the general asymptomatic non-pregnant adult population but stated that screening may be appropriate in selected high-risk groups.[19]

The American Diabetes Association (ADA) recommends screening for type II DM in individuals with one or more risk factors for this condition.[10] The screening test recommended is the fasting blood glucose assay. Routine screening of patients without risk factors is not recommended by the ADA.

Conclusions and Recommendations

Analytic studies have shown no benefit of universal screening for type II adult diabetes mellitus in asymptomatic adults

Screening for DM in asymptomatic non-pregnant adults suffers from two important limitations: the lack of a screening test that combines accuracy with practicality, and the absence of adequate evidence that early detection and treatment improve outcome in asymptomatic persons. Possible, but as yet unproven benefits of early treatment of asymptomatic persons must be weighed against the potential adverse effects of screening (e.g. false positives, labelling) and treatment (e.g. dietary restrictions, medications, risk of hypoglycemic events). In the general population there is fair evidence not to screen for DM (D Recommendation).

In high-risk groups, in which the prevalence is higher, false positive results are likely to be fewer. It may be clinically prudent to consider selective case-finding in these groups, since unrecognized overt diabetes carries the same risks as diagnosed type II diabetes.

Periodic testing of individuals with risk factors for diabetes mellitus, (obesity, older age, family history of diabetes, belonging to a high risk ethnic group) could be a reasonable middle course between screening no one and universal screening. However, there is no evidence that early detection improves outcomes in high-risk groups.

In non-pregnant adults, primary prevention rather than screening may be an important means of preventing diabetes and its complications. Among the many benefits of exercise and weight reduction, for example, are improved glucose tolerance and reduced obesity, important risk factors for diabetes as well as for other serious chronic diseases. Since these healthy behaviours are widely recommended even in the absence of diabetes, patients should be encouraged to adopt these behaviours independent of diabetes screening (see Chapter 47).

Unanswered Questions (Research Agenda)

Evaluating the benefits of primary prevention and screening in high-risk populations is an important research question to resolve.

Evidence

The literature was identified by a MEDLINE search for the English language from 1989 to 1993 using as key words: diabetes non-insulin-dependent or diabetes-gestational and diagnosis, epidemiology and prevention-control. The review was initiated in November 1993 and finalized by the Task Force in January 1994.

Selected References

1. *Report of a Task Force to the Conference of Deputy Ministers of Health* (cat no H39-3/1980E), Health Services and Promotion Branch, Department of National Health and Welfare, Ottawa, 1980

2. *The Canada Health Survey 1976*. Department of Health and Welfare and Statistics Canada, Ottawa, 1978

3. Young TK, Roos NP, Hammerstrand KM: Estimated burden of diabetes mellitus in Manitoba according to health insurance claims: a pilot study. *Can Med Assoc J* 1991; 144: 318-324

4. Brassard P, Robinson E, Lavallée C: Prevalence of diabetes mellitus among the James Bay Cree of northern Quebec. *Can Med Assoc J* 1993; 149: 303-307

5. Harati Y: Diabetic peripheral neuropathies. *Ann Int Med* 1987; 107: 546-559

6. Zinmam B: Preventing the complications of diabetes mellitus. *Can J Diagnosis*, June 1993: 149-159

7. Expert Committee of the Canadian Diabetes Advisory Board: Clinical practice guidelines for the treatment of diabetes mellitus. *Can Med Assoc J* 1992; 147: 697-712

8. Eisenbarth GS, Verge CF, Allen H, *et al*: The design of trials for prevention of IDDM. *Diabetes* 1993; 42: 941-947

9. National Diabetes Data Group: Classification and diagnosis of diabetes mellitus and other categories of glucose intolerance. *Diabetes* 1979; 28: 1039-1057

10. Bourn D, Mann J: Screening for noninsulin dependent diabetes mellitus and impaired glucose tolerance in a Dunedin general practice – is it worth it? *N Z Med J* 1992; 105: 208-210

11. Croxson SC, Absalom S, Burden AC: Fructosamine in diabetes screening of the elderly. *Ann Clin Biochem* 1991; 28: 279-282

12. Guillausseau PJ, Charles MA, Paolaggi F, *et al*: Comparison of HbA1 and fructosamine in diagnosis of glucose-tolerance abnormalities. *Diabetes Care* 1990; 13: 898-900

13. Little RR, England JD, Wiedmeyer HM, *et al*: Relationship of glycosylated hemoglobin to oral glucose tolerance. *Diabetes* 1988; 37: 60-64

14. Singer DE, Coley CM, Samet JH, *et al*: Tests of glycemia in diabetes mellitus. Their use in establishing a diagnosis and treatment. *Ann Int Med* 1989; 110: 125-137

15. Welborn TA, Wearne K: Coronary Heart disease incidence and cardiovascular mortality in Busselton with reference to glucose and insulin concentrations. *Diabetes Care* 1979; 2: 154-160

16. Motala AA, Omar MA, Gouws E: High risk of progression to NIDDM in South-African Indians with impaired glucose tolerance. *Diabetes* 1993; 42: 556-563

17. Harris MI: Undiagnosed NIDDM: clinical and public health issues. *Diabetes Care* 1993; 16: 642-652

18. Jarrett RJ, Keen H, McCartney P: The Whitehall study: ten year follow-up report on men with impaired glucose tolerance with reference to worsening of diabetes and predictors of death. *Diabet Med* 1984; 1: 279-283

19. U.S. Preventive Services Task Force: *Guide to Clinical Preventive Services: an Assessment of the Effectiveness of 169 Interventions*. Williams & Wilkins, Baltimore, Md, 1989: 95-103

Screening for Diabetes Mellitus in the Non-Pregnant Adult

MANEUVER	EFFECTIVENESS	LEVEL OF EVIDENCE <REF>	RECOMMENDATION
Fasting blood glucose	Fasting blood glucose has low sensitivity in asymptomatic low-risk populations.	Cohort studies<11-13> (II-2)	There is fair evidence to exclude screening of the general non-pregnant population in the periodic health examination (D)*
	The efficacy of screening for diabetes mellitus in asymptomatic adults without risk factors has never been demonstrated.	Cohort studies<16,18> (II-2)	

*   Screening in high-risk groups can help to identify relatively more diabetics but there is no
     evidence that they benefit more from treatment due to such early identification.
     High-risk: ethnic groups (native Canadians, Hispanic, Black Americans), obesity,
     strong family history, gestational diabetes or older age.

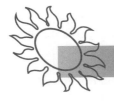

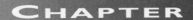

CHAPTER 51

Screening for Thyroid Disorders and Thyroid Cancer in Asymptomatic Adults

By Marie-Dominique Beaulieu

51 Screening for Thyroid Disorders and Thyroid Cancer in Asymptomatic Adults

Prepared by Marie-Dominique Beaulieu, MD, MSc, FCFP[1] drawing from materials prepared for the U.S. Preventive Services Task Force[2]

As in 1990,<1> the Canadian Task Force on the Periodic Health Examination has concluded that there is not enough evidence to recommend the inclusion of screening for thyroid dysfunction (hyperthyroidism and hypothyroidism) in asymptomatic adults. The effectiveness of screening for thyroid cancer has also been poorly evaluated so that neither inclusion nor exclusion of screening for thyroid cancer can be recommended in asymptomatic adults. The line between truly asymptomatic and mildly symptomatic adults may, however, be difficult to draw. Considering the high prevalence of thyroid disease, particularly hypothyroidism in women, and the fact that some studies have shown that affected women may benefit from early treatment, it is recommended that clinicians maintain a high index of suspicion and not hesitate to use immunometric thyroid stimulating hormone (TSH) assays to investigate individuals with vague symptoms that could be related to thyroid dysfunction.

Burden of Suffering

Hyperthyroidism and Hypothyroidism

Overall prevalence of thyroid disorders can reach 8% to 20% in peri-menopausal and elderly women

The definitions of what constitute "asymptomatic" hyperthyroidism and hypothyroidism are far from clear. Overt hyperthyroidism and hypothyroidism are defined as a triad of the classical signs and symptoms of thyroid dysfunction, abnormal TSH levels, and abnormal thyroid function tests (TT4, FT4, etc). Sub-clinical conditions are defined by the presence of abnormal TSH levels, thyroid function test results in the upper or lower normal ranges, and the absence of symptoms. However, the signs and symptoms of hypothyroidism and hyperthyroidism are very vague in nature, insidious, and are often attributed by patients to normal aging. They are not necessarily reported.<2> The vague nature of the symptoms can be misleading; one study showed that 8% of patients with a

---

[1] Associate Professor of Family Medicine, University of Montreal, Montreal, Quebec
[2] By Carolyn DiGuiseppi, MD, MPH, Science Advisor, U.S. Preventive Services Task Force, Washington, D.C.

diagnosis of depression were suffering from undetected hypothyroidism.<3>

Community surveys have reported prevalence rates of overt hyperthyroidism of less than 1.9%, the rates being comparable in elderly populations.<4> If "sub-clinical" cases are included, the prevalence rate can be as high as 2.7%.<4> In a well conducted community study, the annual incidence rate of overt hyperthyroidism was estimated to be 2 to 3 per 1,000 women.<4>

The prevalence of hypothyroidism is three times higher among women than men. The prevalence in an unselected community population of young, middle-aged and elderly individuals is about 1.4% and the estimated annual incidence 1 to 2 per 1,000 women.<4> Surveys of geriatric populations have yielded estimated prevalence rates for overt hypothyroidism of 0.2% to 3%.<5> The reported prevalence of sub-clinical hypothyroidism ranges from 0.9% to 5.2% in the adult population<5> and from 2.6% to 20% in the elderly population.<6>

Thyroid Cancer

Cancer of the thyroid represents 1.5% of cancers in women and 0.5% of cancers in men. In 1990, this cancer was responsible of the death of 113 Canadians, 41 males and 72 females.<7> Cancer of the thyroid includes several cell types: papillary and follicular carcinomas, which are rarely fatal with appropriate treatment, and anaplastic carcinoma, which is one of the most lethal of all cancers. Papillary cancer occurs more frequently in adults younger than 50 years. Anaplastic carcinoma is the more common form of thyroid cancer after the age of 60. An undisputed risk factor is neck radiation.

Thyroid cancer represents 1.5% of all cancers

Maneuver

Hyperthyroidism and Hypothyroidism

The measurement of circulating T4 levels used to diagnose overt thyroid dysfunction is not useful for detecting mild or subclinical conditions in adults. The measurement of basal TSH levels is the most sensitive screening test. The new generation of sensitive immunoradiometric TSH assays can reliably detect a concentration as low as 0.01 mU/L. Normal values range between 0.3 mU/l and 5 mU/l, but some variations around those values are possible in different laboratories. Clinical studies have reported a sensitivity of 80% to 100% and a specificity of nearly 100% for the early detection of subclinical hyperthyroidism and hypothyroidism.<8>

Immunoradiometric TSH assays have a very high sensitivity and specificity

Thyroid Cancer

Neck palpation has
poor test
characteristics

The usual screening test for thyroid cancer is neck palpation. Ultrasonography, scintigraphy and needle aspiration are reserved for diagnostic evaluations. The accuracy of neck palpation varies with the examiner's skill and the size of the mass. Among patients referred for the evaluation of a suspect solitary nodule, the sensitivity and specificity of neck palpation was 63% and 62% compared to ultrasonography. In one study of neck palpation in asymptomatic adults, the sensitivity was 15% and the specificity 100% compared with ultrasonography.[9] Therefore, a negative examination does not exclude the possibility of having a thyroid cancer.

Effectiveness of Screening and Treatment

Hyperthyroidism and Hypothyroidism

The effectiveness of treatment of subclinical hyperthyroidism has never been evaluated. Treatment of hyperthyroidism can be cumbersome and expensive. The choice of a definitive treatment depends on many factors, of which the patient's age and severity of the clinical disease are the most important. Clearly, the treatment strategy is not based solely on laboratory tests. Hence, decisions about how to treat sub-clinical hyperthyroidism rest on evaluation of the clinical impact of the laboratory abnormalities.

There has been no randomized trial (RCT) of the effectiveness of a screening program for sub-clinical hypothyroidism in a completely asymptomatic population. However, there have been two RCTs of the effectiveness of early treatment of sub-clinical hypothyroidism, and there is some evidence concerning the natural history of this condition.

The transition from sub-clinical to overt hypothyroidism does not appear to be inevitable and is estimated to vary from 5% to 8% annually. If both sub-clinical hypothyroidism and asymptomatic autoimmune thyroiditis are present the rate increases to 12-20% annually.[4]

Most experts now consider that an increase in TSH levels above the normal range indicates an insufficiency of circulating hormones.[10] Levels above 10 mU/l are considered as definitely abnormal, and those between 5 mU/l and 10 mU/l are considered as being in the "grey area" in the absence of any symptoms or signs of hypothyroidism.

Treatment of mild and sub-clinical hypothyroidism with T4 replacement therapy has been found to return the TSH and T4 levels to normal and to ameliorate some cardiac function indicators. Improvements in other factors, such as resting heart rate, sodium secretion, serum lipid levels and nerve conduction velocities, have not been found to be statistically or clinically significant.

Two randomized controlled trials of the efficacy of early treatment of sub-clinical hypothyroidism in women have shown that some patients benefited from treatment as their level of well-being increased.[11,12] In addition, treated patients had a statistically significant increase in the systolic interval, an index of cardiac function. However, limitations in the study designs warrant caution in generalizing the results to all perimenopausal and postmenopausal women, especially to very old women, since none of these studies included women above 75 years of age. One study, by Cooper and associates,[11] was conducted in a sample of women previously treated for hyperthyroidism. Though an increase in TSH level revealed a real deficit in thyroid hormone, the likelihood that these women would have developed overt hypothyroidism in the future may have been greater than the usual asymptomatic population.

The second trial by Nyström and collaborators[12] randomly selected 22 of 78 women with confirmed sub-clinical hypothyroidism, identified through a community survey. Treatment conferred a clinical benefit to 25% of the cases. As there were no clinical indices to predict who would respond to treatment, this suggests that three out of four women may have been treated unnecessarily.

Iatrogenic hyperthyroidism has been considered as a potential danger of treatment of sub-clinical hypothyroidism. Iatrogenic hyperthyroidism can precipitate angina or atrial fibrillation in susceptible individuals, namely in the elderly with restricted cardiac reserve. However, this iatrogenic condition can occur in any patient treated for hypothyroidism, and can be avoided by proper monitoring.

Thyroid Cancer

The benefits of early detection of thyroid cancer are not well defined. Five-year survival rates are better for patients with earlier stages of cancer at diagnosis.[13] There have been no controlled trials demonstrating that asymptomatic persons detected by screening have better outcomes than those who sought care because of symptoms. There is no basis on which to conclude that regular neck palpation could have a major effect on the natural history of this infrequent cancer.

Recommendations of Others

Few Canadian organisations have issued recommendations on screening for thyroid diseases. The U.S. Preventive Services Task Force does not recommend screening of asymptomatic adults.[14]

Conclusions and Recommendations

Hyperthyroidism and Hypothyroidism

The effectiveness of screening for thyroid disorders in the general population has not been properly evaluated

There is still insufficient evidence to support the inclusion of screening for hyperthyroidism and hypothyroidism among asymptomatic adults (C Recommendation). However, community surveys and clinical trials have clearly demonstrated that an important proportion of individuals labelled as suffering from subclinical disease in fact had some symptoms. The high prevalence of hypothyroidism among perimenopausal and postmenopausal women warrants a high index of clinical suspicion and liberal use of the sensitive TSH assay in the presence of even vague and subtle complaints. RCTs have shown that such patients can benefit from early treatment. Paradoxically, women over 75 years of aged have been excluded from most studies of the effectiveness of early treatment, but are still the target of screening for many physicians.

Thyroid Cancer

For thyroid cancer, there is no evidence to suggest that regular neck palpation by a physician would have any impact on the outcome of the disease but further evaluation is required (C Recommendation).

Unanswered Questions (Research Agenda)

A well planned randomized controlled trial should evaluate the effectiveness of screening and early treatment of hypothyroidism in apparently asymptomatic women. Such a trial would be most valuable if it could determine effectiveness in very old women as well as in middle-aged and perimenopausal women. The issue of the ideal screening interval should also be clarified.

Evidence

A MEDLINE search between 1989 and 1993 was conducted using the key words: hyperthyroidism and hypothyroidism, with the subheadings screening and prevention and control. Only original articles were considered. The search yielded 12 new articles. Priority was given to the highest levels of evidence according to the CTF methodology.

This review was initiated in December 1992 and recommendations were finalized by the Task Force in January 1994.

Selected References

1. Canadian Task Force on the Periodic Health Examination: The periodic health examination, 1990 update: 1. Early detection of hyperthyroidism and hypothyroidism in adults and screening of newborns for congenital hypothyroidism. *Can Med Assoc J* 1990; 142: 955-961

2. Helfand N, Crapo LM: Screening for thyroid disease. *Ann Intern Med* 1990; 112: 840-849

3. Gold MS, Pottash AC, Extein I: Thyroid dysfunction or depression. *JAMA* 1981; 245: 1919-1925

4. Tunbridge WMG, Evered DC, Hall R, *et al*: The spectrum of thyroid disease in a community: the Whickham survey. *Clin Endocrinol* 1977; 7: 481-493

5. Falkenberg M, Kagedal B, Norr A: Screening of an elderly female population for hypo- and hyperthyroidism by use of a thyroid hormone panel. *Acta Med Scand* 1983; 214: 361-365

6. Parle JV, Franklyn JA, Cross KW, *et al*: Assessment of a screening process to detect patients aged 60 years and over at risk of hypothyroidism. *Brit J Gen Pract* 1991; 41: 414-416

7. *National Cancer Institute of Canada: Canadian Cancer Statistics, 1993*. Toronto, 1993

8. Toft AD: Use of sensitive immunoradiometric assay for thyrotropin in clinical practice. *Mayo Clin Proc* 1988; 63: 1035-1042

9. Brander A, Viikinkoski P, Nickels J, *et al*: Thyroid gland: U.S. screening in a random adult population. *Radiology* 1991; 181: 683-687

10. Sawin CT: Thyroid dysfunction in older persons. *Advanc Intern Med* (Mosby Year Book) 1991; 37: 223-248

11. Cooper DS, Halpern R, Wood LC, *et al*: Thyroxine therapy in subclinical hypothyroidism. A double-blind, placebo-controlled trial. *Ann Intern Med* 1984; 101: 18-24

12. Nyström E, Caidahl K, Fager G, *et al*: A double-blind cross-over 12-month study of L-thyroxine treatment of women with 'subclinical' hypothyroidism. *Clin Endocrinol-Oxf* 1988; 29: 63-76

13. Akslen LA, Haldorsen T, Thoresen SO, *et al*: Survival and causes of death in thyroid cancer: a population based study of 2479 cases from Norway. *Cancer Res* 1991; 51: 1234-1241

14. U.S. Preventive Services Task Force: *Guide to Clinical Preventive Services: an Assessment of the Effectiveness of 169 Interventions*. Williams & Wilkins, Baltimore, Md, 1989: 105-110

Screening for Thyroid Disorders and Thyroid Cancer in Asymptomatic Adults

MANEUVER	EFFECTIVENESS	LEVEL OF EVIDENCE <REF>	RECOMMENDATION
Thyroid disorders (hypothyroidism and hyperthyroidism)			
Clinical examination of postmenopausal women and measurement of serum thyroid-stimulating hormone (TSH) level by immunoradiometric assay	Effectiveness of screening and early treatment has not been evaluated in the general population. Early treatment of hypothyroidism may be beneficial for some women.	Community surveys<4-6> (III) Randomized controlled trials<11,12> (I)	Poor evidence for either inclusion or exclusion of TSH screening (C); due to the high prevalence of thyroid disorders in peri-menopausal women, physicians should maintain a high index of clinical suspicion
Thyroid cancer			
Neck palpation in asymptomatic adults	Effectiveness of screening never evaluated. Poor test characteristics in asymptomatic adults.	Case-series<9,13> (III)	Poor evidence for either inclusion or exclusion of screening for thyroid cancer (C)

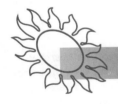

CHAPTER 52

Prevention of Osteoporotic Fractures in Women by Estrogen Replacement Therapy

By Denice S. Feig

Prevention of Osteoporotic Fractures in Women by Estrogen Replacement Therapy

Prepared by Denice S. Feig, MD, FRCPC[1]

There is good evidence to suggest that estrogen therapy slows bone loss in perimenopausal women and fair evidence that estrogen therapy will decrease fractures. In addition, there is fair evidence that estrogen therapy leads to decreased cardiovascular mortality although recent evidence suggests a small increase in the risk of breast cancer. It is therefore recommended that all women be counselled concerning the benefits and possible risks of estrogen replacement therapy (B Recommendation). Decreasing levels of bone mineral density have been associated with increased risk of fracture, however, these predictions remain preliminary. Therefore, widespread bone mineral density screening to identify those at increased risk of fracture is not advised at this time. There may be some merit in performing bone mineral density measurement in selected individual women to assist in decision-making regarding ERT. Note that osteoporosis and diet are discussed briefly in Chapter 49 and the benefits of exercise in Chapter 47.

Burden of Suffering

The most common age-related fractures are those of the distal forearm, vertebrae, and hip. Lifetime risk of Colles' fracture has been estimated to be 15% in white women. These fractures rarely cause death or long-term disability and most need no rehabilitation. Vertebral fractures are the most common of the osteoporotic fractures. The estimated lifetime risk for a 50 year old woman of sustaining a vertebral fracture is 32%. Vertebral collapse is often asymptomatic and found incidentally on x-ray. In others, vertebral fracture may cause back pain which generally lasts a few months and can be managed with bed rest and analgesics. Progressive vertebral collapse can lead in some cases to kyphosis ("Dowager's Hump") and chronic pain. The course of spinal osteoporosis is very unpredictable. The proportion of those who are symptomatic with vertebral deformity or collapse is not known.

Hip fractures are associated with more death, morbidity and medical costs than all other osteoporotic fractures combined. The incidence begins to rise after age 50 but rises dramatically after age 70. A 50 year old white woman whose average life-expectancy is 80 years, has a lifetime hip fracture risk of 15% compared with a 5% risk in men.

---

[1] Assistant Professor of Medicine, University of Toronto, Toronto, Ontario

Hip fracture rates are high in American and European whites, intermediate in oriental populations and low in American Blacks. This may be due to differences seen in peak bone mass achieved.

Mortality rates in the first year following a hip fracture are 12-20% higher than rates in those of similar age and sex who have not sustained a fracture. However, much of the increased mortality may be accounted for by concomitant illness and interventions to prevent hip fracture may not decrease this high mortality. Morbidity following hip fracture is high as well. Of those living at home at the time of fracture who survive the first year, 50% require assistance with walking or with activities of daily living and 15-25% become confined to nursing homes. In the U.S. the cost of acute care attributable to osteoporosis was estimated at U.S. $7-10 billion in 1984.

Maneuver

In order to prevent osteoporotic fractures all perimenopausal women could be treated with estrogen replacement therapy (ERT) or screening strategies could be used to identify those at greatest risk for osteoporosis, using either historical risk factors or bone mineral density measurement.

Effectiveness of Preventive Treatment (ERT)

There is good evidence from randomized controlled trials that in the short-term (≤2 years) use of percutaneous estrogen,[1] oral estrogen[2] or estrogen and progesterone therapy[3] prevents bone loss or may even increase bone mass in perimenopausal women. There is fair evidence that estrogens retard bone loss up to 10 years.[4,5] However, the important issue is whether this decrease in bone loss translates into decreased fracture rates.

There is good evidence that estrogens retard bone loss up to 10 years

Ert and Incidence of Osteoporotic Fractures

There is fair evidence from case-control,[6-10] cohort[11-13] and one randomized controlled study[5] to suggest that ERT prevents osteoporotic fractures, including, most importantly, fractures of the hip (point estimates of relative risk; 0.65-0.79; p<.05).[11,12] Current users and those starting estrogen therapy within 3-5 years of the menopause seem to benefit most.

There is fair evidence that ERT prevents osteoporotic fractures

The optimal duration of use is not known. A recent study found that only women taking ERT for a minimum of 7 years had significantly higher bone mass compared with women who had never used estrogen. There is little information regarding when to discontinue therapy, if at all. Withdrawal of estrogen therapy, even after 10 years of use, leads to the accelerated loss of bone seen in perimenopausal women. The benefit of starting ERT in older women (for example, over 70 years) is unknown since most studies have been based on younger women.

Endometrial Cancer

The increased risk of endometrial cancer due to unopposed estrogen has been demonstrated in both case-control and cohort designs.[14] This risk increases with increasing doses of estrogen and increasing duration of use. This risk appears to be eliminated by the addition of progesterone and in fact, one study showed a significant decrease in risk (incidence in estrogen users 359.1 per 100,000; in estrogen-progesterone users 56.4 per 100,000 and in untreated women 248.3 per 100,000).[15] Many of these studies, however, were based on small numbers of cases.

Breast Cancer

Although recent evidence suggests a small increased risk in breast cancer in women on estrogen replacement, data are conflicting. A recent meta-analysis[16] of case-control studies found an increased relative risk after 15 years. The relative risk of breast cancer in estrogen users was 1.3 (95% confidence interval (CI): 1.2-1.6). Among women with a family history of breast cancer, those who had ever used estrogen replacement had a significantly higher risk (3.4%; 95% CI: 2.0-6.0) than those who had not (1.5%; 95% CI: 1.2-1.7).

Three other meta-analyses have been published to date.[14,17,18] All three found no significant increased risk of breast cancer in women who ever used estrogens. However, Grady et al[14] pooled relative risk estimates from case-control and cohort studies in which women used ERT for 8 years or more and found a summary relative risk of 1.25 (95% CI: 1.04-1.51).

Up until 1987, most cohort studies suggested no increased risk for breast cancer in estrogen users. Since 1987, several large cohort studies have observed a small increased risk of breast cancer.[19-22] Some studies suggest increasing risk with increasing duration of use[20,21] and current use.[21,22] The increased incidence of breast cancer in all these studies may reflect a certain degree of detection bias.

Although there is an increased incidence of breast cancer, breast cancer mortality rates may be lower for estrogen users[22,23] but this may be due to surveillance bias. Further evidence is needed to confirm this finding.

The estimated potential years of life lost (PYLL) to age 85 for women taking estrogen therapy alone for 15 years post-menopause has been calculated assuming that the relative risk of breast cancer was 2.0 (in American studies the RR was 1.3).[24] This was compared with the PYLL from hip fracture. The potential years of life lost from breast cancer was calculated to be 33,000 compared with only 1,200 from hip fracture. However, if breast cancer mortality is in fact unchanged, PYLL from breast cancer would be less than that calculated above.

In conclusion, there is fair evidence to suggest that there is no increased risk of breast cancer when estrogens are taken for a short period (5 years or less). However, ERT may lead to a small increased risk in breast cancer, if taken for more than 10 years. Current users are at higher risk than past users. There is insufficient evidence at present to draw any conclusions regarding the risk of combination therapy although several studies suggest that adding progesterone has no protective effect.[20,25,26]

Cardiovascular Mortality

Five of six prospective cohort studies of cardiovascular mortality in relation to estrogen use published since 1985[27-32] found a decrease in the relative risk of cardiovascular death or morbidity. A recent quantitative overview[33] noted that 15 of the 16 prospective studies published up to 1990 found a decreased relative risk of coronary heart disease among estrogen users, with a combined relative risk of 0.58 (95% CI: 0.48-0.69). In the meta-analysis published by Grady et al[14] a decreased summary relative risk was found for both coronary heart disease (0.65; 95% CI: 0.59-0.71) and cardiac death (0.63; 95% CI: 0.55-0.72) among women who ever used estrogen. Similar studies have shown a decreased overall mortality, likely due to the decreased CV disease. In order to counteract the increased loss of lives from breast cancer one would need a minimum relative risk reduction in ischemic heart disease mortality of at least 0.8 (in women aged 65-85 years).[24] The available evidence indicates that there does appear to be a reduction of at least this magnitude in cardiovascular mortality.

In summary, there is fair evidence to suggest that ERT leads to a decreased rate of cardiovascular (CV) mortality. As much as possible, these studies have made adjustments for baseline characteristics which might confound the findings. A randomized trial would help eliminate possible sources of bias. Another important caveat is based on the fact that most women in these studies used unopposed estrogen therapy. There is reason to believe that the addition of progesterone may lower the HDL and thereby negate the beneficial effects seen on CV mortality.[34] Estrogen therapy is known to have other adverse effects but not with the magnitude of risk of those mentioned above.

There is fair evidence that estrogen users have a decreased rate of cardiovascular mortality

Targeting High-risk Groups for Preventive Therapy

Complex models for risk factor assessment (fractures and decreased bone density) have poor sensitivity and specificity as screening procedures.<35,36> Some studies have examined the possibility of using risk factors as a proxy for bone density measurement. Again, sensitivity and specificity for predicting bone mass were poor.

Bone Mineral Density Measurements to Target High Risk Groups

Case-control studies of bone mineral density (BMD) and fractures have yielded variable results. In general there is considerable overlap between non-fractured and fractured groups.<37,38>

Despite the seemingly poor characteristics of the BMD measurements many experts in the field have compared BMD with procedures such as blood pressure measurement and serum cholesterol determination. They have posed the question, 'can bone density measurement predict RISK of fracture much like hypertension predicts RISK of stroke or cholesterol predicts RISK of cardiovascular events?' To answer this question several investigators, using mainly peripheral bone density measurements, followed patients prospectively over 1.6-10 years and documented non-spine, spine or hip fractures.<39-43> An increased relative risk of fractures was found when comparing those with the highest to those with the lowest bone density measurements. However, in order to predict risk each investigator used different criteria. Where should the "fracture threshold" be? There is no universally accepted level of osteopenia or fracture risk at which it is agreed treatment should be initiated.

Ross and colleages (1987) suggest that the fracture threshold for vertebral fracture should be based on the level at which the fracture risk doubles. This level corresponds to an annual fracture probability of 0.5% and the 95th percentile for fracture incidence cases. At this level approximately 37.5% of perimenopausal women (aged 50-55) would be at increased risk of fracture. For women aged 60-64, over 50% would be at increased risk. This threshold was defined using the Japanese-American population of Hawaii, which may limit its generalizability. As well, the best risk predictor was the density of the os calcis, a measurement unavailable in most Canadian centres.

Most manufacturers and users of bone density technology take the value of 2 SD below the mean for premenopausal women aged 30-45 as the fracture threshold. This level would encompass approximately 15% of women aged 50-55 years old. This threshold has been chosen arbitrarily and is not derived from epidemiological data.

Also, most operators of bone densitometers do not relate the relative risk prediction of their result to the current age and thus the fracture risk of the individual.

Other authors have developed estimates of lifetime fracture risk based on age and the level of femoral bone mineral density. While this model makes intuitive sense, it needs to be evaluated further through longitudinal studies. To date no randomized controlled trials have screened asymptomatic women and demonstrated the efficacy of screening in decreasing fracture rates.

Recommendation of Others

The recommendations of the U.S. Preventive Services Task Force on hormone prophylaxis are currently under review. In 1989, the Task Force recommended against routine screening for decreased bone mass in asymptomatic women but stated that this may be considered in the patient where such information would be used to make decisions regarding ERT.[44] A Consensus Development Conference sponsored by the European Foundation for Osteoporosis and Bone Disease, the National Osteoporosis Foundation and the National Institute of Arthritis and Musculoskeletal and Skin Diseases of the U.S.,[45] recommended that all women at risk for osteoporosis be considered for estrogen therapy, barring contraindications. They also suggested that bone density measurements could aid in predicting risk.

Conclusions and Recommendations

The benefits of estrogen replacement therapy must be weighed against its risks. There is good evidence that estrogen replacement therapy slows the rate of bone loss and fair evidence that estrogen replacement therapy decreases the incidence of fractures. There is also fair evidence that ERT leads to a decreased rate of cardiovascular mortality. This benefit would certainly outweigh the benefit achieved by decreasing fracture risk since the incidence of cardiovascular disease is so great. However, it is not yet known whether this benefit will continue to be seen with combination therapy. The other caveat is the small increase in risk of breast cancer noted in recent studies. It is recommended, therefore, that all women be counselled with regard to the benefits and possible risks of estrogen replacement therapy (B recommendation). Chapters on circulatory disorders (Chapters 53 to 57), tobacco (Chapter 43), physical activity (Chapter 47), and on breast cancer (Chapter 65) may provide useful background information.

Widespread bone mineral density screening is inadvisable at present (D recommendation). There are no universally accepted criteria using bone mineral density measurement to establish a level at which treatment should be instituted. Decreasing levels of bone mineral density are associated with increased risk of fracture. However, true estimates of efficacy can only be obtained by studying perimenopausal women who have been followed for a lengthy period of time. Presently there may be some merit in using bone mineral density measurements in individual women to assist in decision-making regarding ERT.

Unanswered Questions (Research Agenda)

Better quality evidence in terms of a randomized clinical trial would enhance our knowledge regarding the benefits of estrogen therapy in reducing the incidence of both fractures and of cardiovascular deaths. More data are needed regarding the effects of adding progesterone to ERT on breast cancer risk and cardiovascular mortality. More research is needed into the identification of women in the perimenopausal period who are at greatest risk of developing hip fractures. More research is needed in assessing hormone replacement therapy (HRT) benefits in various ethnic groups and in older women. Finally, more research is needed which would assist physicians to assess each individual patient's health risks and benefits so that they could make a more informed decision regarding HRT.

Evidence

A MEDLINE search was performed for articles from 1987 forwards, using the following search terms: osteoporosis, estrogen replacement therapy, synthetic estrogens, evaluation studies, random allocation, double-blind method, drug evaluation, random, cohort studies, clinical trial, menopause, postmenopausal and english. Other evidence was obtained from reference material and content experts. Although men suffer from non-traumatic fractures as well, only studies of women have been included.

This review was initiated in January 1992 and recommendations were finalized in October 1993. Other Task Force recommendations on postmenopausal osteoporosis and related fractures were published in 1988.<46>

Acknowledgements

The author thanks Elaine Wang, MD, CM, FRCPC, Associate Professor, Department of Pediatrics and of Preventive Medicine and Biostatistics, Faculty of Medicine, University of Toronto; Jonathan D. Adachi, BSC, MD, FRCPC, Associate Professor of Medicine, McMaster University, Hamilton, Ontario; Nancy Kreiger, MPH, PhD, Assistant Professor, Department of Preventive Medicine and Biostatistics, University of Toronto, Toronto, Ontario; and Anthony B. Hodsman, MB, FRCPC, Professor, Department of Medicine, University of Western Ontario, London, Ontario.

Selected References

1. Riis BJ, Thomsen K, Strom V, *et al*: The effect of percutaneous estradiol and natural progesterone on postmenopausal bone loss. *Am J Obstet Gynecol* 1987; 156: 61-65

2. Lindsay R, Hart DM, Clark DM: The minimum effective dose of estrogen for prevention of postmenopausal bone loss. *Obstet Gynecol* 1984; 63(6): 759-763

3. Christiansen C, Christensen MS, Transbol I: Bone mass in postmenopausal women after withdrawal of oestrogen/gestagen replacement therapy. *Lancet* 1981; 1(8218): 459-461

4. Nachtigall LE, Nachtigall RH, Nachtigall RD, *et al*: Estrogen replacement therapy I: a 10-year prospective study in the relationship to osteoporosis. *Obstet Gynecol* 1979; 53: 277-281

5. Lindsay R: Prevention of spinal osteoporosis in oophorectomised women. *Lancet* 1980; 2(8205): 1151-1154

6. Kreiger N, Kelsey JL, Holford TR, *et al*: An epidemiologic study of hip fracture in postmenopausal women. *Am J Epidemiol* 1982; 116(1): 141-148

7. Johnson RE, Specht EE: The risk of hip fracture in postmenopausal females with or without estrogen drug exposure. *Am J Public Health* 1981; 71(2): 138-144

8. Paganini-Hill A, Ross RK, Gerkins VR, *et al*: Menopausal estrogen therapy and hip fractures. *Ann Intern Med* 1981; 95: 28-31

9. Weiss NS, Ure CL, Ballard JH, *et al*: Decreased risk of fractures of the hip and lower forearm with postmenopausal use of estrogen. *N Engl J Med* 1980; 303: 1195-1198

10. Hutchinson TA, Polansky SM, Feinstein AR: Post-menopausal oestrogens protect against fractures of hip and distal radius. A case-control study. *Lancet* 1979; 2(8145): 705-709

11. Naessen T, Persson I, Adami HO, *et al*: Hormone replacement therapy and the risk for first hip fracture. A prospective population-based cohort study. *Am Intern Med* 1990; 113: 95-103

12. Kiel DP, Felson DT, Anderson JJ, *et al*: Hip fracture and the use of estrogens in postmenopausal women. The Framingham Study. *N Engl J Med* 1987; 317: 1169-1174

13. Ettinger B, Genant HK, Cann CE: Long-term estrogen replacement therapy prevents bone loss and fractures. *Ann Intern Med* 1985; 102: 319-324

14. Grady D, Rubin SM, Petitti DB, *et al*: Hormone therapy to prevent disease and prolong life in postmenopausal women. *Ann Intern Med* 1992; 117(12): 1016-1037

15. Gambrell RD Jr, Massey FM, Castaneda TA, *et al*: Use of the progestogen challenge test to reduce the risk of endometrial cancer. *Obstet Gynecol* 1980; 55(6): 732-738

16. Steinberg KK, Thacker SB, Smith SJ, *et al*: A meta-analysis of the effect of estrogen replacement therapy on the risk of breast cancer. *JAMA* 1991; 265(15): 1985-1990

17. Armstrong BK: Oestrogen therapy after the menopause-boon or bane? *Med J Australia* 1988; 148: 213-214

18. Dupont WD, Page DL: Menopausal estrogen replacement therapy and breast cancer. *Arch Intern Med* 1991; 151: 67-72

19. Hunt K, Vessey M, McPherson K, *et al*: Long-term surveillance of mortality and cancer incidence in women receiving hormone replacement therapy. *Br J Obstet Gynaecol* 1987; 94: 620-635

20. Bergvist L, Adami HO, Persson I: The risk of breast cancer after estrogen and estrogen-progestin replacement. *N Engl J Med* 1989; 321: 293-297

21. Mills PK, Beeson WL, Phillips RL, *et al*: Prospective study of exogenous hormone use and breast cancer in Seventh-day Adventists. *Cancer* l989; 64: 591-597

22. Colditz GA, Stampfer MJ, Willett WC, *et al*: Type of postmenopausal hormone use and risk of breast cancer: 12-year follow-up from the Nurses' Health Study. *Cancer Causes Control* 1992; 3: 433-439

23. Bergkvist L, Adami H-O, Persson I, *et al*: Prognosis after breast cancer diagnosis in women exposed to estrogen and estrogen-progestogen replacement therapy. *Am J Epidemiol* 1989; 130: 221-228

24. Miller AB: Risk/benefit considerations of antiestrogen / estrogen therapy in healthy postmenopausal women. *Prev Med* 1991; 20: 79-85

25. Persson I, Yuen J, Bergkvist L, *et al*: Combined oestrogen-progestogen replacement and breast cancer risk. [letter] *Lancet* 1992; 340(8826): 1044

26. Nachtigall MJ, Smilen SW, Nachtigall RD, *et al*: Incidence of breast cancer in a 22-year study of women receiving estrogen-progestin replacement therapy. *Obstet Gynecol* 1992; 80: 827-830

27. Bush TL, Barrett-Connor E, Cowan LD, *et al*: Cardiovascular mortality and noncontraceptive use of estrogen in women: results from the Lipid Research Clinics Program Follow-up Study. *Circulation* 1987; 75(6): 1102

28. Criqui M, Suarez L, Barrett-Connor E, *et al*: Postmenopausal estrogen use and mortality. Results from a prospective study in a defined homogenous community. *Am J Epidemiol* 1988; 128(3): 606-614

29. Wilson PW, Garrison RJ, Castelli WP: Postmenopausal estrogen use, cigarette smoking, and cardiovascular morbidity in women over 50. The Framingham study. *N Engl J Med* 1985; 313: 1038-1043

30. Stampfer MJ, Colditz GA, Willett WC, *et al*: Postmenopausal estrogen therapy and cardiovascular disease. *N Engl J Med* 1991; 325: 756-762

31. Henderson BE, Paganini-Hill A, Ross RK: Decreased Mortality in Users of Estrogen Replacement Therapy. *Arch Intern Med* 1991; 151: 75-78

32. Wolf PH, Madans JH, Finucane FF, *et al*: Reduction of cardiovascular disease-related mortality among postmenopausal women who use hormones: evidence from a national cohort. *Am J Obstet Gynecol* 1991; 164: 489-494

33. Stampfer MJ, Colditz GA: Estrogen replacement therapy and coronary heart disease: a quantitative assessment of the epidemiologic evidence. *Prev Med* 1991; 20: 47-63

34. Barrett-Connor E: Estrogen and estrogen-progestogen replacement: Therapy and cardiovascular diseases. *Am J Med* 1993; 95(Suppl 5A): 40S-43S

35. van Hemert AM, Vandenbroucke JP, Birkenhager JC, *et al*: Prediction of osteoporotic fractures in the general population by a fracture risk score. *Am J Epidemiol* 1990; 132(1): 123-135

36. Kleerekoper M, Peterson E, Nelson D, *et al*: Identification of women at risk for developing postmenopausal osteoporosis with vertebral fractures: role of history and single photon absorptiometry. *Bone Miner* 1989; 7: 171-186

37. Pouilles JM, Tremollieres F, Louvet JP, *et al*: Sensitivity of dual-photon absorptiometry in spinal osteoporosis. *Calcif Tissue Int* 1988; 43: 329-334

38. Ott SM, Kilcoyne RF, Chesnut CH: III. Ability of four different techniques of measuring bone mass to diagnose vertebral fractures in postmenopausal women. *J Bone Miner Res* 1987; 2(3): 201-210

39. Wasnich RD, Ross PD, Heilbrun LK, *et al*: Prediction of postmenopausal fracture risk with use of bone mineral measurements. *Am J Obstet Gynecol* 1985; 153: 745-751

40. Hui SL, Slemenda CW, Johnston CC Jr: Baseline measurement of bone mass predicts fracture in white women. *Ann Int Med* 1989; 111: 355-361

41. Gardsell P, Johnell O, Nilsson BE: Predicting fractures in women by using forearm bone densitometry. *Calcif Tiss Int* 1989; 44: 235-242

42. Wasnich RD, Ross PD, Davis JW, *et al*: A comparison of single and multi-site BMC measurements for assessment of spine fracture possibility. *J Nucl Med* 1989; 30: 1166-1171

43. Cummings SR, Black DM, Nevitt MC, *et al*: Appendicular bone denisty and age predict hip fracture in women. *JAMA* 1990; 263(5): 665-668

44. U.S. Preventive Services Task Force: *Guide to Clinical Preventive Services: an assessment of the effectiveness of 169 interventions*. Williams & Wilkins, Baltimore, Md, 1989: 239-243

45. Consensus development conference: diagnosis, prophylaxis, and treatment of osteoporosis. *Am J Med* 1993; 94: 646-650

46. Canadian Task Force on the Periodic Health Examination: The periodic health examination: 2. 1987 update. *Can Med Assoc J* 1988; 138: 618-626

Prevention of Osteoporotic Fractures in Women by Estrogen Replacement Therapy

MANEUVER	EFFECTIVENESS	LEVEL OF EVIDENCE <REF>	RECOMMENDATION
Initial history and physical examination	Early detection of clinical risk factors for osteoporotic fractures have limited sensitivity and specificity.	Cohort studies<35,36> (II-2)	Poor evidence to include in or exclude from periodic health examination (PHE) of asymptomatic people (C)
Single and dual photon absorptiometry, quantitative computed tomography, neutron activation analysis, dual x-ray absorptiometry	Reduced bone mineral content (BMC) and increased fracture risk are correlated but bone mineral density (BMD) does not accurately identify those at risk of fracture and these diagnostic techniques are expensive and not widely available.	Cohort studies<37,38> (II-2)	Fair evidence to exclude from PHE (D)*
Counselling all peri-menopausal women regarding the benefits and risks of estrogen replacement therapy (ERT)**	ERT slows the rate of bone loss.	Randomized controlled trials<1-5> (I)	Fair evidence to include in PHE (B); decisions regarding ERT should be made on an individual basis
	ERT decreases the incidence of osteoporotic fractures.	Randomized controlled trials<5> (I); case-control<6-10> and cohort studies<11-13> (II-2)	
	ERT decreases cardiovascular mortality.	Cohort studies<27-32> (II-2)	
	ERT increases breast cancer risk.	Meta-analyses of case-control studies <14,16-18>; cohort studies<19-25> (II-2)	
	ERT increases risk of endometrial cancer but risk may be eliminated with combination therapy.	Case-control and cohort studies<14,15> (II-2)	

*   Widespread use of bone mineral density measurements is not recommended. However, there may be some merit in using bone mineral measurements in individual women if such measurements will be used in decision-making regarding ERT.

**   There has been no formal evaluation of the effectiveness of counselling as a maneuver.

Circulatory Disorders

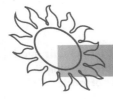

CHAPTER 53

Screening for Hypertension in Young and Middle-Aged Adults

By Alexander G. Logan

Screening for Hypertension in Young and Middle-Aged Adults

Prepared by Alexander G Logan, MD, FRCPC[1]

In 1984 the Task Force recommended that all persons aged 25 or over should receive a blood pressure (BP) measurement during any visit to the physician and that antihypertensive therapy should be limited largely to those with a diastolic pressure of 100 mmHg or greater.<1> These recommendations were based principally on the results of several large scale randomized controlled treatment trials of persons with mild to moderate diastolic hypertension.<2> Since then new data concerning the diagnosis and treatment of hypertension have been published including several randomized controlled trials in the elderly.<3> Important gaps in our knowledge still exist nonetheless; there are, for example, no clinical trial data on the efficacy of treating diastolic hypertension in persons under 21 years of age or isolated systolic hypertension in those under 60 or over 84 years of age. Hypertension in the elderly is addressed in Chapter 79 and prevention of preeclampsia in Chapter 13.

Accurate BP measurement by sphygmomanometer in the physicians' office remains the principal method of diagnosis. There is insufficient evidence to recommend the routine use of echocardiography, self-measurement of BP or ambulatory BP monitoring in diagnosis.<4> While there is good evidence to recommend antihypertensive therapy for young and middle-aged adults with diastolic pressures of 90 mmHg or over, the clinical decision to initiate pharmacologic treatment should take into account the individual's absolute risk for cardiovascular disease, particularly when the average diastolic pressure is in the range of 90 to 99 mmHg and there is no hypertensive target organ damage or other concomitant diseases.<4,5>

Burden of Suffering

Up to 15% of the adult population have definite or established hypertension and an almost equal percentage have labile hypertension

Estimates from several BP surveys over the past decade suggest that up to 15% of the adult population have definite or established hypertension and that an almost equal percentage have labile hypertension characterized by elevations of BP on some, but not all, occasions.<6> Epidemiological and actuarial studies have repeatedly demonstrated that cardiovascular morbidity and mortality are

---

[1] Professor of Medicine, University of Toronto, Toronto, Ontario

substantially higher in hypertensives, compared with normotensives at all ages and in both sexes. Also, the presence of mild hypertension is a powerful predictor of progression to more severe elevations of BP.<7,8> Because hypertension is an important contributor to the principal cardiovascular diseases which account for more than 40% of all deaths in Canada,<9> good BP control will have a major beneficial effect on health care costs.

Epidemiological investigations indicate that with increasing BP levels the excess risk of cardiovascular events in adult men and women increases in a curvilinear manner.<7,8> Hypertension is a major contributor to pressure-related events such as stroke, congestive heart failure and ruptured aortic aneurysm, and a significant risk factor for atheromatous complications such as coronary heart disease and occlusive peripheral arterial disease. Cardiovascular events are as closely linked to systolic as to diastolic pressure elevations, and possibly more so. The absolute risk of cardiovascular disease amongst equally hypertensive individuals varies substantially, depending upon a history of previous cardiovascular disease or the presence of associated risk factors including hypercholesterolemia, cigarette smoking, glucose intolerance, left ventricular hypertrophy, older age, and male gender. Except for individuals with extremely high BP levels, absolute risk is influenced more by these factors than BP level per se.<7> This spectrum of risk is increasingly being taken into account in making treatment decisions,<4,5> since greater benefits in absolute terms are observed among those at higher risk.

Maneuver

The diagnosis of hypertension is the essential starting point in its management. Methods for accurate diagnosis were set out in a consensus report of the Canadian Hypertension Society.<2> The mercury sphygmomanometer is the instrument of choice because of its accuracy and dependability. The aneroid type should be calibrated twice yearly using mercury as the standard. Guidelines for sphygmomanometry include: selection of appropriate cuff size (the rubber bladder should encircle at least 2/3 of the upper arm); measurement should be taken after five minutes of quiet rest, and with the arm bared, supported and positioned at heart level; for screening and diagnosis the seated position should be used; if hypertension is established, subsequent readings should include a lying and standing measurement. The patient should have refrained from smoking or ingesting caffeine 30 minutes before measurement. Two or more readings should be averaged; if the first two differ by more than 5 mm additional readings should be obtained. If an initial BP is mildly elevated in a person not previously known to have hypertension, the BP should be reassessed on at least three occasions over a period of six months. For patients with more severely elevated pressure readings the interval between repeat assessments should be shortened.

Echocardiography, self-measured BP and ambulatory BP monitoring are increasingly being used in the evaluative process and may provide useful information in special circumstances. Nonetheless there is insufficient evidence at the present time to warrant their routine use in diagnosis.[3]

Effectiveness of Prevention

The results of many randomized clinical trials of antihypertensive drug therapy on morbidity and mortality from cardiovascular disease in patients with hypertension of varying severity have been published over the past 30 years.[10] The early trials of antihypertensive therapy demonstrated the efficacy of treating hypertension with initial diastolic BPs of 90 mmHg or higher.[11-15] Detailed analysis of these trials indicated that the benefits of active drug treatment accrued principally to those with more severe hypertension (diastolic pressures of 105 mmHg or over), those with a cardiovascular or renal abnormality at entry, or those who were 50 years of age or older.[16] Consensus recommendations at the time[17] favoured treatment of such individuals and close observation of those with uncomplicated diastolic pressures of 90 to 104 mmHg, initiating drug therapy only when there was clear evidence of a trend of rising BP or of disease progression as demonstrated by adverse changes in target organs (heart, kidneys, and brain).

More recent studies have focused principally on milder forms of diastolic hypertension in young and middle-aged adults,[18-20] the topic of this chapter, and on hypertension in the elderly.[21-24] The major therapeutic trials in mild hypertension were the American Hypertension Detection and Follow-up Program (HDFP), the Australian National Blood Pressure Study (ANBPS), and the British Medical Research Council (MRC) trial.

The HDFP was a community-based, randomized controlled trial that compared the effectiveness of an intensive, supervised program of specified antihypertensive drug treatment ("stepped care" (SC)) with that of routine therapy obtained by referral of patients to their customary source of medical care in the community ("referred care" (RC)).[18] The 10,940 hypertensive men and women, of whom more than 40% were black, were stratified by BP level, with the majority (71.5%) being in the baseline diastolic BP stratum of 90 to 104 mmHg (stratum 1). The age range of participants was 30 to 69 years. Almost one-quarter of stratum 1 participants were receiving antihypertensive medication at the time of stratum designation, indicating that many had a more severe form of hypertension, and a small percentage at entry had left ventricular hypertrophy (3.5%), history of stroke (2.1%), myocardial infarction (4.8%), or diabetes mellitus (7.0%). The difference in mean diastolic BP of 5 mmHg between the SC and RC groups at the end of this 5-year study was associated with a significant reduction in total mortality, the primary end-point, and deaths from all cardiovascular causes. Secondary analyses revealed similar outcomes in stratum 1 participants including those free of end-organ damage and not taking antihypertensive drugs on entry. White women, however, did not appear to benefit from therapy although the difference in the percentage of individuals receiving treatment between the SC and RC groups was smallest in this subgroup. Because the HDFP did not include an untreated control group, some maintain that the source of care and other factors unrelated to hypertension control were largely responsible for the difference in outcomes. This viewpoint was supported by the marked reduction in deaths from non-cardiovascular causes in the SC group, a finding not observed in the actively treated group in other similar trials.[19,20]

The ANBPS was a randomized, placebo-controlled, single-blind trial involving 3,427 white men and women aged 30 to 69 years with untreated diastolic BPs (phase V) of 95 to 109 mmHg and systolic BPs under 200 mmHg.[19] Participants were virtually free of any cardiovascular disease at entry (0.4% had previous myocardial infarction) and had no diabetes mellitus, stroke history or electrocardiographic evidence of myocardial ischemia. The in-trial average diastolic BP was 5.6 mmHg lower in the actively treated than in the control group and this difference resulted in a significant reduction in trial end-points (death from any cause and non-fatal cardiovascular events). Actively treated women had significantly fewer trial end-points than those in the control group.[25] The number needed to treat for 5 years to prevent one cardiovascular event was 44.

In the British MRC trial, 17,354 men and women, aged 35 to 64 years, having an untreated mean phase vs. diastolic BP of 90 to 109 mmHg and systolic BP under 200 mmHg and free of significant cardiovascular disease (about 2% had left ventricular hypertrophy, electrocardiographic Q wave abnormalities or stroke history) or diabetes mellitus, were randomized in a single-blind fashion to receive active treatment or placebo.[20] The extent of separation between average diastolic pressures in actively treated and control groups was 5 to 6 mmHg. Active treatment significantly reduced the trial end-points (death from any cause and non-fatal cardiovascular events). The rates of stroke and of all cardiovascular events were significantly reduced but treatment had no effect on coronary events. Deaths from all causes were reduced in men on treatment but slightly increased in women. There were no other differences in outcomes by gender. The number needed to treat for 5 years to prevent one cardiovascular event was 141.

Quantitative meta-analyses of the results of these and other smaller trials of anti-hypertensive therapy have been reported[10,26] and the findings compared with data from several prospective observational studies on the effects on stroke and on coronary heart disease of prolonged BP differences of the same size.<10> A reduction in diastolic BP of 5 to 6 mmHg, the observed effect of active treatment in the randomized trials, resulted in a 42% reduction in fatal and nonfatal strokes (95% confidence interval (CI): 33% to 50%) and a 14% reduction in all coronary heart disease (95% CI: 4% to 22%). The expected decline in stroke incidence based on observational data for such a BP reduction was estimated to be 35% to 40%; thus the benefits of therapy were fully realized within three years, the average duration of the clinical trials. In sharp contrast the benefits for coronary heart disease were less than the predicted reduction of 20% to 25% from prospective observational studies. Several explanations for this apparent discrepancy have been posited including a delay in the full attainment of benefit of sustained BP reduction on a predominantly atherosclerotic disease process, adverse effects of treatment, and chance. New data suggest that the type of drug therapy is not responsible for the failure to obtain full coronary heart disease benefit from BP lowering.<22>

Treatment of Hypertension

Diuretics and beta-adrenergic blockers were the two major classes of drugs used as first-line treatment in most of the major outcome trials. Medications were generally given in a stepwise sequence with maximum dosage of a drug being prescribed at each step before the agent at the next step was added to achieve the treatment goal. A variety of antihypertensive agents was introduced as additional therapy including reserpine, alpha-methyldopa, guanethidine, hydralazine and clonidine, agents which are no longer commonly prescribed.

Fortunately the incidence of serious or life-threatening drug reactions in these trials was rare. Less serious side effects, however, were common, resulting in discontinuation of randomized treatment (almost 20% by the fifth year in the British MRC trial<20>) or a substantial increase in patient discomfort (difference in subjective complaints of approximately 15% between active treatment and placebo groups<12>). In some instances the symptoms were predictable adverse effects associated with a particular class of drug but more often they represented a patient's idiosyncratic reaction to a drug.

Benefits from treatment are probably related to lowering blood pressure per se rather than to any specific property of antihypertensive agents

None of the trials employed the newer classes of antihypertensive agents (calcium entry blockers, angiotensin converting enzyme inhibitors, or alpha-adrenergic blockers) or the now common treatment approach of sequential monotherapy. These therapeutic innovations were introduced to reduce drug-related side effects and to circumvent the adverse metabolic consequences of older classes of drugs. The newer agents have been shown to be as effective as diuretics and beta-blockers in lowering BP,<27,28> are well tolerated by most patients, and appear to provide substantial advantages in specific patient groups.<28,29> Nonetheless there are insufficient data on the long-term benefits and risks of these drugs and the comparative advantages over substantially less expensive 'older' agents to recommend them as first-line drug treatment. From available evidence it seems likely that the magnitude of benefit from treatment is related to lowering BP per se rather than to any specific property of the various antihypertensive agents. Given the importance of this issue, however, new information is urgently needed.

Several nonpharmacologic measures including weight reduction in overweight subjects, moderation in alcohol consumption, increased physical activity and sodium restriction particularly in sodium-sensitive individuals have been shown in relatively short studies to lower BP in hypertensive patients.<30> No data exist, however, on whether these short-term changes in BP translate into less cardiovascular morbidity and mortality. Generally non-pharmacologic interventions are less effective than drug treatment in lowering BP and their effects on quality of life is quite variable.<31,32> Some measures such as weight loss improve elements of quality of life, whereas others such as sodium restriction may make them worse.<32> Despite the absence of evidence on the long-term safety, acceptability and effectiveness of nonpharmacologic therapy, they are considered a useful starting point for treatment and viewed as important adjuncts to drug therapy.<30>

Decision to Initiate Drug Treatment

There is a continuum of cardiovascular risk associated with level of BP that extends well down into the arbitrarily defined normal BP range, beginning for systolic above 110 mmHg and for diastolic above 70 mmHg.<33> Evidence on the benefits of antihypertensive therapy comes from clinical trials in which treatment categories were defined by BP level alone.<11-15,18-24> The results indicate that young and middle-aged patients (ages 21 to 64 years) with diastolic BPs of 90 mmHg or over will benefit from antihypertensive drug therapy.<10> Despite this demonstration there has been general reluctance to use BP level alone as the sole determinant for drug treatment in persons whose average diastolic pressure is in the range of 90 to 99 mmHg.<4,5,34-37> In these instances the presence of other cardiovascular disease risk factors or concomitant diseases strongly influences the decision to initiate drug therapy. Factors generally taken into account include left ventricular hypertrophy, or cardiovascular, cerebrovascular or peripheral vascular disease. In addition patients with renal disease, diabetes mellitus, or hypercholesterolemia, or who smoke cigarettes are at substantial risk for morbid or fatal cardiovascular events and should be more aggressively treated. In low-risk individuals, on the other hand, treatment has focused principally on non-pharmacologic measures to which drug therapy is added in the event of progression to more severe hypertension or the development of hypertension-related target organ damage.

This modification of treatment decisions based on epidemiological risk is theoretically attractive and has been adopted in some manner or other by most groups formulating guidelines for clinical practice.<4,5,34-37> Nonetheless this treatment strategy has not been formally evaluated and past experiences with multifactorial intervention trials of primary prevention of cardiovascular disease in high risk subjects generally have been disappointing.<38-40>

Recommendations of Others

The primary goal of treatment in most guidelines is a diastolic blood pressure below 90 mmHg

Guidelines of most other groups identify two threshold pressures, one for the diagnosis of hypertension, which for diastolic pressure is 90 mmHg or higher and for systolic pressure, 140 mmHg or higher, and one for the initiation of drug treatment based on BP level alone.<4,5,30,34-37> The drug treatment threshold for diastolic BP alone differs considerably amongst the guidelines being 90,<30> 95,<35-37> or 100 mmHg.<4> Most guidelines suggest that factors other than BP should influence the decision to begin drug treatment of patients with pressures between the thresholds for diagnosis and routine treatment of hypertension.<4,5,34-37> There are few differences amongst the guidelines on factors that interact with hypertension to increase the likelihood of cardiovascular risk and include older age, male gender, smoking cigarettes, hypercholesterolemia, diabetes, hypertensive target organ damage, and the presence of cardiovascular disease. Most guidelines recommend diuretics or beta-blockers as initial drug therapy for patients in whom there are no specific contradictions;<5,30,34-37,41> the World Health Organization/International Society of Hypertension guidelines suggest, however, that any particular class of antihypertensive agent may be chosen.<35> The primary goal of treatment in most guidelines is a diastolic BP below 90 mmHg,<4,30,34-37> and even lower levels in certain situations such as the presence of renal disease in diabetic patients.<30,35,42> All guidelines recommend a more individualized therapeutic approach in special circumstances<4,5,30,34-37> although even here the American Joint National Committee guidelines still tend to favour diuretics and beta-blockers as initial therapy in most instances.<30>

The Preventive Services Task Force recommends that BP be measured regularly in all persons aged 3 and above.<43>

Conclusions and Recommendations

There is fair evidence to measure BP in young and middle-aged adults (B Recommendation). Case-finding should be considered in all persons aged 21 to 64 years; individual clinical judgment should be exercised in all other cases. Accurate BP measurement by sphygmomanometer in the physicians' office remains the principal method of diagnosis. There is insufficient evidence to recommend the routine use of echocardiography, self-measurement of BP or ambulatory BP monitoring in diagnosis.

While there is good evidence to recommend antihypertensive therapy for young and middle-aged adults (ages 21 to 64 years) with diastolic pressures of 90 mmHg or over (A Recommendation), the clinical decision to introduce pharmacologic treatment should take into account a person's absolute risk for cardiovascular disease, particularly when the average diastolic pressure is in the range of 90 to 99 mmHg and there is no hypertensive target organ damage or other concomitant diseases. There is insufficient evidence to evaluate therapy in persons 1) with elevated pressure aged under 21 years; or 2) with isolated systolic hypertension defined as a systolic pressure of 140 mmHg or higher and diastolic pressure less than 90 mmHg.

Unanswered Questions (Research Agenda)

Important gaps in our knowledge on the management of hypertension still exist. With respect to diagnosis, the role of echocardiography, self-measurement of BP and ambulatory BP monitoring needs to be defined. For example, if persons who demonstrate the 'white-coat' phenomenon were found not to be at increased risk for cardiovascular disease events, treatment of up to a quarter of the hypertensive population might be avoided. Equally the early detection of left ventricular hypertrophy by echocardiography or the demonstration of increasing left ventricular mass may enhance the specificity of therapeutic intervention.

The benefits and risks of treating diastolic hypertension in persons under 21 years of age, or isolated systolic hypertension in those under 60 or over 80 years of age still needs to be demonstrated. Furthermore large-scale trials of non-pharmacologic measures with clinical endpoints need to be conducted both in persons with hypertension and in those at risk to develop hypertension in the future.

Future management approaches will likely involve genetic testing to detect persons at risk for hypertension. Identification of genetic susceptible individuals should enhance selectivity of primary prevention strategies and raises the possibility of gene therapy.

Evidence

A MEDLINE search was conducted using a MESH heading hypertension and the subheadings complications, diagnosis, drug therapy, epidemiology, prevention and control, and therapy for primary papers published from January 1966 to March 1994. A search was also carried out for review articles published between 1984 and 1994. References from these papers were reviewed to identify relevant articles. This review was initiated in October 1993 and recommendations were finalized by the Task Force in March 1994.

Selected References

1. Canadian Task Force on the Periodic Health Examination: The periodic health examination: 2. 1984 update. *Can Med Assoc J* 1984; 130: 1278-1285

2. Logan AG: Report of the Canadian Hypertension Society's consensus conference on the management of mild hypertension. *Can Med Assoc J* 1984; 131: 1053-1057

3. Carruthers SG, Larochelle P, Haynes RB, *et al*: Report of the Canadian Hypertension Society Consensus Conference: 1. Introduction. *Can Med Assoc J* 1993; 149: 289-293

4. Haynes RB, Lacourciere Y, Rabkin SW, *et al*: Report of the Canadian Hypertension Society Consensus Conference: 2. Diagnosis of hypertension in adults. *Can Med Assoc J* 1993; 149: 409-418

5. Jackson R, Barham P, Bills J, *et al*: Management of raised blood pressure in New Zealand: a discussion document. *BMJ* 1993; 307: 107-110

6. Joffres MR, Hamet P, Rabkin SW, *et al*: Prevalence, control and awareness of high blood pressure among Canadian adults. Canadian Heart Health Surveys Research Group. *Can Med Assoc J* 1992; 146: 1997-2005

7. Dawber TR: The Framingham Study. The epidemiology of atherosclerotic disease. Cambridge: Harvard University Press, 1980

8. Society of Actuaries: Build and blood pressure study. Society of Actuaries, Chicago, 1959

9. Nicholls E, Nair C, MacWilliam L, *et al*: Cardio-vascular Disease in Canada (addendum to cat 82-544), Statistics Canada and Dept. of National Health and Welfare, Ottawa, 1988

10. Collins R, Peto R, MacMahon S, *et al*: Blood pressure, stroke, and coronary heart disease. Part 2, Short-term reductions in blood pressure: overview of randomized drug trials in their epidemiological context. *Lancet* 1990; 335: 827-838

11. Veterans Administration Cooperative Study Group on Antihypertensive Agents: 1. Results in patients with diastolic blood pressures averaging 115 through 129 mmHg. *JAMA* 1967; 202: 1028-1034

12. Veterans Administration Cooperative Study Group on Antihypertensive Agents: Effects of treatment on morbidity in hypertension: II. Results in patients with diastolic blood pressure averaging 90 through 114 mmHg. *JAMA* 1970; 213: 1143-1152

13. Wolff FW, Lindeman RD: Effects of treatment in hypertension: Results of a controlled study. *J Chron Dis* 1966; 19: 227-240

14. Hypertension-Stroke Co-operative Study Group: Effect of antihypertensive treatment on stroke recurrence. *JAMA* 1974; 229: 409-418

15. Smith WM: Treatment of mild hypertension. Results of a ten-year intervention trial. U.S. Public Health Service Hospitals Cooperative Study Group. *Circulation* 1977; 40 (suppl 1): 98-105

16. Veterans Administration Cooperative Study Group on Antihypertensive Agents: Effects of treatment on morbidity in hypertension: III. Influence of age, diastolic pressure and prior cardiovascular disease; further analysis of side-effects. *Circulation* 1972; 45: 991-1004

17. Report of the Ontario Council of Health: Hypertension 1977, Ontario Council Health, Toronto, 1977

18. Hypertension Detection and Follow-up Program Cooperative Group: Five-year findings of the Hypertension Detection and Follow-up Program. 1. Reduction in mortality of persons with high blood pressure, including mild hypertension. *JAMA* 1979; 242: 2562-2571

19. Report by the Management Committee. The Australian Therapeutic Trial in Mild Hypertension. *Lancet* 1980; 1: 1261-1267

20. Medical Research Council Working Party: MRC trial of treatment of mild hypertension: principal results. *Br Med J Clin Res Ed* 1985; 291: 97-104

21. Amery A, Birkenhager W, Brixko P, *et al*: Mortality and morbidity results from the European Working Party on High Blood Pressure in the Elderly trial. *Lancet* 1985; 1: 1349-1354

22. SHEP Cooperative Research Group: Prevention of stroke by antihypertensive drug treatment in older persons with isolated systolic hypertension. *JAMA* 1991; 265: 3255-3264

23. Dahlof B, Lindholm LH, Hansson L, *et al*: Morbidity and mortality in the Swedish trial in Old Patients with Hypertension (STOP-Hypertension). *Lancet* 1991; 338: 1281-1285

24. MRC Working Party: Medical Research Council trial of treatment of hypertension in older adults: principal results. *BMJ* 1992; 304: 405-412

25. The Management Committee of the Australian National Blood Pressure Study: Prognostic factors in the treatment of mild hypertension. *Circulation* 1984; 69: 668-676

26. MacMahon SW, Cutler JA, Furberg CD, *et al*: The effects of drug treatment for hypertension on morbidity and mortality from cardiovascular disease: a review of randomized controlled trials. *Prog Cardiovasc Dis* 1986; 24 (3 suppl 1): 99-118

27. Fletcher AE, Bulpitt CJ, Chase DM, *et al*: Quality of life with three antihypertensive treatments. Cilazapril, atenolol, nifedipine. *Hypertension* 1992; 19: 499-507

28. The Treatment of Mild Hypertension Research Group: The treatment of mild hypertension study. A randomized, placebo-controlled trial of a nutritional-hygienic regimen along with various drug monotherapies. *Arch Intern Med* 1991; 151: 1413-1423

29. Lewis EJ, Hunsicker LG, Bain RP, *et al*: The effect of angiotensin-converting-enzyme inhibition on diabetic nephropathy. *N Engl J Med* 1993; 329: 1456-1462

30. National High Blood Pressure Education Program: The fifth report of the Joint National Committee on Detection, Evaluation, and Treatment of High Blood Pressure. *Arch Intern Med* 1993; 153: 154-183

31. Neaton JD, Grimm RH Jr, Prineas RJ, *et al*: Treatment of mild hypertension study. Final results. *JAMA* 1993; 270: 713-724

32. Wassertheil-Smoller S, Oberman A, Blaufox D, *et al*: The trial of antihypertensive interventions and management (TAIM) study. Final results with regard to blood pressure, cardiovascular risk, and quality of life. *Am J Hypertens* 1992; 5: 37-44

33. Neaton JD, Wentworth D: Serum cholesterol, blood pressure, cigarette smoking, and death from coronary heart disease. Overall findings and differences by age for 316,099 white men. Multiple Risk Factor Intervention Trial Research Group. *Arch Intern Med* 1992; 152: 56-64

34. Alderman MH, Cushman WC, Hill MN, *et al*: International round table discussion of national guidelines for the detection, evaluation, and treatment of hypertension. *Am J Hypertens* 1993; 6: 974-981

35. Guidelines Subcommittee of the WHO/ISH Mild Hypertension Liaison Committee: 1993 guidelines for the management of mild hypertension. Memorandum from a World Health Organization/International Society of Hypertension meeting. *Hypertension* 1993; 22: 392-403

36. Sever P, Beevers G, Bulpitt C, *et al*: Management guidelines in essential hypertension: report of the second working party of the British Hypertension Society. *BMJ* 1993; 306: 983-987

37. Whitworth JA, Clarkson D, Dwyer T, *et al*: The management of hypertension: a consensus statement. *Med J Aust* 1994; 160(Suppl 21): S1-S16

38. Multiple Risk Factor Intervention Trial Research Group: Multiple Risk Factor Intervention Trial: Risk factor changes and mortality results. *JAMA* 1982; 248: 1465-1477

39. Wilhelmsen L, Berglund G, Elmfeldt D, *et al*: The multifactor primary prevention trial in Goteborg, Sweden. *Eur Heart J* 1986; 7: 279-288

40. Strandberg TE, Salomaa VV, Naukkarinen VA, *et al*: Long-term mortality after 5-year multifactorial primary prevention of cardiovascular diseases in middle-aged men. *JAMA* 1991; 266: 1225-1229

41. Ogilvie RI, Burgess ED, Cusson JR, *et al*: Report of the Canadian Hypertension Society Consensus Conference: 3. Pharmacologic treatment of essential hypertension. *Can Med Assoc J* 1993; 149: 575-584

42. Dawson KG, McKenzie JK, Ross SA, *et al*: Report of the Canadian Hypertension Society Consensus Conference: 5. Hypertension and diabetes. *Can Med Assoc J* 1993; 149: 821-826

43. U.S. Preventive Services Task Force: *Guide to Clinical Preventive Services: an Assessment of the Effectiveness of 169 Interventions.* Williams & Wilkins, Baltimore, Md, 1989: 23-27

Screening for Hypertension in Young and Middle-Aged Adults

MANEUVER	EFFECTIVENESS	LEVEL OF EVIDENCE <REF>	RECOMMENDATION
Measurement of blood pressure (BP) level	Average of at least two readings on each of at least three occasions over a period of six months. Although not evaluated for its effectiveness, case-finding should be considered in all persons aged 21 to 64 years; individual clinical judgment should be exercised in all other cases	Expert opinion* (III)	Fair evidence to include in periodic health examination (PHE) (B)
Pharmacologic treatment of hypertension	Therapy for hypertension should be based on type and level of BP elevation and age		
	a) persons aged 21 to 64 years with diastolic pressures of 90 mmHg or higher — treatment lowers risk of stroke, cardiac events and death.	Randomized controlled trials<18-20> (I)	Good evidence to treat (A)
	b) persons with elevated diastolic pressure under age 21 years; there is no evidence of benefit to treatment.	Expert opinion (III)	Insufficient evidence to include in or exclude from PHE (C)
	c) persons with isolated systolic hypertension defined as a systolic pressure of 140 mmHg or higher and diastolic pressure less than 90 mmHg; there is no evidence of benefit to treatment.	Expert opinion (III)	Insufficient evidence to include in or exclude from PHE (C)

*   High prevalence, effective detection maneuver and efficacious treatment

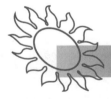

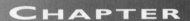

CHAPTER

54

Lowering the Blood Total Cholesterol Level to Prevent Coronary Heart Disease

By Alexander G. Logan

Lowering the Blood Total Cholesterol Level to Prevent Coronary Heart Disease

Prepared by Alexander G. Logan, MD, FRCPC[1]

In 1979 the Canadian Task Force on the Periodic Health Examination concluded that there was insufficient evidence to include or exclude screening for hyperlipidemia (elevated cholesterol or triglyceride level above arbitrarily defined normal ranges) as part of the periodic health examination.

In the ensuing 10 years there was a dramatic increase in knowledge about and general interest in cholesterol. The Task Force has re-examined the evidence published subsequent to its 1993 update<1> and again finds insufficient evidence to recommend routine cholesterol screening but endorses case-finding in men 30-59 years old, corresponding to the group where drug therapy has been shown to be effective.

Burden of Suffering

Although the death rate from coronary heart disease (CHD) in Canada has decreased by almost 40% over the past 15 years, cardiovascular disease, the primary cause of premature death in most industrialized countries, still accounts for more than 40% of all deaths in Canada. Most of these deaths were from CHD.

An increased blood cholesterol level, specifically a high low-density lipoprotein (LDL) cholesterol, is closely linked to the severity of atherosclerosis in the coronary arteries and is a major risk predictor of clinical CHD.<2,3> In addition, there is a continuous, graded relation over most of the serum cholesterol range.<3> There is also increasing evidence from epidemiologic studies that other cholesterol subfractions (high-density lipoprotein cholesterol (HDL-C), very low-density lipoprotein cholesterol (VLDL-C)), the carrier apolipoproteins of cholesterol and α-lipoprotein) may help to predict the risk of myocardial infarction.<4> Several studies suggest an independent and inverse association between levels of HDL-C and risk for CHD<5> and HDL-C and triglyceride levels are independent predictors of CVD death in women.<4>

Recent data on risk factors for cardiovascular disease in Canada come from heart health surveys in each province between 1986 and 1990 involving over 20,000 men and women aged 18 to 74 years. Among men and women the prevalence rates of a total plasma

---

[1] Professor of Medicine, University of Toronto, Toronto, Ontario

cholesterol level of 6.20 mmol/L or more were 18% and 17% respectively, an LDL-C level of 4.10 mmol/L or more 16% and 14%, an HDL-C level below 0.90 mmol/L 13% and 4%, and a triglyceride level of 2.30 mmol/L or more 20% and 11%.

The prevalence rates of hypercholesterolemia and CHD are higher among older people;[6,7] menopause has also been associated with a major increase in serum total cholesterol concentration (19% over an 8-year period).[8] Among older people the gradient of CHD risk with increasing total cholesterol levels is flatter, but risk has been shown to be significant for both elderly women and men in large studies[9] although in some reports it disappears after 64 years of age. While the strength of the association between cholesterol and CHD may decline with age, absolute excess risk does not[9] given the almost ten-fold difference in the incidence rate of death from CHD in men 65 years or older and men under 65.

As people become very old, however, the relation between total cholesterol and longevity appears to change. Several studies, including very elderly women and men, reported higher death rates in those with lower cholesterol levels or among those with the greatest decline in cholesterol levels.[10] It may be that those who survive to a very advanced age are no longer susceptible to elevated total cholesterol levels or that a low cholesterol concentration in the very old is simply a marker of chronic noncardiac disease. The benefits of therapy for this group are questionable.

Although the risk of CHD is strongly related to the serum total cholesterol level, at any level of cholesterol the risk varies widely depending on the presence of other risk factors. For example, in the Framingham Heart Study it was found that a 45-year-old man with a serum cholesterol level of 7.40 mmol/L, an elevated systolic pressure, electrocardiographic evidence of left ventricular hypertrophy and glucose intolerance who smokes is 12 times more likely to have cardiovascular disease over an 8-year period than a man of the same age with the same cholesterol level who is free of the other risk factors. In contrast, over 8 years the risk for a 45-year-old man with a serum cholesterol level of 8.00 mmol/L but no other risk factors would be 2.4 times that of a man with the same risk profile whose cholesterol level is normal (5.40 mmol/L). Excess body weight in white American men has been associated with deleterious changes in the lipoprotein profile.[11] Such evidence was the basis for several trials of multifactorial interventions to prevent cardiovascular disease.[12,13]

In the context of routine clinical practice the use of the serum total cholesterol level to predict future CHD events in individual patients is not straightforward. In familial hypercholesterolemia (FH), for example, the clinical expression of CHD can occur at very different ages, even among siblings with closely matched cholesterol levels. Lower cutoffs have been proposed for screening close relatives of

Serum cholesterol level discriminates poorly between people destined to have symptomatic CHD and those who will remain symptom-free

confirmed FH cases.<14> In the Framingham cohort the distribution of serum cholesterol levels in men under the age of 50 years who had CHD was very similar to that in subjects who remained disease-free; the average cholesterol level in the former group was only 6.30 mmol/L. In the Pooling Project more than 40% of asymptomatic men aged 40 to 59 years who experienced their initial CHD event during an 8.6-year follow-up period had a serum cholesterol level of less than 6.30 mmol/L, and about 88% of those with a higher level had no clinical signs of CHD. Thus, the serum cholesterol level is a poor discriminator between people destined to have symptomatic CHD and those who will remain symptom-free. It is this weak predictive power that has been a source of concern about recommending universal screening.

Maneuver

Screening

The nonfasting measurement of blood total cholesterol is widely recommended as an initial screening tool to detect hypercholesterolemia.<15,16> This relatively low cost test is widely available and reflects mainly the LDL-C level (about 70% of total cholesterol in blood is transported in LDL). Repeat measurements may be carried out without substantially increasing the economic burden of cholesterol screening. Because of analytic and biologic variability<17> and test characteristics (indirect indicator of LDL-C level), there will be a substantial number of false positive and false negative results.

False positive results can be lessened by repeated measurement of total cholesterol or by selective lipoprotein analysis

The rate of false positive results can be lessened by repeated measurement of the total cholesterol level which will reduce biologic variability or by selective lipoprotein analysis which will identify individuals with high levels of protective HDL (usually in women). The rate of false negative results may be reduced by lowering the level of total cholesterol for retesting or by adding lipoprotein analysis to initial cholesterol testing. The latter approach, for example, would identify individuals with low HDL levels who are at increased risk for CHD, but would also increase costs, introduce greater analytic and biologic variability,<18> and reduce accessibility to high-quality analytic procedures.

Some authorities have recommended including a non-fasting measurement of HDL-cholesterol in screening for lipid disorders<15> because of the association of a low HDL level with CHD mortality and morbidity even amongst subjects without elevated total cholesterol. Apart from greater analytic and biologic variability of HDL determinations<17,18> and increased cost there are few clinical trial data linking changes in plasma concentration of this or other lipid fractions to reductions in the CHD death rate. The effects of labelling a person as having hypercholesterolemia have been considered by several groups and there appear to be few or no adverse consequences.<19,20>

Treatment Approaches

Dietary and pharmacologic interventions have been used to lower LDL-cholesterol levels. The dietary approach derives from observations that the typical North American diet is too high in total fat (35% to 40% of total energy intake), cholesterol (more than 500 mg/d) and total kilojoules and too low in the ratio of polyunsaturated to saturated fatty acids (PS ratio) and fibre-rich carbohydrates.<15>

Key elements in current dietary recommendations are to: 1) reduce the intake of total fat to 30% of the total energy intake and the saturated fatty acids to below 10% of the total energy intake; 2) increase the intake of complex carbohydrates and either cis-monounsaturated or polyunsaturated fatty acids; and 3) restrict the number of kilojoules for overweight people.<15,16,21> Lowering of the dietary cholesterol intake to less than 300 mg/d is also advocated, although the additive effect of this change on the plasma cholesterol and lipoprotein concentrations against the recommended background diet is controversial and may be small. When compared with the average North American diet, these dietary changes can reduce the plasma total cholesterol level by about 14%, the LDL-C level by 16% and the HDL-C level by 3% in healthy, noninstitutionalized people, although a recent trial in free-living individuals produced only a 5% reduction in total cholesterol.<22>

The evidence for a favourable effect of short-term dietary manipulations on blood lipids in controlled settings is compelling, but the long-term effectiveness in asymptomatic outpatients has generally been disappointing. Net reductions in total cholesterol level of 1-13% have been reported in various populations with the largest reductions occurring in patients with symptomatic CHD<23,24> or patients with diets very high in fat. The disappointing results have been attributed generally to poor dietary compliance and sustained contact appears to be a critical element in maintaining a good response. Several other factors appear to influence the magnitude of the cholesterol response to dietary changes including baseline cholesterol level, weight change, level of physical activity, presence or treatment of other risk factors, and alcohol intake.

Several classes of lipid-lowering drugs are available. The bile acid sequestrants (cholestyramine and colestipol) and nicotinic acids or niacin have been studied extensively in clinical trials, and their long-term safety has been established.<15> Typically, these agents lower the total cholesterol and LDL-C levels by 10% to 15% in usual practice settings. Their acceptability, however, has been limited by the hardships related to their use, their lack of palatability and the high incidence rate of side effects, which include gastrointestinal distress, pruritus and severe flushing.

The fibric acid derivatives (clofibrate and gemfibrosil) have also been extensively evaluated in long-term clinical trials and are particularly effective in lowering elevated triglyceride levels. They also lower the total cholesterol and LDL-C levels by 10% to 15%, and gemfibrozil, at least, increases the HDL-C level by about 10%.[25,26] Of the two drugs gemfibrozil is preferred because of its better safety record.[15]

Probucol lowers total cholesterol level in part by reducing HDL-C level, the cardioprotective lipid fraction. The drug, however, has an antioxidant action that may inhibit LDL oxidation and retard atherosclerosis. Estrogens may lower LDL-C by 15% and raise HDL-C by about 15%. Some authorities suggest women consider estrogen before other cholesterol-lowering drugs,[15] although their influence on the incidence of uterine and breast cancer is still uncertain (see Chapter 52).

The most significant advance in the treatment of hypercholes-terolemia is the introduction of 3-hydroxy-3-methylglutaryl-coenzyme A (HMG CoA) reductase inhibitors such as lovastatin into clinical practice. Unlike other lipid lowering agents this class of agent is well-tolerated, very effective in lowering cholesterol levels, and widely accepted. Clinical studies have reported reductions in LDL-C levels by as much as 40%.[27] Adverse effects including a rise in liver or muscle enzymes appear to be uncommon. The possibility that drugs of this class produce cancer, lens opacity, sleep disturbance and other health problems has not been excluded, since the long-term safety of these agents has not yet been established.

Primary Prevention Trials

Since the early 1960s six single-factor controlled clinical trials aimed at reducing the incidence rate of CHD among mostly asymptomatic middle-aged men through the reduction of serum cholesterol levels have been reported: the Lipid Research Clinics (LRC) Coronary Primary Prevention trial,[28] the Helsinki Heart Study,[25] the WHO Clofibrate Trial,[26,29] Upjohn's Colestipol Study (UCS),[30] the Los Angeles Veterans Diet Study (LAVDS)[31] and the Minnesota Coronary Survey (MCS).[32] Recently a major report on the efficacy and safety of lovastatin in patients with hypercholesterolemia (EXCEL) has been published[27] and the findings are included in this assessment of primary prevention trials.

The main features of the primary prevention trials are summarized in Table 1. In brief, the trials enrolled predominantly middle-aged men without any clinical evidence of CHD. There were, however, exceptions. About half of the participants in the LAVDS were 65 years or older, and roughly an equal proportion of study subjects in the UCS, MCS, and EXCEL were women. In addition, a sizeable minority of the subjects in the LAVDS, UCS and EXCEL had clinical signs of CHD. In the WHO trial 2% of the enrollees reported that they had angina pectoris, and men with a positive exercise test result but no other manifestations of CHD were not excluded from the LRC trial. The mean baseline total cholesterol levels were elevated only in the drug trials as the presence of hyperlipidemia was not a criterion for entry into the diet studies. Each drug trial used a different cholesterol-lowering agent, whereas in the two dietary trials polyunsaturated fatty acids were substituted for saturated fatty acids as the primary therapeutic maneuver leaving total fat intake unchanged.

The quality of the UCS was the poorest of the intervention studies. It had no uniform criteria for CHD, no double-blinding and a high withdrawal rate. The other four drug studies were of comparable and high quality. The two dietary intervention studies had quality scores between those of the UCS and the other three drug studies. The results of data aggregation were not altered by excluding the UCS from the analysis.

The intermediate measure of effectiveness, alterations in the blood lipid levels, is presented in Table 2. The mean net reduction in the blood total cholesterol level ranged from 9 to 23% in the drug studies, and 14% in the diet trials. The direction of change in the triglyceride levels in the studies in which it was measured was consistent with the known effects of the interventions on this blood lipid.

The data in men from the primary prevention trials were combined and published in a Task Force report on cholesterol lowering.[1] Several points emerged. First, there was a consistent and significant reduction in the number of non-fatal cardiac events in the actively treated group (odds ratio (OR) 0.74, 95% confidence interval (CI): 0.64 to 0.85) and a slight, but insignificant, fall in the number of cardiac deaths (OR 0.90, 95% CI: 0.71 to 1.14). These benefits were offset by a significant increase in the rate of death from non-cardiac causes (OR 1.19, 95% CI: 1.03 to 1.39), which resulted in a slight but insignificant excess in total mortality. Cholesterol lowering was associated with consistent and significant increases in the number of violent deaths (OR 1.78, 95% CI: 1.17 to 2.72) and events of gallbladder disease (OR 1.69, 95% CI: 1.28 to 2.23), and a less consistent and borderline significant increase in the number of deaths from cancer (OR 1.41, 95% CI: 1.05 to 1.89). These small excesses of cancer and trauma deaths have been attributed to chance.[33]

Since this publication the results of a trial examining the short-term efficacy and safety of lovastatin have appeared which included data on 3,390 women with moderate primary hypercholes-terolemia.[27] In light of increasing recognition of the importance of preventing CHD in women, the data of all primary prevention trials including EXCEL and the two older studies, UCS[30] and MCS[32], that enrolled women were reanalyzed using standard meta-analytic techniques. Data on 38,940 study subjects were pooled (Tables 3 and 4). Surprisingly cardiac deaths were not reduced in the drug trials of cholesterol lowering (OR 1.00, 95% CI: 0.80 to 1.26) and only slightly so when the data of the drug and diet trials were combined (OR 0.99, 95% CI: 0.83 to 1.18). As noted before[1] cholesterol-lowering was associated with a significant increase in non-cardiac deaths (OR 1.17, 95% CI: 1.03 to 1.34) and the increase in total mortality (OR 1.10, 95% CI: 0.99 to 1.22) approached but did not reach conventional levels of significance (p=0.082). There was a significant increase in deaths from cancer (OR 1.30, 95% CI: 1.02 to 1.66) and a non-significant increase in deaths from violence. These increases were observed in both the drug and diet trials.

Other meta-analyses of primary prevention randomized trials of cholesterol-lowering produced conclusions that were similar to those conducted by the Task Force.[34,35] Law and colleagues, however, in an analysis that included subjects with and without known ischemic heart disease, reached different conclusions.[36] In their report which combined the results of both primary and secondary prevention trials there was a significant reduction in CHD, a non-significant reduction in all-cause mortality, and a non-significant rise in non-cardiac deaths. The difference in findings and conclusions may well be explained by the inclusion of secondary prevention trials in their pooled analysis. Unlike primary prevention trials where less than one-half of deaths were cardiac in origin, the cause of death in these trials were largely from CHD (on average greater than 85%). Thus there is little "opportunity" to die from a non-cardiac cause.

Observational Studies

International studies have revealed that the proportion of the total energy intake derived from fat and the degree of saturation of that fat are strongly and positively correlated with the level of serum cholesterol and the rate of death from CHD. Evidence from several sources including studies of Japanese immigrants to Hawaii and Finnish families adopting a southern European diet suggest that international differences are dietary in origin rather than merely reflecting genetic variability. The importance of other differences between communities, however, such as the presence of diseases or cultural or socio-economic factors that influence food habits and health outcomes in communities cannot be excluded as possible explanations for observed associations.

Cohort studies conducted within communities have also demonstrated an association between CHD and dietary constituents.[37-42] The risk of death from CHD is positively related to the baseline level of dietary scores, inversely related to the intake of polyunsaturated fatty acids and fibre, and positively related to the dietary intake of cholesterol and saturated fatty acids. There are several caveats to these observations. First, these relations often remained statistically significant even after adjustment for the serum total cholesterol level and other variables. Second, the subjects enrolled in the cohort diet studies were largely adult men aged 30 to 69 years, thus, limiting, at least potentially, the generalizability of the results to adult women, the elderly, children, and young adults. Finally, the dose-response relation of dietary scores and CHD risk is not linear, as might be predicted.<37,38>

Recommendations of Others

Diet therapy has been advocated by the Canadian Consensus Conference on Cholesterol<16>, the U.S. National Cholesterol Education Program,<15> and the American Heart Association<21> as first-line treatment for hypercholesterolemia. Candidates for drug therapy are restricted generally to patients with severe forms of hypercholesterolemia or multiple CHD risk factors.

The Canadian Cholesterol Consensus Conference<16> recommended case-finding of adults 18 years of age and older with particular attention being given to those with cardiovascular disease risk factors, family history of CHD, or clinically apparent cardiovascular disease. Testing should be repeated every 5 years if blood lipids are normal. If total cholesterol is between 5.2 and 6.2 mmol/L, lipoprotein analysis should be done.

In 1993 the U.S. National Cholesterol Education Program recommended that HDL-C determinations (and in some cases TG level measurement) accompany measurements of total cholesterol when healthy individuals are being assessed for CHD risk.<15> Emphasis was placed on screening those at higher risk of CHD based on total cholesterol measurement or other known risk factors, in locations where accuracy of measurement, appropriate counselling and follow-up can be assured – at least 2 and preferably 3 samples taken in the fasting state at least 1 week apart.

More selective screening strategies have been proposed that entail the use of prescreen information to focus cholesterol screening on people at increased risk for CHD. Information on risk factors for CHD would be obtained during the course of clinical evaluation, as proposed by the Toronto Working Group on Cholesterol Policy,<43> or by questionnaire. Although the ability of a risk assessment to identify people with a high total cholesterol level has not been formally evaluated, experience with the questionnaire method indicates that almost 25% of those with hypercholesterolemia were not identified. This case-finding strategy is built on the premise that people at increased risk because of other CHD risk factors have more to gain from treatment. The results of multifactorial trials of primary prevention of cardiovascular disease in high-risk subjects, however, generally have not supported this assumption, despite favourable responses to interventions on risk factors.

The recommendations of the U.S. Preventive Services Task Force are currently under review.

Conclusions and Recommendations

Screening

For reasons of cost and convenience, measurement of the total cholesterol level should be the initial screening test, even though it may not always accurately reflect the LDL-C concentration. Although nonfasting total cholesterol levels are marginally higher than fasting values, the inconvenience of demanding only fasting samples markedly outweighs the minimal gain in diagnostic accuracy.

Case-finding should be directed to all men aged 30 to 59 years who present to their physician's office for any reason, individual clinical judgement being exercised in all other circumstances. This selective form of case-finding stresses the importance of the link between the detection of hypercholesterolemia and the favourable effect of lowering the cholesterol level on the incidence rate of CHD in this group. Cholesterol testing should be considered when other CHD risk factors are present such as smoking, hypertension, or diabetes mellitus, or when there is a strong family history of hypercholesterolemia or premature CHD. People with an initial total cholesterol level above 6.2 mmol/L should undergo another nonfasting test in 1 to 8 weeks.

The optimum frequency of repeat testing for people with a total cholesterol level of 6.2 mmol/L or less is unknown, but a prudent approach might be to have another test done within 5 years. Because the effectiveness of cholesterol screening has not been evaluated, the value of measuring the blood total cholesterol level is based on expert opinion (C Recommendation).

Dietary Modifications

There is no strong evidence that the dietary changes currently being advocated<15,16,21> as the initial therapeutic intervention will reduce the risk of CHD in the general population or in high-risk groups. On the other hand, there is level I evidence that dietary intervention used in conjunction with a smoking cessation program significantly lowers the incidence rate of CHD in normotensive middle-aged men at high risk because of marked hypercholesterolemia (serum total cholesterol level of 7.50 to 9.80 mmol/L) and cigarette smoking. Previous dietary trials,<31,32> although successful in reducing the incidence rate of CHD in men, substituted polyunsaturated fatty acids for saturated fatty acids as the primary treatment strategy, an intervention now considered potentially harmful.<15,21>

A stepped dietary intervention program, as recommended by several expert groups,<15,16,21> should be the initial therapeutic intervention for all men aged 30 to 59 years with a serum total cholesterol level above 6.85 mmol/L or an LDL-C level above 4.90 mmol/L. Evidence for this approach comes largely from randomized controlled trials of drug treatment of hypercholesterolemia in which dietary therapy was used to identify men whose cholesterol levels were highly sensitive to diet.<25,28> People with a total cholesterol level of 6.20 to 6.85 mmol/L or an LDL-C level of 4.15 to 4.90 mmol/L may also benefit from a therapeutic diet, although supporting clinical data for this recommendation are weaker. Drug therapy should be considered only in those who have failed to respond to an adequate dietary trial. The exceptions to this approach are patients with a severely elevated serum total cholesterol level. To classify people as having an abnormal cholesterol level necessitating drug treatment, the average of three determinations of the total cholesterol level, or the average of two determinations of the total cholesterol level and at least one measurement of the LDL-C level must be calculated.

Drug Therapy

There is level I evidence that a reduction of elevated serum cholesterol levels in otherwise healthy men through the use of lipid-lowering drugs will reduce the incidence rate of CHD, particularly nonfatal myocardial infarction.<25,26,28-30> This favourable outcome is offset, however, by an increase in the rate of death from noncardiac causes, which results in a slight but insignificant increase in the overall death rate. Without a reduction of the overall death rate the basis to treat elevated cholesterol levels rests on whether death or disability from CHD is considered a worse fate than death or disability from other causes.

Currently the efficacy and short-term safety of drug treatment in the primary prevention of CHD have only been adequately determined in middle-aged men with hypercholesterolemia.<25,26,28-30> The Task Force therefore recommends this form of treatment in asymptomatic men aged 30 to 59 years with a mean serum total cholesterol level persistently above 6.85 mmol/L or an LDL-C level above 4.50 mmol/L after an adequate trial of intensive dietary therapy for at least 6 months. There is fair evidence to support this approach (B Recommendation) since the long-term safety of lipid-lowering drugs is unknown and a favourable impact on the overall death rate has not been established.

The decision to extend drug treatment to other people with a serum total cholesterol level above 6.85 mmol/L or an LDL-C level

The long-term safety of lipid lowering drugs and their impact on overall death rate have not been established

above 4.50 mmol/L must take the following issues into consideration. There are no efficacy trials involving elderly people, children or young adults, and the limited data available on adult women do not support therapeutic intervention.<30,32> The significant excess in the rate of death from noncardiac causes and the increase in total mortality noted in meta-analyses of primary prevention trials of cholesterol-lowering cannot be ignored in people at lower risk. Therefore, a grade C Recommendation (indicating insufficient evidence to include or exclude this approach) was considered appropriate until more compelling data become available.

The decision to offer drug treatment to people with a blood total cholesterol level of 6.85 mmol/L or less or an LDL-C level of 4.50 mmol/L or less is even more complex.

If it is assumed that the positive relation of blood total cholesterol to the risk of CHD is curvilinear in all segments of the population, the potential benefit of cholesterol lowering becomes progressively less with as the baseline cholesterol level gets lower. For example, among MRFIT participants a reduction of the total cholesterol level by 1.29 mmol/L from a baseline level of 7.76 mmol/L would hypothetically lower the absolute risk of CHD by 50%; however, the same reduction would lower the risk by 25% if the initial level was 6.47 mmol/L and by only 8% if the initial level was 5.17 mmol/L. For women and elderly people the benefits would be significantly less, since the gradient of CHD risk is much less steep.

A related issue is the number of people who must be treated (NNT) in order to prevent one critical event. From the LRC trial the number of patients with hypercholesterolemia needed to be treated for 5 years to prevent one CHD event (fatal or nonfatal) was 89. Because the rate of baseline events is lower among people at low and moderate risk the NNT would be substantially higher. If it is estimated that the average rate is 25% of that in the high-risk group and that the same relative risk reduction were achieved with therapy, a rough estimate of the NNT for 5 years to prevent one CHD event would be 356 in this group. Thus, the benefits of therapy would be marginal.

Given the uncertainties about the long-term safety of the available lipid-lowering drugs, the primary mode of treatment will likely be dietary. Apart from the aforementioned lack of data on the efficacy and safety of this intervention, credence to use data from drug studies to make dietary recommendations rests on the assumption that the mode of cholesterol lowering is less important than the actual blood total cholesterol level achieved. This premise, although reasonable, does not negate the possibility that the beneficial effects of drug treatment on the rate of CHD events may, at least in part, be independent of changes in the cholesterol level.

On the basis of these considerations the Task Force concluded that there was insufficient evidence to include or exclude a stepped fat-modified therapeutic diet to which a cholesterol-lowering drug would be added if the dietary response was deemed inadequate (grade C Recommendation).

General Dietary Advice

There is fair evidence (B Recommendation) to support dietary advice for men aged 30 to 69 years since the lowering of their total fat, saturated fat and cholesterol intake and a modest increase in the intake of polyunsaturated fat are associated with decreased CHD rates. Because of the lack of similar evidence for women, the elderly, children and young adults a grade C Recommendation is appropriate. For more information on nutritional counselling in adults see Chapter 49.

Unanswered Questions (Research Agenda)

The potential health impact of lowering the cholesterol level should be greater for elderly people than for younger people, assuming that a change in this risk factor would affect disease incidence in this target population. This assumption, however, remains unproved and needs to be formally evaluated in a properly conducted randomized controlled trial.

Future investigations toward the ideal diet should focus on ways to raise the plasma HDL-C concentration while reducing the LDL-C level, leaving the plasma triglyceride level unchanged and ensuring palatability. Furthermore, the adverse effects of labelling a person as having hypercholesterolemia, need to be systematically studied.

Evidence

A MEDLINE search was conducted using the MESH heading cholesterol and the subheadings complications, diagnosis, drug therapy, epidemiology, prevention and control and therapy for articles published from 1979 through 1991. Pertinent references from these studies as well as references from recent review articles were examined.

The Mantel-Haenszel method was used to obtain an overall estimate of benefits and risks of lowering the cholesterol level in primary prevention trials; the iterative method of Gart was used to compute 95% confidence intervals (CIs) for these estimates. The significance of the summary measure of treatment effect was judged by means of the uncorrected Mantel-Haenszel χ^2 test with 1 degree of freedom; the consistency of effect was assessed by means of the Breslow-Day χ^2 test. Only data for men were considered in the analysis, because data for women were limited and generally reported in summary form.

This review was initiated in June 1993 to update the Task Force report<1> published in 1993 and recommendations were finalized by the Task Force in June 1994; only new references or evidence that was crucial to the recommendations are cited below and readers are referred to the 1993 publication for a full citation list.

Selected References

1. Canadian Task Force on the Periodic Health Examination: The periodic health examination, 1993 update: 2. Lowering the blood total cholesterol level to prevent coronary heart disease. *Can Med Assoc J* 1993; 148: 521-538

2. Consensus Conference: Lowering blood cholesterol to prevent heart disease. *JAMA* 1985; 253: 2080-2086

3. Neaton JD, Wentworth D: Serum cholesterol, blood pressure, cigarette smoking, and death from coronary heart disease. Overall findings and differences by age for 316,099 white men. Multiple Risk Factor Intervention Trial Research Group. *Arch Intern Med* 1992; 152: 56-64

4. Bass KM, Newschaffer CJ, Klag MJ, *et al*: Plasma lipoprotein levels as predictors of cardiovascular death in women. *Arch Intern Med* 1993; 153: 2209-2216

5. Gordon DJ, Probstfield JL, Garrison RJ, *et al*: High-density lipoprotein cholesterol and cardiovascular disease. Four prospective American studies. *Circulation* 1989; 79: 8-15

6. Sempos CT, Cleeman JI, Carroll MD, *et al*: Prevalence of high blood cholesterol among US adults. An update based on guidelines from the second report of the National Cholesterol Education Program Adult Treatment Panel. *JAMA* 1993; 269: 3009-3014

7. Johnson CL, Rifkind BM, Sempos CT, *et al*: Declining serum total cholesterol levels among US adults. The National Health and Nutrition Examination Surveys. *JAMA* 1993; 269: 3002-3008

8. van Beresteijn EC, Korevaar JC, Huijbregts PC, *et al*: Perimenopausal increase in serum cholesterol: a 10-year longitudinal study. *Am J Epidemiol* 1993; 137: 383-392

9. Dyer AR, Stamler J, Shekelle RB: Serum cholesterol and mortality from coronary heart disease in young, middle-aged, and older men and women from three Chicago epidemiologic studies. *Ann Epidemiol* 1992; 2: 51-57

10. Pekkanen J, Nissinen A, Vartiainen E, *et al*: Changes in serum cholesterol level and mortality: a 30-year follow-up. The Finnish cohorts of the Seven Countries Study. *Am J Epidemiol* 1994; 139: 155-165

11. Denke MA, Sempos CT, Grundy SM: Excess body weight: an underrecognized contributor to high blood cholesterol levels in white American men. *Arch Intern Med* 1993; 153: 1093-1103

12. Gomel M, Oldenburg B, Simpson JM, *et al*: Work-site cardiovascular risk reduction: a randomized trial of health risk assessment, education, counselling, and incentives. *Am J Public Health* 1993; 83: 1231-1238

13. Gibbins RL, Riley M, Brimble P: Effectiveness of a programme for reducing cardiovascular risk for men in one general practice. *BMJ* 1993; 306: 1652-1656

14. Williams RR, Hunt SC, Schumacher MC, *et al*: Diagnosing heterozygous familial hypercholesterolemia using new practical criteria validated by molecular genetics. *Am J Cardiol* 1993; 72: 171-176

15. Expert Panel on Detection, Evaluation, and Treatment of High Blood Cholesterol in Adults. Summary of the second report of the National Cholesterol Education Program (NCEP) expert panel on Detection, Evaluation, and Treatment of High Blood Cholesterol in Adults. *JAMA* 1993; 269: 3015-3023

16. Canadian Consensus Conference on Cholesterol: Final Report. The Canadian Consensus Conference on the Prevention of Heart and Vascular Disease by Altering Serum Cholesterol and Lipoprotein Risk Factors. *Can Med Assoc J* 1988; 139(11 Suppl): 1-8

17. McQueen MJ, Henderson AR, Patten RL, *et al*: Results of a province-wide quality assurance program assessing the accuracy of cholesterol, triglycerides, and high-density lipoprotein cholesterol measurements and calculated low-density lipoprotein cholesterol in Ontario, using fresh human serum. *Arch Pathol Lab Med* 1991; 115: 1217-1222

18. Smith SJ, Cooper GR, Myers GL, *et al*: Biological variability in concentrations of serum lipids: sources of variation among results from published studies and composite predicted values. *Clin Chem* 1993; 39(6): 1012-1022

19. Irvine MJ, Logan AG: Is knowing your cholesterol number harmful? *J Clin Epidemiol* 1994; 47: 131-145

20. Havas S, Reisman J, Hsu L, *et al*: Does cholesterol screening result in negative labeling effects? Results of the Massachusetts Model Systems for Blood Cholesterol Screening Project. *Arch Intern Med* 1991; 151: 113-119

21. Nutrition Committee, American Heart Association: Dietary guidelines for healthy American adults. *Circulation* 1986; 74: 1465A-1468A

22. Hunninghake DB, Stein EA, Dujovne CA, *et al*: The efficacy of intensive dietary therapy alone or combined with lovastatin in outpatients with hypercholesterolemia. *N Engl J Med* 1993; 328: 1213-1219

23. Ornish D, Brown SE, Scherwitz LW: Can lifestyle changes reverse coronary heart disease? *Lancet* 1990; 336:129-133

24. Singh RB, Rastogi SS, Verma R, *et al*: Randomized controlled trial of cardioprotective diet in patients with recent acute myocardial infarction. Results of one year follow-up. *BMJ* 1992; 304: 1015-1019

25. Frick MH, Elo O, Haapa K, *et al*: Helsinki Heart Study: primary-prevention trial with gemfibrozil in middle-aged men with dyslipidemia. Safety of treatment, changes in risk factors, and incidence of coronary heart disease. *N Engl J Med* 1987; 317: 1237-1245

26. Report from the Committee of Principal Investigators: A co-operative trial in the primary prevention of ischaemic heart disease using clofibrate. *Br Heart J* 1978; 40: 1069-1118

27. Bradford RH, Shear CL, Chremos AN, *et al*: Expanded clinical evaluation of lovastatin (EXCEL) study results. I. Efficacy in modifying plasma lipoproteins and adverse event profile in 8,245 patients with moderate hypercholesterolemia. *Arch Intern Med* 1991; 151: 43-49

28. The Lipid Research Clinics Coronary Primary Prevention Trial results: I. Reduction in incidence of coronary heart disease. *JAMA* 1984; 251: 351-364

29. Heady JA, Morris JN, Oliver MF: WHO clofibrate/cholesterol trial: clarifications. *Lancet* 1992; 340: 1405-1406

30. Dorr AE, Gundersen K, Schneider JC Jr, *et al*: Colestipol hydrochloride in hypercholesterolemic patients-effect on serum cholesterol and mortality. *J Chronic Dis* 1978; 31: 5-14

31. Dayton S, Pearce ML, Hashimoto S, *et al*: A controlled clinical trial of a diet high in unsaturated fat in preventing complications of atherosclerosis. *Circulation* 1969; 40(Suppl II): 1-63

32. Frantz ID Jr, Dawson EA, Ashman PL, *et al*: Test of effect of lipid lowering by diet on cardiovascular risk. The Minnesota Coronary Survey. *Atherosclerosis* 1989; 9: 129-135

33. MacMahon S: Lowering cholesterol: effects on trauma death, cancer death and total mortality. *Aust NZ J Med* 1992; 22: 580-582

34. Muldoon MF, Manuck SB, Matthews KA: Lowering cholesterol concentrations and mortality: a quantitative review of primary prevention trials. *BMJ* 1990; 301: 309-314

35. Holme I: An analysis of randomized trials evaluating the effect of cholesterol reduction on total mortality and coronary heart disease incidence. *Circulation* 1990; 82: 1916-1924

36. Law MR, Thompson SG, Wald NJ: Assessing possible hazards of reducing serum cholesterol. *BMJ* 1994; 308: 373-379

37. Shekelle RB, Shryock AM, Paul O, *et al*: Diet, serum cholesterol, and death from coronary heart disease. The Western Electric Study. *N Engl J Med* 1981; 304: 65-70

38. Kushi LH, Lew RA, Stare FJ, *et al*: Diet and 20 year mortality from coronary heart disease. The Ireland-Boston Diet-Heart Study. *N Engl J Med* 1985; 312: 811-818

39. Shekelle RB, Stamler J: Dietary cholesterol and ischaemic heart disease. *Lancet* 1989; 1: 1177-1179

40. McGee DL, Reed DM, Yano K, *et al*: Ten-year incidence of coronary heart disease in the Honolulu Heart Program. Relationship to nutrient intake. *Am J Epidemiol* 1984; 119: 667-676

41. Kromhout D, Booschieter EB, Coulander CL: The inverse relation between fish consumption and 20-year mortality from coronary heart disease. *N Engl J Med* 1985; 312: 1205-1209

42. Kushi LH, Kottke TE: Dietary fat and coronary heart disease: evidence of a causal relation. In Goldbloom RB, Lawrence RS (eds): *Preventing Disease: Beyond the Rhetoric*. Springer-Verlag, New York, 1990: 385-400

43. Toronto Working Group on Cholesterol Policy: Asymptomatic hypercholesterolemia: a clinical policy review. *J Clin Epidemiol* 1990; 43: 1029-1121

Table 1: Main characteristics of trials of primary prevention of coronary heart disease

Study[1]	LRC	HHS	WHO	UCS	EXCEL	LAVDS	MCS
No. of patients enrolled	3,806	4,081	10,627	2,278	8,245	846	9,057
% of male patients	100	100	100	48	59	100	49
Mean duration of trial, yr	7.4	5.3	5.3	1.9	0.92	3.5	1.1
Mean age of patients (and range), yr	47.8 (35-59)	47.3 (40-55)	45.9 (30-59)	53.9 (>17)	55.8 (18-70)	65.5 (50-89)	– (>17)
Baseline level, mmol/L							
Total Cholesterol	7.50	7.00	6.40	8.13	6.67	6.00	5.40
LDL-C	5.60	4.90	–	–	4.65	–	–
HDL-C	1.20	1.20	–	–	1.16	–	–
Non-HDL-C	–	5.80	–	–	–	–	–
Triglycercides	1.80	2.00	–	2.38	1.75	–	1.30
Intervention+	Choles	Gemfib	Clofib	Colest	Lovast	Δ P:S	Δ P:S
Mean blood pressure, mmHg	121/80	141/90	135/87	133/83	(39.6)§	136/78	–
% of patients who smoked	37	36	56	–	18	70	–
People with diabetes included?	No	Yes	Yes	Yes	Yes	–	–
% of patients with prior MI	0	0	0	6	18	7	–
Atherosclerotic heart disease or angina	0	0	2	25	29	18	–

[1] LRC = Lipid Research Clinics Coronary Primary Prevention Trial (28), HHS = Helsinki Heart Study (25), WHO = World Health Organization Clofibrate Trial (26, 29), UCS = Upjohn's Colestipol Study (30), EXCEL = Expanded Clinical Evaluation of Lovastatin (27), LAVDS = Los Angeles Veterans Diet Study (31), MCS = Minnesota Coronary Survey (32); LDL-C = low-density lipoprotein cholesterol, HDL-C = high density lipoprotein cholesterol, MI = myocardial infarction; + Choles = Cholestyramine, Gemfib = Gemfibrozil, Clofib = Clofibrate, Colest = Colestipol, Lovast = Lovastatin, Δ P:S = change in polyunsaturated:saturated fat ratio in diet; § % of patients with hypertension.

Table 2: Change from baseline in blood lipid and lipoprotein levels after intervention

Trial	Lipid; change in level, %			
	Total Cholesterol	LDL-C	HDL-C	Triglycerides
LRC[1]	− 9	−13	+ 3	+ 5
HHS	−10	−10	+10	−35
WHO	− 9	–	–	–
UCS	−10	–	–	–
EXCEL	−23	−32	+ 8	−15
LAVDS	−13	–	–	–
MCS	−14	–	–	−10

[1] Abbreviations the same as in Table 1

Table 3: Number of deaths by treatment status in asymptomatic adult men and women

Trial	No. of patients	Cardiac	Noncardiac	Total	Cancer[2]	Violence[2]
Drug Therapy						
LRC[1]						
Treated	1,906	32	36	68	16	11
Control	1,900	44	27	71	15	4
HHS						
Treated	2,051	14	31	45	11	10
Control	2,030	19	23	42	11	4
WHO						
Treated	5,331	91	145	236	75	24
Control	5,296	77	104	181	55	25
UCS						
Treated	1,149	14[†]	18	37	2[‡]	2[‡]
Control	1,129	16[†]	17	48	2[‡]	0[‡]
EXCEL						
Treated	6,582	28	5	33	0	0
Control	1,663	3	0	3	0	0
TOTAL						
Treated	17,019	179	235	419[¶]	104	47
Control	12,018	159	171	345[¶]	83	33
Dietary Therapy						
LAVDS						
Treated	424	41	133	174	33[§]	–
Control	422	50	127	177	20[§]	–
MCS						
Treated	4,541	61	208	269	23	33
Control	4,516	54	194	248	20	28
TOTAL						
Treated	4,965	102	341	443	56	33
Control	4,938	104	321	425	40	28
Overall Total						
Treated	21,984	281	576	862[¶]	160	80
Control	16,956	263	492	770[¶]	123	61

Header note: Cause; Number of deaths

1   Abbreviations the same as in Table 1
2   Included in deaths from noncardiac causes
†   Denominator includes only men without history of coronary heart disease at entry (372 in treatment group and 385 in control group)
‡   Only data on men reported
§   A total of 31 deaths from cancer in the treatment group and 17 in the control group occurred during the diet phase; however, a follow-up report included 5 deaths from other types of cancer (1)
¶   Number of deaths from cardiac and noncardiac causes does not add up to total because in the UCS trial cardiac-related deaths in men with a history of coronary heart disease were not included in the category of death from cardiac causes

Table 4: Effects of lowering the cholesterol level on cause-specific and overall death rates in asymptomatic adult men and women

Cause; Odds Ratio (and 95% Confidence Interval)

Trial	Cardiac	Noncardiac	Total	Cancer	Violence
Drug Therapy					
LRC	0.72 (0.44-1.17)	1.43 (0.79-2.27)	0.95 (0.67-1.36)	1.06 (0.50-2.27)	2.75 (0.81-10.2)
HHS	0.73 (0.35-1.53)	1.34 (0.75-2.38)	1.06 (0.68-1.66)	0.99 (0.40-2.45)	2.48 (0.72-9.39)
WHO	1.18 (0.86-1.62)	1.40 (1.07-1.82)	1.31 (1.07-1.60)	1.36 (0.94-1.96)	0.95 (0.53-1.73)
UCS	0.87 (0.40-1.89)	1.04 (0.51-2.13)	0.75 (0.47-1.18)	0.98[1] (0.10-9.73)	5.00[1] (.26->99)
EXCEL	2.36 (0.69-9.76)	2.78 (0.20->99)	2.79 (0.82-11.4)	[2]	[2]
TOTAL	1.00 (0.80-1.26)	1.35 (1.10-1.65)	1.15 (0.99-1.65)	1.25 (0.92-1.68)	1.41 (0.89-2.25)
Dietary Therapy					
LAVDS	0.80 (0.50-1.26)	1.06 (0.78-1.44)	0.96 (0.73-1.28)	1.70 (0.93-3.13)	[2]
MCS	1.13 (0.77-1.65)	1.07 (0.87-1.31)	1.08 (0.90-1.30)	1.14 (0.60-2.17)	1.17 (0.69-2.00)
TOTAL	0.97 (0.73-1.30)	1.07 (0.90-1.26)	1.05 (0.90-1.22)	1.41 (0.92-2.18)	1.17 (0.69-2.00)
Overall Total	0.99 (0.83-1.18)	1.17 (1.03-1.34)	1.10 (0.99-1.22)	1.30 (1.02-1.66)	1.30 (0.92-1.84)

[1] Only data on men reported.
[2] Indeterminant as no events occurred (EXCEL) or reported separately (LAVDS).

Lowering the Blood Cholesterol Level to Prevent Coronary Heart Disease

MANEUVER	EFFECTIVENESS	LEVEL OF EVIDENCE <REF>	RECOMMENDATION
Measurement of blood total cholesterol level	Average of three or more readings accurately reflects "true" level if measured in standardized laboratory. Although not evaluated for its effectiveness, screening should be considered in all men aged 30 to 59 years; individual clinical judgement should be exercised in all other cases.	Expert opinion<2,15,16> (III)	Insufficient evidence to include or exclude from periodic health examination (PHE) (C)
Stepped fat-modified diet to which a cholesterol-lowering drug is added if response is inadequate (mean total cholesterol level of more than 6.85 mmol/L or LDL-C level of more than 4.50 mmol/L)	For men 30 to 59 years old with a mean total cholesterol level of more than 6.85 mmol/L or an LDL-C level of more than 4.90 mmol/L treatment is efficacious in reducing incidence of CHD.	Randomized controlled trials<25-32> (I)	Fair evidence to include in PHE (B)*
	For all other asymptomatic individuals the value of treatment has not been demonstrated.	Expert opinion<2,15,16> (III)	Insufficient evidence to include in or exclude from PHE (C)
General dietary advice on fat (especially saturated fat) and cholesterol intake	For men 30 to 69 years decreased intake of total fat, saturated fat and cholesterol is associated with decreased incidence of CHD.	Prospective cohort studies<37-42> (II-2)	Fair evidence to include in PHE (B)
	For all others value of such advice has not been demonstrated.	Expert opinion<42> (III)	Insufficient evidence to include in or exclude from PHE (C)

* Long-term safety of lipid-lowering drugs is unknown, and a favourable impact on the overall death rate has not been established.

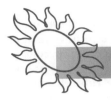

CHAPTER **55**

Screening
for Abdominal
Aortic Aneurysm

By Christopher Patterson

55 Screening for Abdominal Aortic Aneurysm

Prepared by Christopher Patterson, MD, FRCPC[1]

*T*he prevalence of abdominal aortic aneurysm (AAA) rises sharply with age. Risk factors include male sex, a positive family history of aneurysm, smoking, hypertension and other vascular risk factors. Small aneurysms enlarge slowly, but probably as an exponential function. Symptoms occur late, and rupture may be the first indication of disease. Elective surgery has a mortality of less than 5%, rupture carries a mortality of 50 to 70% even when surgery is performed. Abdominal palpation is sensitive for large aneurysms. Abdominal ultrasound is sensitive and specific for aneurysms of all sizes. While there is insufficient evidence to recommend for or against screening with physical examination or ultrasound, the prudent physician may choose to include a targeted physical examination for aneurysm in males over age 60 in the periodic health examination.

Burden of Suffering

Abdominal aortic aneurysm, a localized abnormal dilatation of the aorta, is usually due to atherosclerotic changes affecting the arterial intima. It is defined as a dilatation of the aorta greater than 3 cm or 150% of the aortic diameter at the diaphragm (usually 2 cm in men aged 65-74 years). Most commonly AAA arise below the renal arteries, and remain asymptomatic for many years. Symptoms may occur from pressure effects on adjacent structures, (e.g. causing back pain or abdominal throbbing), from embolization of intramural thrombus, or in association with other vascular complaints such as intermittent claudication. As the aneurysm enlarges the incidence of rupture increases, particularly in saccular aneurysms. The characteristic presentation of rupture includes excruciating back pain, hypovolemic shock and pulsatile abdominal mass. The classic triad is present in approximately 70% of cases reaching hospital. Aortic rupture is a surgical emergency of the most urgent type, and even with surgery, mortality rates of 50 to 70% are common.

The prevalence of aneurysms is related to age and vascular risk factors. It is more common in men and in those with a positive family history. In community surveys, the prevalence of AAA is reported to be between less than 1%<1> and 5.4%.<2> In hospital outpatient clinics dealing with hypertension, vascular or cardiac disorders, the prevalence is between 5.3 and 21%.<3,4>

Prevalence of abdominal aortic aneurysm is 1-5% in community surveys; up to 20% in older men with vascular problems

[1] Professor and Head, Division of Geriatric Medicine, McMaster University, Hamilton, Ontario

The incidence of aneurysm has been estimated at 52 per 100,000 per annum in men aged 55-64 years[5] and 499 per 100,000 per annum in men over 80 years.[6] There are approximately 520 hospital separations and 270 deaths annually from AAA in Canada.[7]

Maneuver

For screening or case finding there are two practical detection measures, physical examination and ultrasound.

The accuracy of physical examination depends on many factors such as the skill of the examiner, the size of the aneurysm, and habitus of the individual. Where the prevalence of aneurysm is between 5 and 10%, sensitivity is from 22-50%, with specificity of 71-94%. Where the prevalence of large AAA is high, in settings such as preoperative vascular clinics, the sensitivity is above 80%, with high specificity.[8-10] There is evidence to suggest that examination specifically seeking aneurysm is significantly more sensitive than routine palpation.

Abdominal examination is 80% sensitive for detection of large (surgical) abdominal aortic aneurysm

Abdominal ultrasound is an ideal technique for detecting AAA and estimating its size. Sensitivity approaches 100% in detecting AAA in the presence of a pulsatile abdominal mass.[10] Ultrasound may overestimate the size of an aneurysm compared to intraoperative measurement. Technical problems arise with ultrasound when the patient is obese or if there is excessive intestinal gas at the time of examination. In one study there was inadequate visualization of the aorta in 18%.[11] In most case series failure to visualize the aorta occurred in only a few percent. Community studies have demonstrated poor compliance rates in screening programs: less than 60%[2] and less than 50%.[11]

The only community-based screening program to describe outcome was recently published from Norway. Two thousand six hundred and fifty-four males over 60 years were invited to attend for ultrasound screening for a modest fee (150 Norwegian krona). One thousand two hundred and fifty-six (47%) complied and 92 aneurysms were detected – 7.3% of attendees. Of these 92, 69 were smaller than 4.0 cm and 23 were 4.0 cm or larger. Seventeen of these underwent elective surgery within 18 months of screening, with elective surgery within 18 months of screening, with no mortality and no serious complications.[11]

Effectiveness of Screening and Treatment

The natural history of a small aneurysm is gradual enlargement, with an increasing risk of rupture as the size increases. For aneurysms less than 5 cm, the mean growth rate lies between 0.17 and 0.48 cm per year. In a community based retrospective study, no aneurysm less than 3.5 cm had ruptured by 8 years; between 3.5 and 4.9 cm, 5% had ruptured by 9 years, and for those greater than 5 cm 25% had ruptured by 8 years.<12> In several series of untreated AAA, survival at one year was between 59 and 84%, at 2 years between 44 and 58%, and at 5 years less than 20%. Modelling studies suggest that mean expansion rate is an exponential function.<13>

Elective surgical mortality is less than 5%; mortality of ruptured abdominal aortic aneurysm, even with surgery, is usually 50%

While correction of risk factors, particularly hypertension, may play a role in slowing the enlargement of aneurysm, the only definitive treatment for AAA is replacement graft. Most centres now perform elective AAA replacement graft with a surgical mortality of less than 5%.<8> Mortality is increased by large aneurysm size, impaired renal function, blood loss greater than 4 units, and the presence of coronary artery disease.<14> If operation is delayed until symptoms are present but before rupture has occurred, mortality of the procedure is 5-33%. In the presence of aortic rupture, surgical mortality remains extremely high, in many cases exceeding 50%. Following successful surgery, subsequent mortality is strongly influenced by coexistent disease. When there is no coexistent disease the survival curve does not differ significantly from that of age-matched controls. Subsequent mortality is higher in hypertensives and those with vascular disease.<15>

When an aneurysm smaller than 5 cm is detected, the recommended approach includes serial ultrasound (at 3-6 monthly intervals) and treatment of hypertension and other risk factors.<16> A clinical trial is underway to determine whether beta-adrenergic blocking drugs slow the rate of enlargement of small AAA. If an aneurysm greater than 5 cm is detected, referral to a vascular surgeon is indicated, providing the patient is suitable for surgery.

Cost Effectiveness

Several cost effectiveness analyses of screening for AAA have been published.<17> The most recent simulation was based upon screening a cohort of 10,000 men between the ages of 60 and 80 years.<18> It was concluded that using the "most probable" values for the simulation parameters, a single screen by abdominal palpation followed by abdominal ultrasound for positive screens is estimated to gain 20 life-years at a cost of US$ 28,741 per life-year. A single ultrasound screen gains 57 life-years at a cost of US$ 41,550 per life-year. A repeat ultrasound screen after five years gains one additional life-year at a cost of US$ 906,769.

Recommendations of Others

Oboler and Laforce recommend abdominal examination for aneurysm in men over age 60 as a prudent maneuver.<19>

Conclusions and Recommendations

Population screening for AAA produces a very low yield of aneurysms of sufficient size to warrant consideration of surgical treatment. While physical examination is insensitive for small aneurysms, sensitivity to detect aneurysms large enough to be considered for surgery is as high as 80-90%. As the prevalence and incidence of AAA is age and sex dependent, targeted physical examination of the abdomen for men over the age of 60 may be considered a prudent maneuver, although there is insufficient evidence to recommend for or against inclusion in the periodic health examination (C Recommendation). While ultrasound screening is more sensitive and specific than physical examination, it is more expensive, and community studies have demonstrated poor compliance with the maneuver. There is therefore poor evidence for or against a recommendation to screen for AAA using ultrasound (C Recommendation). Ultrasound should be reserved for those where any suspicious pulsation is detected by examination, or if the abdominal aorta is impalpable due to obesity. In the older male smoker with hypertension, claudication, evidence of other vascular disease, or a positive family history of AAA, a more liberal policy of case finding with ultrasound could be considered. Costs of screening with ultrasound are substantially higher than physical examination.

Unanswered Questions (Research Agenda)

The following have been identified as research priorities:

1. To determine in the primary care setting, the characteristics of physical examination for the detection of AAA of different sizes using ultrasound as the gold standard.

2. To determine the natural history of small aortic aneurysms discovered by screening, using serial ultrasound.

3. To define and quantify risk factors for the development rapid growth and rupture of AAA.

4. To determine the value of ultrasound screening for AAA in high risk individuals.

5. To determine the best method of disseminating the risks and benefit of surgery in elective and symptomatic situations.

Evidence

The literature was identified with a MEDLINE search of the years 1980 to October 1991 by exploding the terms aortic aneurysm and aorta, abdominal, costs and cost analysis, and decision making, and a MEDLINE search from 1991 to 1993 with the major headings aortic aneurysm and mass screening.

This review was initiated in October 1993 and updates a report published in 1991.<8> Recommendations were finalized by the Task Force in January 1994.

Selected References

1. Lindholm L, Ejlertsson G, Forsberg L, *et al*: Low prevalence of abdominal aortic aneurysm in hypertensive patients. A population-based study. *Acta Med Scand* 1985; 218: 305-310

2. Collin J, Araujo L, Walton J, *et al*: Oxford screening programme for abdominal aortic aneurysm in men aged 65 to 74 years. *Lancet* 1988; 2: 613-615

3. Allen PI, Gourevitch D, McKinley J, *et al*: Population screening for aortic aneurysms. [letter] *Lancet* 1987; 2: 736

4. Thurmond AS, Semler HJ: Abdominal aortic aneurysm: incidence in a population at risk. *J Cardiovasc Surg Torino* 1986; 27: 457-460

5. Castleden WM, Mercer JC: Abdominal aortic aneurysms in Western Australia: descriptive epidemiology and patterns of rupture. *Br J Surg* 1985; 72: 109-112

6. Melton LJ 3d, Bickerstaff LK, Hollier LH, *et al*: Changing incidence of abdominal aortic aneurysms: a population-based study. *Am J Epidemiol* 1984; 120: 379-386

7. Hill G: Data presented at International Workshop on abdominal aortic aneurysms. 1989. January 20-21st, Ottawa

8. Canadian Task Force on the Periodic Health Examination: The periodic health examination, 1991 Update: 5. Screening for abdominal aortic aneurysm. *Can Med Assoc J* 1991; 145: 783-789

9. Brewster DC, Darling C, Raines JK: Assessment of abdominal aortic size. *Circulation* 1977; 56: 164-169

10. Gomes MNH, Shellinger D, Hufragel CA: Abdominal aortic aneurysms: diagnostic review and new technique. *Ann Thorac Surg* 1979; 27: 478-479

11. Kullmann G, Wolland T, Krohn CD, *et al*: [Ultrasonography for early diagnosis of abdominal aortic aneurysm.] *Tidsskr Nor Laegeforen* 1992; 112: 1825-1826

12. Nevitt MP, Ballard DJ, Hallet JW Jr: Prognosis of abdominal aortic aneurysms. A population-based study. *N Engl J Med* 1989; 321: 1009-1114

13. Bergqvist D, Bengtsson H: Should screening for abdominal aortic aneurysms be advocated? *Acta Chir Scand Suppl* 1990; 555: 89-97

14. Amundsen S, Skjaerven R, Trippestad A, *et al*: Abdominal aortic aneurysms – a study of factors influencing postoperative mortality. Norwegian Aortic Aneurysm Trial. *Eur J Vasc Surg* 1989; 3: 405-409

15. Roger VL, Ballard DJ, Hallet JW Jr, *et al*: Influence of coronary artery disease on morbidity and mortality after abdominal aortic aneurysmectomy: a population-based study, 1971-1987. *J Am Coll Cardiol* 1989; 14: 1245-1252

16. Lederle FA: Management of small abdominal aortic aneurysms. [editorial] *Ann Intern Med* 1990; 113: 731-732

17. Bengtsson H, Bergqvist D, Jendteg S, *et al*: Ultrasonographic screening for abdominal aortic aneurysm: analysis of surgical decisions for cost-effectiveness. *World J Surg* 1989; 13: 266-271

18. Frame PS, Fryback DG, Patterson C: Screening for abdominal aortic aneurysm in men ages 60 to 80 years. A cost-effectiveness analysis. *Ann Intern Med* 1993; 119: 411-416

19. Oboler SK, LaForce FM: The periodic physical examination in asymptomatic adults. *Ann Intern Med* 1989; 110: 214-226

Screening for Abdominal Aortic Aneurysm

MANEUVER	EFFECTIVENESS	LEVEL OF EVIDENCE <REF>	RECOMMENDATION
Abdominal palpation	Physical examination is a sensitive procedure for detecting large abdominal aortic aneurysms (AAA).	Case series<8-10> (III)	Poor evidence to include or exclude in periodic health examination of asymptomatic individuals (C)
	Surgical resection and replacement grafts prevent rupture.	Case series<8> (III)	
Abdominal ultrasound	Ultrasound is highly sensitive and specific for detection of AAA.	Cohort<11> II-2	Poor evidence to include or exclude in periodic health examination of asymptomatic individuals (C) but screening may be considered for individuals at high risk*

* High-risk individuals are: males over the age of 60 who are smokers with hypertension, claudication, evidence of other vascular disease or a positive family history of AAA.

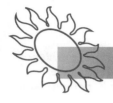

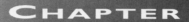

CHAPTER

56

Acetylsalicylic Acid and the Primary Prevention of Cardiovascular Disease

By Geoffrey Anderson

Acetylsalicylic Acid and the Primary Prevention of Cardiovascular Disease

Prepared by Geoffrey Anderson, MD, PhD[1]

A series of clinical trials has provided convincing evidence that acetylsalicylic acid (ASA) can significantly reduce the incidence of vascular events and related deaths in patients with a history of symptomatic vascular disease, including previous myocardial infarction, unstable angina, stroke and transient ischemic attack.<1,2> The drug's beneficial effects in preventing premature illness and death in symptomatic patients have led to interest in the possible benefits of preventing vascular disease in people without previous symptoms. Case-control and cohort studies have raised the possibility that ASA reduces the risk of cardiovascular disease by about 20%.<3> This chapter reviews the results of recent studies and makes recommendations regarding the appropriate use of ASA in asymptomatic patients.

Burden of Suffering

In 1989 an estimated 80,858 deaths from circulatory disease occurred in Canada; this resulted in 362,235 potential life-years lost. An estimated 49,148 deaths were due to coronary artery disease and 14,232 to stroke. Coronary artery disease was the leading cause of death among men 40 years of age or more and among women 60 years or more. In 1987 there were 77,790 deaths due to circulatory disease, for a death rate of 324 per 100,000 among men and 283 per 100,000 among women. The rate of death from cardiovascular disease begins to increase about 10 years earlier among men than among women, but eventually nearly as many women as men die from such disease (36,794 vs. 40,977 in 1987).

The overall rate of death from cardiovascular disease has shown a relatively stable decrease since the 1950s

The overall rate of death from cardiovascular disease has shown a relatively stable decrease since the 1950s. The rates among men and women 35 to 90 years of age are expected to decrease from 780 and 415 per 100,000 respectively (1982-86 data) to 655 and 310 per 100,000 respectively by the year 2000. The age-standardized rates of death from stroke among Canadians over 65 years of age decreased by more than 60% among women and 50% among men between 1951 and 1986, but hospital morbidity rates from 1971 to 1984 did not reflect the same rate of decline. Each year in Canada about 50,500 patients are admitted to hospital for treatment of acute myocardial infarction.

---

[1] Senior Scientist, Institute for Clinical Evaluative Sciences in Ontario (ICES) and Associate Professor, Department of Health Administration, University of Toronto, Toronto, Ontario

In 1987-88 there were 8.9 million hospital patient-days for diseases of the circulatory system. In addition, circulatory disease accounts for 25% of all disability pensions paid by the Canada Pension Plan before age 65.

Over 40% of deaths from coronary artery disease are sudden, and half of the sudden deaths occur in people without a history of overt disease. Reduction of the incidence of sudden death in asymptomatic people will require the use of effective primary prevention strategies.

Effectiveness of Prevention

The results of two large randomized clinical trials of the effects of ASA in males without symptomatic cardiovascular disease have been published<4-7> and the results of a large prospective cohort study of ASA use in women was published recently.<8>

The British Aspirin Trial

This trial was undertaken in Britain from 1978 to 1984.<4> The study subjects were recruited in two stages. All male physicians residing in Britain in 1951 were contacted and asked to participate. The total sample was 5,139 out of about 20,000 physicians contacted. The authors stated that most of those contacted but not recruited were willing to participate but were ineligible because they had a history of symptomatic vascular disease or were unable to take ASA. All physicians over 79 years of age were excluded. About 50% of the subjects were less than 60 years old, and about 15% were between 70 and 79.

Two-thirds (3,429) of the subjects were randomly allocated to the experimental group and were asked to take 500 mg of ASA daily. The remaining 1,710 physicians constituted the control group and were asked to avoid the use of ASA. The two groups were similar in terms of several risk factors for cardiovascular disease, although the control group had a mean systolic blood pressure (BP) that was on average 1 mmHg lower than the mean pressure in the experimental group (p=0.05).

Follow-up was excellent, 99% of the surviving physicians completed the final questionnaire. The study provided some 30,000 man-years of observation. The results were analyzed according to which study group the physicians were assigned to and not their actual use of ASA. After 1 year 19% of the physicians in the experimental group had stopped taking ASA, and by the end of the 6-year trial compliance with the treatment regimen had decreased to 55%. In the control group about 10% of the physicians were taking ASA regularly by the end of the trial.

The main outcomes of the trial are presented in Table 1. There were no statistically significant differences in the rates of fatal or non-fatal myocardial infarction between the two groups. However, given the small number of poor outcomes the confidence interval (CI) for the estimated differences is wide. The experimental group had a significantly lower rate of transient ischemic attacks than the control group, but there was no significant difference in either the total rate of strokes or of deaths from stroke. Further analysis indicated a significantly higher rate of disabling strokes in the experimental group than in the control group. Differences in the rates of vascular and nonvascular events and total deaths were not significant. Detailed subgroup analysis indicated the rate of death from endocardial disease and acute respiratory disease was significantly lower in the experimental group. The experimental group also had a significantly lower rate of migraines and musculoskeletal disorders but a higher rate of peptic ulcers.

The U.S. Aspirin Trial

This study began in 1982 and ended in early 1988.[5-7] Recruitment letters were sent to all 261,248 male physicians in the U.S. aged 40 to 84 years; 112,528 responded, and 59,285 agreed to participate. Physicians were excluded if they reported a history of myocardial infarction, stroke, transient ischemic attack, important health problems, current routine use of ASA or contraindications to the use of ASA. This left 33,223 eligible physicians. After an 18-week pretrial compliance study 22,071 physicians were found to be compliant and were randomly assigned to an experimental group (11,037) or a control group (11,034). The participants were blinded to their allocation: those in the experimental group were asked to take a pill containing 325 mg of ASA every second day, and those in the control group were asked to take a placebo pill every second day. About 75% of the participants were less than 60 years of age, and only 7% were 70 or older.

At the end of the trial the vital status of all the participants was known, and 99.7% of the surviving physicians had completed the final questionnaire. The study provided slightly more than 110,000 man-years of observations.

The results were analyzed according to the group to which the physicians had been allocated. At the end of the trial 86% of those in the experimental group and 14% in the control group were taking ASA or another platelet-active drug.

The main results of this trial[6] are summarized in Table 2. There was a significant decrease in the rates of fatal and nonfatal myocardial infarction in the experimental group. ASA had no significant effect on the rates of fatal and nonfatal stroke, although the rates were higher in the experimental group. Further analysis of the stroke data indicated a relative risk (RR) of 2.14 for confirmed hemorrhagic stroke in the experimental group; however, this difference failed to reach conventional levels of significance (95% CI: 0.96 to 4.77, p=0.06). ASA had no significant effect on the overall cardiovascular death rate or the all-cause death rate. A separate analysis involving the 21,738 physicians who did not have angina pectoris at the beginning of the trial revealed no significant effect of ASA on the incidence of angina pectoris (RR 1.10 in the experimental group; 95% CI: 0.84 to 1.36).[7]

Compared with the control group, the experimental group had a higher rate of bleeding problems such as bruising, hematemesis and melena (RR 1.32; 95% CI: 1.25 to 1.40, p<0.0001). The experimental group also had a higher incidence of transfusion (RR 1.75; 95% CI: 1.09 to 2.69, p=0.02).

Subgroup analysis indicated that the beneficial effect of ASA on the incidence of myocardial infarction was greater among the subjects who were 50 years of age or older and those with lower cholesterol levels than among the others.

The Nurses' Health Study

The Nurses' Health Study[8] established a cohort of 121,700 female nurses aged 30 to 55 years in 1976. The analyses included 6 years of follow-up for the cohort with a total of 475,265 persons-years of data for fatal outcomes and 459,696 person-years of data for nonfatal outcomes. The follow-up rate for nonfatal outcomes was 96.7%. The authors estimated that the follow-up for fatal events was more than 98%. The cohort was divided into 4 exposure groups based on survey responses: 1) 0 aspirin per week; 2) 1-6 aspirin per week; 3) 7-14 aspirin per week; and 4) 15 or more aspirin per week. Relative risks were computed as the rate of events in each exposure category divided by the rate in the reference category (no aspirin per week). All relative risks were age-adjusted and controlled for the effects' cardiovascular risk factors.

The main results of the trial are summarized in Table 3. There was a statistically significant reduction in relative risk for nonfatal MI and coronary artery deaths combined in the group taking 1 to 6 aspirin per week compared to the no aspirin group. Women aged 50 years and more and women with coronary risk factors had the largest risk reductions. The relative risk for nonfatal MI alone was 0.68 (95% CI: 0.49-0.93) in this exposure group. The relative risk for strokes, cardiovascular deaths and total deaths were each less than 1.0 for the group exposed to 1 to 6 aspirin per week, but none of these lower relative risks was statistically significant.

Overview

The two randomized controlled ASA trials were conducted in populations of male physicians. Although the inclusion of physicians may have improved the quality of self-reported information the generalizability of the results to other populations has to be questioned. On one hand, physicians may be more compliant with long-term therapy than members of the general public. On the other hand, the subjects in the two studies may have been "healthier" than asymptomatic men in other populations. In the U.S. study the overall rate of death from cardiovascular disease was 15% of that expected in a general population of white men with the same age distribution.

Decrease in incidence of fatal myocardial infarction did not translate into a decrease in cardiovascular disease death rate

The U.S. trial did show a significant decrease in the incidence of both fatal and nonfatal myocardial infarction. The decrease in the incidence of fatal myocardial infarction did not translate into a decrease in the overall rate of death from cardiovascular disease; this was because of death from other causes, most notably stroke and "sudden death". As Sempos and Cooper[9] pointed out, the rate of sudden death noted in the U.S. study was much higher than that found in the general population, and if diagnosed cases of sudden death are included in the category of myocardial infarction, then there is no longer a significant decrease in the incidence of fatal myocardial infarction in the experimental group.

The British trial showed a statistically significant decrease in the incidence of transient ischemic attacks in the experimental group. This did not translate into a significant decrease in the incidence of either fatal or nonfatal stroke. The U.S. study did not report on the impact of ASA therapy on transient ischemic attacks.

When assessing the benefits of long-term therapy in previously asymptomatic patients it is important to consider carefully the impact of side effects. The two studies showed a higher incidence of adverse effects, including peptic ulcer and bleeding disorders, in the experimental groups than in the control groups. They also indicated that ASA therapy may be related to an increased incidence of hemorrhagic stroke. The routine use of ASA may have some unexpected beneficial effects, such as a decreased incidence of migraines and musculoskeletal disorders.

Although the two studies differed with regard to the age distribution of the physicians, dosage of ASA, compliance rate and some of the details of causes of death, it has been suggested that it would be useful to combine the results. Analysis of the combined data[10] indicated a significant reduction of 33% in the incidence of nonfatal myocardial infarction among those taking ASA ($p<0.0001$). There was no significant change in the incidence of nonfatal stroke or death from stroke or myocardial infarction; however, there was a significant increase in the incidence of disabling stroke among those taking ASA ($p=0.016$).

A recent overview of antiplatelet therapy concluded that there was no clear evidence on the balance of risks and benefits of antiplatelet therapy in primary prevention among low risk subjects.<11> To try to balance the effects on myocardial infarction and stroke Jonas<12> analyzed the U.S. trial data that applied quality-of-life values to the main outcomes (i.e., death, nonfatal myocardial infarction and major or minor stroke). This analysis indicated that the lost quality of life over the 5-year follow-up was not significantly different in the experimental group from that in the control group. Although these results are based on specific assumptions regarding the quality of various health states they do indicate the importance of balancing benefits against risks.

The prospective cohort study in women indicated a lower rate of fatal and nonfatal MI in those who reported using 1 to 6 aspirin per week compared to those who reported no aspirin use. There was no statistically significant association between aspirin use and cardiovascular deaths or total deaths.

Recommendations of Others

The recommendation of the U.S. Preventive Services Task Force on low-dose aspirin therapy is currently under review.

Conclusions and Recommendations

Given the available information there is no clear evidence that routine use of ASA in asymptomatic men leads to a reduction in the rates of death from all causes, from cardiovascular disease or from myocardial infarction (when sudden deaths are taken into account). The benefit of ASA therapy observed in the decreased incidence of myocardial infarction needs to be balanced against the potential adverse effects, particularly disabling stroke, that may be related to hemorrhagic properties of ASA.

There is no evidence from the U.S. Aspirin trial to indicate that ASA therapy is particularly effective in reducing the incidence of myocardial infarction among asymptomatic people who may have risk factors for ischemic heart disease (i.e., smoking, hypertension or a family history of myocardial infarction).

The evidence is not strong enough to support a recommendation that routine ASA therapy be used or not be used for the primary prevention of cardiovascular disease in asymptomatic men (C Recommendation). The Nurses' Health Study is a large cohort study that suggests that regular use of 1 to 6 aspirin a week may be associated with lower rates of MI in women. The study did not reveal a significant association of aspirin use with a lower risk of death. This evidence is not strong enough to support a recommendation of routine ASA therapy to prevent heart disease in women

(C Recommendation). The decision on whether to prescribe ASA should be made on an individual basis after the benefits of decreased risk of ischemic cardiovascular events have been balanced against the potential risks associated with prolonged ASA use.

Evidence

The evidence was identified using a MEDLINE search for the period 1991 to March 1993 with the MESH headings: aspirin and cardiovascular diseases.

This review was initiated in March 1993 and updates a report with a full reference list (except for the Nurses' Health study) that was published in 1991.<13> Recommendations were finalized by the Task Force in March 1994.

Selected References

1. Antiplatelet Trialists' Collaboration: Secondary prevention of vascular disease by prolonged antiplatelet treatment. *BMJ* 1988; 296: 320-331

2. Hennekens CH, Buring JE, Sandercock P, *et al*: Aspirin and other antiplatelet agents in the secondary and primary prevention of cardiovascular disease. *Circulation* 1989; 80: 749-756

3. Hennekens CH, Buring JE: Aspirin and cardiovascular disease. *Bull NY Acad Med* 1989; 65: 57-68

4. Peto R, Gray R, Collins R, *et al*: Randomized trial of prophylactic daily aspirin in British male doctors. *BMJ* 1988; 296: 313-316

5. Steering Committee of the Physicians' Health Study Research Group: Preliminary report: findings from the aspirin component of the ongoing Physicians' Health Study. *N Engl J Med* 1988; 318: 262-264

6. Steering Committee of the Physicians' Health Study Research Group: Final report on the aspirin component of the ongoing Physicians' Health Study. *N Engl J Med* 1989; 321: 129-135

7. Manson JE, Grobbee DE, Stampfer MJ, *et al*: Aspirin in the primary prevention of angina pectoris in a randomized trial of United States physicians. *Am J Med* 1990; 89: 772-776

8. Manson JE, Stampfer MJ, Colditz GA, *et al*: A prospective study of aspirin use and primary prevention of cardiovascular disease in women. *JAMA* 1991 266(4): 521-527

9. Sempos CT, Cooper RS: The Physicians' Health Study: aspirin for the primary prevention of myocardial infarction. [letter] *N Engl J Med* 1988; 318: 924-925

10. Hennekens CH, Peto R, Hutcheson GB, *et al*: An overview of the British and American aspirin studies. [letter] *N Engl J Med* 1988; 318: 923-924.

11. Antiplatelet Trialists' Collaboration: Collaborative overview of randomized trials of antiplatelet treatment. Part 1: prevention of death, myocardial infarction and stroke by prolonged antiplatelet therapy in various categories of patients. *Br Med J* 1994; 308: 81-106

12. Jonas S: The Physicians' Health Study: a neurologist's concern. *Arch Neurol* 1990; 47: 1352-1353

13. Canadian Task Force on the Periodic Health Examination: The periodic health examination, 1991 update: 6. Acetylsalicylic acid and the primary prevention of cardiovascular disease. *Can Med Assoc J* 1991; 145: 1091-1095

Table 1: Main Outcomes of the British Aspirin Trial[4]

Event	Group; rate per 10,000 man-years		Relative Risk
	Experimental	Control	
Fatal			
Myocardial infarction	47.3	49.6	0.95
Stroke	16.0	12.7	1.26
All vascular causes	78.6	83.5	0.94
All non vascular causes	64.8	76.0	0.85
All causes	143.5	159.5	0.90
Nonfatal			
Confirmed myocardial infarction	42.5	43.3	0.98
Confirmed stroke	32.4	28.5	1.14
Confirmed transient ischemic attack	15.9	27.5	0.58[1]

[1] $0.01 < p < 0.05$.

Table 2: Main Outcomes of the U.S. Aspirin Trial[6]

Event	Group; rate per 10,000 man-years[1]		Relative Risk[2]
	Experimental	Control	
Fatal			
Myocardial infarction	1.8	5.1	0.31[3]
Stroke	1.8	1.3	1.44
All cardiovascular causes	14.8	15.1	0.96
All noncardiovascular causes	22.6	24.2	0.93
All causes	39.5	41.4	0.96
Nonfatal			
Myocardial infarction	23.6	39.2	0.59[4]
Stroke	20.0	16.7	1.20

[1] Calculated from data reported in reference 8.
[2] Data taken directly from reference 8.
[3] $p < 0.005$.
[4] $p < 0.00001$.

Table 3:   Main Outcomes of the Nurses' Health Study[8]

Event	Combined Adjusted Relative Risk Aspirin per week			
	0	1-6	7-14	≥ 15
Non fatal Myocardial infarction and Fatal Coronary Heart Disease (95% CI)	1.0	0.75[1] (0.58-0.99)	1.20 (0.84-1.69)	0.89 (0.63-1.27)
Total Strokes (95% CI)	1.0	0.99 (0.71-1.36)	0.83 (0.49-1.42)	1.26 (0.79-1.83)
Cardiovascular Deaths (95% CI)	1.0	0.89 (0.59-1.33)	1.05 (0.58-1.90)	1.09 (0.64-1.85)
Total Deaths (95% CI)	1.0	0.86 (0.72-1.03)	1.14 (0.89-1.47)	0.97 (0.76-1.23)

[1] $p < 0.05$

Acetylsalicylic Acid and the Primary Prevention of Cardiovascular Disease

MANEUVER	EFFECTIVENESS	LEVEL OF EVIDENCE <REF>	RECOMMENDATION
Daily low-dose intake of ASA	No clear evidence that routine use in asymptomatic men will reduce the rate of death from all causes, or from cardiovascular disease or myocardial infarction (MI); a reduced rate of nonfatal MI needs to be balanced against potential adverse effects (hemorrhage and disabling stroke).	Randomized controlled trials<4-7> (I)	Weak evidence to use or not to use routine ASA therapy for the primary prevention of cardiovascular disease in asymptomatic men and women (C)
	No clear evidence that routine use of ASA in women reduces the rate of death from all causes or from cardiovascular disease; routine use may be associated with a decreased risk of MI.	Prospective cohort study<8> (II-2)	

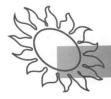

CHAPTER 57

Asymptomatic Carotid Disease

By Ariane Mackey, Robert Côté
and Renaldo N. Battista

Asymptomatic Carotid Disease

Prepared by Ariane Mackey, MD, FRCPC[1], Robert Côté, MD, FRCPC[2] and Renaldo N. Battista, MD, ScD, FRCPC[3]

In 1984 the Canadian Task Force did not recommend screening for cervical bruits in the context of a periodic health examination. There is currently no compelling data to recommend neck auscultation to detect a carotid bruit or noninvasive testing for carotid artery disease in asymptomatic patients with the ultimate objective of preventing stroke. Neck bruits are insensitive, non-specific markers for carotid stenosis. They are mostly considered, when present, as a general indicator of systemic atherosclerosis. Population-based studies show no increase in ipsilateral ischemic stroke in persons with asymptomatic neck bruits. Furthermore, among asymptomatic patients with carotid stenosis who do develop cerebrovascular symptoms most will have transient ischemic attacks (TIAs) rather than unheralded strokes. For most of these symptomatic patients efficacious stroke prevention interventions are available.

The role of prophylactic carotid endarterectomy or medical intervention such as antiplatelet drugs for asymptomatic patients is still undefined, whatever the degree of stenosis or clinical circumstance (incidental finding or preoperative assessment).

Patients with established risk factors for vascular disease should, however, be educated as to the symptoms of TIA and stroke, and their risk factors should be managed appropriately, especially control of blood pressure (Chapter 53) and cessation of smoking (Chapter 43).

Burden of Suffering

Stroke is one of the leading causes of mortality in Canada. It accounts for 7% of deaths; the overall stroke mortality rate is 55 and 44 per 100,000 annually in men and women respectively and reaches 885 and 768 per 100,000 in the elderly over 75 years of age.[1] In Canada, about 50,000 new strokes occur each year and the estimated prevalence of stroke survivors is 208,000.[2] Stroke-related neurological disability has a major impact on the patient, family

---

[1] Fellow (Cerebro-Vascular), Division of Neurology, Department of Medicine, Montreal General Hospital, Montreal, Quebec
[2] Division of Clinical Epidemiology, Montreal General Hospital and Assoicate Professor of Neurology and Neurosurgery, McGill University, Montreal, Quebec
[3] Director, Division of Clinical Epidemiology, Montreal General Hospital, McGill University, Montreal, Quebec

members and caretakers; among survivors, 17% will remain institutionalized and 25% to 50% will need moderate to total assistance for activities of every day living.<2> The annual cost of stroke in Canada, including hospital costs and loss of productivity, is estimated to be $1.5 billion.

Extracranial carotid artery disease however plays a relatively minor role as an underlying cause of stroke. Indeed, cerebral ischemic infarcts constitute 70-85% of all strokes, about three-quarters of these are in the carotid territory and of those only 20 to 50% are associated with carotid stenosis.<3>

The prevalence of neck bruits in the normal adult population is about 3-4%. It increases with age reaching 8% in people over 75 years.<4,5> According to some population-based studies the prevalence of bruits also increases with hypertension, diabetes and female gender. In patients undergoing coronary artery bypass graft (CABG) or peripheral vascular reconstruction (PVR) asymptomatic bruits occur in approximately 10-20% of cases respectively.

Since cervical bruits inadequately predict the presence and degree of carotid disease, more recent studies have focused rather on the severity of arterial lesions based on non-invasive testing. In neurologically asymptomatic individuals, the prevalence of significant carotid artery stenosis ranges between 4% and 30% depending on the type of population studied. The presence and severity of extracranial carotid disease and stenosis increases with age, hypertension and peripheral and coronary vascular disease.

Stroke Risk

Population studies<4,5> have reported that patients with asymptomatic neck bruits are at increased risk for stroke: slightly more than 2% per year in the Evans County study (7.5 fold increase for men and 1.6 fold increase for women) and in the Framingham study the two year incidence of stroke was 3% in men and 4% in women, a 2 to 3 fold increased risk. In these studies, the presence of a bruit did not predict the type (thromboembolic, cardioembolic, lacunar or hemorrhagic) or the hemispheric location of the stroke. Most of the strokes either occurred in a different vascular territory or their presumed cause was unrelated to the carotid stenosis itself.

In more recent years, non-invasive imaging (ultrasonography), has shown that the risk of neurological events is directly correlated with the severity of carotid stenosis (Figure 1).<6-12> It has also been observed that rapid progression of carotid bifurcation plaque may herald a significant risk of stroke.<6,13> Correlation with plaque morphology such as ulceration or intraplaque hemorrhage as well as correlation with other risk factors is less well defined.

In a Canadian prospective referral population study of 696 patients with asymptomatic bruits followed on average for 3.5 years,[7] the annual stroke rate was 1.3% in patients with equal or less than 50% stenosis[4] and 3.3% in those with greater than 50% stenosis. Ipsilateral stroke rate was 2.5% in patients with >50% stenosis. Other prospective studies of large populations of patients with asymptomatic bruits have shown similar results;[6,8-10,13] the overall risk of stroke is 1 to 2% annually, that is approximately three times the likelihood of having an ischemic stroke in an age- and sex-matched population without bruits.[11]

Cardiac Risk (Myocardial Infarction and Cardiac Death)

In the study[4] by Norris and colleagues,[7] the annual rate of cardiac ischemic events and cardiac death was 9.9% in those with ≤ 50% stenosis and 14.8% in those with >50% stenosis. Similarly, in most surveys on asymptomatic carotid bruit or stenosis the major risk is cardiac, not cerebrovascular.[4,5,7] However this depends on the type of population studied and their initial cardiac status; in another ongoing prospective study,[10] in which patients with heart conditions requiring the obligatory use of aspirin were excluded, neurological events were more frequent among patients with asymptomatic bruits.

Maneuver

Auscultation

Neck bruits do not reliably predict the presence or absence of underlying occlusive carotid disease

Neck bruits do not reliably predict presence or absence of underlying occlusive carotid disease. Cervical bruits may be due to other causes such as transmitted cardiac murmurs, anatomic variations, tortuosity, and hyperdynamic states.

Studies looking at the relationship between carotid bruit and corresponding stenosis have used different methodologies which limits comparability (populations with different prevalence of vascular disease, interobserver variability among clinicians about auditory characteristics of the bruit, different methods of imaging and different definition of carotid lesion severity). Depending on the method of assessment, the predictive value of a carotid bruit for ipsilateral moderate to severe stenosis ranges from approximately 16% to 75%.[3,12,14-17] Patients with asymptomatic bruits are less likely to have an underlying stenosis than patients with symptomatic bruits

---

[4] What is defined as a 50% stenosis (measured by maximal diameter reduction) is referred to, in this study, as 75% stenosis (measured by percentage reduction in the cross-sectional area of the carotid lumen).

(cerebrovascular accident (CVA) or TIA).[3,18] According to some,[3] among patients with asymptomatic neck bruits, 17% had a >75% stenosis, while in patients with both carotid stroke and bruits, 60% had a >75% stenosis. Conversely, many patients with a high grade stenosis do not have a cervical bruit.[15,17,19,20]

Non-Invasive Testing

The most reliable non-invasive test used to evaluate the extracranial carotid arteries is Duplex scanning which combines two ultrasound techniques: a pulsed echo or B-mode ultrasound which can detect anatomic abnormalities and a Doppler ultrasound which provides functional information about blood flow. When compared to angiography, the test has been found to have a sensitivity (to detect >50% stenosis) of approximately 85% (range 82% to 100%) and a specificity ranging between 81% and 100%.[6,21] Information from the B-mode component of the Duplex is used to assess location and extension of atherosclerosis including minimal disease not causing changes in blood flow. It can also determine morphological characteristics of the plaque suggestive of intraplaque hemorrhage or ulceration, however the importance of these changes in the pathogenesis of cerebral ischemia remains controversial. These abnormalities appear to represent markers of the severity of the stenosis and plaque instability rather than playing a direct role in the pathogenesis of TIAs and stroke. Information from the Doppler component of the duplex scan provides blood flow information used to measure the degree of stenosis, which seems more relevant from a clinical viewpoint.

Carotid Doppler ultrasound is a reasonable and less expensive alternative providing an overall accuracy for lesions with a greater than 50% stenosis of 90% with a sensitivity of 87% to 89% and specificity of 92% to 97%.[21,22] A recent report from the North American Symptomatic Carotid Endarterectomy Trial (NASCET) has documented a specificity of 60% for Doppler ultrasound in detecting high-grade carotid stenosis and has suggested that angiography be required for accurate determination of operability. The lower specificity reported in this study results from an angiographical measurement approach that underestimates the degree of carotid stenosis when compared to the standard measurement approach used in most other studies. Also, determining the operability of lesions is not relevant in the context of asymptomatic carotid disease given that surgery is of unproven value.

Magnetic resonance angiography, another non-invasive but more expensive and less widely available method of imaging is not used routinely to screen persons with asymptomatic bruits.

Effectiveness of Prevention

Identification and Management of Risk Factors

Identification and treatment of hypertension as well as cessation of smoking are recommended for the prevention of cerebrovascular disease even in the absence of carotid stenosis (see Chapters 53 and 43). These are well established risk factors for stroke, as well as predictors for carotid artery atherosclerosis. Treatment of hypertension and cessation of smoking significantly reduces the incidence of cerebrovascular accidents.

The relation of blood lipids and lipoproteins to the occurrence of atherothrombotic brain infarction remains unclear. In a meta-analysis combining the results of ten studies, Qizilbash and associates[23] found the relative risk of stroke (mostly ischemic) to be 1.3 (95% confidence interval: 1.11-1.54) among patients with hypercholesterolemia (≥220 mg/dl). Serum lipid levels have also been related to carotid artery atherosclerosis, however, it is not clear whether reduction of cholesterol levels has any effect on the cervical or intracranial atherothrombotic process, or on stroke risk. In middle aged men, lowering serum cholesterol does not reduce stroke mortality or morbidity according to a recent meta-analysis of thirteen randomized controlled trials (also see Chapter 54). Nevertheless, hypercholesterolemia should be managed appropriately especially considering it's relationship to coronary artery disease.

Medical Management

Pharmacological management of patients with asymptomatic carotid disease has not been properly studied

Pharmacological management for patients with asymptomatic carotid disease has not been properly studied. Two primary prevention studies in healthy physicians assessing the effect of aspirin on occurrence of occlusive vascular events did not show any reduction of incidence in ischemic strokes (see Chapter 56). In those studies, no systematic neck auscultation or non-invasive testing was undertaken.

A prospective, randomized, double blind study looking at the efficacy of ASA 325 mg a day compared to placebo in preventing occurrence of vascular events in asymptomatic patients with significant (≥50%) stenosis is currently underway.[24]

Therapies directed at regression of atheroma are also being assessed. Antiplatelets agents have been proven beneficial in reducing recurrent neurological events in symptomatic patients.[25] However, these results do not necessarily apply to asymptomatic persons especially when one considers their lower level of risk for ischemic events and the small but definite risk of hemorrhagic complications due to chronic aspirin use.

Prophylactic Carotid Endarterectomy

A) In Otherwise Healthy Individuals

There have been several case reports on the possible benefits of prophylactic carotid endarterectomy (CE) in asymptomatic individuals with carotid stenosis, however most of these small series have serious methodological flaws which make their results difficult to interpret. Three prospective randomized clinical trials have been published. One was terminated early because of higher than expected morbidity in the surgical group;[26] another had a complex design and many methodological inadequacies and gave no conclusions regarding the potential benefit of CE in patients with >90% stenosis.[27] In the third study[28] 444 men with asymptomatic stenosis >50% determined by angiography, were followed for an average of 47.9 months. The study showed no protective effect of surgery on the combined incidence of stroke and death though the incidence of ipsilateral neurological events (CVA and TIA) in the surgical group was 8% compared to 20.6% in the medical group. Indeed, the benefit of (CE) in asymptomatic patients should depend on stroke prevention and not only on reducing the number of TIAs since surgical intervention has recently been proven beneficial in patients with TIA or minor strokes and stenosis of between 70-99%.[29,30] It is hoped that the Asymptomatic Carotid Artery Stenosis Study (ACASS),[31] an ongoing randomized trial of CE in asymptomatic stenosis, will shed light on this still unresolved issue. Since the incidence of ipsilateral ischemic stroke is low[7,8,10] and considering that the morbidity-mortality of CE for asymptomatic lesions ranges from approximately 1 to 4.5%, and recognizing the inherent risk of intra-arterial angiography, prophylactic CE cannot be systematically recommended and remains of unproven benefit in this clinical context.

B) In Patients Undergoing Major Vascular Surgery

The question of whether prophylactic CE safely lowers the risk of perioperative stroke in asymptomatic patients with severe carotid stenosis undergoing major vascular surgery has not been addressed directly by a prospective randomized trial. In a recent prospective study of 358 patients undergoing CABG or PVR, none of 53 patients who had a >50% carotid stenosis, suffered an ipsilateral perioperative stroke.[32] According to others, patients with symptomatic coronary heart disease or peripheral vascular disease undergoing vascular surgery, in whom a carotid bruit or stenosis has been detected have a greater risk of stroke. However the exact incidence of thromboembolic events secondary to the stenotic process itself remains uncertain since perioperative strokes may be caused by a variety of pathogenetic mechanisms including embolism from the heart (thrombus, arrhythmias etc) or aorta and abnormalities of coagulation. Therefore, preoperative screening using neck auscultation and/or

Performance of preventive carotid surgery in asymptomatic patients cannot be presently justified

cervical ultrasonography of patients undergoing vascular surgery may fail to identify many who are at higher risk of sustaining strokes. Considering the above, and the fact that adding CE to a major vascular procedure often increases the risk of cardiac and cerebral complications and death,<33,34> performance of preventive carotid surgery in those asymptomatic patients cannot be justified at present.

Recommendations of Others

The recommendations of the U.S. Preventive Services Task Force on screening for cerebrovascular disease are currently under review.

The American College of Physicians also does not recommend routine diagnostic testing for carotid artery disease in patients with asymptomatic bruits. Concerning CE, they state that the procedure is "of most inappropriate use" in unselected asymptomatic patients with carotid artery abnormalities. However, they feel that CE may be indicated in patients with other risk factors for stroke, who have a high degree of stenosis (70% or greater), particularly when the contralateral artery is occluded and if surgery can be done at low risk. No recommendation was made regarding prophylactic CE before CABG.

A consensus report from the Asymptomatic Carotid Atherosclerosis Study Group concluded that baseline non-invasive evaluation of the carotid arteries was appropriate in persons considered to be at high risk for extracranial carotid artery disease. Those included patients with carotid bruits, with a strong family history of coronary and/or cerebrovascular disease and candidates for major vascular surgery.

The Ad Hoc Committee of the Joint Council of the Society for Vascular Surgery and the North American Chapter of the International Society for Vascular Surgery has recommended that patients with asymptomatic carotid artery diameter reduction of 75% or greater who are otherwise healthy and have a projected life expectancy greater than 5 years, should be considered for surgery if the operative morbidity and mortality is less than 3%.

Conclusions and Recommendations

Asymptomatic carotid stenosis is generally associated with systemic atherosclerosis and its known complications such as myocardial infarction, stroke and peripheral vascular disease. Identification and management of risk factors associated with these conditions is mandatory as well as patient education explaining the symptoms of TIAs, which would then require further evaluation and specific intervention, either medical or surgical. Screening the population for cervical bruits and stenoses would identify only a relatively small fraction of individuals at high risk for stroke or TIA. It could be a cost effective procedure if it led to prevention of a substantial number of strokes without further risk to the patient, but since the efficacy of any specific prophylactic method, medical or surgical, remains unproven, (in fact C and D Recommendations, respectively) routine auscultation or non-invasive testing of carotids in unselected individuals cannot be systematically recommended at the present time (D Recommendation). However, in centers where prospective trials are ongoing, screening of asymptomatic patients is highly encouraged.

Unanswered Questions (Research Agenda)

Whether pharmacological or surgical therapy is safe and beneficial in asymptomatic persons with carotid bruits or stenosis is currently under investigation.<24,31> When those answers become available, firmer recommendations regarding screening, for asymptomatic bruits or stenosis and, in some patients, for periodic non-invasive testing to detect rapidly progressing stenosis might be made. Other areas of interest include identification of subgroups of patients who have inadequate collateral circulation and may be at higher risk of sustaining an ipsilateral ischemic stroke. This aspect is being studied using techniques such as single photon emission computed tomography (SPECT) and transcranial Doppler. Carotid angioplasty might also have a role in asymptomatic patients. This, of course, will depend on the risk/benefit ratio of the procedure which is currently being assessed in a randomized, multicenter trial in patients with symptomatic and asymptomatic cerebrovascular disease – the Carotid and Vertebral Artery Transluminal Angioplasty Study (CAVATAS).

Evidence

The literature was identified with a MEDLINE search for the years 1988 to August 1993 using the following key words: asymptomatic neck bruits (cervical bruit or carotid bruit), carotid stenosis, carotid artery disease, carotid ultrasound, duplex sonography, stroke risk factors, carotid endarterectomy.

This review was initiated in January, 1993 and recommendations were finalized by the Task Force in January, 1994. A technical report with a full reference list is available upon request.

Acknowledgements

We would like to thank Ms. Diane Telmosse for her excellent secretarial assistance.

Selected References

1. Heart and Stroke Foundation of Canada: *Cardiovascular Disease in Canada.* 1993

2. Mayo NE: Epidemiology and recovery. *In*: Physical medicine and rehabilitation: state of the art reviews. Philadelphia: Hanley & Belfus, 1993; 7: 1-25

3. Zhu CZ, Norris JW: Role of carotid stenosis in ischemic stroke. *Stroke* 1990; 21: 1131-1134

4. Heyman A, Wilkinson WE, Heyden S, *et al*: Risk of stroke in asymptomatic persons with cervical arterial bruits: a population study in Evans County, Georgia. *N Engl J Med* 1980; 302: 838-841

5. Wolf PA, Kannel WB, Sorlie P, *et al*: Asymptomatic carotid bruit and risk of stroke. The Framingham Study. *JAMA* 1981; 245: 1442-1445

6. Roederer GO, Langlois YE, Jager KA, *et al*: The natural history of carotid arterial disease in asymptomatic patients with cervical bruits. *Stroke* 1984; 15: 605-613

7. Norris JW, Zhu CZ, Bornstein NM, *et al*: Vascular risks of asymptomatic carotid stenosis. *Stroke* 1991; 22: 1485-1490

8. Meissner I, Wiebers DO, Whisnant JP, *et al*: The natural history of asymptomatic carotid artery occlusive lesions. *JAMA* 1987; 258: 2704-2707

9. Autret A, Pourcelot L, Saudeau D, *et al*: Stroke risk in patients with carotid stenosis. *Lancet* 1987; 1: 888-890

10. Mackey A, Côté R, Abrahamowicz M, *et al*: Outcome of patients with asymptomatic bruits. *Neurology* 1993; 43: A351 [abstract]

11. Wiebers DO, Whisnant JP, Sandok BA, *et al*: Prospective comparison of a cohort with asymptomatic carotid bruit and a population-based cohort without carotid bruit. *Stroke* 1990; 21: 984-988

12. AbuRahma AF, Robinson PA: Prospective clinicopathophysiologic follow-up study of asymptomatic neck bruit. *Am Surg* 1990; 56: 108-113

13. Hennerici M, Hulsbomer HB, Hefter H, *et al*: Natural history of asymptomatic extracranial arterial disease. Results of a long term prospective study. *Brain* 1987; 110: 777-791

14. Lusiani L, Visona A, Castellani V, *et al*: Prevalence of atherosclerotic lesions of the carotid bifurcation in patients with asymptomatic bruits: an echo-Doppler (duplex) study. *Angiology* 1985; 36: 235-239

15. Chambers BR, Norris JW: Clinical significance of asymptomatic neck bruits. *Neurology* 1985; 35: 742-745

16. Floriani M, Giulini SM, Bonardelli S, *et al*: Value and limits of "critical auscultation" of neck bruits. *Angiology* 1988; 39: 967-972

17. Ingall TJ, Homer D, Whisnant JP, *et al*: Predictive value of carotid bruit for carotid atherosclerosis. *Arch Neurol* 1989; 46: 418-422

18. Goldman L, Koller RL, Lebow SS, *et al*: Cervical bruits: clinical correlated of stenosis. *Angiology* 1991; 42: 491-497

19. Kuller LH, Sutton KC: Carotid artery bruit: Is it safe to and effective to auscultate the neck? *Stroke* 1984; 15: 944-947

20. Caplan LR: Carotid artery disease. *N Engl J Med* 1986; 315: 886-888

21. Feussner JR, Matchar DB: When and how to study the carotid arteries. *Ann Int Med* 1988; 109: 805-818

22. Bornstein NM, Chadwick LG, Norris JW: The value of carotid Doppler ultrasound in asymptomatic extracranial arterial disease. *Can J Neurol Sci* 1988; 15: 378-393

23. Qizilbash N, Duffy SW, Warlow C, *et al*: Lipids are risk factors for ischaemic stroke: overview and review. *Cerebrovas Dis* 1992; 2: 127-136

24. The Asymptomatic Cervical Bruit Study Group: Natural history and effectiveness of aspirin in asymptomatic patients with cervical bruits. *Arch Neurol* 1991; 48: 683-686

25. Antiplatelet Trialists' Collaboration: Collaborative overview of randomized trials of antiplatelet treatment. Part 1: prevention of death, myocardial infarction and stroke by prolonged antiplatelet therapy in various categories of patients. *Br Med J* 1994; 308: 81-106

26. Mayo Asymptomatic Carotid Endarterectomy Study Group: Results of a randomized controlled trial of carotid endarterectomy for asymptomatic carotid stenosis. *Mayo Clin Proc* 1992; 67: 513-518

27. The CASANOVA Study Group: Carotid surgery versus medical therapy in asymptomatic carotid stenosis. *Stroke* 1991; 22: 1229-1235

28. Hobson RW, Weiss DG, Fields WS, *et al*: Efficacy of carotid endarterectomy for asymptomatic carotid stenosis. *N Engl J Med* 1993; 328: 221-227

29. North American Symptomatic Carotid Endarterectomy Trial Collaborations: Beneficial effect of carotid endarterectomy in symptomatic patients with high grade carotid stenosis. *N Engl J Med* 1991; 325: 445-453

30. European Carotid Surgery Trialist Collaboration Group: MRC European Carotid Surgery Trial: interim results for symptomatic patients with severe (70-99%) or mild (0-29%) carotid stenosis. *Lancet* 1991; 337: 1235-1243

31. The Asymptomatic Carotid Atherosclerosis Study Group: Study design for randomized prospective trial of carotid endarterectomy for asymptomatic atherosclerosis. *Stroke* 1989; 20: 844-849

32. Gerraty RP, Gates PC, Doyle JC: Carotid stenosis and perioperative stroke risk in symptomatic and asymptomatic patients undergoing vascular or coronary surgery. *Stroke* 1993; 24: 1115-1118

33. Brener BJ, Brief DK, Alpert J, *et al*: The risk of stroke in patients with asymptomatic carotid stenosis undergoing cardiac surgery: a follow-up study. *J Vasc Surg* 1987; 5: 269-279

34. Bass A, Krupski WC, Dilley RB, *et al*: Combined carotid endarterectomy and coronary artery revascularisation: a sobering review. *Isr J Med Sci* 1992; 28: 27-32

Figure 1

TIA and Stroke

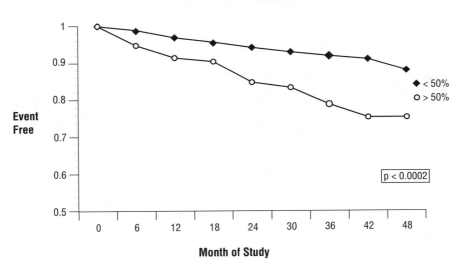

Adapted from reference <27> the Kaplan-Meir curves indicate the incidence of neurological conditions among patients with asymptomatic stenosis >50% (n=314) and among patients with asymptomatic stenosis <50% (n=363).

Asymptomatic Carotid Disease

MANEUVER	EFFECTIVENESS	LEVEL OF EVIDENCE <REF>	RECOMMENDATION
Neck auscultation	Insensitive and non-specific marker for underlying carotid stenosis. Positive predictive value ranging from 16-75%.	Descriptive studies<14-20> (III)	Fair evidence not to include in periodic health examination of asymptomatic individuals (D)
Medical therapy	No actual evidence for effectiveness or ineffectiveness of medical therapy (antiplatelets) in patients with asymptomatic carotid bruit or stenosis.	One controlled randomized trial in progress<24> (II-2)	Insufficient evidence to include or exclude in treatment of those with asymptomatic carotid disease (C)
Carotid endarterectomy (CE)	Presently, evidence is not conclusive regarding preventive effect of CE on occurrence of fatal and non-fatal stroke in asymptomatic individuals with carotid stenosis but CE is associated with severe morbidity or mortality of 1-4.5%.	Randomized controlled trials<26-28> (I)	Fair evidence not to use carotid endarterectomy to treat those with asymptomatic carotid stenosis (D)

Other Infectious Diseases

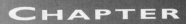

CHAPTER

58

Screening
for HIV
Antibody

By Elaine E. L. Wang

Screening for HIV Antibody

Prepared by Elaine E. L. Wang, MD, CM, FRCPC[1]

Human immunodeficiency virus (HIV) antibody screening may reduce the incidence of acquired immunodeficiency syndrome (AIDS) through counselling to prevent HIV transmission and may delay the onset of AIDS through treatment of asymptomatic HIV-positive patients.

Burden of Suffering

By October 7, 1991, 5,349 AIDS cases had been reported in Canada, including 63 pediatric cases. Sixty four percent of affected adults were ages 20 to 39 years. Sixty percent had died. Under reporting by up to 20% may result from efforts to maintain patient confidentiality and the complexity of the reporting procedure. HIV seroprevalence is 0.3 to 0.6 per 1,000 among pregnant women and 2-3 times higher among urban women.<1-5>

Behaviours that increase risk of HIV infection include having many sexual partners, receiving anal intercourse, sharing needles during injection drug use and receiving blood or blood products prior to introduction of universal HIV antibody screening by blood banks. Homosexual or bisexual men, prostitutes, injection drug users, people receiving blood products between 1978 and 1985, sexual contacts of people with HIV infection and people from countries with a high HIV prevalence are at high risk. Of all cases reported in Canada, 78% were associated with homosexual or bisexual activity only, 1.4% with injection drug use only, and 3.5% with both. 95% of AIDS cases belonged to an identified risk group.

Maneuver

Deciding who should undergo HIV antibody screening is complex and difficult. There are problems with both the frequency with which physicians ask the necessary questions and the quality of responses. A sexual history was routinely obtained by less than half of physicians recently surveyed. Seropositivity rates vary within identified risk groups (related to factors such as race, income, recent injections, or injections in "shooting galleries" within the injection drug use group). Barriers to obtaining accurate information may include worries about self-incrimination, illiteracy, race or ethnic background, language and socioeconomic status.<6> Risk factors were acknowledged in less than 60% of HIV-positive parturient women;<7-10> targeted screening

---

[1] Associate Professor of Pediatrics and of Preventive Medicine and Biostatistics, University of Toronto, Toronto, Ontario

(e.g. premarital testing or in sexually transmitted disease (STD) clinics) has low sensitivity and specificity. The addition of counselling did not improve the sensitivity of questionnaires in identifying seropositive women.<11> Increased patient acceptance of routine testing and the poor accuracy of targeted screening suggest that routine screening is preferable to targeted screening if an elevated seroprevalence rate is suspected in any population.<6-8,10,12>

However, a complete sexual and drug-use history should be obtained for all patients as part of a clinical assessment. The contents of such a history are described in guidelines from the Canadian Medical Association and other groups.

Once a decision is made to screen, informed consent must be obtained, and counselling must be provided before the test and after receipt of the results – an important component of the testing procedure. Maintaining confidentiality is likely to increase the acceptance of testing, although it has not been studied.

Screening for HIV infection currently involves detection of antibodies. The first step requires one of a number of commercially available enzyme-linked immunosorbent assay (ELISA) kits. These are highly sensitive but their specificity is reduced by cross-reactions with components other than HIV antigens. ELISA is easy to perform and inexpensive. If the results are repeatedly positive, the second step involves a more specific confirmatory test, such as the Western blot, radioimmunoprecipitation or immunofluorescence assay. These confirmatory tests are labour intensive and costly. The combined sensitivity of the two tests approaches 100%. However, the trauma to a single individual falsely identified as seropositive may offset the advantage to those who are truly seropositive. The higher the prevalence, the more true positives are identified for every false positive; acceptable prevalence rates to justify screening have not been defined.

The sensitivity and specificity of ELISA combined with a confirmatory test approaches 100% for identifying HIV infection

False negative results after combined testing with ELISA and the Western blot technique may occur because of the delay in antibody development after HIV exposure. This period is usually less than 6 months. A false negative result may falsely reassure people in whom antibody has not yet developed. Testing should be repeated after 6 months in seronegative people whose behaviour put them at risk.

In neonates inaccurate results may occur if only the antibody but not the virus is passed to the neonate or because of poor antibody response.<13-15> Thus, viral DNA detection through a polymerase chain reaction or virus isolation is required for diagnosis. False-positives may also result from errors in specimen identification or contamination in the laboratory.

The screening test is not accurate for detecting infection in neonates

Effectiveness of Prevention and Treatment

Risks of Screening

Implications of HIV seropositivity go beyond the infection and relate to behaviours that increase the risk of infection. Being identified as a homosexual man may subject a person to discrimination and prejudice. Behaviours such as illicit injection drug use and prostitution place the seropositive person at risk for legal prosecution. Discrimination in employment, housing, education, health insurance and access to medical care have also occurred among those identified as HIV positive. Rejection by family and friends reduces needed support. Depression and anger are more common in subjects aware of their serologic status than in those unaware of it.<16>

Whether patients who have been engaging in high-risk behaviour are reassured and encouraged to continue these behaviours after receiving a negative test result is unknown but unlikely. Studies of counselling suggest a reduction in behaviour known to transmit the virus, although this reduction is often greater among HIV-positive than HIV-negative people.<16-20>

Benefits of Screening

In asymptomatic people with a history of risk factors, knowledge of being truly seronegative may provide a great deal of relief and influence future plans regarding marriage, children, employment, insurance and protection of sexual partners.

Drug therapy has also been shown to be beneficial. Zidovudine (AZT) delays the onset of AIDS in people with asymptomatic HIV infection with a CD4 lymphocyte count of less than 0.5×10^9/L.<21>

Therapy with zidovudine and *P. carinii* pneumonia prophylaxis of HIV-positive asymptomatic individuals delays the onset of AIDS

Optimism about early AZT therapy must be tempered by several considerations. The drug must be given to 100 patients for a year to delay the onset of opportunistic infection in 4 patients. Data are not available on important outcomes such as survival, quality of life and adverse effects. Studies of HIV isolates in treated patients are showing drug resistance. Few data are available for injection drug users, women who have acquired HIV infection heterosexually or children;<21-23> the generalizability of the results to these populations is questionable. In a study involving symptomatic people there was no difference in survival between those given early AZT therapy and those given late therapy despite a delay in the onset of AIDS.<24> More information is needed on long-term efficacy and toxic effects of AZT. The finding that treatment of asymptomatic HIV infection can delay the development of AIDS suggests that the CD4 count should be monitored until it reaches a level at which AZT treatment should be started.

In a randomized trial,<25> the risk of *P. carinii* pneumonia was reduced by 70% by aerosol pentamidine prophylaxis in asymptomatic patients with a CD4 count less than 0.2×10^9/L and in patients with AIDS or advanced symptomatic HIV infection who had not had *P. carinii* pneumonia. Several trials of primary prophylaxis with other similar agents are under way. Previous trials have demonstrated the efficacy of trimethoprim-sulfamethoxazole in other immunocompromised populations.

Screening for and management of concurrent infectious diseases such as tuberculosis (see Chapter 62), fungal infections or parasitic infections may be altered by knowledge of HIV seropositivity. Most recommendations for primary prophylaxis or treatment of these conditions are based on expert opinion, recognizing that conventional management is less efficacious in HIV-positive patients than in HIV-negative subjects.

Efficacy of Counselling

Counselling on high-risk sexual practices or on the use of condoms is expected to increase desired behaviours and decrease the spread of HIV infection. Cohort studies involving homosexual men, have shown a statistically significant reduction in risk behaviour among those aware of their seropositive status.<16-18,26-28> These studies have been criticized because of the highly selected nature of the participants and because of difficulties in measuring and validating sexual behaviour. Studies of counselling people with hemophilia and injection drug users have shown reduction in risk behaviour but have the same design flaws.<20,29-33> Nonetheless, one can conclude that counselling probably reduces but does not eliminate unsafe sexual practices.

Screening of Pregnant Women

Screening of pregnant women is a special situation because the risk of vertical transmission to the fetus is about 30%. One might expect that women found to be seropositive would opt for an elective abortion. However, two studies involving injection drug users showed that seropositive women had the same rate of pregnancy and therapeutic abortion as seronegative women. Nevertheless, knowledge of seropositivity may result in: 1) avoidance of certain obstetric maneuvers (e.g., amniocentesis, chorionic villus sampling and fetal monitoring) that may increase the risk of HIV transmission; 2) earlier diagnosis of associated illnesses that might otherwise be attributed to pregnancy; 3) avoidance of breast feeding, which may be a vehicle for HIV transmission; and 4) earlier treatment of infected infants.

Recommendations of Others

The U.S. Centers for Disease Control (CDC) recommends screening people in identified risk groups, including those with STDs. In 1985 the CDC also recommended screening and counselling for women in high-risk groups to prevent perinatal HIV transmission. Testing and counselling should also be offered to woman who request testing. Testing was not recommended for women at low risk because of difficulties in interpreting the results. In addition, it was recommended that patients being treated for tuberculosis be counselled and undergo HIV antibody testing because of the implications for management. Trimethoprim-sulfamethoxazole or aerosol pentamidine prophylaxis for *P. carinii* pneumonia has been recommended for adults with a CD4 count of less than 0.2×10^9/L and trimethoprim-sulfamethoxazole prophylaxis for children with a CD4 count 20% or more below the normal age-specific count.<34,35>

In 1989, the U.S. Preventive Services Task Force<36> concluded that there was fair evidence to recommend screening in a high-risk population and in pregnant women but no evidence to either include or exclude screening in a low-risk population.

Conclusions and Recommendations

Obtaining a history of sexual behaviour and injection drug use and offering counselling has limited sensitivity for identifying HIV-positive people in the general population, but is likely to increase detection of risk behaviours. Its inclusion in the periodic health examination of asymptomatic people in the general population is based on expert opinion (C Recommendation).

Recommendations for HIV antibody screening must consider characteristics of the screening maneuver, particularly sensitivity and specificity, and the availability of treatment for asymptomatic seropositive people. There is insufficient evidence to recommend the inclusion or exclusion of HIV antibody screening among pregnant women (C Recommendation). Because the prevalence of HIV infection is lower in Canada than in the U.S. the generalizability of the results of U.S. studies is questionable. Even with excellent test characteristics the positive predictive value cannot be perfect with a low prevalence rate. Screening should be considered for those in large cities because of the low sensitivity of targeted screening and better compliance with routine screening.

HIV antibody screening should be offered to people with high-risk behaviours or those in high-risk groups because of good evidence of the effectiveness of early treatment in delaying the development of AIDS and the efficacy of aerosol pentamidine prophylaxis (A Recommendation). However, labelling is a problem, and there is no information about the long-term effects of treatment.

Cohort studies suggest that testing followed by counselling may reduce the spread of HIV infection among injection drug users and homosexual men.

There is fair evidence to recommend HIV antibody screening for neonates of HIV-positive women (B Recommendation); however, antibody screening is not specific or sensitive for infection, and other diagnostic tests, such as the viral DNA polymerase chain reaction or virus isolation, must be done. Follow-up and vaccinations will be different for seropositive children.

There is insufficient evidence to recommend the inclusion or exclusion of HIV antibody screening in low-risk populations (C Recommendation). The harm caused by false positive results must be weighed against any treatment benefits gained by the few seropositive people identified.

Unanswered Questions (Research Agenda)

Strategies to improve the identification of people who should undergo testing need to be evaluated. Although the results of initial studies of pamphlets are discouraging, the efficacy of cheaper alternatives to individual counselling should be considered.

The appropriate frequency of screening needs to be studied further.

Although public education on needle-exchange programs, counselling on condom use and counselling of seropositive people reduce high-risk behaviour they do not eliminate it. Therefore, further studies in this area are needed.

Studies of AZT and other antiviral agents, either alone or in combination, should include patient populations other than homosexual men to determine the generalizability of the results. Such studies should examine the optimal point at which treatment should be started and the long-term effects of therapy. The incremental improvement in efficacy with the use of an immunomodulator should also be studied.

Evidence

The literature was identified with a MEDLINE search to September 1991 using the following MESH headings: HIV antibody tests, AIDS, and sex-education, sex-counselling, sex-behaviour, attitude, screening, truth-disclosure, counselling, and patient education.

This review was initiated in June 1988 and recommendations were finalized by the Task Force in November 1991. A report with a full reference list was published in September 1992.<37>

Acknowledgements

The task force thanks Alfred O. Berg, MD, MPH, Professor and Associate Chair, Department of Family Medicine, University of Washington, Seattle, Washington; Abbyann Lynch, Director of Bioethics, Hospital for Sick Children, Toronto, Ontario, and Martin Schechter, MD, FRCPC, Department of Health Care and Epidemiology, University of British Columbia, Vancouver, British Columbia for reviewing the manuscript.

Selected References

1. Hoff R, Berardi VP, Weiblen BJ, *et al*: Seroprevalence of human immunodeficiency virus among childbearing women. *N Engl J Med* 1988; 318: 525-530

2. Schechter MT, Ballem PJ, Buskard NA, *et al*: An anonymous seroprevalence survey of HIV infection among pregnant women in British Columbia and the Yukon Territory. *Can Med Assoc J* 1990; 143: 1187-1192

3. Hankins CA, Laberge C, Lapointe N, *et al*: HIV infection among Quebec women giving birth to live infants. *Can Med Assoc J* 1990; 143: 885-893

4. Coates RA, Frank JW, Arshinoff R, *et al*: The Ontario HIV seroprevalence study of childbearing women: results from the first year of testing. *Clin Invest Med* 1992; 15: 1-7

5. Peckham CS, Tedder RS, Briggs M, *et al*: Prevalence of maternal HIV infection based on unlinked anonymous testing of newborn babies. *Lancet* 1990; 335: 516-519

6. Lifson AR, Chiasson MA, Stoneburner RL: Screening for HIV infection in sexually transmitted disease clinics. *N Engl J Med* 1988; 319: 242-243

7. Landesman S, Minkoff H, Holman S, *et al*: Serosurvey of human immunodeficiency virus infection in parturients. Implications for human immunodeficiency virus testing programs of pregnant women. *JAMA* 1987; 258: 2701-2703

8. Barbacci MB, Dalabetta GA, Repke JT, *et al*: Human immunodeficiency virus infection in women attending an inner-city prenatal clinic: ineffectiveness of targeted screening. *Sex Transm Dis* 1990; 17: 122-126

9. Fehrs LJ, Hill D, Kerndt PR, *et al*: Targeted HIV screening at a Los Angeles prenatal/family planning health center. *Am J Public Health* 1991; 81: 619-622

10. Lindsay MK, Feng TI, Peterson HB, *et al*: Routine human immunodeficiency virus infection screening in unregistered and registered inner-city parturients. *Obstet Gynecol* 1991; 77: 599-603

11. Wenstrom KD, Zuidema LJ: Determination of the seroprevalence of human immunodeficiency virus infection in gravidas by non-anonymous versus anonymous testing. *Obstet Gynecol* 1989; 74: 558-561

12. Human immunodeficiency virus infection in the United States: a review of current knowledge. *MMWR* 1987; 36: 1-48

13. Pizzo PA: Pediatric AIDS: problems within problems. *J Infect Dis* 1990; 161: 316-325

14. Husson RN, Comeau AM, Hoff R: Diagnosis of human immunodeficiency virus infection in infants and children. *Pediatrics* 1990; 86: 1-10

15. Walter EB, McKinney RE, Lane BA, *et al*: Interpretation of western blots of specimens from children infected with human immunodeficiency virus type 1: implications for prognosis and diagnosis. *J Pediatr* 1990; 117(2 Pt 1): 255-258

16. McCusker J, Stoddard AM, Mayer KH, *et al*: Effects of HIV antibody test knowledge on subsequent sexual behaviors in a cohort of homosexually active men. *Am J Public Health* 1988; 78: 462-467

17. Schechter MT, Craib KJP, Willoughby B, *et al*: Patterns of sexual behavior and condom use in a cohort of homosexual men. *Am J Public Health* 1988; 78: 1535-1538

18. Van Griensven GJP, de Vroome EMM, Tielman RAP, *et al*: Effect of human immunodeficiency virus (HIV) antibody knowledge on high-risk sexual behavior with steady and nonsteady sexual partners among homosexual men. *Am J Epidemiol* 1989; 129: 596-603

19. Van Griensven GJP, De Vroome EMM, Tielman RAP, *et al*: Impact of HIV antibody testing on changes in sexual behavior among homosexual men in the Netherlands. *Am J Public Health* 1988; 78: 1575-1561

20. Robertson JR, Skidmore CA, Roberts JJK: HIV infection in intravenous drug users: a follow-up study indicating changes in risk-taking behaviour. *Br J Addict* 1988; 83: 387-391

21. Volberding PA, Lagakos SW, Koch MA, *et al*: Zidovudine in asymptomatic human immunodeficiency virus infection. A controlled trial in persons with fewer than 500 CD4-positive cells per cubic millimeter. *N Engl J Med* 1990; 322: 941-949

22. Pedersen C, Sandstrom E, Petersen CS, *et al*: The efficacy of inosine pranobex in preventing the acquired immunodeficiency syndrome in patients with human immunodeficiency virus infection. *N Engl J Med* 1990; 322(25): 1757-1763

23. Leibovitz E, Rigaud M, Pollack H, *et al*: *Pneumocystis carinii* pneumonia in infants infected with the human immunodeficiency virus with more than 450 CD4 T lymphocytes per cubic millimeter. *N Engl J Med* 1990; 323(8): 531-533

24. Hamilton JD, Hartigan PM, Simberkoff MS, *et al*: A controlled trial of early versus late treatment with zidovudine in symptomatic human immunodeficiency virus infection. Results of the Veterans Affairs cooperative study. *N Engl J Med* 1992; 326: 437-443

25. Hirschel B, Lazzarin A, Chopard P, *et al*: A controlled study of inhaled pentamidine for primary prevention of *Pneumocystis Carinii* pneumonia. *N Engl J Med* 1991; 324: 1079-1083

26. Fox R, Odaka NJ, Brookmeyer R, *et al*: Effect of HIV antibody disclosure on subsequent sexual activity in homosexual men. *AIDS* 1987; 1: 241-246

27. Frazer IH, McCamish M, Hay I, *et al*: Influence of human immunodeficiency virus antibody testing on sexual behaviour in a "high-risk" population from a "low-risk" city. *Med J Aust* 1988; 149: 365-368

28. van Griensven GJP, de Vroome EMM, Goudsmit JAAP, *et al*: Changes in sexual behaviour and the fall in incidence of HIV infection among homosexual men. *BMJ* 1989; 298: 218-221

29. Kim HC, Raska K, Clemow L: Human immunodeficiency virus infection in sexually active wives of infected hemophilic men. *Am J Med* 1988; 85: 472-476

30. Laurian Y, Peynet J, Verroust F: HIV infection in sexual partners of HIV-seropositive patients with hemophilia. *N Engl J Med* 1989; 320: 183

31. Casadonte PP, Des Jarlais DC, Friedman SR, *et al*: Psychological and behavioral impact among intravenous drug users of learning HIV test results. *Int J Addict* 1990; 25(4): 409-426

32. Martin GS, Serpelloni G, Galvan U, *et al*: Behavioural change in injecting drug users: evaluation of an HIV/AIDS education programme. *AIDS Care* 1990; 2: 275-279

33. McKeganey N: Being positive: drug injectors' experiences of HIV injection. *Br J Addict* 1990; 85: 1113-1124

34. Centers for Disease Control: Guidelines for prophylaxis against *Pneumocystis carinii* pneumonia for persons infected with human immunodeficiency virus. *MMWR-Morb-Mortal-Wkly Rep* 1989; 38(Suppl 5): 1-9

35. Centers for Disease Control: Guidelines for prophylaxis against *Pneumocystis carinii* pneumonia for children infected with human immunodeficiency virus. *MMWR* 1991; 40(RR-2): 1-13

36. U.S. Preventive Services Task Force: *Guide to Clinical Preventive Services: as Assessment of the Effectiveness of 169 Interventions.* Williams & Wilkins, Baltimore, Md, 1989: 139-146, 331-339

37. Canadian Task Force on the Periodic Health Examination: The periodic health examination, 1992 update: 3. HIV antibody screening. *Can Med Assoc J* 1992; 147: 867-876

Screening for HIV Antibody

MANEUVER	EFFECTIVENESS	LEVEL OF EVIDENCE <REF>	RECOMMENDATION
Obtaining history of sexual practices and injection drug use and counselling people in the general population	Limited sensitivity for identifying HIV-positive people but may be offered for patient education; it is more sensitive than if history were not obtained.	Expert opinion <6, 11, 12> (III)	Poor evidence to include in or exclude from periodic health examination (PHE) of asymptomatic people (C)
	Reduces but does not eliminate high-risk activities in high-risk populations.	Cohort studies <16-20, 26-33> (II-2)	
Voluntary screening with an enzyme-linked immunosorbent assay (ELISA) and confirmatory test; repeat test after 6 months fo seronegative people at high risk*	Combination of ELISA and Western blot technique has almost 100% sensitivity and specificity.		
	High-risk groups:* AIDS development was delayed with early treatment if CD4 count was less than $0.5 \times 10^9/L$; labelling is a problem.	Randomized controlled trials <21, 25> (I)	Good evidence to include offer of screening in PHE of asymptomatic people at high risk (A)*
	Pregnant women: Low rate of HIV infection in Canada raises concerns about poor positive predictive value; should be considered in large cities, where rate is highest.	Cohort studies <1-5, 7-11> (II-2)	Poor evidence to include in or exclude from PHE of asymptomatic pregnant women (C)
	Infants of HIV-positive women: Risk of vertical transmission is 20-50% but usual screening methods are not sensitive or specific enough.	Cohort studies <13-15> (II-2)	Fair evidence to include in PHE of children of HIV-positive women (B)

High-risk groups include homosexual and bisexual men, prostitutes, injection drug users, people with sexually transmitted diseases, people receiving blood products between 1978 and 1985, sexual contacts of HIV-positive people and people from countries with a high prevalence rate of HIV infection.

(Continued on next page)

Screening for HIV Antibody (concl'd)

MANEUVER	EFFECTIVENESS	LEVEL OF EVIDENCE <REF>	RECOMMENDATION
Voluntary screening with an enzyme-linked immunosorbent assay (ELISA) and confirmatory test	**People at low risk:** False positive results may outweigh benefit of treating the few seropositive people identified.	Expert opinion (III)	Poor evidence to include in or exclude from PHE of asymptomatic people at low risk (C)

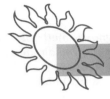

CHAPTER 59

Prevention
of
Gonorrhea

By Brenda L. Beagan and Elaine E. L. Wang

Prevention of Gonorrhea

Prepared by Brenda L. Beagan, MSc[1] and Elaine E. L. Wang MD, CM, FRCPC[2]

Despite the development of different diagnostic methods, Gram stain and culture of urethral or vaginal smears remain the methods of choice for diagnosing infection with Neisseria gonorrheae. The prevalence of this organism in asymptomatic individuals is so low that screening should be considered only in high-risk groups. These include individuals under age 30 years with at least 2 sexual partners in the previous year or age ≤16 years at first intercourse, prostitutes, and sexual contacts of individuals known to have a sexually transmitted disease (STD). Of greater note is the increase in penicillin-resistant organisms necessitating changes in antibiotic management. Previous studies have shown that treatment is efficacious.

Burden of Suffering

In 1992, gonorrhea was the second most frequently reported notifiable disease in Canada. However, the incidence of the disease, which peaked at 56,336 cases in 1981, has decreased steadily to 9,045 cases in 1992.<1> In 1987, 15-29 year-olds accounted for 78% of all reported cases in Canada. In 1988, the rate for females 15-19 years old surpassed that in both males and females aged 20-24 due to less of a decline in the younger female group.

In the U.S., gonorrhea was the most frequently reported sexually transmitted disease with 24% to 30% of cases occurring in adolescents. Rates per 100,000 dropped from 573 to 327 cases in males and 356 to 230 cases in females between 1981 and 1991.<2> The highest rate of 1,044 cases per 100,000 is currently in adolescent girls 15-19 years. U.S. rates are highest in black adolescents – the proportion with infection varying regionally from 3.5% to 7.3%. Although gonorrhea is a reportable disease, it is possible that some of the differences result from differential reporting or detection at private physicians' offices versus publically funded clinics. In the former setting, treatment may be administered without laboratory confirmation of infection. This, in turn, may lead to decreased reporting.

While the overall incidence of gonorrhea has been declining, the proportion of gonorrhea organisms that are antibiotic-resistant has been increasing. The first cases of penicillinase-producing *Neisseria*

[1] Formerly Research Associate, Canadian Task Force on the Periodic Health Examination, Department of Pediatrics, Dalhousie University, Halifax, Nova Scotia
[2] Associate Professor of Pediatrics and of Preventive Medicine and Biostatistics, University of Toronto, Toronto, Ontario

gonorrhoeae (PPNG) in Canada and the United States were reported in 1976.<3,4> Only 0.5% of all reported gonorrhea cases in Canada in 1985 were caused by PPNG, compared to 5.5% in 1989, an 11-fold increase.<3> There were PPNG outbreaks in both Ontario and Quebec in 1988.<5> The number of reported cases of PPNG increased from 591 in 1988 to 1046 in 1989.<3> The proportions are highest in Quebec (9.9%) and Ontario (8.6%),<3> where rates are well above the hyperendemic cut-off of 3.0%.<6> Preliminary figures for Ontario and British Columbia for the first half of 1990 show that the percentage of reported cases of gonorrhea due to PPNG has doubled since 1989 in these two provinces.<3,6,7> There have been several major outbreaks of PPNG in several centers in the United States.<4,8,9>

In the U.S., the proportion increased from less than 1% in 1985 to 7% in 1989. In one survey of resistance patterns during 1991, 32% of *N. gonorrheae* were penicillin or tetracycline resistant.<10> However, this survey was conducted in a sentinel system for early detection of resistant bacteria and is therefore an overestimate of the national problem.

Gonococcal infection may be symptomatic, asymptomatic and/or complicated and may involve various anatomical sites. The majority of patients have anogenital and/or pharyngeal infection. Local complications may include epididymitis, lymphangitis, penile edema and urethral stricture in men, and salpingitis or pelvic inflammatory disease in women, as well as systemic complications in men or women, including disseminated gonococcal infection, endocarditis and meningitis. Over 90% of pharyngeal infections are asymptomatic. Women and unborn children carry the major physical impact of gonorrhea in the Western world. Compared with the relatively inconsequential acute gonorrhea in males, gonococcal infections in females lead much more frequently to hospitalization and surgery. Pelvic inflammatory disease (PID), a serious complication of 10-20% of gonococcal infections, can result in serious medical sequelae such as infertility, ectopic pregnancy, and chronic pelvic pain. (PID is also discussed in the Chapter 46 on preventing unintended pregnancy in adolescents). More than 80% of the total cost of gonococcal infections in the U.S. health care system in 1976 went for care necessitated by gonococcal PID.

Maneuver

Given the overall low infection rates, screening of the general population is inappropriate. Several studies have examined risk factors for infection, including a family practice based Canadian study.<11> In this study, two factors were found to be predictive of infection in asymptomatic patients after adjustment in a logistic model: history of contact with a case of STD and age less than 30 years.

In another study in Boston, culture specimens for gonorrhea were obtained from 1,441 obstetric and gynecology patients receiving routine pelvic examinations.<12> Information on sexual history and symptoms was obtained through a self-administered, 50-item questionnaire. Twenty-five (1.7%) women had positive cultures for gonorrhea. Multivariate analysis showed five factors were independently associated with gonococcal infection: partners with gonorrhea or urethral discharge (Odds Ratio = 5.7), endocervical bleeding induced by swab (OR = 4.6), age at first intercourse ≤16 (OR = 4.2), payment by Medicaid (OR = 2.8), and low abdominal or pelvic pain (OR = 2.6). Race was not an independent risk factor. The authors calculated that the risk of infection for a woman with one or more risk factors was 2.5%, compared to 0.2% for a woman with no risk factors.

A group in Cleveland devised a diagnostic index for estimating the probability of cervical infection with either gonorrhea or chlamydia.<13> The index, developed from examining and questioning 190 gynecologic patients, identified three independent predictors of cervical infection: age, purulent vaginal discharge, and high-risk sexual contact (a new partner in the prior 6 months, or a partner with a suspected genital infection). Points were assigned to the variables based on their multiple regression logistic coefficients, as follows: age <20 years – 2 points; age 20-29 years, 1 point; and 1 point each for purulent vaginal discharge and high-risk sexual contact. When the diagnostic index was tested on 588 women, the rate of cervical infection was directly associated with the index scores (p<0.001), with infection occurring in 28% of women with 3 or 4 points, 7% of women with 2 points, 3% of women with 1 point, and 0% of women with 0 points.

Gram stain and culture remain the most widely available and accurate method to identify *N. gonorrheae*

The standard diagnostic tests for gonorrhea are culture and Gram stain of clinical specimens. However, they have some limitations. The specificity of stained smears is 95-100% at all anatomical sites, and its diagnostic sensitivity for urethral specimens from males with acute symptomatic gonorrhea is high, ranging from 90-95%.<14> The Gram stain is relatively insensitive in asymptomatic males (50-70%), for female anogenital infections (45-70%), and for all pharyngeal and rectal infections.

Bacterial cultures have superior diagnostic sensitivity for female anogenital gonorrhea, male asymptomatic gonorrhea, and all pharyngeal gonococcal infections. In women, single endocervical cultures are estimated to have a sensitivity of 80-95%. Culture procedures may be limited by the inhibition of growth by antibiotics in the selective culture medium, such as the failure to detect vancomycin-susceptible strains using the usual culture medium. Also, results may be unsatisfactory if clinical specimens are inadequate or if the medium is not quality controlled, stored, inoculated, incubated and transported properly.

More recently developed diagnostic maneuvers include serological tests to detect serum antigonococcal antibodies, tests for specific endotoxins, enzymes or fatty acids, demonstration of gonococcal antigens using enzyme immunoassays or DNA hybridization techniques. Alternatives to Gram stain and culture have not been studied in an asymptomatic population. Studies in symptomatic individuals with urethral or vaginal discharge may not be generalizable to a population visiting their physician who do not have such complaints.

Serology, which was developed for population screening, is not accurate enough for detection.[3] Similarly, tests for gonococcal bacterial products are also insufficiently accurate when compared with bacterial culture.

Enzyme immunoassays for detection of gonococcal antigens in male urethral specimens have a sensitivity and specificity of 95% or more. These immunoassays also have a very high accuracy when performed on urine as compared with male urethral specimens.[4] Because obtaining urine specimens for diagnosis is substantially less uncomfortable, this diagnostic method may be of use in screening if accuracy is as high in asymptomatic men. However, the sensitivity and specificity of this test on specimens taken from the female genital tract range from 60% to 100% and 70% to 98%, respectively.[5]

Assays based on DNA hybridization techniques are limited to laboratories with molecular diagnostic capabilities. Sensitivity and specificity of this method were found to be greater than 97% and 99%, respectively.[6,8] Again, the accuracy of this method compared with culture is higher for male urethral specimens than for female cervical specimens. This methodology, however, will not shorten time for diagnosis to a clinically significant degree. Furthermore, diagnostic tests which reveal the presence or absence of N. gonorrheae do not give information about antibiotic susceptibility.

Effectiveness of Prevention and Treatment

Antibiotics for Treatment of Uncomplicated Gonorrhea

Early detection of gonorrhea in asymptomatic persons may prevent the development of complications, through antibiotic treatment. It may also facilitate the notification of sexual contacts.

If N. gonorrheae is susceptible to penicillin, oral amoxicillin remains the drug of choice for management, because it is relatively inexpensive. In areas with a high frequency of resistant N. gonorrheae, however, alternative agents are now the first line drugs. In general, these newer agents are substantially more expensive than amoxicillin. In uncontrolled trials, ceftriaxone had an average cure rate of 99.2%;

the cure rate for four different quinolones ranged from 93.3% to 100%, with an average of 99.5%. Numerous clinical trials have now been conducted comparing the efficacy of a number of quinolones to intramuscular ceftriaxone. The advantage of the quinolones and cefixime, another third generation cephalosporin, is that they may be administered orally. No significant difference has been observed with single-dose oral agents compared with ceftriaxone.[9,15] Because the efficacy rate of treatment of uncomplicated gonorrhea should be at least 95%, recommendations to evaluate new treatments rigorously have been made.[16]

Impact of Educational Interventions

Three controlled trials have examined the impact of an educational intervention at the initial STD visit on treatment behavior and compliance. Giving patients educational pamphlets on gonorrhea did not increase the overall follow-up rate in men, compared to a control group, but did increase the rate of follow-up attendance in women.[17] In one U.S. study, 340 men diagnosed with gonorrhea were given either routine counselling about medication and follow-up, or an intensive educational counselling session based on six compliance-enhancing strategies.[18] Compliance with taking medication was not affected, but the educational intervention increased the follow-up attendance rate from 66% in the control group to 71% in the experimental group (p=0.05). Similarly, a ten-minute soap-opera style educational videotape which was randomly shown or not shown to 902 men diagnosed with gonorrhea did not affect the patients' willingness to contact all their sexual partners, but did increase the rate of attendance for follow-up, from 43.3% in the control group to 53.5% in the experimental group (p<0.003).[19]

Prevention Maneuvers

Primary prevention through avoiding exposure is the best means of controlling the spread of gonorrhea and other STDs. Condoms, used properly, may reduce the risk of infection and transmission. There is epidemiological and case-control evidence that consistent condom use does reduce the frequency of gonorrhea.[20] There are also indications that condom use may be increasing, at least in selected populations. However, there are no data on the frequency or causes of either user failure or product failure.

There has also been a general assumption, and some epidemiological evidence, that spermicidal preparations help to prevent gonococcal infections. However, large-scale well-designed studies have been lacking. A recent randomized, double-blind, placebo-controlled trial of 818 women has clearly shown benefit from the use of a vaginal gel containing Nonoxynol-9.[21] The study, which had a six-month follow-up rate of 78% (n=636, spermicide group, 317; placebo group,

319), found that the relative rate of gonococcal infection in the spermicide group was 0.75 (90% confidence limits, 0.58 and 0.96). Among women reporting at least 50% compliance, the relative rate was reduced to 0.61 (p=0.0031; 95% confidence limits, 0.42 and 0.87). (Also see Chapter 46).

Recommendations of Others

In 1989, the U.S. Preventive Services Task Force recommended that routine cultures for gonorrhea be performed in high-risk groups, including prostitutes, persons with multiple sexual partners or whose partner has multiple sexual partners, persons with a history of repeated episodes of gonorrhea, and sexual contacts of persons with gonorrhea.<22> Specific treatment regimens were not addressed.

The U.S. Centers for Disease Control recommend that all cases should be diagnosed or confirmed by culture, to facilitate a system of antibiotic susceptibility testing. Their recommended treatment regimen for uncomplicated urogenital or rectal infection is a single intramuscular dose of Ceftriaxone 250 mg, plus Doxycycline 100 mg orally twice daily for 7 days to treat for presumptive coexisting chlamydial infection.

The Laboratory Centre for Disease Control in Canada recommends ceftriaxone as a preferred treatment plus tetracycline or doxycycline (for *Chlamydia trachomatis*).<23> Alternatives to ceftriaxone have been listed as spectinomycin, ciprofloxacin, cefixime or cefuroxime axetil. In areas with active monitoring for resistance and resistance levels below 3%, oral amoxicillin or ampicillin with probenecid may replace ceftriaxone. High-risk groups for screening include sexual contacts of cases, sexually active adolescents, children who have been sexually abused and their siblings, and adults with two or more of the following risk factors: age under 25, ≥2 sexual partners in the previous year, a new sexual partner within the previous two months, a history of STD, non-use of contraception or use of non-barrier methods, and anal intercourse with a high-risk partner. They also strongly recommend screening for women who are pregnant, seeking an abortion, or being seen for insertion of an IUD.

Conclusions and Recommendations

Abstinence is the most effective way to prevent transmission of STDs. There is also fair evidence to support the use of condoms. Given the effectiveness of counselling, educational pamphlets and educational videotape in improving compliance with clinic follow-up, there is fair evidence to provide counselling or educational materials to prevent the spread of gonorrhea (B Recommendation).

The low prevalence rate of infection with *N. gonorrheae* would make mass screening of the general population an inefficient intervention (D Recommendation). However, screening should be performed in certain populations: 1) individuals under 30 years, particularly adolescents, with at least 2 sexual partners in the previous year; 2) prostitutes; 3) sexual contacts of individuals known to have a sexually transmitted disease; and 4) age ≤16 years at first intercourse (A Recommendation). The frequency with which such screening should take place has not been examined, but subjects are presumably at risk when they continue behaviours that place them at increased risk, such as prostitution.

Intramuscular ceftriaxone or oral quinolones, cefuroxime axetil, and cefixime should be used as initial therapy unless there is epidemiologic information indicating that the patient is unlikely to be infected with a resistant strain of *N. gonorrheae*. An effective agent against *C. trachomatis* should be initiated at the same time because of the high frequency of co-infection.

Because of the high rates of penicillin resistance, treatment of gonorrhea should be initiated with ceftriaxone, cefixime or a quinolone

Unanswered Questions (Research Agenda)

The test characteristics of newer diagnostic methods, particularly less invasive urine tests, should be studied in asymptomatic subjects. These would be more acceptable specimens for mass screening. Whereas, current management of patients attending sexually transmitted disease clinics includes initiation of treatment prior to laboratory confirmation, rapid tests may be particularly helpful when screening asymptomatic individuals. A trial of early initiation of antibiotics compared with specific therapy in subjects with proven infections is indicated in this setting. More information is needed on the most efficient frequency of screening. Methods to increase the wearing of condoms need to be studied, particularly since condoms may prevent the transmission of many infectious pathogens in addition to *N. gonorrheae*. Diligent surveillance with culture and susceptibility testing in sentinel sites continues to be needed to provide warning about the development of resistance to newer anti-infective agents. As new drugs become available, clinical trials should determine their efficacy with more resistant organisms.

Evidence

A MEDLINE search was conducted using the major MESH heading Gonorrhea, with the subheadings Complications, Diagnosis, Drug Therapy, Epidemiology, Prevention and Control, Therapy, and Transmission, for the years 1981 to January 1994. Relevant articles identified through the search were reviewed, with emphasis on screening and treatment. Pertinent references from these studies were also reviewed, along with references from recent review articles. In general, priority was placed on articles that dealt with trials, rather than editorials, case reports, letters or commentaries. Only published articles were reviewed. This review was initiated in November 1991 and recommendations were finalized by the Task Force in March 1994.

Selected References

1. Notifiable Diseases Summary. *Canada Communic Dis Rep* 1993; 19-11: 84

2. Webster LA, Berman SM, Greenspan JR: Surveillance for gonorrhea and primary and secondary syphilis among adolescents, United States – 1981-1991. *MMWR* 1993; 42: 1-11

3. *Canada Dis Wkly Rep* 1991; 17: 49-50

4. Gorwitz RJ, Nakashima AK, Moran JS, *et al*: Sentinel surveillance for antimicrobial resistance in Neisseria gonorrhoeae-United States, 1988-1991. The gonococcal isolate surveillance project study group. *MMWR CDC Surveillance Summaries* 1993; 42: 29-39

5. Allard R, Robert J, Turgeon P, *et al*: Predictors of asymptomatic gonorrhea among patients seen by private practitioners. *Can Med Assoc J* 1985; 133: 1135-1139, 1146

6. Phillips RS, Hanff PA, Wertheimer A, *et al*: Gonorrhea in women seen for routine gynecologic care: Criteria for testing. *Am J Med* 1988; 85: 177-182

7. Rosenthal GE, Mettler G, Pare S, *et al*: A new diagnostic index for predicting cervical infection with either *Chlamydia trachomatis* or *Neisseria gonorrhoeae*. *J Gen Intern Med* 1990; 5: 319-326

8. Goh BT, Varia KB, Ayliffe PF, *et al*: Diagnosis of gonorrhea by gram-stained smears and cultures in men and women: Role of the urethral smear. *Sex Transm Dis* 1985; 12: 135-139

9. Beebe JL: Physician utilization of a gonococcal antibody screening test. *Sex Transm Dis* 1983; 10: 195-197

10. Papapetropoulou M, Detorakis J, Arkoulis A, *et al*: Screening for asymptomatic gonorrhea in males: A comparison of four techniques. *J Chemother* 1990; 2: 37-39

11. Lieberman RW, Wheelock JB: The diagnosis of gonorrhea in a low-prevalence female population: Enzyme immunoassay versus culture. *Obstet Gynecol* 1987; 69: 743-746

12. Vlaspolder F, Mutsaers JA, Blog F, *et al*: Value of a DNA probe assay (Gen-Probe) compared with that of culture for diagnosis of gonococcal infection. *J Clin Microbiol* 1993; 31: 107-110

13. Hale YM, Melton ME, Lewis JS, *et al*: Evaluation of the PACE 2 Neisseria gonorrheae assay by three public health laboratories. *J Clin Microbiol* 1993; 31: 451-453

14. Handsfield HH, McCormack WM, Hook EW, *et al*: A comparison of single-dose cefixime with ceftriaxone as treatment for uncomplicated gonorrhea. The gonorrhea treatment study group. *N Engl J Med* 1991; 325: 1337-1341

15. Smith BL, Mogabgab WJ, Dalu ZA, *et al*: Multicenter trial of fleroxacin versus ceftriaxone in the treatment of uncomplicated gonorrhea. *Am J Med* 1993; 94(3A): 81S-84S

16. Handsfield HH, McCuchan JA, Corey L, *et al*: Evaluation of new anti-infective drugs for the treatment of uncomplicated gonorrhea in adults and adolescents. Infectious Diseases Society of America and the Food and Drug Administration. *Clin Infect Dis* 1992; 15 Suppl: S123-S130

17. Bewley S: Who defaults after treatment for gonorrhoea? Randomised controlled study of effect of an educational leaflet. *Genitourin Med* 1988; 64: 241-244

18. Blonna R, Legos P, Burlack P: The effects of an STD educational intervention on follow-up appointment keeping and medication-taking compliance. *Sex Transm Dis* 1989; 16: 198-200

19. Solomon MZ, deJong W: The impact of a clinic-based educational videotape on knowledge and treatment behavior of men with gonorrhea. *Sex Transm Dis* 1988; 15: 127-132

20. Condoms for prevention of sexually transmitted diseases. *MMWR* 1988; 37: 133-137

21. Louv WC, Austin H, Alexander WJ, *et al*: A clinical trial of Nonoxynol-9 for preventing gonococcal and chlamydial infections. *J Infect Dis* 1988; 158: 518-523

22. U.S Preventive Services Task Force: *Guide to Clinical Preventive Services: An Assessment of the Effectiveness of 169 Interventions.* Williams & Wilkins, Baltimore, Md, 1989: 135-137, 331-336

23. Interim guidelines for the treatment of uncomplicated gonococcal infection. *Can Med Assoc J* 1992; 146: 1587-8, 1591-1592

Prevention of Gonorrhea

MANEUVER	EFFECTIVENESS	LEVEL OF EVIDENCE <REF>	RECOMMENDATION
Counselling, educational pamphlets, educational videotape	Counselling and educational materials result in no increase in compliance with medications or willingness to inform sexual contacts, but increase compliance with clinic follow-up.	Randomized controlled tirals<17-19> (1)	Fair evidence to provide counselling to prevent spread of gonorrhea (B)
	Abstinence prevents transmission of sexually transmitted disease (STD) and use of condoms reduces STD transmission	Case-control study<20> (11-2)	
Screening for *N. gonorrheae* with Gram stain and culture of cervical or urethral smear	Screening the general population has low yield. Yield higher with increased prevalence in high-risk* subpopulation.	Cohort studies<5-7> (11-2)	Fair evidence not to screen the general population (D); good evidence to screen those at high-risk* (A)
	Good evidence that treatment of patients with gonorrhea with ceftriaxone, oral cephalosporins, or quinolones results in >95% eradication.	Randomized controlled trials<14-16> (1)	

High-risk groups include: individuals under age 30 years with at least 2 sexual partners in the previous year or age ≤16 years at first intercourse, prostitutes, sexual contacts of individuals known to have a sexually transmitted disease.

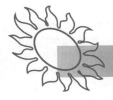

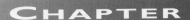

CHAPTER **60**

Screening for Chlamydial Infection

By H. Dele Davies

Screening for Chlamydial Infection

Prepared by H. Dele Davies, MD, MSc, FRCPC[1]

In 1984, the Canadian Task Force on the Periodic Health Examination found that there was fair evidence to support exclusion of routine screening of the general population for chlamydial infections (D Recommendation), poor evidence to support inclusion or exclusion of screening for high risk groups (C Recommendation), and fair evidence to support screening of pregnant women (B Recommendation).<1> After review of the literature published subsequently, the Task Force now recommends screening for both high-risk groups and pregnant women (B Recommendations) but not for the general population (D Recommendation). The basis of these recommendations includes:

1. *The burden of illness caused by asymptomatic chlamydial infections and their sequelae is high;*

2. *Currently available screening tests are accurate, reliable and cost effective for high-risk groups;*

3. *Effective treatment is available; and*

4. *Earlier detection leads to improved health outcome, consisting of prevention of symptomatic disease in high risk non-pregnant women and men and improved outcome of pregnancy.*

Burden of Suffering

At highest risk for chlamydial infection are sexually active young women with new or multiple partners in the preceding year

Infection with *Chlamydia trachomatis* is the most common sexually transmitted disease (STD) in North America, causing two to five times more infections than *Neisseria gonorrhea*. In Canada, the incidence is 216 per 100,000 population.<2> Most infections in females (60-80%) are asymptomatic, but the disease spectrum includes mucopurulent cervicitis (MPC), endometritis, salpingitis, the urethral syndrome, proctitis, post-abortal pelvic sepsis and perihepatitis. In numerous case-control and cohort studies chlamydial infection has been associated with the long-term complications of pelvic inflammatory disease (PID), infertility and ectopic pregnancy. Serologic studies suggest that 64% or more of tubal infertility and 42% of ectopic pregnancies are attributable to chlamydial infection. Screening in different female populations in Canada have shown carrier rates of 1% to 25%. In Canada the women at highest risk for chlamydial infection are those who are sexually active and aged 15-19 years, followed by

---

[1] Assistant Professor of Microbiology, of Infectious Diseases and of Pediatrics, University of Calgary, Calgary, Alberta

20-25 years.<2> Other factors associated with increased risk of infection include: intercourse with 2 or more partners per year or a new partner in the preceding year, low socioeconomic class, use of non barrier contraception, intermenstrual bleeding, cervical friability and purulent discharge on examination. Infection rates in pregnant women range from 5% to 25%. In prospective cohort studies, 11% to 44% of infants born to mothers infected with chlamydia developed conjunctivitis and 11-20% developed pneumonia<3-6> during the first year of life.

In males, the spectrum of disease due to *C. trachomatis* includes urethritis, epididymitis, prostatitis and occasionally proctitis or proctocolitis via homosexual transmission. Up to 50% of reported cases of non-gonococcal urethritis and 31% of cases of acute epididymitis are due to *C. trachomatis*. One percent to 21% of all men may be asymptomatic carriers and act as a reservoir for spread. Younger age, multiple sexual partners in the preceding year, and a history of gonorrhea in the past year are associated with increased likelihood of chlamydial infections in males.

Maneuver

There is no simple, inexpensive laboratory test for diagnosing *C. trachomatis* infections, and different anatomical sites require different screening tests. In adult females, examination with a speculum and endocervical swabs are the appropriate methods. In prepubertal females, the immature vagina is the genital site of infection with *C. trachomatis* and *N. gonorrhea*. Thus, a speculum examination to obtain a cervical specimen is both unnecessary and potentially traumatic.

Cervical swab for chlamydial culture has an estimated sensitivity of 75% to 90%, and a specificity of 100% but test time is 2-3 days. Cotton tipped aluminum and rayon tipped plastic swabs are superior to calcium alginate or cotton tipped wooden swabs for maximum yield of culture. This mode of diagnosis of *C. trachomatis* is expensive and time consuming, and requires technical expertise unavailable to most clinical laboratories. Cytologic testing using Giemsa or other methods is 95-100% sensitive for detecting conjunctivitis, but has low sensitivity for diagnosis of genital infections. Direct fluorescent antibody (DFA) testing using fluorescein-conjugated monoclonal antibodies and enzyme-linked immuno-assays (EIA) are the most widely used non-culture techniques for diagnosing cervical infections in clinical practice. DFA test time ranges from 15 minutes to 1 hour while EIA requires from 3-5 hours. They are not recommended for use on throat and rectal specimens from sexually abused children because chlamydia may cross react with bacterial flora giving false positive results. DFA sensitivity is 70-100% and specificity is 85-98% when compared to culture of cervical and urethral specimens in women.<7-9> The

Culture is the diagnostic standard but EIA, DFA or nucleic acid probes are adequate for most routine screening

sensitivity and positive predictive value of DFA decrease significantly as the prevalence of chlamydia in the population decreases. EIA has a sensitivity of 67-98% for cervical infections and specificity can be increased from 85% to almost 100% by the use of confirmatory blocking antibody assays.<10>

In men, *C. trachomatis* infections have traditionally been diagnosed by culture, DFA or EIA on urethral swabs. However, in contrast to women, testing of first void urine (FVU) specimens gives a yield that approaches that of urethral swabs. This represents a non-invasive alternative for chlamydial screening.<11,12>

Polymerase chain reaction (PCR) testing of cervical specimens in women and FVU specimens in men is 95% – 100% sensitive and almost 100% specific and its use may become more widespread with the availability of commercial kits.<13,14> Nucleic acid probes are about 95% sensitive and 98 – 100% specific when compared to culture, are available in 2-4 hours, and like EIA can be used for large volumes of samples, but are currently limited by high cost.

Effectiveness of Screening and Treatment

Although effective treatment is available for chlamydial infections, no controlled studies have demonstrated that screening of non-pregnant men or women leads to reduction in complications.

No controlled trials demonstrate that screening men or non-pregnant women reduces long-term complications

Treatment of C. Trachomatis

Tetracyclines are the drugs of choice for treatment of *C. trachomatis* infections in non-pregnant females and in males.<15,16> The recommended dosage is 500 mg by mouth, four times a day for 7 days or doxycycline 100 mg by mouth, two times a day for 7 days.

Traditionally, erythromycin 500 mg by mouth, four times a day for 7 days has been recommended for pregnant women and for those in whom tetracycline is contraindicated. Erythromycin is curative in 90% or more of patients who are able to take it.<17> The major drawback of the 2 g dose is the high incidence of gastrointestinal side effects. Amoxicillin 500 mg by mouth, three times a day for 7 days was shown in a recent double-blind randomized trial to be equal in efficacy to erythromycin, but with fewer dropouts due to side effects.

More recently, introduction of azithromycin has raised the prospect of single dose therapy. In prospective studies,<18-21> a single 1 g dose of oral azithromycin was as effective as 100 mg of doxycycline given twice a day for 7 days in eradicating uncomplicated urogenital *C. trachomatis* infections in men and women. Side-effects (mainly gastrointestinal) were mild and of equal frequency in both treatment groups. Azithromycin is licensed in the United States but is not currently available in Canada. Ofloxacin 300 mg twice a day for

7 days is also efficacious for treatment of uncomplicated infections in non-pregnant women,[22] but is expensive for first line usage.

Studies of Screening for Chlamydia in Pregnancy and Outcome

Five published studies have assessed the outcome in screened pregnant women.[23-27] The first study[23] was retrospective cohort in nature with a 5.8% incidence of chlamydial infection among 5,875 pregnant women screened with DFA during their first prenatal visits and then every 2 to 3 months. Infected patients who were successfully treated with erythromycin had significantly lower rates of premature delivery (2.87%) compared to those who failed therapy (13.92%) and those who were negative for chlamydia (11.89%). There were also significantly lower rates of premature rupture of membranes (PROM), premature contractions, and small for gestational age (SGA) infants in those successfully treated compared with those who failed treatment. Similarly, in a prospective cohort study[24] involving 11,554 women screened with culture at their first prenatal visit, 1,110 were treated with erythromycin, 1,323 were left untreated and 9,111 were not infected. PROM and SGA babies were twice as common in the untreated group compared with the treated and uninfected groups. There was also a four-fold improvement in perinatal mortality in the treated compared to the untreated group.

The third study[27] provided weak evidence of improved outcome of screening. During their third trimester, 1,082 women were cultured for *C. trachomatis*. Eighty five (7.8%) were positive for chlamydia, and erythromycin therapy (500 mg twice a day for 10 days) was prescribed for 38 of these women. There were no complications in the treated women compared with complications in 5 of 47 untreated women (chorioamnionitis, endometritis, post partum fever, and a growth retarded infant). Only 37 infants from the original 85 (41%) were available for follow-up. In all these positive studies, the main value of screening may have been due to other effects of erythromycin and not necessarily the eradication of chlamydia. Erythromycin in the 3rd trimester for women infected with *Ureaplasma urealyticum* and *Mycoplasma hominis* also reduced the incidence of low birth weight infants and increased mean birth weights.[28]

A fourth study[25] of poorer quality found no difference in incidence of infant pneumonia and conjunctivitis in treated and untreated women screened for chlamydia from a high prevalence (26%) population. This study was limited by small sample size (199 women) and by the possibility of other confounding factors in untreated women. A final prospective cohort study[26] involved 184 pregnant women screened for chlamydia by culture at their first prenatal visit and treated with erythromycin at 36 weeks gestation. Seventy-seven women (42%) were lost from the study; only 83 infants had complete follow-up. Using chlamydial disease as end point, 2 treated infants had pneumonia and 1 had conjunctivitis (3/59 or 5% total complication rate), compared with infants of 4 untreated women with pneumonia and 1 with conjunctivitis (5/24 or 21% total complication rate).

Thus, three cohort studies[23,24,27] have provided fair (Level II) evidence for screening and intervention leading to better outcome for some perinatal complications. Of the remaining two smaller studies,[25,26] one supported, but the other did not support screening.

Contact Tracing

Contact tracing is an integral part of attempts at chlamydia control. In most studies, men are more efficient in transmitting *C. trachomatis* to their female partners with spread 40-64% of the time, whereas women transmit the infection to their male partner 21-35% of the time.[29-33] However, given the efficiency of transmission, and despite difficulties in tracing partners, treatment of contacts may be more cost effective than screening.

Costs and Economic Evaluations

Chlamydial infections are estimated to cost over U.S. $2.2 billion a year in the U.S.[34] Infections in women account for over 79% of this cost.

Economic evaluations support chlamydial screening of asymptomatic persons under specific conditions. Phillips *et al*[35] used decision analysis to estimate the clinical and economic implications of testing for cervical infection caused by *C. trachomatis* in asymptomatic women during routine gynecologic visits. A strategy of no routine testing was compared with one involving routine cultures or use of non-culture tests (DFA or EIA). They concluded that the use of the non-culture tests would reduce overall costs if the prevalence of infection was 7% or greater, and routine cultures if the prevalence was 14% or more.

In Canada, Estany *et al*[36] calculated that screening with DFA or EIA in women would be cost effective if the prevalences of chlamydial infection by each method exceeded 6% and 7% respectively. The mean cost of DFA and EIA was estimated at $11. Sensitivity analysis showed that the two most important factors in cost savings were the probability of developing PID and the cost of the test. Sellors *et al*[37] recently determined that selective screening of sexually active young women with EIA is an effective and efficient strategy for detecting chlamydia. Their model was based on average cost of $8.66 for culture and $9.33 for EIA. Nettleman *et al*[38] estimated that DFA testing of all pregnant women would be cost effective if the test cost less than U.S. $6.30 or the prevalence of infection exceeded 6%.

Recommendations of Others

In 1989 the U.S. Preventive Services Task Force[39] recommended routine screening for asymptomatic persons at high risk of infection, and at the first prenatal visit for pregnant women in high-risk categories. These recommendations are currently being reviewed. The Canadian Expert Interdisciplinary Advisory Committee on Sexually Transmitted Diseases in Children and Youths[15] suggested more extensive screening, but many of their screening recommendations were intended for detection of STDs other than chlamydia. Children recommended for screening by this committee included sexual contacts of people with proven or suspected urethritis or other STDs, sexual contacts of high-risk adults, pregnant adolescents, male and female prostitutes, street youth, users of illicit drugs, young women undergoing therapeutic abortion, those with a history of previous STDs, children and siblings of children who have been sexually abused, and neonates with one or both parents known to have urethritis, cervicitis, PID, epidydimitis or other STDs.

More recently, the Centers for Disease Control have suggested screening women with MPC, sexually active women <20 years of age, women 20-24 years of age who are inconsistent in their use of barrier contraceptives or having new or more than one sex partner during the last 3 months.[40]

Conclusions and Recommendations

Although there is sufficient evidence linking chlamydial infections to many complications, there is currently insufficient evidence in males and non-pregnant females to show that screening is effective in preventing these complications. Thus routine screening is not recommended in the general population (D Recommendation). However, the high burden of illness caused by chlamydia and favourable economic evaluation studies suggest that screening of certain populations at high risk for asymptomatic chlamydial infection may be useful to try and prevent symptoms and to reduce overall cost of infection (B Recommendation). These high risk groups are – sexually active females less than 25 years old, new partner or two partners in preceding year, cervical friability, use of non-barrier contraception and women symptomatic with mucopurulent discharge or intermenstrual bleeding. Although the benefits may be related to treatment with erythromycin, there is fair evidence (Level II-2) that screening of pregnant women leads to improvements in pregnancy outcome (B Recommendation).

Unanswered Questions (Research Agenda)

A prospective, well designed randomized community trial of screening for chlamydial infections in two similar asymptomatic populations for development of complications is warranted.

Evidence

The literature was identified with a MEDLINE search conducted by exploding the major MESH heading Chlamydial trachomatis with the subheadings complications, diagnosis, drug therapy, economics, epidemiology, etiology, history, microbiology, mortality, prevention and control, therapy, and transmission, for the years 1983 through 1993.

This review was initiated in June 1992 and the recommendations finalized by the task force in October 1992.

Acknowledgements

The Task Force would like to acknowledge the help of Robert C. Brunham, MD, FRCPC, Professor and Head, Department of Medical Microbiology, University of Manitoba, Winnipeg, Manitoba, John W. Sellors, MSc(DME), MD, CCFP, FCFP, Associate Clinical Professor, McMaster University, Hamilton, Ontario and Paul R. Gully, MB, ChB, FFCM, FRCPC, Chief, Division of STD control, Health Protection Branch, Health Canada, Ottawa, Ontario for very useful comments on the technical report.

Selected References

1. Canadian Task Force on the Periodic Health Examination: The periodic health examination. *Can Med Assoc J* 1984; 130: 1278-1285

2. Gully P: Chlamydial infection in Canada. *Can Med Assoc J* 1992; 147(6): 893-896

3. Frommell GT, Rothenberg R, Wang S, *et al*: Chlamydial infection of mothers and their infants. *J Pediatr* 1979; 95: 28-32

4. Schachter J, Grossman M, Sweet RL, *et al*: Prospective study of perinatal transmission of *Chlamydia trachomatis*. *JAMA* 1986; 255(24): 3374-3377

5. Schachter J, Grossman M, Holt J, *et al*: Prospective study of chlamydial infections in neonates. *Lancet* 1979; 2(8139): 377-380

6. Hammerschlag MR, Anderka M, Semine D, *et al*: Prospective study of maternal and infantile infection with *Chlamydia trachomatis*. *Pediatrics* 1979; 64(2): 142-148

7. Forbes BA, Bartholoma N, McMillan J, *et al*: Evaluation of a monoclonal antibody test to detect chlamydia in cervical and urethral specimens. *J Clin Microbiol* 1986; 23(6): 1136-1137

8. Shafer M-A, Vaughan E, Lipkin ES, *et al*: Evaluation of fluorescein-conjugated monoclonal antibody test to detect *Chlamydia trachomatis* endocervical infections in adolescent girls. *J Pediatr* 1986; 108(5 Pt 1): 779-783

9. Stamm WE, Harrison HR, Alexander ER, *et al*: Diagnosis of *Chlamydia trachomatis* infections by direct immunofluorescence staining of genital secretions. *Ann Intern Med* 1984; 101(5): 638-641

10. Moncada J, Schachter J, Bolan G, *et al*: Confirmatory assay increases specificity of the chlamydiazyme test for *Chlamydia trachomatis* infection of the cervix. *J Clin Microbiol* 1990; 28: 1770-1773

11. Sellors J, Mahony J, Jang D, *et al*: Rapid, on site diagnosis of chlamydia urethritis in men by detection of antigens in urethral swabs and urine. *J Clin Microbiol* 1991; 29: 407-409

12. Chernesky M, Castriciano S, Sellors J, *et al*: Detection of *Chlamydia trachomatis* antigens in urine as an alternative to swabs and cultures. *J Infect Dis* 1990; 161: 124-126

13. Mahony JB, Luinstra KE, Sellors JW, *et al*: Confirmatory polymerase chain reaction testing for *Chlamydia trachomatis* in first – void urine from asymptomatic and symptomatic men. *J Clin Microbiol* 1992; 30(9): 2241-2245

14. Jaschek G, Gaydos CA, Welsh LE, *et al*: Direct detection of *Chlamydia trachomatis* in urine specimens from symptomatic and asymptomatic men by using a rapid polymerase chain reaction assay. *J Clin Microbiol* 1993; 31(5): 1209-1212

15. Health and Welfare Canada: Canadian guidelines for screening for *Chlamydia trachomatis* infection. *Can Dis Wkly Rep* 1989; 15(S5): 1-12

16. Centers for Disease Control: 1989 sexually transmitted diseases guidelines. *MMWR* 1989; 38(S-8): 1-43

17. Linnemann CC Jr, Heaton CL, Ritchey M: Treatment of *Chlamydia trachomatis* infections: comparison of 1- and 2-g doses of erythromycin daily for seven days. *Sex Transm Dis* 1987; 14(2): 102-106

18. Lassus A: Comparative studies of azithromycin in skin and soft-tissue infections and sexually transmitted infections by Neisseria and Chlamydia species. *J Antimicrob Chemother* 1990; 25(Suppl A): 115-121

19. Steingrimsson O, Olafsson JH, Thorarinsson H, *et al*: Azithromycin in the treatment of sexually transmitted disease. *J Antimicrob Chemother* 1990; 25(Suppl A): 109-114

20. Johnson RB: The role of azalide antibiotics in the treatment of Chlamydia. *Am J Obstet Gynecol* 1991; 164(6 Pt 2): 1794-1796

21. Martin DH, Mroczkowski TF, Dalu ZA, *et al*: A controlled trial of a single dose of azithromycin for the treatment of chlamydial urethritis and cervicitis. *N Engl J Med* 1992; 327: 921-925

22. Hooton TM, Batteiger BE, Judson FN, *et al*: Ofloxacin versus doxycycline for treatment of cervical infection with *Chlamydia trachomatis. Antimicrob Agents Chemother* 1992; 36(5): 1144-1146

23. Cohen I, Veille J-C, Calkins BM: Improved pregnancy outcome following successful treatment of chlamydial infection. *JAMA* 1990; 263(23): 3160-3163

24. Ryan GJ, Abdella TN, McNeeley SG, *et al*: *Chlamydia trachomatis* infection in pregnancy and effect of treament on outcome. *Am J Obstet Gynecol* 1990; 162(1): 34-39

25. Black-Payne C, Ahrabi MM, Bocchini JA, *et al*: Treatment of *Chlamydia trachomatis* identified with Chlamydiazyme during pregnancy. Impact on perinatal complications and infants. *J Reprod Med* 1990; 35(4): 362-367

26. Schachter J, Sweet RL, Grossman M, *et al*: Experience with the routine use of erythromycin for chlamydial infections in pregnancy. *N Engl J Med* 1986; 314: 276-279

27. McMillan JA, Weiner LB, Lamberson HV, *et al*: Efficacy of maternal screening and therapy in the prevention of chlamydia infection of the newborn. *Infection* 1985; 13(6): 263-266

28. McCormack WM, Rosner B, Lee YH, *et al*: Effect on birth weight of erythromycin treatment of pregnant women. *Obstet Gynecol* 1987; 69: 202-207

29. Cates W, Wasserheit J: Genital chlamydial infections: epidemiology and reproductive sequelae. *Am J Obstet Gynecol* 1991; 164(6 Pt 2): 1771-1781

30. Stamm WE, Koutsky LA, Beneditti JK, *et al*: *Chlamydia trachomatis* urethral infections in men. *Ann Intern Med* 1984; 100: 47-51

31. Lycke E, Lowhagen GB, Hallhagen G, *et al*: The risk of transmission of genital *Chlamydia trachomatis* infection is less than that of genital Neisseria gonorrhoeae infection. *Sex Transm Dis* 1980; 7: 6-10

32. Leka T, Patrick K, Benenson AS: *Chlamydia trachomatis* urethritis in university men: risk factors and rates. *J Am Board Fam Pract* 1990; 3: 81-86

33. Fish AN, Fairweather DV, Oriel JD, *et al*: *Chlamydia trachomatis* infection in a gynecology clinic population: identification of high-risk groups and the value of contact tracing. *Eur J Obstet Gynecol Reprod Biol* 1989; 31: 67-74

34. Washington AE, Johnson RE, Sanders LL Jr: *Chlamydia trachomatis* infections in the United States. What are they costing us? *JAMA* 1987; 257(15): 2070-2072

35. Phillips RS, Aronson MD, Taylor WC, *et al*: Should tests for *Chlamydia trachomatis* cervical infection be done during routine gynecologic visits? An analysis of the costs of alternative strategies. *Ann Intern Med* 1987; 107(2): 188-194

36. Estany A, Todd M, Vasquez M, *et al*: Early detection of genital chlamydial infection in women: an economic evaluation. *Sex Transm Dis* 1989; 16(1): 21-27

37. Sellors JW, Pickard L, Gafni A, *et al*: Effectiveness and efficiency of selective vs. universal screening for chlamydial infection in sexually active young women. *Arch Intern Med* 1992; 152: 1837-1844

38. Nettleman M, Bell T: Cost-effectiveness of prenatal testing for *Chlamydia trachomatis. Am J Obstet Gynecol* 1991; 164(5 Pt 1): 1289-1294

39. U.S. Preventive Services Task Force: *Guide to Clinical Preventive Services: an Assessment of the Effectiveness of 169 Interventions.* Williams & Wilkins, Baltimore, Md, 1989: 147-150

40. Centers for Disease Control: Recommendations for the prevention and management of *Chlamydia trachomatis* infections, 1993. *MMWR* 1993; 42(RR-12): 1-39

Screening for Chlamydial Infection

MANEUVER	EFFECTIVENESS	LEVEL OF EVIDENCE <REF>	RECOMMENDATION
Screening for chlamydia (culture or polymerase chain reaction (PCR) for all sites; or direct fluorescent antibody (DFA) for genitourinary (GU), conjunctival (CJ), rectal and nasopharyngeal sites; enzyme-linked immuno-assays (EIA) for GU or CJ specimens; DNA probes for GU specimens) and treatment (erythromycin for pregnant women; tetracyclines or azithromycin for non-pregnant women and men)	**Pregnant Women** Erythromycin treatment of screened women leads to some improved perinatal and postnatal outcomes for children.	Cohort studies<23-27> (11-2)	Fair evidence to support screening and treating pregnant women (B)
	High-Risk Group* Available screening tests are accurate and reliable.	Cohort studies: DFA<7-9> EIA<10>, and PCR<13, 14> (11-2)	Fair evidence to support screening of high-risk groups (B)*
	Treatment is effective in eliminating chlamydia. No studies show that screening leads to reduction of complications.	Randomized controlled trials<15-21> (I)	
	Economic evaluation studies suggest that screening high-risk populations may prevent symptoms and reduce overall cost of infection.	Modelling<35-38>	
	General Population Available screening tests are accurate and reliable but have poor positive predictive value and economic viability when prevalence is low. There have been no studies demonstrating that screening and early detection leads to reduction in complications.	Modelling<35-38>	Fair evidence to support exclusion of routine screening in the general population (D)

*   High risk groups are: sexually active females less than 25 years old, or women with new or multiple partners in the preceding year, who use non-barrier contraception, or who have cervical friability, mucopurulent discharge or intermenstrual bleeding.

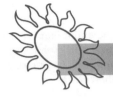

CHAPTER 61

Prevention
of
Influenza

By R. Wayne Elford and Michael Tarrant

Prevention of Influenza

Prepared by R. Wayne Elford, MD, CCFP, FCFP[1] and Michael Tarrant, MD, CCFP, FCFP[2]

In 1979, the Canadian Task Force on the Periodic Health Examination reviewed the evidence then available and concluded that there was good evidence for high-risk groups such as persons over 65 years of age or those with a chronic debilitating disease to receive yearly vaccinations for influenza (A Recommendation).<1> There was fair evidence for not vaccinating the general population who are not at risk (D Recommendation).

Review of new evidence has moderated the strength of these earlier recommendations. Nevertheless, there is still fair evidence for annual vaccination of selected high-risk populations and health care providers but insufficient evidence to recommend for or against vaccination of the general population under 65 years of age. There is good evidence, however, to provide outreach to high-risk groups and to use amantadine chemoprophylaxis among high-risk individuals in contact with an index case.

Burden of Suffering

Influenza is the most important acute viral respiratory illness that causes adults to seek medical care

Influenza is the most important acute respiratory illness that causes adults to seek medical care. Influenza A and B viruses are responsible, but mutate with great regularity, resulting in new strains and subtypes of virus that cause new epidemics almost annually. Current theories of influenza viral epidemiology have not explained fully the persistence, seasonality, and explosiveness of outbreaks over large geographical areas. Excess mortality in the general population is one of the hallmarks of an influenza epidemic. The age group over 65 years accounts for over 95% of the mortality associated with influenza. The increased mortality and morbidity among persons over 65 years, is mostly due to the higher prevalence of chronic heart and lung diseases in the elderly. The peak occurrence of hospitalizations of persons with acute respiratory disease, usually pneumonia, coincides with the peak of influenza virus activity each year. The magnitude of the problem is compounded when the increase in sick-leave in health care providers coincides with peak periods of hospitalization. The

---

[1] Professor and Director of Research and Faculty Development, Department of Family Medicine, University of Calgary, Calgary, Alberta
[2] Associate Professor of Family Medicine, University of Calgary, Calgary, Alberta

excess cost of sick-leave among those of working age during influenza epidemic years exceeds that for all other acute illnesses.<2>

Maneuver

The proper use of inactivated (killed-virus) vaccine is the mainstay of prophylaxis. The traditional intramuscular routes of vaccination may soon be replaced by less invasive approaches. Ingestion of subunit-killed influenza vaccine in the form of enteric-coated capsules stimulates local synthesis of secretory IgA antibody. A comparative study suggests that protection against mucosal infection by respiratory viruses correlates better with level of surface IgA antibody than with serum antibody.

From a prevention viewpoint, the value of early detection is primarily for the purpose of surveillance and the resulting ability to implement intervention maneuvers in high-risk populations, thereby reducing the explosiveness of epidemic outbreaks in local regions.

Clinical Detection

Practically, whenever the epidemiological evidence suggests a high prevalence of influenza virus in the community, any febrile (>38°C) respiratory illness accompanied by prostration, myalgia, headache and cough is likely to be diagnosed as influenza by community practitioners.<3>

Isolation of the Virus

Inoculation of cell cultures with nasopharyngeal washes, throat/nasopharyngeal swabs and daily observation for cytopathic effects remains the gold standard for detection of influenza.<4>

Serological

Over a two week interval, a fourfold rise in antibody titre following natural influenza virus infection and/or artificial induction with vaccine can be detected with a complement fixation test using nucleoprotein or a haemaglutination inhibition (HAI) test. Because most laboratories stock only "generic" strains of the group A and B influenza virus antigens, the antibody response for specific strains of naturally occurring virus is detected variably from season to season.

Rapid Diagnostic Kit

Smears of nasopharyngeal secretions can now be examined for respiratory viruses using rapid immunofluorescence techniques. A positive result on a "Directigen Flu A test" has a positive predictive value of 62.6% compared to virus isolation and a negative predictive value of 100% when used in a controlled laboratory setting (if the rapid diagnostic kit is negative, virus isolation culture is negative 100% of the time).<4> The test produces results in less than 15 minutes and is available in community (non-laboratory) centre environments as an adjunct to clinical diagnosis. However, the reliability of the test in the hands of non-laboratory trained personnel in the community environment is still unknown.

Effectiveness of Prevention

On the basis of clinical trials, vaccines have been shown to be 70-80% effective in reducing both the occurrence of the disease and the associated mortality in normal subjects when the vaccine and the epidemic strain are closely matched.<5> Because efficacy of the vaccine is proven, it would be unethical to withhold the vaccine pending further clinical trials. Therefore, grade I evidence for high risk populations will never be obtained. There is fair (grade II-2) evidence for providing annual influenza vaccination for high-risk population groups such as the institutionalized elderly, persons with chronic heart and or pulmonary conditions,<6> diabetics,<7> and immunocompromised individuals including HIV infected.<8> Directing the use of the vaccine to those most likely to have fatal complications of influenza is the most effective way to diminish mortality.<9,10>

Public Awareness

Surveillance permits the correct virus strains to be incorporated annually into each new vaccine. The World Health Organization (WHO) utilizes two reference laboratories, in Atlanta and London, to monitor global patterns and receive reports of influenza activity through surveillance systems developed in collaboration with regional and local health departments in countries world wide. The wide fluctuation in vaccine use from year to year suggests that increasing public awareness through community health education could improve herd immunity among the general population. A number of well designed field trials have demonstrated that the influenza vaccination rate in non-institutionalized high risk patients can be significantly increased by introducing outreach strategies in the primary care physician's office.<11,12> These study findings have led to specific proactive health education programs that encourage vaccination of high risk patients and health care providers in many acute care hospitals, ambulatory care settings, and chronic care facilities. However, minimal reduction in clinical symptoms was documented in a randomized trial of vaccination of health care providers.<13>

Isolation

Crowding, as occurs in institutionalized populations, greatly enhances the spread of the influenza virus. Early detection and protocol-directed isolation approaches to reduce transmission will ameliorate a more severe outbreak of influenza. This process has limited practicability in real institutional management other than restricting visitation to high-risk individuals during periods of epidemic activity.

Annual Vaccination

Even in high-risk populations the benefit from influenza vaccination is highly variable, because of poor vaccine antigenic match, poor compliance with obtaining vaccination and poor antibody response rates among the elderly. In both Canada and the U.S., the public health services have established a policy objective of immunizing 60% of high risk persons with influenza vaccine annually and make the vaccine available for this group free of charge.<14> Split vaccines have been chemically treated to reduce pyogenic components and are the type that should be used in children under 13 years. In the elderly, however, live-attenuated vaccines have not been shown to offer an advantage over inactivated vaccines in terms of inducing serum or secretory antibodies or immunologic memory. There is a paucity of evidence suggesting that the frequency of adverse reactions to vaccination should constitute a deterrent to patient compliance with influenza vaccination.<15> The chief problem associated with the influenza vaccine is the failure to use it.

The chief problem associated with the influenza vaccine is the failure to use it

Antiviral Prophylaxis/Pharmacotherapy

Randomized trials have proven the efficacy of amantadine in the prevention of influenza illness by restricting the replication of the influenza A virus.<16> It, however, is not effective against influenza B virus which is responsible for approximately 20% of epidemics. Used therapeutically within 48 hours of onset of symptoms, it usually shortens the course of influenza A illness by up to 50%.<17> Elderly patients with congestive heart failure, high serum creatinine, and multiple underlying diagnoses have a significant incidence (40%) of attributable adverse reactions to amantadine. The most common gastrointestinal and central nervous symptoms are dose-related and disappear promptly when the drug is discontinued. Amantadine is best considered as a supplement to vaccination for the prophylaxis of influenza A. Studies have shown that when unvaccinated high-risk patients are encountered after an index case of acute influenza has been identified in the community, the most appropriate management is to vaccinate and then administer amantadine for two weeks so as to provide protection while antibody production is induced.

Amantadine is best considered a supplement to vaccination for the prophylaxis of influenza A

Recommendations of Others

The National Advisory Committee of the Bureau of Communicable Disease Epidemiology, Department of Health and Welfare Canada recommends that intramuscular administration of split or whole-virus vaccines be given annually to: 1) people at high risk; 2) people capable of transmitting influenza to those at high risk; and 3) other people who provide essential community services. Additionally they recommend amantadine prophylaxis for the control of influenza A outbreaks among residents of institutions, and as an adjunct to late vaccination in people at high risk. Amantadine is also recommended for treatment in order to reduce the severity and shorten the duration of influenza A in healthy adults.<18>

The Immunization Practices Advisory Committee (ACIP) of the U.S. Department of Health and Human Services strongly recommends the use of influenza vaccine for any person greater than 6 months who – because of age or underlying medical condition – is at increased risk for complications of influenza. After underscoring that chemoprophylaxis is not a substitute for vaccination, they recommend the use of amantadine for preventing illness and for the symptomatic treatment in order to reduce the duration and severity of systemic symptoms.<9>

In 1989, the U.S. Preventive Services Task Force<19> also recommended vaccinating high-risk groups (A Recommendation); this recommendation is currently being reviewed. The U.S. Public Health Service has established a policy objective of vaccinating 60% of high risk persons with influenza vaccine annually. A 1991 consensus conference in Canada established the goal of vaccinating 70% of high-risk persons. Both countries now make the vaccine available for this group free of charge.

Conclusion and Recommendations

Even though good (grade I) evidence exists for the efficacy of influenza vaccination in the general population, directing the use of the vaccine to those who are most likely to have fatal complications of influenza is the most effective way to diminish mortality. There is fair (grade II-2) evidence for providing annual influenza vaccination for high-risk population groups such as the institutionalized, elderly, persons with chronic heart and/or pulmonary conditions, diabetics or the immunocompromised (B Recommendation). There is fair evidence to immunize health care providers (B Recommendation). There is also good (grade I) evidence that the influenza vaccination rate in the non-institutionalized high-risk patients can be increased significantly by introducing outreach strategies (A Recommendation). There is fair (grade II-1) evidence from studies performed in controlled laboratory settings that the use of a rapid diagnostic kit for diagnosis of influenza

A virus infections has high specificity and negative predictive value, and therefore could be useful in the early detection of influenza A infections. There is good (grade I) evidence that early daily administration of amantadine to high risk persons and to unvaccinated persons exposed to influenza A virus during an outbreak of influenza reduces the spread of the infection (A Recommendation).

Unanswered Questions (Research Agenda)

The epidemiology of patterns of spread of the influenza virus over large geographical areas remains enigmatic. The pathogenesis (e.g. serum sickness vs. viremia) of clinical prostration manifestations of influenza illness is still unclear. In the elderly, there is considerable room for improvement of vaccine efficacy, possibly through different modes of administration and/or enhancement of antibody response rates. There is a need for field trials using "Rapid Diagnostic Kit" detection in order to determine the reliability of out-of-laboratory use in community office setting, and the effectiveness of early treatment with amantadine.

Evidence

The MEDLINE search strategy for this review identified articles for the years 1981-1992 using the following MESH headings: influenza virus, influenza vaccination, influenza chemo-prophylaxis and produced 115 citations. The list of citations was refined by excluding reviews, editorials, commentaries and animal studies, and expanded by the addition of key references contained in the bibliography of the medline articles. In the situation where multiple articles on the same topic existed, the more recent articles and those with the most rigorous design were retained in the selected bibliography.

This review was initiated in April 1992 and recommendations were finalized by the Task Force in June 1993.

Selected References

1. Canadian Task Force on the Periodic Health Examination: The periodic health examination. *Can Med Assoc J* 1979; 121: 1193-1254

2. Glezen WP, Decker M, Perrotta DM: Survey of underlying conditions of persons hospitalized with acute respiratory disease during influenza epidemics in Houston, 1978-1981. *Am Rev Respir Dis* 1987 Sept; 136(3): 550-555

3. Canadian Communicable Disease Surveillance System: Disease specific definitions and surveillance methods. Bureau of Communicable Disease Epidemiology, Laboratory Centre for Disease Control, Health and Welfare Canada, *Can Dis Wk Rep* 1991; 17 (S-3)

4. Waner JL, Todd S, Shalaby H, *et al*: Comparison of Directigen Flu-A with viral isolation and direct immunofluorescence for the rapid detection and identification of influenza A virus. *J Clin Microbiol* 1991; 29(3): 479-482

5. Douglas RG Jr: Prophylaxis and treatment of influenza. *N Engl J Med* 1990; 322(7): 443-450

6. Cartter ML, Renzullo PO, Helgerson SD, *et al*: Influenza outbreaks in nursing homes: how effective is influenza vaccine in the institutionalized elderly? *Infect Control Hosp Epidemiol* 1990; 11(9): 473-478

7. Diepersloot RJ, Bouter KP, Hoekstra JB: Influenza infection and diabetes mellitus. Case for annual vaccination. *Diabetes Care* 1990; 13(8): 876-882

8. Huang KL, Ruben FL, Rinaldo CR JR, *et al*: Antibody responses after influenza and pneumococcal immunization in HIV-infected homosexual men. *JAMA* 1987; 257(15): 2047-2050

9. Prevention and Control of Influenza: recommendations of the Immunization Practices Advisory Committee. Morbidity and Mortality Weekly Report. *JAMA* 1993; 269(14): 1778-1779

10. Prevention and Control of Influenza: Recommendations of the Immunization Practices Advisory Committee. *MMWR Morb Mortal Wkly Rep* 1992; 41(RR-9): 1-17

11. Gerace TM, Sangster JF: Influenza vaccination: a comparison of two outreach strategies. *Fam Med* 1988; 20(1): 43-45

12. Hutchison BG: Effect of computer-generated nurse/physician reminders on influenza immunization among seniors. *Fam Med* 1989; 21(6): 433-437

13. Weingarten S, Staniloff H, Ault M, *et al*: Do hospital employees benefit from the influenza vaccine? A placebo-controlled clinical trial. *J Gen Intern Med* 1988; 3(1): 32-37

14. Fedson DS: The influenza vaccination demonstration project: an expanded policy goal. *Infect Control Hosp Epidemiol* 1990; 11(7): 357-361

15. Margolis KL, Nichol KL, Poland GA, *et al*: Frequency of adverse reactions to influenza vaccine in the elderly. A randomized, placebo-controlled trial. *JAMA* 1990; 264(9): 1139-1141

16. Sears SD, Clements ML: Protective efficacy of low dose amantadine in adults challenged with wild-type influenza A virus. *Antimicrob Agents Chemother* 1987; 31(10): 1470-1473

17. VanVoris LP, Betts RF, Hayden FG, *et al*: Successful Treatment of Naturally Occurring Influenza A. *JAMA* 1981; 245: 1128-1131

18. Statement on Influenza Vaccination for the 1992-93 Season. *Can Med Assoc J* 1992; 147(5): 673-676

19. U.S. Preventive Services Task Force: *Guide to Clinical Preventive Services: an Assessment of the Effectiveness of 169 Interventions*. Williams & Wilkins, Baltimore, Md, 1989: 363-368

Prevention of Influenza

MANEUVER	EFFECTIVENESS	LEVEL OF EVIDENCE <REF>	RECOMMENDATION
Annual immunization with influenza vaccine	**High-risk groups:*** Reduces incidence and severity of disease.	Analytic cohort studies<6-8> (II-2)	Fair evidence to immunize high-risk groups (B)*
	Health care providers: Minimal reduction of clinical symptoms.	Randomized controlled trial<13> (I)	Fair evidence to immunize health care providers (B)
	General population <65yrs: Efficacious but effectiveness debatable.	Expert opinion<10>** (III)	Insufficient evidence to include or exclude (C)
Outreach to high-risk groups	Nurse/physician reminders and letter or telephone contact with elderly increases the vaccination rate.	Randomized controlled trials<11,12> (I)	Good evidence to include (A)
Rapid diagnostic test use in suspected cases	Good negative predictive value.	Trial without randomization<4>*** (II-1)	Insufficient evidence to include or exclude (C)
Amantadine chemoprophylaxis of high-risk or unvaccinated individuals around index case	Reduces incidence of symptomatic infection from influenza A virus.	Randomized controlled trial<16> (I)	Good evidence to include (A)

*   High-risk groups include: institutionalized people, those over age 65 years or those with a chronic debilitating illness (chronic heart or pulmonary disease, diabetes mellitus or who are immunocompromised).

**   Not considered cost effective.

*** Studies have only been performed in laboratory settings.

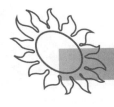

CHAPTER 62

Screening and Isoniazid Prophylactic Therapy for Tuberculosis

By Sharon L. Walmsley

Screening and Isoniazid Prophylactic Therapy for Tuberculosis

Prepared by Sharon L. Walmsley MD, FRCPC[1]

Tuberculosis remains a major worldwide health problem with at least 10 million new cases and 3 million deaths estimated to occur annually. In 1979, the Canadian Task Force on the Periodic Health Exam<1> recommended Bacille Calmette-Guérin (BCG) immunization and chemoprophylaxis of unimmunized tuberculin-positive individuals from high risk-groups (A Recommendation) but not for the general population (E Recommendation). With the changing epidemiology of tuberculosis in North America and concerns about the risk of drug-induced hepatitis, the value of screening for tuberculosis and of isoniazid (INH) chemoprophylactic therapy as part of the periodic health examination was re-examined. The Task Force concludes that screening by tuberculin skin testing should be offered to persons at high risk of infection, but is not recommended for the general population. INH chemoprophylactic therapy is recommended for household contacts of active cases of tuberculosis. It is also recommended for persons with positive tuberculin skin tests who have documented skin test conversion, radiographic lesions suggestive of inactive but previously untreated tuberculosis, who are under 35 years of age, or those with an underlying medical condition which predisposes them to reactivation (especially HIV infection) regardless of age.

Burden of Suffering

The number of cases of active tuberculosis in Canada has been decreasing gradually over the past few decades, and in the past few years has plateaued, with 1,995 cases (7.5 per 100,000) reported in 1990.<2> For individuals born in Canada, most reported cases occur in the very young and in those of advancing age. Among the Canadian-born, rates are ten times higher for the aboriginal group. Proportionally, more active cases occur in immigrants to Canada, with the highest rates reported in those immigrating from areas where tuberculosis is endemic, including Africa, Asia, Central America and certain countries in South America and the Caribbean.

Death rates from tuberculosis have also declined. In Canada in 1990, 129 persons with tuberculosis died (0.6 per 100,000 population)

Proportionally more cases of tuberculosis occur in immigrants from areas endemic for tuberculosis and in Canadian-born aboriginals

[1] Assistant Professor, Department of Medicine and Microbiology, University of Toronto, Toronto, Ontario

and in 60 cases, tuberculosis was the cause of, or a significant contributor to death.

Most new cases of tuberculosis are pulmonary. Persons infected with large inocula (i.e. following household exposure to a cavitary case) and those with increased susceptibility to infection (e.g. children less than 5 years) are at higher risk of acquiring infection. In 90% of exposed persons, host defenses contain the primary infection, but the individual develops a positive tuberculin skin test. In the absence of preventive measures 5-15% will develop reactivation tuberculosis during their lifetime, the risk being greatest during the first two years following exposure. From observational studies, certain groups have been identified to be at an increased risk of reactivation, although in many cases the exact level of risk is not well defined. In patients with silicosis, head and neck cancer, jejunoileal bypass or in those who require hemodialysis, the relative risk is reported to be increased 10-30 times over that of the baseline population. The relative risk for patients with low body weight or nutritional deficiency, diabetes mellitus, or gastrectomy is reported to be increased 2-5 times. Persons infected with HIV are now recognized to be at the highest risk of reactivation with rates reported at 8-9% per year in recent studies. Other groups identified to be at increased risk are those with other immunosuppressive disorders (hematologic malignancies), those requiring immunosuppressive therapy for malignant or non-malignant conditions, patients requiring high dosages of corticosteroids over prolonged periods, the urban poor, persons living in shelters, intravenous drug users and alcoholics.

Maneuver

The Mantoux tuberculin skin test is the gold standard screening test to identify infection with the human tubercle bacillus. For testing, 0.1 ml of PPD-T (standardized purified protein derivative, Connaught Laboratories) containing 5 TU (tuberculin units) is injected intracutaneously into the dorsal (volar) surface of the forearm. The 1 TU and 250 TU tuberculins are not biologically standardized and are not recommended for routine use. The injection is made intradermally and a discrete wheal 6-10 mm in diameter should be produced in all cases. Tuberculin tests should be read at 48-72 hours. The basis of reading is the transverse diameter in millimetres of the induration (not the erythema) which can be determined by inspection and palpation or by the ball point pen method.[2]

---

[2] The pen method of tuberculin interpretation is performed as follows: Using a medium ball point pen, a line is drawn from a point 5 to 10 mm away from the margin of the skin induration towards its center, until resistance is felt to further movement. The procedure is repeated on the opposite side and in a right angle axis. The average of the measurements in the two axes is recorded.

The cut-off point for the interpretation of a positive test was derived from multiple population surveys comparing the reaction size in patients with or without presumed exposure and development of subsequent active disease. There is no clear point of separation between a positive and a negative test. Defining a positive reaction becomes increasingly difficult as the prevalence of cross-reactions with atypical mycobacteria increases and true infections due to *Mycobacterium tuberculosis* become less frequent. These observations have led experts to recommend use of different cut-off values for different population groups.[3] For individuals at very high risk of reactivation, including contacts of infectious cases, and persons with HIV infection, the recommended cut point is 5 mm. For persons not likely to be exposed, who reside in geographic areas where infection with atypical mycobacterium is common (i.e. the United States), the cut off is increased to 15 mm. For those with an intermediate risk, such as those living in or immigrating from endemic areas, or those areas where cross reactions with atypical mycobacteria are less common (i.e. Canada) an intermediate level of 10 mm is used. It should be noted that most patients who receive BCG vaccination as children, lose their cutaneous hypersensitivity reaction to tuberculin within 5 years. Therefore, a significant reaction more likely represents true exposure to tuberculosis especially in the setting of a recent exposure.

Another problem with tuberculin skin testing is inter- and intra-observer variation in the interpretation of test results.[4] Agreement is highest when the results are clearly positive (>15 mm) or clearly negative (<5 mm), with more inter-observer variation (mean 6 mm) when more readings are in the 5-14 mm range. This degree of variation can result in incorrect labelling. Some patients with compromised immune systems (especially those infected with HIV who have low CD4 counts) may be anergic. These individuals are unable to mount a skin test response to injected antigens (including tuberculin) despite previous exposure, and may be incorrectly labelled as negative.

The tuberculin skin test is a safe procedure. Purified protein derivative (PPD) does not sensitize nor activate a latent reaction. A few (1-2%) exquisitively sensitive persons with positive tests may respond with a severe local reaction with ulceration or vesiculation, regional adenopathy and fever. These reactions are typically self-limited, but painful, and may be reduced with intralesional steroids. Localized allergic reactions including wheal and flare and localized rash may occur in 2-3% of patients particularly those with a history of atopy. These reactions tend to occur in the first few hours, are self-limited, and do not correlate with the tuberculin response. Anaphylaxis or death have not been reported.

For persons with positive reactions it is imperative to rule out active disease by clinical history, chest radiograph and the appropriate laboratory investigations. Once active infection is ruled out, it is important to explain to the patient that a positive reaction implies a subclinical infection with tuberculosis and the risk for subsequent reactivation to active disease, but that the individual does not have active disease nor are they infectious to others.

Effectiveness of Prevention

The main purpose of chemoprophylaxis is to prevent reactivation of a latent infection to clinical disease. It is important prior to the initiation of chemoprophylaxis that active TB is excluded. The only drug which has been studied extensively for chemoprophylaxis is Isoniazid (INH). More than 20 clinical trials evaluating the role of chemoprophylaxis in tuberculosis are reported in the literature. Despite the multitude of methodological flaws of these early studies, including 1) non-random allocation; 2) inclusion of previously treated cases; 3) use of other therapies in combination with INH; 4) historical controls; 5) randomization by groups (families, hospital wards), but analysis by individuals; and 6) the inclusion of active cases, all but one of these trials has shown a significant benefit for INH prophylaxis. The best studies demonstrating effectiveness of INH prophylaxis in different patient groups are outlined below:

The risk:benefit ratio of INH prophylaxis varies with age, likelihood of a true positive test, the time since exposure, underlying medical conditions and risk of reactivation

Positive Tuberculin Skin Test <35 Years

During a routine skin testing program (1958-1966) in San Francisco public school students with a large immigrant population,<5> a non-randomized comparative study evaluated INH prophylaxis. Over a 1-2 year follow up, 1 of 2,910 children in the INH-treated group (0.34 per 1,000) and 25 of 1,192 on no treatment (20.9 per 1,000) developed active tuberculosis. Although demonstrating a highly statistical and clinical benefit of INH prophylaxis, there is concern about the comparability of the two groups, with racial differences noted between the treatment and control groups. Other reasons for not choosing treatment may also have been associated with increased risk of tuberculosis in controls. There is fair evidence to support prophylaxis in this setting, especially for children.

Positive Tuberculin Skin Test > 35 Years

27,924 patients from 39 U.S. Mental Institutions were randomly allocated by ward to receive INH or placebo.<6> During the medication year, 21 of 12,326 (1.7 per 1,000) patients assigned placebo and 4 of 12,884 (0.3 per 1,000) assigned INH developed active tuberculosis, with 17 of the 25 patients who developed tuberculosis having had an abnormal chest x-ray on entry. Although this is a statistically significant reduction in cases, the clinical significance and generalizability of the results are uncertain. The crowding and institutionalization would likely have increased the risk of disease. Other biases in the study weaken the strength of the observations. The Task Force feels there is insufficient evidence to recommend routine prophylaxis for all adults >35 years with a positive tuberculin skin test.

Although no controlled studies have been performed, INH prophylaxis is strongly recommended (by expert opinion) for patients with medical conditions that increase the risk of reactivation of tuberculosis, regardless of age.[16]

HIV Infected Patients

From 1986-89, 118 asymptomatic HIV positive persons in Haiti were randomized to receive INH prophylaxis with vitamin B6 or B6 alone for 12 months.[7] Eleven of sixty (18%) patients in the B6 group developed active tuberculosis over the study period in contrast to four of 62 who received INH and B6, p=0.03. This is consistent with a reduction from 7.5 to 2.2 cases per 100-person years. There is good evidence to support the use of INH prophylaxis in patients with HIV infection.

Household Contacts of Active Cases

The Tuberculosis Program of the U.S. Public Health Service studied INH prophylaxis in household contacts of new active pulmonary cases in the U.S. and Puerto Rico between 1957 and 1960.[8] The groups were similar in age and race distribution. Two thirds of all participants <20 years were randomized to receive INH or placebo for one year. Pulmonary or extrapulmonary tuberculosis developed in 78 of 12,594 (6.5 per 1,000) placebo recipients versus 18 of 12,439 (1.5 per 1,000) INH recipients.

A similar household-based study in Japan failed to show a benefit of INH prophylaxis[9] although there was a trend toward decreased tuberculosis in the INH treated group (8 per 1,142) compared to the control group (11 per 1,096). Poor compliance and the small sample size were the most likely reasons for the lack of significant effect.

The Task Force concludes there is good evidence to support the role of INH chemoprophylaxis in household contacts of active cases of tuberculosis.

Tuberculin Skin Test Converters

Recruits of the Royal Netherlands Navy whose skin tests converted to positive following exposure to an active case of pulmonary tuberculosis were randomized to receive INH (n=133) or placebo (n=128) for one year.[10] During the treatment year, 9 cases of tuberculosis developed in the placebo recipients (70 per 1,000) in contrast to 1 case in the INH group (7.5 per 1,000), a significant difference.

INH prophylaxis was evaluated in a cohort of nursing home patients with tuberculin skin test conversion.<11> Tuberculosis developed in 1 of 605 converters receiving INH (1.6 per 1,000) and in 45 of 757 (59 per 1,000) receiving no treatment. This was clinically and statistically significant.

The Task Force concludes that there is good evidence to recommend INH prophylaxis in skin test converters regardless of age.

PPD Positive, Old Fibrotic Scar on Chest Radiograph

The International Union Against Tuberculosis (IUAT) performed a European multi-center, double-blind, placebo-controlled trial of INH prophylaxis in patients with a positive PPD and an old fibrotic scar on chest x-ray.<12> Of the 27,830 patients enrolled (median age 50 years), 6,953 were randomized to receive INH for 12 weeks, 6,965 INH for 24 weeks, 6,919 INH for 52 weeks and 6,990 patients were randomized to placebo. Over the 5 year study, active pulmonary tuberculosis developed in 97 placebo recipients (14.3 per 1,000), 76 patients on INH for 12 weeks (11.3 per 1,000), 34 patients on 24 weeks of INH (5.0 per 1,000) and 24 patients on 52 weeks of INH (3.6 per 1,000). This represents a 60% reduction in cases for patients receiving a 6 month course and approximately 90% reduction for patients receiving a 12 month course of INH. An additional 181 patients were removed from the trial as suspected cases of tuberculosis (either extra-pulmonary tuberculosis, or pulmonary tuberculosis without positive culture) but it is not reported how many of these patients received INH. Based on this study the Task Force feels there is fair evidence to support the use of INH prophylaxis in this setting.

Duration of Therapy

Most studies evaluating INH chemoprophylaxis have utilized a one year course of therapy, and this is the duration recommended by the Task Force. A cost analysis study has suggested that a 24 week regime was more cost effective.<13>

Alternative Regimes

There have been case reports of failed INH chemoprophylaxis for patients infected with INH-resistant organisms. There is no study available to recommend alternative agents in this setting. Expert opinion suggests that Rifampin and Ethambutol, Rifampin and INH or Pyrazinamide containing regimes should be considered.

Compliance

Compliance remains an important barrier to effective chemoprophylaxis. In the clinical trials cited above, compliance ranged from 50-75% through one year of preventive therapy. In a study involving Canadian aboriginals, compliance was improved by a program of daily observed prophylaxis and education but was not sustained after observation was discontinued.<14>

Adverse Events of Screening and Treatment

Prophylaxis with INH has been associated with many adverse events, including hypersensitivity reactions, INH-induced lupus-like syndrome, peripheral neuropathy, gastrointestinal distress, and central nervous system abnormalities ranging from memory loss to psychosis or seizures. The most significant and potentially dose-limiting side effect is hepatitis. Fifteen percent of patients will experience a transient asymptomatic increase in their liver transaminases on treatment. Clinical hepatitis is much less common and is rarely fatal, particularly when recommendations for surveillance are followed.

The best prospective study to determine the incidence of INH hepatitis documented 236 suspected cases among 13,838 receiving prophylaxis.<15> Of these cases, 92 were classified as probably INH-related and 82 possibly INH-related by an expert panel. The case rates appeared to increase with age, with rates for probable cases <20 years (0 per 1,000), 20-34 years (3 per 1,000), 35-49 (12 per 1,000), 50-64 years (23 per 1,000) and >64 years (8 per 1,000). The rates also varied with race, with the highest rates occurring in Orientals (18 per 1,000) in contrast to 11.4 per 1,000 in whites and 7.1 per 1,000 for blacks. The rate for those who drank alcohol (14.1 per 1,000) was double that of non-drinkers and the rate for daily drinkers (26.5 per 1,000) was even higher. In the IUAT trial, the risk of INH-related hepatitis was 0.5%, with a mortality rate of 14 per 100,000.<12>

Other disadvantages of chemoprophylaxis include the inconvenience of daily medication over a one year period and the need to attend regular clinic visits. The cost of the program, and demands on staff for screening and follow-up must also be considered.

Recommendations of Others

The American Thoracic Society (ATS) has recently published new guidelines.<7> They propose the same groups for tuberculin testing as the Canadian Task Force but use "recent contacts" rather than "household contacts" of new cases. The high risk group for reactivation infection, also includes medically underserviced populations, persons resident in long-term care facilities, nursing homes, mental institutions and correctional institutions. They do not recommend prophylaxis for patients with positive tuberculin skin test and fibrotic lesions on chest radiographs, but rather recommend that these patients be treated with multi-drug regimes as for active disease. They recommend INH prophylaxis for all patients with known or suspected HIV infection and a positive PPD.

The Centers For Disease Control in Atlanta also recommend routine skin testing of all persons at high risk, including the homeless.[17]

The Canadian Thoracic Society has also developed new guidelines (personal communication, Dr. M. Fitzgerald). They recommend that given the low frequency of infection with atypical mycobacteria, that the 10 mm cut-off be used for the general Canadian population.

In 1989, the U.S. Preventive Services Task Force recommended skin testing for patients at increased risk for tuberculosis.[18] In addition, they recommend following the ATS guidelines for prophylaxis.

The American Academy of Pediatrics Redbook recommends annual testing of high-risk children, including those who are black, Hispanic, Asian, American Indian, Native Alaskan, the socioeconomically deprived, those living in neighbourhoods where case rates are above the national average, children or their parents who themselves have immigrated from high risk areas of Asia, Africa, the Middle East, Latin America or the Caribbean, households where there have been active cases and those with underlying medical risk factors.[19] Annual testing is not recommended for low-risk groups but skin testing in these low-risk children is recommended at 12-15 months, 4-6 years, and 14-16 years. INH is recommended for all infants, children and young adults up to 35 years of age with positive PPD for 9 months. No justification is given for the duration.

Conclusions and Recommendations

Tuberculosis screening should be offered to persons in Canada at high risk of infection with the tubercle bacillus, including immigrants from endemic areas, Canadian-born aboriginals, close contacts of active cases, persons with abnormal chest radiographs consistent with healed tuberculosis, and persons with underlying medical conditions which increase their likelihood of reactivation of tuberculosis if infected, including those with HIV infection, silicosis, hemodialysis patients, those with immunosuppressive conditions or therapy, intravenous drug users, diabetes, gastrectomy patients or those with gastrointestinal bypass surgery, and the nutritionally deficient (A Recommendation). Routine screening is not recommended for the general population (E Recommendation). INH prophylaxis for twelve months is recommended for household contacts of active cases of tuberculosis (A Recommendation) and for persons with positive tuberculin skin tests who have documented skin test conversion

(A Recommendation), chest radiographic lesions suggestive of inactive tuberculosis (B Recommendation), HIV infection (A Recommendation) and for patients under 35 years of age with a positive tuberculin test (B Recommendation). Prophylactic therapy is not recommended for persons with positive skin tests over the age of 35 years (C Recommendation) unless they have a medical condition associated with an increased risk of reactivation where prophylaxis is recommended (A Recommendation).

Unanswered Questions (Research Agenda)

A number of areas continue to be of concern regarding the detection of infected persons and the use of prophylaxis. Priorities that need to be addressed include the development of: 1) more effective, less toxic, shorter duration preventive treatments; 2) ways to improve compliance with chemoprophylaxis; 3) effective vaccines; 4) better studies to determine the true incidence of reactivation tuberculosis in patients with isolated positive tuberculin skin tests with no other risk factors; 5) the true relative risks for reactivation in those patients with various underlying medical disorders; and 6) chemoprophylactic measures for patients infected with INH resistant strains.

Evidence

The literature was identified with a MEDLINE search with the use of the main MESH heading "tuberculosis" and the subheadings "tuberculin skin test", "prevention and control" and "isoniazid" for articles presented from 1966 through 1992. Indices of the American Review of Respiratory Diseases and Tubercle were screened from 1960-1992 for articles with emphasis on screening and treatment.

This review was initiated in August 1992 and the recommendations were finalized by the Task Force in January 1994.

Acknowledgements

The Task Force thanks Sam Akor, BSc, MB, ChB, MCommH, MA, Director/DMOH, Rural Health Training School, Kintempo, Ghana for his work on the preliminary report. Helen Holden MD, FRCPC, FCCP, Valley Regional Hospital, Kentville, Nova Scotia, Richard Menzies, MD, MSc, FRCPC, Assistant Professor, McGill University and Montreal Chest Hospital, Montreal, Quebec and Mark Fitzgerald, MD, FRCPC, Assistant Professor, University of British Columbia and Department of Respiratory Medicine, Vancouver General Hospital, Vancouver, British Columbia are thanked for reviewing the draft report.

Selected References

1. Canadian Task Force on the Periodic Health Examination: The periodic health examination. *Can Med Assoc J* 1979; 121: 1193-1254

2. Statistics Canada: Tuberculosis Statistics, 1990. *Health Reports* 1992; 4(2 Suppl 10): 1-14

3. Screening for tuberculosis and tuberculous infection in high-risk populations. The use of preventative therapy for tuberculous infection in the United States. Recommendations of the Advisory Committee for Elimination of Tuberculosis. *MMWR* 1990; 39(RR-8): 1-12

4. Longfield JN, Margileth AM, Golden SM, *et al*: Interobserver and method variability in tuberculin skin testing. *Pediatr Infect Dis* 1984; 3(4): 323-326

5. Curry FJ: Prophylactic effect of isoniazid in young tuberculin reactors. *New Engl J Med* 1967; 277(11): 562-567

6. Ferebee SH, Mount FW, Murray FJ, *et al*: A controlled trial of isoniazid prophylaxis in mental institutions. *Am Rev Respir Dis* 1963; 88(2): 161-17

7. Pape JW Jean SS, Ho JL: Effect of isoniazid prophylaxis on the incidence of active tuberculosis and progression of HIV infection. *Lancet* 1993; 342: 268-272

8. Mount FW, Ferebee SH: The effect of isoniazid prophylaxis on tuberculosis morbidity among household contacts of previously known cases of tuberculosis. *Am Rev Respir Dis* 1962; 85: 821-827

9. Bush O, Sigimoto M, Fujii Y, *et al*: Isoniazid prophylaxis in contacts of persons with known tuberculosis. Second Report. *Am Rev Respir Dis* 1965; 92: 732-740

10. Veening GJ: Long term isoniazid prophylaxis: Controlled trial on INH prophylaxis after recent tuberculin conversion in young adults. *Bull Un Int Tuberc* 1968; 41: 169-171

11. Stead WW, Lofgren JP, Warren E, *et al*: Tuberculosis as an endemic and nosocomial infection among the elderly in nursing homes. *New Engl J Med* 1985; 312(23): 1483-1487

12. International Union Against Tuberculosis Committee on Prophylaxis: Efficacy of various durations of isoniazid preventative therapy for tuberculosis: five years of follow-up in the IUAT trial. *Bull World Health Organization* 1982; 60(4): 555-564

13. Snider DE Jr., Caras GJ, Koplan JP: Preventative therapy with isoniazid. Cost-effectiveness of different durations of therapy. *JAMA* 1986; 255: 1579-1583

14. Wobeser W, To T, Hoeppner VH: The outcome of chemoprophylaxis on tuberculosis prevention in the Canadian Plains Indian. *Clin Invest Med* 1989; 12(3): 149-153

15. Kopanoff DE, Snider DE, Caras GJ: Isoniazid-related hepatitis: A US Public Health Service Cooperative Surveillance study. *Am Rev Respir Dis* 1978; 117: 991-1001

16. American Thoracic Society: Control of tuberculosis in the United States. *Am Rev Respir Dis* 1992; 146: 1623-1633

17. Prevention and control of tuberculosis in US communities with at-risk minority populations. Prevention and control of tuberculosis among homeless persons. Recommendations of the Advisory Council for the Elimination of Tuberculosis. *MMWR Morb Mortal Wkly Rep* 1992; 41(RR-5): 1-23

18. U.S. Preventive Services Task Force: *Guide to Clinical Preventive Services: an Assessment of the Effectiveness of 169 Interventions.* Williams & Wilkins, Baltimore, Md, 1989: 125-128, 370-372

19. Peter G (ed): *Report of the Committee of Infectious Diseases.* 22nd Edition, American Academy of Pediatrics, 1991

Screening and Isoniazid Prophylactic Therapy for Tuberculosis

MANEUVER	EFFECTIVENESS	LEVEL OF EVIDENCE <REF>	RECOMMENDATION
Mantoux tuberculin test	**Detection** The test is safe and identifies individuals with infection; some interobserver variation in interpretation and false positives may occur due to cross reactions with a typical bacteria or Bacille Calmette-Guérin (BCG) vaccination.	Cohort and case-control studies<3,4> (II-2)	Good evidence to support screening individuals at high-risk* (A) and good evidence not to screen individuals from the general population (E)
Isoniazid (INH) chemoprophylactic therapy	**Intervention** INH prophylaxis is effective in preventing active cases of tuberculosis for patients with positive skin test result but has been associated with adverse side effects including hepatitis.	Randomized controlled trials: household contacts<8,9>, skin test converters<10,11> fibrotic scars on chest radiographs <35 yrs<5> and >35 yrs co-infection with HIV<6,7> (I); expert opinion: persons with underlying medical conditions increasing risk of reactivation <16> (III)	Good evidence to recommend INH prophylaxis to household contacts and skin test converters and persons with underlying medical conditions like HIV that increase the risk of reactivation of infection (A); fair evidence to recommend INH prophylaxis for those aged <35 years or individuals with fibrotic scars on chest x-ray (B); poor evidence to recommend for or against prophylaxis for those aged over 35 years (C)

* High-risk groups include immigrants from endemic areas (Africa, Asia, Central America and certain countries in South America and the Caribbean), Canadian-born aboriginals, close contacts of active cases, persons with abnormal chest radiographs consistent with healed tuberculosis, and persons with underlying medical conditions which increase their likelihood of reactivation of tuberculosis if infected (those with silicosis, jejunoileal by-pass, hemodialysis, gastrectomy, malnutrition, intravenous drug users, alcohol abusers and especially those with known or suspected infection with HIV).

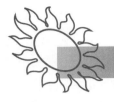

CHAPTER 63

Screening for Human Papillomavirus Infection

By J. Kenneth Johnson

63

Screening for Human Papillomavirus Infection

Prepared by J. Kenneth Johnson, MD[1]

The Canadian Task Force on the Periodic Health Examination has not issued prior recommendations on screening for Human Papilloma Virus (HPV), although clear recommendations have been made for cervical cancer screening (see Chapter 73). HPV is of increasing interest because evidence linking HPV infection and increased risk for cancer of the cervix has been accumulating. This report reviews the evidence for and against HPV screening in asymptomatic women and concludes that screening should not be done since therapy is ineffective and potentially harmful.

Burden of Suffering

HPV commonly exists in a subclinical form (only about 10% of those infected have visible condylomata)

Much of the epidemiology of HPV remains to be determined, and precise estimates of incidence and prevalence are not available. Condylomata acuminata (proliferative HPV) is reportable in the United Kingdom, where it is the most frequently diagnosed viral sexually transmitted disease (STD). Data from STD clinics in the U.K. and Australia indicate a prevalence of genital warts of 4-13% in clinic attenders. These data are based on visible condylomata and considerably underestimate prevalence, since HPV commonly exists in a subclinical form (only about 10% of those infected have visible condylomata, while 20% have lesions demonstrable by colposcopy or magnifying lens). A large Canadian study of a screening program for cervical cancer in the late 1970s showed that 1.69% of 234,715 women had signs of cervical HPV on cytological examination. In a population-based study of 63,115 Finnish women aged 20-65 years, the estimated lifetime risk of infection with HPV was calculated to be 79%. HPV prevalence varies widely from 0.8% to 88% depending on the groups studied. Rates in STD clinics, for sexually active adolescents and sexual contacts of women with HPV all show higher prevalence. Those with more lifetime sexual partners and younger women (in their teens and twenties) are at significantly greater risk for HPV infection.

Over 60 separate serotypes of HPV have been identified to date. HPV-16 and HPV-18 are most closely associated with risk for genital cancers. Numerous epidemiological studies, with or without viral typing, have confirmed the connection between HPV infection and cervical cancer, as well as the correlation between the presence of

[1] Research Associate, Department of Preventive Medicine and Biostatistics, University of Toronto, Toronto, Ontario, 1992

HPV and increasing grade of disease.<1-11> A study by Meisels and Morin in Quebec found evidence of HPV (koilocytosis) on Pap smear in 1.69% of over 234,000 women screened, while HPV was found in 25.6% of Pap smears showing either dysplasia or neoplasia.<12>

In Canada in 1993 approximately 1,300 new cases of invasive carcinoma of the cervix were diagnosed, and about 400 deaths were expected to occur from this disease. The yearly overall cost of invasive disease and death in Canada from cervical cancer has been estimated at 180 to 270 million dollars.

The natural history of untreated HPV infection is not well understood, since different studies have reported different outcomes. In a Finnish prospective study, a cohort of 343 women was followed for a mean of 18.7 months. Twenty-five percent of lesions regressed spontaneously, while 61% remained unchanged and 14% progressed to carcinoma.<13> In a cohort of 100 women followed in the U.K. for a minimum of 19 months, 11 showed spontaneous regression, 64% no change, and 26% progressed to cervical intraepithelial neoplasia (CIN) type 3.<5> Two hundred and thirty-five women with mild to moderate cervical dysplasia and HPV infection were followed in Canada for up to 24 months without treatment.<14> Nine (5.5%) patients showed progression, 134 (57%) converted to normal cytology, and the rest were unchanged during follow-up. Although the likelihood of progression of HPV infection is most consistently associated with presence of HPV-16<15-17> some studies have failed to demonstrate such a relationship<18> and the importance of HPV typing in screening is therefore unclear.

Maneuver

Until recently, HPV infections have been most commonly diagnosed by simple visual inspection or with the aid of a hand lens. For proliferative lesions, this is a highly specific but very insensitive technique. Application of 3-5% acetic acid to the area allows visualization of some other features of HPV, and with the addition of colposcopy can improve the sensitivity of clinical examination. However, visible proliferative lesions are less likely to be caused by HPV types associated with a greater risk of cancer.

Visible proliferative lesions are less likely to be caused by HPV types associated with greater risk of cancer

Pap smears have been used to identify changes related to HPV infection but are only moderately sensitive (15%).<19> Pap smears are also unable to distinguish the types of HPV with any acceptable degree of accuracy. In a population-based screening program for cervical cancer, the sensitivity of cytology for HPV infection was estimated at 19%. A small study (21 women) in the U.S. attempted to determine the sensitivity and specificity of cytology and colposcopy relative to hybridization techniques in diagnosing HPV infection.<20> Pap smear sensitivity was 57% when equivocal smears were scored as negative for HPV, with specificity of 50%, but 100% sensitive when equivocal smears were considered positive for HPV. Colposcopy had a sensitivity of 100% but specificity of only 10-20%. Reid et al compared cervical cytology, cervicography and/or DNA hybridization for HPV as screening techniques for cervical cancer among 1,012 women.<21> Pap smears had a sensitivity of 52.2%. No single technique succeeded in identifying all of the abnormalities, but the best (96%) sensitivity was achieved by retesting only those women with an initial high-grade cytologic abnormality or positive cervicography results. In the cohort study of Koutsky et al,<3> 27 of the 28 women who developed CIN 2/3 had cytological evidence of CIN 2/3 as well as a positive HPV DNA test, and the 28th woman had CIN 1 on cytology prior to biopsy.

Papillomavirus group-specific antigen can be detected by immunohistochemical staining of cell or tissue samples, but has low specificity and is unable to differentiate between HPV types. The correlation between presence of antigen and clinical outcome is poor.<15,22>

Southern blot and dot blot methods were developed using biopsy material (although they may now use 'non-invasive' cervical/vaginal scrapings) and are based on identifying viral DNA separated from cellular DNA through gel electrophoresis. The method is not well-suited to mass screening because it is time-consuming, labour-intensive, and consequently relatively expensive. Hybridization assays are relatively new methods for detection of HPV and are limited by as-yet poorly defined sensitivity and specificity and problems of interpretation, at least partly related to adequacy of sampling technique.<15,11,20,21,23,24> In situ hybridization is less sensitive than the other DNA identification techniques; the filter in situ method may have a higher incidence of false-positive reactions. The polymerase chain reaction (PCR) is extremely sensitive but may also have a significant false-positive rate.

Effectiveness of Early Detection and Treatment

There is no effective therapy for HPV infection that is specific or consistently produces long-term success

There is no effective therapy for HPV infection that is specific or consistently produces long-term success. Many types of physical or chemically destructive agents (conization,<25> cryosurgery, lasers, salicylic acid, cantharidin, bi- and trichloroacetic acid), as well as chemotherapeutic agents (podophyllin, 5-fluorouracil, bleomycin) have been used for treating common warts or genital condylomata. The success rate for all of these therapies has been discouraging. For example, a randomized controlled clinical trial of patient-administered Podophyllotoxin (one of the active lignans present in podophyllin resin) showed complete clearing of penile warts in 53.3% of 34 patients, but 100% recurrence in all the patients who returned after 16 weeks for follow-up.<26> High recurrence rates of visible genital warts are typical of almost all studies with sufficiently long follow-up.

Two therapeutic approaches that have had somewhat better results are interferon therapy<27-29> and CO2 laser vaporization.<30-33> Although the 'cure' rates are generally better than are usually seen with the older therapies, a significant recurrence rate remains in most studies as well as a good 'cure' rate in untreated subjects, suggesting that no treatment may be a reasonable approach in many circumstances.

It should be emphasized that the goal of treatment may vary between individuals. Complete or permanent elimination of visible condylomata may not matter if the main concern is cancer detection or prevention. Older chemical treatments may be more acceptable to some patients than the newer, more invasive and expensive techniques such as laser vaporization. Currently, no therapy exists for non-visible (latent) HPV infection, and the value of detecting such latent infections through screening is unclear. Potential harmful effects include morbidity of testing and treatment, financial cost of the testing and therapeutic load and labelling of otherwise healthy individuals as STD patients.

Recommendations of Others

A Canadian workshop on cervical cancer screening held in 1989 found that there was insufficient evidence to routinely add specific tests for HPV to screening for cervical cancer.

Conclusions and Recommendations

The present screening recommendations for cervical cancer do not include specific testing for HPV infection beyond the recommendations for Pap smear screening. Current criteria for recall testing are appropriate for balancing false negative and false positive rates for Pap smears alone as a screening procedure. Addition of further diagnostic testing to the present routine would add little to the effort to reduce cervical cancer incidence. Further testing would, however, increase monetary costs considerably, stretch the existing system beyond its capacity (especially with a rapid increase in referrals for colposcopy), and likely create considerably more morbidity in terms of quality of life for many persons screened, without adding established benefit. For specific HPV screening procedures, given the prevailing imprecision of diagnostic testing for HPV, uninterpretable risk of significant disease, and generally ineffective treatments for HPV infection, there is fair evidence to exclude HPV screening from the routine periodic health examination (D Recommendation).

Unanswered Questions (Research Agenda)

The following have been identified as research priorities:

1. To refine a diagnostic method which will be sensitive and specific, non-invasive and appropriate for large-scale screening purposes to identify the type of HPV present or to predict which lesions are likely to progress.

2. To define more precisely the incidence of HPV infections in the general population.

3. To assess the risks associated with specific HPV genotypes for progression to genital cancers.

4. To identify co-factors which influence HPV transmission and which may promote carcinomatous changes in cervical lesions.

5. To develop effective methods of treating HPV infection.

6. To develop immunological therapies for HPV, especially regarding a possible vaccine.

7. To assess the efficacy of screening for HPV, including assessment of cost effectiveness of such a program.

Evidence

A literature search using MEDLINE was conducted from 1966 to June 1993, using the key words: papillomavirus, cervix neoplasms, mass screening, prospective studies, prevalence, sensitivity, specificity, human and female.

This review was initiated in January 1992 and recommendations were finalized by the Task Force in June 1992. A technical report (1993) with a full reference list is available upon request.

Acknowledgements

The Task Force thanks Dr. George H. Anderson, Head, Cytology Laboratories, British Columbia Cancer Agency, Vancouver, British Columbia; Máire A. Duggan, MB FRCPC, Foothills Hospital, Calgary, Alberta; and Dr. Paul R. Gully, MB, ChB, FFCM, FRCPC, Chief, Division of STD Control, Health Canada, Ottawa, Ontario for reviewing the draft report.

Selected References

1. de Villiers E-M, Wagner D, Schneider A, *et al*: Human papillomavirus infections in women with and without abnormal cervical cytology. *Lancet* 1987; 2: 703-706

2. Van Den Brule AJ, Walboomers JM, Du Maine M, *et al*: Difference in prevalence of human papillomavirus genotypes in cytomorphologically normal cervical smears is associated with a history of cervical intraepithelial neoplasia. *Int J Cancer* 1991; 48(3): 404-408

3. Koutsky LA, Holmes KK, Critchlow CW, *et al*: A cohort study of the risk of cervical intraepithelial neoplasia grade 2 or 3 in relation to papillomavirus infection. *N Engl J Med* 1992; 327: 1272-1278

4. Mitchell H, Drake M, Medley G: Prospective evaluation of risk of cervical cancer after cytological evidence of human papilloma virus infection. *Lancet* 1986; 1: 573-575

5. Campion MJ, McCance DJ, Cuzick J, *et al*: Progressive potential of mild cervical atypia: prospective cytological, colposcopic, and virological study. *Lancet* 1986; 2: 237-240

6. Pagano R, Chanen W, Rome RM, *et al*: The significance of human papilloma virus atypia ('wart virus infection') found alone on cervical cytology screening. *Aust N Z J Obstet Gynaecol* 1987; 27(2): 136-139

7. Ritter DB, Kadish AS, Vermund SH, *et al*: Detection of human papillomavirus deoxyribonucleic acid in exfoliated cervicovaginal cells as a predictor of cervical neoplasia in a high-risk population. *Am J Obstet Gynecol* 1988; 159(6): 1517-1525

8. Reeves WC, Brinton LA, Garcia M, *et al*: Human papillomavirus infection and cervical cancer in Latin America. *New Engl J Med* 1989; 320(22): 1437-1441

9. Borst M, Butterworth CE, Baker V, *et al*: Human papillomavirus screening for women with atypical Papanicolaou smears. *J Reprod Med* 1991; 36(2): 95-99

10. Rader JS, Rosenzweig BA, Spirtas R, *et al*: Atypical squamous cells. A case-series study of the association between papanicolaou smear results and human papillomavirus DNA genotype. *J Reprod Med* 1991; 36(4): 291-297

11. Schiffman MH, Bauer HM, Hoover RN, *et al*: Epidemiologic evidence showing that human papillomavirus infection causes most cervical intraepithelial neoplasia. *J Nat Cancer Inst* 1993; 85: 958-964

12. Meisels A, Morin C: Human papillomavirus and cancer of the uterine cervix. *Gynecol Oncol* 1981; 12(2 Pt 2): S111-S123

13. Syrjanen K, Vayrynen M, Saarikoski S, *et al*: Natural history of cervical human papillomavirus (HPV) infections based on prospective follow-up. *Br J Obstet Gynecol* 1985; 92: 1086-1092

14. Carmichael JA, Maskens PD: Cervical dysplasia and human papillomavirus. *Am J Obstet Gynecol* 1989; 160: 916-918

15. Koutsky, LA, Galloway DA, Holmes KK: Epidemiology of genital human papillomavirus infection. *Epidemiol Rev* 1988; 10: 122-163

16. Schiffman MH: Recent progress in defining the epidemiology of human papillomavirus infection and cervical neoplasia. *J Nat Cancer Inst* 1992; 84(6) 394-398

17. Reeves WC, Rawls WE, Brinton LA: Epidemiology of genital papillomaviruses and cervical cancer. *Rev Infect Dis* 1989; II(3): 426-439

18. Kitchener HC, Neilson L, Burnett RA, *et al*: Prospective serial study of viral change in the cervix and correlation with human papillomavirus genome status. *Br J Obstet Gynecol* 1991; 98(10): 1042-1048

19. Schneider A, Meinhardt G, de Villiers E-M, *et al*: Sensitivity of the cytologic diagnosis of cervical condyloma in comparison with HPV DNA hybridization studies. *Diagn Cytopathol* 1987; 3: 250-255

20. Spitzer M, Brandsma JL, Steinberg B, *et al*: Detection of conditions related to human papillomavirus. Comparison of cytology, colposcopy, histology, and hybridization. *J Reprod Med* 1990; 35(7): 697-703

21. Reid R, Greenberg MD, Lorincz A, *et al*: Should cervical cytologic testing be augmented by cervicography or human papillomavirus deoxyribonucleic acid detection? *Am J Obstet Gynecol* 1991; 164: 1461-1471

22. Cecchini S, Iossa A, Grazzini G: Estimate of clinical human papillomavirus infection prevalence in a population-based screening. *Cervix Lower Fem Genit Tract* 1988; 6(3): 213-217

23. de Villiers E-M: Laboratory techniques in the investigation of human papillomavirus infection. *Genitourin Med* 1992; 68: 50-54

24. Wilbur DC, Stoler MH: Testing for human papillomavirus: basic pathobiology of infection, methodologies, and implications for clinical use. *Yale J Biol Med* 1991; 64: 113-125

25. Yliskoski M, Saarikoski S, Syrjanen K: Conization for CIN associated with human papillomavirus infection. *Arch Gynecol Obstet* 1991; 249(2): 59-65

26. Kirby P, Dunne A, King DH, *et al*: Double-blind randomized clinical trial of self-administered podofilox solution versus vehicle in the treatment of genital warts. *Am J Med* 1990; 88: 465-469

27. Eron LJ, Judson F, Tucker S, *et al*: Interferon therapy for condylomata acuminata. *N Engl J Med* 1986; 315: 1059-1064

28. Yliskoski M, Cantell K, Syrjanen K, *et al*: Topical treatment with human leukocyte interferon of HPV 16 infections associated with cervical and vaginal intraepithelial neoplasias. *Gynecol Oncol* 1990; 36(3): 353-7

29. Dunham AM, McCartney JC, McCance DJ, *et al*: Effect of perilesional injection of alpha-interferon on cervical intraepithelial neoplasia and associated human papillomavirus infection. *J R Soc Med* 1990; 83(8): 490-492

30. Ferenczy A, Mitao M, Nagai N, *et al*: Latent papillomavirus and recurring genital warts. *N Engl J Med* 1985; 313: 784-788

31. Riva JM, Sedlacek TV, Cunnane MF, *et al*: Extended carbon dioxide laser vaporization in the treatment of subclinical papillomavirus infection of the lower genital tract. *Obstet Gynecol* 1989; 73: 25-30

32. Shafi MI, Finn C, Luesley DM, *et al*: Carbon dioxide laser treatment for vulval papillomatosis (vulvodynia). *Br J Obstet Gynaecol* 1990; 97(12): 1148-1150

33. Ruge S, Felding C, Skouby SO, *et al*: CO2-laser vaporization of human papillomavirus (HPV)-induced abnormal cervical smears. A simple and effective solution to a recurrent clinical problem. *Clin Exp Obstet Gynecol* 1991; 18(2): 99-101

Screening for Human Papillomavirus Infection

MANEUVER	EFFECTIVENESS	LEVEL OF EVIDENCE <REF>	RECOMMENDATION
Human Papillomavirus (HPV) screening (added to Pap smear screening for cervical cancer*) using any of the following diagnostic tests: Visual inspection, Pap smear, Colposcopy/cervicography HPV group-specific antigen, DNA probe, Dot blot, Southern Blot or polymerase chain reaction	HPV is associated with increased risk and grade of cervical cancer.	Cohort<3-6> and case-control<8,11> studies (II-2)	Fair evidence to exclude from periodic health examination (D)
	The natural history of untreated HPV infection is poorly understood and there is no effective therapy that produces long-term success.	Randomized controlled trials<26-29,33> (I); cohort studies<27> (II-2); case series<24> (III) for various therapies	
	HPV diagnostic maneuvers have poor test characteristics or are invasive, costly or inadequately studied. Adverse effects of screening include: morbidity of testing and treatment, associated costs and labelling. Adding HPV screening to screening protocols for cervical cancer has not been studied.	Case Series<3,11,15, 19-24> (III)	

* The Task Force recommends Pap smear screening (B Recommendation), see Chapter 73.

Neoplasms

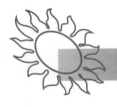

CHAPTER 64

Interventions Other than Smoking Cessation to Prevent Lung Cancer

By Brenda J. Morrison

Interventions Other than Smoking Cessation to Prevent Lung Cancer

Prepared by Brenda J. Morrison, PhD[1]

The primary prevention of lung cancer through smoking cessation must be the long-term goal of preventive health care. However, many people who have overcome their addiction to tobacco or who have reduced their tobacco use are still at risk for lung cancer because of the number of years that they did smoke. Therefore, this chapter examines primary and secondary preventive interventions other than the modification of smoking behaviour. Lower rates of lung cancer are associated with some components of diet; however, there is no evidence that physician counselling on diet influences behavior. There is fair to good evidence that screening for lung cancer using sputum cytology and/or chest radiography are not effective screening maneuvers.

Burden of Suffering

In Canada lung cancer is the most common cause of death from cancer among men and ranks second among women. In 1993 there were an estimated 19,100 new cases of lung cancer and 16,300 deaths due to lung cancer in Canada. An estimated 202,000 potential years of life were lost due to lung cancer in Canada in 1989. Although the mortality rate is levelling off among men it continues to increase among women. If this trend among women continues the number of deaths from lung cancer will surpass the number from breast cancer by the year 2000. In the United States lung cancer is the leading cause of cancer deaths (130,000 annually) and 150,000 new cases are diagnosed each year. The 5-year survival rate is only 13%; this is the poorest prognosis for cancer of any site other than the pancreas. Important risk factors for lung cancer include the use of tobacco, exposure to environmental tobacco smoke, exposure to radon gas and occupational exposure to certain carcinogens. Tobacco alone is responsible for over 80% of all cases.

Maneuver

Counselling on dietary prevention of lung cancer has not been studied. However, 20 dietary studies indicate that consumers of fruits and vegetables containing high levels of carotene are at lower risk.

---

[1] Professor of Health Care and Epidemiology, University of British Columbia, Vancouver, British Columbia

Effectiveness of Prevention and Treatment

Dietary Intervention

The review of 4 prospective dietary studies,[1-4] 11 retrospective case-control dietary studies[5-15] and 5 prospective serum studies[16-22] published before 1989, provided moderately strong evidence that one or more of the carotenoids protects against lung cancer. The diets among the various study groups were diverse, since the investigations were carried out in several countries. In general, smokers who consume a diet low in ß-carotene have a risk of lung cancer 1.5 to 2.0 times higher than those on a diet high in ß-carotene. The same degree of apparent protection has recently been observed in a large study of non-smokers, for those whose diets included a large amount of green vegetables or fresh fruit.

Individuals who frequently consume fruits and vegetables with high carotenoid content have significant reduction of lung cancer risk

The apparently protective effect is not large, but this probably reflects a substantial underestimate because of the errors in dietary reporting and recall and the crudeness of the assay procedures for carotenoids.[6] The results of the earlier studies suggested that ß-carotene is the active agent, but more recent investigations[23-30] imply that other constituents such as lutein, lycopene and/or indoles may also be involved. A recent Finnish randomized controlled trial[31] of ß-carotene and alpha-tocopherol supplementation found an 18% increase in the lung cancer rate (95% confidence interval (CI): 3-36%) among male smokers 50-69 years of age assigned to receive 20 mg of ß-carotene per day. Studies of retinol, synthetic retinoids and alpha-tocopherol are also being carried out.

Dietary supplementation trials with retinol, ß-carotene, synthetic retinoids and tocophenol are in progress

Early Detection

Three large randomized controlled trials have evaluated the effectiveness of screening by chest radiography and sputum cytology in reducing the rate of death from lung cancer. After 5 to 11 years of follow-up they showed no significant benefit resulted from such screening.[32-34] Two of the trials[32,33] tested the benefit of frequent cytologic examination (every 4 months), and the third[34] compared the benefit of frequent cytologic and radiographic examinations (every 4 months) with a recommendation for annual chest radiography. In the first two trials the lung cancer detection rates in the study and control groups were almost identical, and the mortality rates were not significantly different. In the third trial the mortality rates were also very similar, being slightly higher in the study group; however, the detection rate was significantly higher in the study group (p<0.001). The latter difference could have resulted from either a defective randomization procedure or from overly zealous reporting of abnormalities detected by chest radiography. Given the care that

Screening with sputum cytology or chest x-ray does not reduce lung cancer mortality

had apparently been taken in the study design and implementation<34> the latter explanation seems more likely.

Recommendations of Others

The U.S. Preventive Services Task Force<35> does not recommend routine chest radiography or sputum cytology for asymptomatic persons but focuses on counseling about the use of tobacco products for all persons. Their dietary guidelines, currently being reviewed, indicate that patients should be encouraged to eat a variety of foods with emphasis on the consumption of whole grain products and cereals, vegetables and fruits.

Conclusions and Recommendations

Smokers and ex-smokers should be advised to eat a diet rich in green leafy vegetables and fruit (a portion once daily on average). There is no evidence of the effectiveness of physician counselling in inducing dietary changes; however, there is fair evidence to support an increase in intake of such vegetables and fruit to prevent lung cancer. In view of the results of the recent Finnish trial, physicians might be well advised to counsel their patients against the use of ß-carotene supplements.

Cytologic examination of sputum has been clearly shown to be an ineffective screening method for reducing the rate of death from lung cancer. There is good evidence to exclude cytologic screening of sputum from the periodic health examination of asymptomatic people (E Recommendation).

Three chest radiographic examinations per year apparently confer no advantage over one. This observation, together with the manifest ineffectiveness of sputum cytologic screening, indicates that there is fair evidence to recommend that the annual chest radiographic examination be eliminated from the periodic health examination of asymptomatic people (D Recommendation).

Unanswered Questions (Research Agenda)

The positive protective effect of dietary factors against lung cancer and other malignancies requires further investigation and proof of causality.

Evidence

The literature was identified with a MEDLINE search up to March 1993 using the following MESH headings: lung neoplasms, diet, mass screening, mass chest X-ray, smoking, human.

This review was initiated in March 1993 and updates a report published in 1990.<36> Recommendations were finalized by the Task Force in October 1993.

Acknowledgements

The Task Force thanks Dr. Steven Woolf, MD, MPH, Science Advisor, U.S. Preventive Services Task Force, Washington, DC and Assistant Clinical Professor, Department of Family Practice, Medical College of Virginia, Richmond, VA, USA for reviewing the literature on lung cancer.

Selected References

1. Kvale G, Bjelke E, Gart J: Dietary habits and lung cancer risk. *Int J Cancer* 1983; 31: 397-405

2. Hirayama T: Diet and cancer. *Nutr Cancer* 1979; 1: 67-81

3. Shekelle R, Liu S, Raynor W, *et al*: Dietary vitamin A and risk of cancer in the Western Electric Study. *Lancet* 1981; 2: 1185-1190

4. Paganini-Hill A, Chao A, Ross RK, *et al*: Vitamin A, beta-carotene and the risk of cancer: a prospective study. *J Natl Cancer Inst* 1987; 79: 443-448

5. MacLennan R, DaCosta J, Day N, *et al*: Risk factors for lung cancer in Singapore Chinese, a population with high female incidence rates. *Int J Cancer* 1977; 20: 854-860

6. Gregor A, Lee P, Roe F, *et al*: Comparison of dietary histories in lung cancer cases and controls with special reference to vitamin A. *Nutr Cancer* 1980; 2: 93-97

7. Doll R, Bradford Hill A: Mortality in relation to smoking: ten years observations of British doctors. *Br Med J* 1964; 1: 1399-1410

8. Mettlin C, Graham S, Swanson M: Vitamin A and lung cancer. *J Natl Cancer Inst* 1979; 62: 1435-1438

9. Hinds MW, Kolonel LN, Hankin JH, *et al*: Dietary vitamin A, carotene, vitamin C and risk of lung cancer in Hawaii. *Am J Epidemiol* 1984; 119: 227-237

10. Wu AH, Henderson BE, Pike MC, *et al*: Smoking and other risk factors for lung cancer in women. *J Natl Cancer Inst* 1985; 74: 747-751

11. Samet JM, Skipper BJ, Humble CG, *et al*: Lung cancer risk and vitamin A consumption in New Mexico. *Am Rev Respir Dis* 1985; 131: 198-202

12. Byers TE, Graham S, Haughey BP, *et al*: Diet and lung cancer risk: findings from the Western New York Diet Study. *Am J Epidemiol* 1987; 125: 351-363

13. Pisani P, Berrino F, Macaluso M, *et al*: Carrots, green vegetables and lung cancer: a case-control study. *Int J Epidemiol* 1986; 15: 463-468

14. Pastorino U, Pisani P, Berrino F, *et al*: Vitamin A and female lung cancer: a case-control study on plasma and diet. *Nutr Cancer* 1987; 10: 171-179

15. Bond G, Thompson F, Cook R: Dietary vitamin A and lung cancer: results of a case-control study among chemical workers. *Nutr Cancer* 1987; 9: 109-121

16. Stahelin H, Rosel F, Buess E, *et al*: Cancer, vitamins and plasma lipids: prospective Basel study. *J Natl Cancer Inst* 1984; 73: 1463-1468

17. Willett WC, Polk BF, Underwood BA, *et al*: Relation of serum vitamins A and E and carotenoids to the risk of cancer. *N Engl J Med* 1984; 310: 430-434

18. Colditz GA, Stampfer MJ, Willett WC: Diet and lung cancer. A review of the epidemiologic evidence in humans. *Arch Intern Med* 1987; 147: 157-160

19. Katrangi N, Kaplan LA, Stein EA: Separation and quantitation of serum beta-carotene and other carotenoids by high performance liquid chromatography. *J Lipid Res* 1984; 25: 400-406

20. Menkes MS, Comstock GW, Vuilleumier JP, *et al*: Serum beta-carotene, vitamins A and E, selenium, and the risk of lung cancer. *N Engl J Med* 1986; 315: 1250-1254

21. Wald NJ, Thompson SG, Densem JW, *et al*: Serum beta-carotene and subsequent risk of cancer: results from the BUPA study. *Br J Cancer* 1988; 57: 428-433

22. Nomura AM, Stemmermann GN, Heilbrun LK, *et al*: Serum vitamin levels and the risk of cancer in specific sites in men of Japanese ancestry in Hawaii. *Cancer Res* 1985; 45: 2369-2372

23. Fraser GE, Beeson WL, Phillips RL: Diet and lung cancer in California Seventh-day Adventists. *Am J Epidemiol* 1991; 133(7): 683-693

24. Jain M, Burch JD, Howe GR, *et al*: Dietary factors and risk of lung cancer: Results from a case-control study, Toronto, 1981-1985. *Int J Cancer* 1990; 45: 287-293

25. LeMarchand LL, Yoshizawa CN, Kolonel LN, *et al*: Vegetable consumption and lung cancer risk: a population-based case-control study in Hawaii. *J Natl Cancer Inst* 1989; 81: 1158-1164

26. Swanson CA, Mao BL, Li JY, *et al*: Dietary determinants of lung-cancer risk: results from a case-control study in Yunnan province, China. *Int J Cancer* 1992; 50: 876-880

27. Knekt P, Järvinen R, Seppänen R, *et al*: Dietary antioxidants and the risk of lung cancer. *Am J Epidemiol* 1991; 134: 471-479

28. Candelora EC, Stockwell HG, Armstrong AW, *et al*: Dietary intake and risk of lung cancer in women who never smoked. *Nutr Cancer* 1992; 17(3): 263-270

29. Chow WH, Schuman LM, McLaughlin JK, *et al*: A cohort study of tobacco use, diet, occupation, and lung cancer mortality. *Cancer Causes Control* 1992 May; 3(3): 247-254

30. Kalandidi A, Katsouyanni K, Voropoulou N, *et al*: Passive smoking and diet in the etiology of lung cancer among non-smokers. *Cancer Causes Control* 1990; 1: 15-21

31. The Alpha-Tocopherol, Beta Carotene Cancer Prevention Study Group: The effect of vitamin E and beta carotene on the incidence of lung cancer and other cancers in male smokers. *N Engl J Med* 1994; 330: 1029-1035

32. Melamed MR, Flehinger BJ, Zaman MB, *et al*: Screening for early lung cancer. Results of the Memorial Sloan-Kettering study in New York. *Chest* 1984; 86: 44-53

33. Ball WC, Frost JK, Tockman MS, *et al*: Screening for lung cancer: the effect of 5-7 years of periodic roentgenographic and cytologic examinations on detection survival and mortality from lung cancer. [abstract] *Am Rev Respir Dis* 1985; 131: A84

34. Fontana RS, Sanderson DR, Woolner LB, *et al*: Lung cancer screening: the Mayo program. *J Occup Med* 1986; 28: 746-750

35. U.S. Preventive Services Task Force: *Guide to Clinical Preventive Services: an Assessment of the Effectiveness of 169 Interventions*. Williams & Wilkins, Baltimore, Md, 1989: 67-75

36. Canadian Task Force on the Periodic Health Examination: The periodic health examination, 1990 update: 3. Interventions to prevent lung cancer other than smoking cessation. *Can Med Assoc J* 1990; 143(4): 269-272

Interventions Other than
Smoking Cessation to Prevent Lung Cancer

MANEUVER	EFFECTIVENESS	LEVEL OF EVIDENCE <REF>	RECOMMENDATION
Advice to follow a diet high in green leafy vegetables and fruit	Risk of lung cancer is about 2.0 times higher among smokers whose diet is low in green leafy vegetables and fruit than among those who eat more of them. No evidence regarding effectiveness of physician counselling in inducing dietary changes.	Cohort and case-control studies<1-30> (II-2)	Fair evidence to advise smokers to eat an average of seven portions of green leafy vegetables or fruit per week (B)
Sputum cytology	Frequent cytologic examination of sputum does not significantly change detection and mortality rates.	Randomized controlled trials<31-33> (I)	Good evidence to exclude from periodic health examination of asymptomatic people (E)
Chest radiography	Frequent screening by chest radiography improves detection rate but does not significantly change mortality rate.	Randomized controlled trial<33> (I)	Fair evidence to exclude from periodic health examination of asymptomatic people (D)

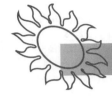

CHAPTER

Screening for Breast Cancer

By Brenda J. Morrison

Screening for Breast Cancer

Prepared by Brenda J. Morrison, PhD[1]

Screening by clinical examination and mammography is recommended for women age 50 to 69; the basis for this recommendation is that seven randomized controlled trials (RCTs), using one or both of these modalities, have shown a survival benefit in this age group.<1> However, although more than 150,000 women between the ages of 40 and 49 were enrolled in these trials no significant decrease in breast cancer mortality was demonstrated for them. As a consequence it is now recommended that women younger than 50 not be screened, whereas in 1986 the Task Force found insufficient evidence to make a recommendation for this age group.<2>

Some cohort studies<3-6> suggest a decreased mortality for women who practice breast self-examination (BSE), but the biases implicit in this type of study make it impossible to make a positive recommendation with regard to the teaching and practice of BSE. This recommendation remains unchanged from that made in 1986.<2>

Burden of Suffering

Breast cancer is the third most common cause of death in women in Canada and excluding skin cancer is the most common cancer in women in Canada.<7> There were an estimated 16,300 new cases of breast cancer in Canada in 1993 and an estimated 5,400 deaths. Over the last 20 years the incidence rate has increased by about 15% whereas the mortality has remained relatively stable.<8>

Within Canada, there is an east-west gradient with lower rates in the east. Risk factors for breast cancer include hormonal, dietary and hereditary factors. Early menarche, late menopause and delayed first pregnancy are associated with higher risk. There is some evidence linking high intake of dietary fat to risk of breast cancer; family history, obesity, alcohol use, ionizing radiation and post-menopausal estrogen replacement therapy (see Chapter 52) have also been associated with increased risk, while the evidence for oral contraceptives is more controversial.

---

[1] Professor, Department of Health Care and Epidemiology, University of British Columbia, Vancouver, British Columbia

Maneuver

There are three maneuvers to be considered. They are clinical examination of the breasts, mammography, and self-examination of the breasts. Some of the seven RCTs carried out these screening maneuvers in combination, and some separately; the prescribed frequencies of the mammographic screenings varied from 12 to 33 months. The sensitivities and specificities of detection varied widely between the trials[1] depending on the maneuver(s) that were employed, the length of the interval between screenings, the underlying incidence of the disease and the method of calculating estimates of the screening proficiency. For sensitivity the range was 46-88%; for specificity, it was 82-99.9%. In the Canadian trial the sensitivity, using the ratio of screen-detected cases to all cases, of annual mammography plus clinical examination was 88% in women 50-59 and 81% in the women 40-49. Specificity, using surgical biopsy as the definition of a positive case, ranged from 96.5% to 99.9%. For the younger women, the ratio of benign biopsy to malignant biopsy was about 9:1 on the first screen, dropping to 6:1 on later screens.[9] For women 50 and over, it was about 5:1 on the initial screen, dropping to 3:1 for later screens.[10]

Effectiveness of Prevention and Treatment

Clinical Examination and Mammography

The seven screening trials enrolled women whose age at entry ranged from 40 to 74. In three of the trials individuals were the unit of randomization; in the the other four the units were neighbourhood or practice clusters. The four trials which were located in Sweden investigated only the benefits of mammography.

Clinical Examination and Mammography for Women Aged Over 50 years

The original trial, that of the Health Insurance Plan (HIP) of New York,[11] demonstrated a significant mortality reduction with a relative risk (RR) of 0.45 five years after entry in women aged 50 to 59.[12] After nine years this rose to 0.67.[13] The combined Swedish trials,[14] after 7 to 12 years of follow-up,[1] also showed a significant benefit extending to the age of 69 (RR=0.71). The Edinburgh trial[15] at 10 years of follow-up produced a non-significant benefit (RR=0.85). Compliance in this trial was poor though and the study and control groups were found to differ on factors that could have affected survival. The Canadian trial,[10] which in the 50-59 year old age group looked only at the benefits of mammography over and above that of annual clinical examination, found an improved survival rate

Screening by mammography has resulted in reduced mortality for 50-69 year olds

(RR=0.97), but at 7 years of follow-up the improvement was not statistically significant.

Clinical Examination and Mammography for Women Aged 40-49 years

Most interest in breast screening has centered about benefit for the 40-49-year-old women. In this age group the HIP showed a non-significant decrease in mortality (RR=0.95) five years after entry.<12> At nine years this had dropped to 0.81 but it was still not significant.<13> However, the number of women in the group was not large and consequently the power of the test was low. Because of these two factors the Task Force in its 1986 report gave a C Recommendation for the 40-49 year olds.<2> Now with seven trials reporting, and two of them, the Swedish Two County trial and the Canadian trial,<9> having large numbers of compliant enrollees, there is now a considerable amount of evidence. None of the trials showed a significant benefit. The relative risks ranged from 0.51 to 1.36. In the five trials that had reported early age-specific follow-up, increased mortality occurred in this younger age group in all of the studies (in the Malmo trial the younger age group was composed of women 45-54). In the HIP the excess of deaths disappeared after 3 years but in the other trials it lasted for seven or eight years. Of all the trials, the Canadian study showed the greatest excess, RR=1.36 (95% confidence interval: 0.84-2.21); this was after seven years of follow-up. This is not really surprising since the Canadian trial was the only one of the seven which was an efficacy trial and the results of efficacy trials are expected to be more extreme than those of effectiveness trials.

At present plans are being made to organize and carry out a RCT in Europe and the U.S. of 1.5 million women age 40-42, who will be followed for 10 years.<16>

Breast Self-Examination (BSE)

Before the introduction of mass screening programs, the vast majority of tumours were reputed to have been detected by the women themselves. As a consequence of this, breast self-examination was and is advocated by various bodies and organizations in the hopeful expectation that early detection will result in improved survival. Five studies<2,17-20> have shown an association between the practice of BSE and factors associated with better survival, such as stage, tumour size or axillary node involvement, but other studies have shown no benefit.<21-23>

Four studies compared the survival rates from breast cancer in women who had been taught or practiced BSE and in those who had not been instructed or did not practice it. Foster looked at those who had performed it regularly with those who had not. At five years the respective rates were 75% and 57% (p<0.0002). Locker compared all those invited to attend an instructive course in BSE with an historical group of cases. The latter had slightly better survival despite having poorer prognostic indicators. However, after seven years of follow-up those in the instructed group who attended had a significantly lower mortality in contrast with those who did not attend (p<0.001).

Le Geyte compared those who practiced BSE with those who had never been taught it. After 6 years of follow-up the respective survival rates were 73.1% and 66.1% (p=0.07). Kuroishi compared those who had found their cancer by self-examination with those who had found theirs by chance. After five year the follow-up rates were significantly different (p<0.001) but at ten years the difference was no longer significant, suggesting that the apparent improvement was due to lead-time bias. The results of all of these studies could have been distorted by lead-time, length-time and self-selection bias.

Recommendations of Others

In 1992 the U.S. Preventive Services Task Force (USPSTF) called for annual clinical breast examinations after age 40, mammography every 1 to 2 years beginning at age 50 and early screening of women at increased risk for breast cancer.[24] These recommendations are currently under review. The differences between our recommendations and the USPSTF could be accounted for by the recent publication of longer follow-up results from several of the trials.

Conclusions and Recommendations

Since all of the trials demonstrated a mortality reduction in the 50-69 age group, the Task Force recommends breast screening for women of this age (A Recommendation). Because the relative contributions of mammography and clinical examination have not yet been fully ascertained, both manuevers are recommended. Also, since from the limited data available it is not possible to deduce confidently if biennial screening is as effective as annual screening, the Task Force advises that annual screening be maintained. Wherever possible, screening should be done at centers dedicated to this purpose.

In view of the absence of a significant benefit and the possibility that screening and intervention might be causing harm, the Task Force recommends that until further evidence is available, women age 40-49 not be screened (D Recommendation).

The evidence is not strong enough to make a clear recommendation on teaching breast self-examination; there is insufficient evidence to either include or exclude such teaching in periodic health examinations for women (C Recommendation).

Unanswered Questions (Research Agenda)

Isolation of a gene (or genes) for familial breast cancer may soon be accomplished

In 1990 a gene responsible for a sizeable proportion of familial breast cancer, possibly 45%, and 80% of familial ovarian cancer,<25> was localized by genetic linkage on the long arm of chromosome 17.<26> The gene, BRCA1, has not yet been isolated but some screening, by means of linkage, is being performed on high risk women.<27-29> Two other genes relating to breast cancer have also been localized<30> ESR and p53 (associated with the Li-Fraumeni syndrome). It is estimated that inherited susceptibility occurs in 1 in 200 women in the U.S. and may be responsible for about 10-15% of premenopausal breast cancer. BRCA1 and p53 appear to be autosomal dominants and relate most strongly to premenopausal breast cancer. The penetrance of the BRCA1 gene has been estimated to be at least 50% by age 50 and 80% by age 80, and that for the p53 gene, slightly higher. At present identification requires blood samples from many members of a family, including those who have developed the disease, but in the near future these genes will be isolated and cloned. Then individuals carrying the genes will be able to be identified by a simple blood test. This scientific breakthrough is a mixed blessing for those found to have the gene, but for those who are found to be negative the knowledge will bring substantial relief. Centres presently carrying out this screening have set up intensive counselling programs for sessions prior and subsequent to testing and disclosure.

Unlike the situation with Huntington's Chorea, "preventive" strategies (preventive in terms of breast and ovarian cancer) are presently available. They are bilateral mastectomy and oophorectomy, or medication with tamoxifen. These are radical measures; nevertheless, many women who consider themselves at high risk are prepared to undergo these treatments. No randomized trials of the efficacy of prophylactic mastectomy or oophorectomy have been carried out specifically in the women carrying these genes, but there is some evidence that both of these measures have reduced the risk in women who have undergone them. A large RCT is being carried out on tamoxifen at present.<31> Screening for these breast cancer genes will probably be the first widespread presymptomatic genetic test for adults in general medical practice.<25>

Evidence

The evidence reviewed was identified from the collection of the author and using a MEDLINE search in November 1993 using the key words: breast neoplasms, mass screening, guideline, familial or genetic markers.

This review was initiated in March 1993 and recommendations were finalized by the Task Force in January 1994.

Selected References

1. Fletcher SW, Black W, Harris R, *et al*: Report of the International Workshop on Screening for Breast Cancer. *J Natl Cancer Inst* 1993; 85(20): 1644-1656

2. Canadian Task Force on the Periodic Health Examination: The periodic health examination: 2. 1985 update. *Can Med Assoc J* 1986; 134: 724-729

3. Foster RS Jr, Constanza MC: Breast self-examination practices and breast cancer survival. *Cancer* 1984; 53: 999-1005

4. Locker AP, Caseldine J, Mitchell AK, *et al*: Results from a seven-year programme of breast self-examination in 89,010 women. *Br J Cancer* 1989; 60: 401-405

5. Le Geyte M, Mant D, Vessey MP, *et al*: Breast self examination and survival from breast cancer. *Br J Cancer* 1992; 66: 917-918

6. Kuroishi T, Tominaga S, Ota J, *et al*: The effect of breast self-examination on early detection and survival. *Jpn J Cancer Res* 1992; 83: 344-350

7. Statistics Canada: Cancer in Canada. *Health Reports* 1992; 4 (3 Suppl 8): Catalogue No. 82-003S12. Ottawa

8. Band PR, Gaudette LA, Hill GB, *et al*: The making of the Canadian cancer registry: cancer incidence in Canada and its regions, 1969 to 1988. Catalogue No. C52-42/1992. Bureau of Chronic Disease Epidemiology, Health and Welfare. Ottawa

9. Miller AB, Baines CJ, To T, *et al*: Canadian National Breast Screening Study: 1. Breast cancer detection and death rates among women aged 40 to 49 years. *Can Med Assoc J* 1992; 147: 1459-1476

10. Miller AB, Baines CJ, To T, *et al*: Canadian National Breast Screening Study: 2. Breast cancer detection and death rates among women aged 50 to 59 years. *Can Med Assoc J* 1992; 147: 1477-1488

11. Shapiro S, Venet W, Strax P, *et al*: Selection, follow-up, and analysis in the Health Insurance Plan Study: A randomized trial with breast cancer screening. *National Cancer Institute Monograph* No. 67, 1985, NIH Publication No. 85-2713. Department of Health and Human Services

12. Shapiro S, Venet W, Strax P, *et al*: Ten- to fourteen-year effect of screening on breast cancer mortality. *J Natl Can Inst* 1982; 69: 349-355

13. Shapiro S: Evidence on screening for breast cancer from a randomized trial. *Cancer* 1977; 39: 2772-2782

14. Nystrom L, Rutqvist LE, Wall S, *et al*: Breast cancer screening with mammography: overview of Swedish randomized trials. *Lancet* 1993; 341: 973-978

15. Roberts MM, Alexander FE, Anderson TJ, *et al*: Edinburgh trial of screening for breast cancer: mortality at seven years. *Lancet* 1990; 335: 241-246

16. Eckhardt S, Badellino F, Murphy GP: UICC meeting on breast-cancer screening in pre-menopausal women in developed countries. *Int J Cancer* 1994; 56: 1-5

17. Greenwald P, Nasca PC, Lawrence CE, *et al*: Estimated effect of breast self-examination and routine physician examinations on breast cancer mortality. *N Engl J Med* 1978; 299: 271-273

18. Huguley CM Jr, Brown RL: The value of breast self-examination. *Cancer* 1981; 47: 989-995

19. Feldman JG, Carter AC, Nicastri AD, *et al*: Breast self-examination, relationship to stage of breast cancer at diagnosis. *Cancer* 1981; 47: 2740-2745

20. Mant D, Vessey MP, Neil A, *et al*: Breast self examination and breast cancer stage at diagnosis. *Br J Cancer* 1987; 55: 207-211

21. Smith EM, Francis AM, Polissar L: The effect of breast self-exam practices and physician examinations on extent of disease at diagnosis. *Prev Med* 1980; 9: 409-417

22. Senie RT, Rosen PP, Lesser ML, *et al*: Breast self- examination and medical examination related to breast cancer stage. *Am J Public Health* 1981; 71: 583-590

23. Philip J, Harris WG, Flaherty C, *et al*: Breast self- examination: clinical results from a population-based prospective study. *Br J Cancer* 1984; 50: 7-12

24. Woolf SH: United States Preventive Services Task Force recommendations on breast cancer screening. *Cancer* 1992; 69: 1913-1918

25. Biesecker BB, Boehnke M, Calzone K, *et al*: Genetic counseling for families with inherited susceptibility to breast and ovarian cancer. *JAMA* 1993; 269: 1970-1974

26. Hall JM, Lee MK, Newman B, *et al*: Linkage of early-onset familial breast cancer to chromosome 17q21. *Science* 1990; 250: 1684-1689

27. Easton DF, Bishop DT, Ford D, *et al*: Genetic linkage analysis in familial breast and ovarian cancer: results from 214 families. *Am J Hum Genet* 1993; 52: 678-701

28. Houlston RS, Lemoine L, McCarter E, *et al*: Screening and genetic counselling for relatives of patients with breast cancer in a family clinic. *J Med Genet* 1992; 29: 691-694

29. Lynch HT, Watson P, Conway TA, *et al*: DNA screening for breast/ovarian cancer susceptibility based on linked markers. *Arch Intern Med* 1993; 153: 1979-1987

30. King M-C, Rowell S, Love SM: Inherited breast and ovarian cancer. What are the risks? What are the choices? *JAMA* 1993; 269: 1975-1980

31. Nayfield SG, Karp JE, Ford LG, *et al*: Potential role of tamoxifen in prevention of breast cancer. *J Natl Cancer Inst* 1991; 83: 1450-1459

Screening for Breast Cancer

MANEUVER	EFFECTIVENESS	LEVEL OF EVIDENCE <REF>	RECOMMENDATION
Clinical examination and mammography, women aged 50-69 years	Routine clinical examination and mammography reduces mortality from breast cancer. Optimum frequency of screening has not been determined.	Randomized controlled trials<1> (I)	Good evidence for screening women aged 50-69 years annually by clinical examination and mammography (A)
Clinical examination and mammography, women aged 40-49 years	Routine clinical examination and mammography has not consistently been shown to reduce mortality from breast cancer.	Randomized controlled trials<1> (I)	Contradictory evidence regarding benefits and risks of clinical examination and mammography but fair evidence to exclude from periodic health examination of asymptomatic women aged 40-49 years (D)
Teaching breast self-examination (BSE)	Increased survival and other indicators of early detection demonstrated but studies subject to bias.	Cohort and case-control studies <3-6,17-23> (II-2)	Inadequate evidence that the practice of BSE improves survival; insufficient evidence to include or exclude from the periodic health examination (C)

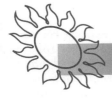

CHAPTER **66**

Screening
for
Colorectal
Cancer

By Michael J. Solomon and Robin S. McLeod

Screening for Colorectal Cancer

Michael J. Solomon, MB, BCH, BAO (Hons), FRACS[1] and Robin S. McLeod, MD, FRCSC FACS[2]

In 1989, the Canadian Task Force on the Periodic Health Examination (CTF)<1> and the U.S. Preventive Services Task Force<2> reviewed the available evidence and concurred that there was no evidence to include or exclude Hemoccult fecal occult blood screening, sigmoidoscopy or colonoscopy in the asymptomatic population over the age of 40 years. With the recent publication of new evidence, the CTF has updated but basically not changed its recommendations. There is evidence that annual rehydrated Hemoccult fecal occult blood screening has a small but significant cancer-specific mortality benefit after more than 10 years of annual screening but not with biennial screening (every two years). However, the high false positivity and poor sensitivity of the technique make this a poor method for detecting colorectal cancer. There is limited evidence for potential improvement in survival with screening sigmoidoscopy. The cost and poor compliance of colonoscopic screening make this an unfeasible strategy. Thus, there is insufficient evidence to support the inclusion or exclusion of fecal occult blood, sigmoidoscopic or colonoscopic screening of asymptomatic individuals over the age of 40 years. There is fair evidence to support screening with colonoscopy of individuals with Cancer Family Syndrome.

Burden of Suffering

Colorectal cancer remains a leading cause of mortality in the western world. In Canada there were an estimated 16,000 new cases and 6,300 deaths due to colorectal cancer in 1993. Colorectal cancer is the second most common cancer in Canada, accounting for more than 14% of cancers in both sexes.<3> Rates in Canada are among the highest in the world, particularly in men and there appears to be a slight east-west gradient across the country, with lower rates in the Pacific and Prairies; rates are substantially lower in the North.<3>

Several groups of individuals have been identified as being at high risk for colorectal cancer. People with ulcerative colitis or familial polyposis are at higher risk but they are not members of the asymptomatic, otherwise healthy target population of the periodic health examination and they are specifically excluded. Risk factors for

---

[1] Director of Research, University of Sydney, Department of Colorectal Surgery, Royal Prince Alfred Hospital, Newtown, NSW, Australia
[2] Associate Professor of Surgery, University of Toronto, Toronto, Ontario

colorectal cancer include familial and genetic factors, and possibly low physical activity, alcohol consumption, high dietary fat and meat intake and low intake of fibre and vegetables.[3] Age is a risk factor as less than 2% of cases occur in people under the age of 40. By the age of 50 the risk of colorectal cancer is 18 to 20 times that for a 30-year-old person, and it continues to double about every 7 years.[1]

Maneuver

The most common protocol followed in colorectal cancer screening is a multiphase screen using fecal occult blood testing in the first phase followed by colonoscopy or sigmoidoscopy combined with barium enema for those patients who are occult blood positive. The Hemoccult test detects the peroxidase-like activity of hemoglobin. Several other methods of fecal analysis have been developed although none have been rigorously assessed in randomized controlled trials for screening. Hemoquant detects the porphyrin-like moiety of hemoglobin, while immunochemistry employing a high titre of monospecific antisera to intact human hemoglobin has also been used. Recent evidence suggests Hemoquant is only equally or even less sensitive than Hemoccult for cancer detection.[4] An alternative to the multiphase screen is a uniphase periodic screen with sigmoidoscopy or colonoscopy alone.

Effectiveness of Prevention

Multiphase Screening in Asymptomatic Individuals With Hemoccult

Four large randomized controlled trials and one non-randomized controlled trial have assessed the value of screening with Hemoccult.[5-9] There are fairly consistent data from these trials showing that in asymptomatic individuals over 40 years of age there is a 1-2 per 1,000 probability that a cancer will be detected if subjects are offered multiphase screening. Of those who comply, this increases to 2-3 per 1,000. However, the chance of detecting a cancer is approximately equal to the chance of missing a cancer (interval cancer). Although cancers detected by screening are more likely to be at an earlier stage of disease, to date the evidence from 3 trials demonstrates no improved overall survival.[5,6,9] One trial has shown a definite, statistically significant improvement in cancer-specific mortality[5] for annual but not biennial Hemoccult and two trials have shown a decreased cancer-specific mortality in the screened group but the differences were not statistically significant.[6,9] The high false positive rate, especially with rehydrated Hemoccult slides, would require full colonic evaluation in up to 10% of the screened population at each screen. The poor sensitivity of annual (49%) and

Hemoccult provides a small cancer-specific benefit at a high potential cost with 50% of cancers missed

biennial (38%) screening and high number of false positives limits the feasibility of Hemoccult screening. The statistically significant cancer specific mortality benefit in one study and the trend in 2 studies represents a risk reduction of 28-32%. While this may seem impressive, in absolute terms this represents a survival benefit of 1-3 per 1,000 patients but requires repeated annual screens for more than 10 years. During this period, more than a thousand colonoscopic examinations would have been required as a result of false positives.

The prevalence of colorectal cancer in the screened compared to control groups with longer follow-up periods should determine whether the detection and removal of adenomas has had any effect. There is no evidence from these trials that the detection and removal of adenomas has decreased the prevalence of colorectal cancer in the screened populations. Thus, to date there is direct evidence that screening with Hemoccult has a clinically small but statistically significant cancer specific mortality benefit for annual screening but not biennial screening. In view of the insensitivity, high false positivity (9.8%), limited feasibility and small clinical benefit of Hemoccult screening the C recommendation has not been altered.

Uniphase Screening of Asymptomatic Individuals With Sigmoidoscopy

Sigmoidoscopy is potentially a good screening test but requires further evaluation

The results of one randomized controlled trial are widely quoted as specifically addressing the question of whether sigmoidoscopy alone is of value in screening asymptomatic individuals for cancer.<10> Unfortunately the design of the Kaiser Multiphase Evaluation Study raises more questions than it answers and has led to several conflicting reports. Only two descriptive studies with adequate follow-up (Grade III evidence) have been performed.<11,12> These have shown encouraging results in favour of sigmoidoscopy but without an unscreened control group the effects of volunteer, lead-time and length-time bias cannot be measured.

In a case-control study reported by Selby and colleagues,<13> patients who had fatal colorectal cancers were reviewed retrospectively and compared to matched controls to determine the proportion of patients in each group who had had a rigid sigmoidoscopy in the preceding 10 years. Of the fatal cases 8.8% compared to 24.2% of controls had sigmoidoscopy performed within the preceding 10 years (p<0.001). Although this study suggests that patients with fatal colorectal cancers were less likely to have had rigid sigmoidoscopy in the preceding 10 years compared with matched controls, in fact only 12 of 868 (1%) control patients had adenomas detected and removed at the time of sigmoidoscopy. This suggests that the observed difference may have been due to intrinsic differences between the case and control groups since the intervention which should explain the benefit (i.e. polypectomy) was performed in such a small proportion of patients in the control group. Screening sigmoidoscopy per se without any consequent therapeutic procedure should not decrease mortality.

A second case-control study published by Newcomb and coworkers[14] compared each member of a health plan who died of large bowel cancer (cases) to 3 matched control subjects who were members of the same health plan. Approximately 70% of the control subjects had a screening sigmoidoscopy compared with only 11% of the cases (Odds ratio (OR) 0.21; 95% confidence interval 0.08-0.52). However, these authors failed to report the number of subjects in whom a polyp was detected and treated at screening sigmoidoscopy. As pointed out previously, screening sigmoidoscopy without any resulting therapeutic intervention should not decrease mortality. It is impossible, therefore, to evaluate the specific impact sigmoidoscopy had on cancer mortality in this study. Furthermore, the OR of having a proximal cancer was 0.36 in subjects who had not had a screening sigmoidoscopy. Although this difference was not statistically significant (possibly because of a Type II error), it suggests that the subjects who had a screening sigmoidoscopy were intrinsically different with a lower risk for the development of large bowel cancers since the risk of cancer in the more proximal bowel should be unaltered by screening sigmoidoscopy.

The evidence to date suggests that 1 or 2 cancers per 1,000 individuals may be detected by sigmoidoscopy and these cancers may be detected at an earlier stage. However, there is no available information on the sensitivity, specificity or predictive values of sigmoidoscopy. The figures from uncontrolled studies[11,12] and from two case-control studies[13,14] suggest that survival may have been improved, but evidence from one controlled trial suggests that the improved mortality rates may have been due to volunteer bias rather than the screening procedure itself.[10] Flexible sigmoidoscopy may be preferable to rigid sigmoidoscopy as it examines the more proximal colon than the rigid instrument and thus detects more lesions and it is more acceptable than the rigid sigmoidoscope despite the widespread use of rigid sigmoidoscopy in the studies discussed. Bowel perforations only occur at a rate of 1.4 per 10,000 sigmoidoscopies in asymptomatic individuals and it is thus a relatively safe procedure although flexible sigmoidoscopy does require a more qualified examiner.

Uniphase Screening of Asymptomatic Individuals With Colonoscopy

Only the results of small case series (Grade III evidence) in asymptomatic individuals over the age of 50 years with no family history of colorectal cancer have been reported.[15,16] Because there were no control groups or follow-up, there is no direct evidence for or against the effectiveness of colonoscopic screening of asymptomatic individuals. Although colonoscopy is accepted as the best method for detecting both polyps and cancers, poor patient compliance and acceptability and cost make this an impractical method of screening the asymptomatic population. In addition, there is a relatively high complication rate. The reported risk of perforation following diagnostic colonoscopy ranges from 0.3-0.8%, following polypectomy 0.5-1.0% and the risk of bleeding following polypectomy 1.4-2.0%.

Screening High-Risk Groups

Patients with a family history of colorectal carcinoma or previously treated colorectal cancer or adenomas continue to be a dilemma as regards screening. At present, guidelines are derived from descriptive studies with survival benefits of screening extrapolated from the possible higher risk of developing malignancy rather than from evidence that screening is effective.

In the cancer family syndrome, the risk of an adenocarcinoma (uterine, stomach, breast, ovarian and colorectal) developing in a first degree relative approaches 50%[17] and as cancer family syndrome patients have a higher proportion of right-sided colon cancers, periodic screening with colonoscopy would thus be wise in this group. However, when to start and at what intervals to repeat the procedure has not been determined.

The value of screening individuals with one or two first degree relatives with colorectal cancer is controversial. Rozen *et al* screened 471 asymptomatic first degree relatives of patients with colorectal cancer with Hemoccult tests and sigmoidoscopy and compared the results to those in a group of 457 asymptomatic volunteers with no family history of colorectal cancer.[18] There was a threefold increase in the prevalence of neoplasia (both polyps and cancers) in the group with a family history of colorectal cancer. However, only 2 invasive cancers were detected in the study group (cancer detection rate 0.004) compared with 1 in the control group (cancer detection rate 0.002). The study group had a threefold increase in colonoscopic examinations despite no significant difference in the rate of positive Hemoccult tests or sigmoidoscopy. This diagnostic suspicion bias may explain some of the difference in the detection rate of neoplasia.

Several historical case-control studies in the past have reported an association between a family history of colorectal cancer and a 2-4 times increased risk of colorectal cancer.[19,20] No attempt to exclude cancer family syndrome cases or to confirm the accuracy of the family history in cases and controls by medical or pathology records was performed in these studies ("family information bias"). Thus, there is little evidence to confirm or refute an increased prevalence of neoplasms or increased mortality nor to justify a different approach to screening for individuals with only one or two relatives with colorectal cancer compared with the population with no family history, despite widespread encouragement to do so. In the large population of individuals with a first degree relative with colorectal cancer a better understanding of the genetic predisposition for colorectal cancer may identify smaller subgroups with a cancer prevalence that justifies the cost and adverse effects of colonoscopic screening. On the other hand, the development of a screening test that is much more sensitive than Hemoccult or more acceptable than colonoscopy may potentially benefit both these individuals and asymptomatic individuals with no family history of colorectal cancer.

The recurrence of polyps in those who have had previous polypectomy is approximately 33%. Because of the perceived increased risk of cancer in these individuals, periodic colonoscopy has been recommended for all patients who have had colorectal adenomas or carcinomas removed previously.[1] More recent evidence suggests that this should be limited to: previous carcinomas, tubular adenomas that are >10 mm and tubulo-villous or villous adenomas.[21] Periodic colonoscopy for patients with other adenomas may be unwarranted. The recently reported National Polyp Study was a multicentre randomized controlled study of surveillance colonoscopy after polypectomy for adenomas.[22] The results suggest there is no significant difference in the detection of clinically important colorectal neoplasms when colonoscopy is performed both 1 and 3 years after polypectomy as compared with a single 3 year follow-up colonoscopy. Further evaluation is required.

Recommendations of Others

The recommendations of the U.S. Preventive Services Task Force on screening for colorectal cancer are currently under review. The American Cancer Society revised it's recommendations in 1992 and recommends annual screening with Hemoccult combined with flexible sigmoidoscopy every 3-5 years.[23] The National Cancer Institute recommends a uniphase periodic screen with sigmoidoscopy alone as an alternative to the multiphase screen.[24]

Conclusions and Recommendations

Ultimately, a screening test more sensitive than Hemoccult, less costly and invasive than colonoscopy, and which screens the entire colorectum is necessary. Certainly the significant burden of illness of colorectal cancer and the improvement in survival with earlier stage detection make the development of such a test a high research priority. Furthermore, efforts directed at identification of different risk groups and development of different strategies for these groups may be appropriate. The true cancer family syndrome patients have a

The small benefit demonstrated by an insensitive test has shown that screening in colorectal cancer can potentially alter survival

higher risk of colorectal cancer and a higher incidence of right sided colon cancer, thus colonoscopy rather than sigmoidoscopy is recommended. There is fair evidence to support the use of colonoscopy (B Recommendation) and fair evidence not to use multiphasic fecal output screening (D Recommendation) or sigmoidoscopy (D Recommendation) for this group based on expert opinion. It is recommended that individuals with a family history of only 1 or 2 relatives with colorectal cancer be screened no differently than asymptomatic individuals older than 40 years.

There is direct evidence that screening with Hemoccult has a clinically small but statistically significant cancer-specific mortality benefit for annual screening but not biennial screening. In view of the insensitivity, high false positivity, limited feasibility and small clinical benefit of Hemoccult screening the C Recommendation has not been altered – there is insufficient evidence to include or exclude Hemoccult screening in the periodic health examination of individuals over age 40 years.

Two case-control studies have demonstrated an association between improved survival for colorectal cancer and sigmoidoscopy, however, in one study there was no therapeutic intervention (only 1% had removal of adenomas) to account for the survival benefit. In the other, data regarding the frequency of polyps and polypectomy in those having sigmoidoscopy were not reported. Thus differences in survival may have been due to inherent differences in the two groups. Therefore, there is no new evidence to change the recommendation of screening with sigmoidoscopy or insufficient evidence to support inclusion or exclusion of sigmoidoscopy in the periodic health examination (C Recommendation). There is also insufficient evidence to recommend for or against screening with colonoscopy in the general population (C Recommendation).

Unanswered Questions (Research Agenda)

The following have been identified as research priorities:

1. Identification of genetic and environmental risk factors for more accurate determination of true high-risk groups.

2. Development of a screening maneuver more sensitive than Hemoccult and more acceptable than colonoscopy for examination of the whole colorectum.

3. A randomized controlled trial of flexible sigmoidoscopy in asymptomatic individuals older than 40 years.

4. Acceptability of colonoscopy versus flexible sigmoidoscopy.

Evidence

Articles assessing screening for colorectal neoplasia were retrieved by a MEDLINE search from 1966 to June 1993 using the Mesh headings Screening, colorectal neoplasia and limited to English. This review was initiated in January 1992 and recommendations finalized by the Task Force in June 1993. The technical report was published in 1994.<25>

Acknowledgements

The Task Force thanks Dr. Charles Erlichman, MD, ABOncol FRCPC, Associate Professor of Medicine, University of Toronto, Toronto, Ontario, and Dr. Paul Belliveau, MD, FRCFc, CSPQ, FACS, Associate Professor of Surgery, McGill University, Montreal, Quebec. The views expressed here are those of the Task Force and do not necessarily reflect those of reviewers.

Selected References

1. Canadian Task Force on the Periodic Health Examination: The periodic health examination: 2. 1989 update. *Can Med Assoc J* 1989; 141: 205-216

2. U.S. Preventive Services Task Force: *Guide to Clinical Preventive Services: an Assessment of the Effectiveness of 169 Interventions*. Williams & Wilkins, Baltimore, Md, 1989: 47-55

3. Canadian Council of Cancer Registries, Health and Welfare Canada, Statistics Canada: The Making of the Canadian Cancer Registry: Cancer incidence in Canada and its regions, 1969 to 1988. Minister of Supply and Services Canada, (Cat. No. C52-42/1992; ISBN 0-660-54887-9), 1993; 45-46

4. Ahlquist DA, Wieand HS, Moertel CG, *et al*: Accuracy of fecal occult blood screening for colorectal neoplasia. A prospective study using Hemoccult and HemoQuant tests. *JAMA* 1993; 269: 1262-1267

5. Mandel JS, Bond JH, Church TR, *et al*: Reducing mortality from colorectal cancer by screening for fecal occult blood. *N Engl J Med* 1993; 328: 1365-1371

6. Jensen BM, Kronborg O, Fenger C: Interval cancers in screening with fecal occult blood test for colorectal cancer. *Scand J Gastroenterol* 1992; 27: 779-782

7. Kewenter J, Bjork S, Haglind E, *et al*: Screening and rescreening for colorectal cancer. A controlled trial of fecal occult blood testing in 27,700 subjects. *Cancer* 1988; 62: 645-651

8. Hardcastle JD, Thomas WM, Chamberlain J, *et al*: Randomised, controlled trial of fecal occult blood screening for colorectal cancer. Results for first 107,349 subjects. *Lancet* 1989; 1: 1160-1164

9. Winawer SJ, Schottenfeld D, Flehinger BJ: Colorectal cancer screening. *J Natl Cancer Inst* 1991; 83(4): 243-253

10. Selby JV, Friedman GD: Sigmoidoscopy in the periodic health examination of asymptomatic adults. *JAMA* 1989; 261: 595-601

11. Gilbertsen VA, Nelms JM: The prevention of invasive cancer of the rectum. *Cancer* 1978; 41: 1137-1139

12. Hertz REL, Deddish MR, Day E: Value of periodic examinations in detecting cancer of the colon and rectum. *Postgrad Med* 1960; 27: 290-294

13. Selby JV, Friedman GD, Quesenberry CP, *et al*: A case-control study of screening sigmoidoscopy and mortality from colorectal cancer. *N Engl J Med* 1992; 326: 653-657

14. Newcomb PA, Norfleet RG, Storer BE, *et al*: Screening sigmoidoscopy and colorectal cancer mortality. *J Natl Cancer Inst* 1992; 84: 1572-1575

15. Johnson DA, Gurney MS, Volpe RJ, *et al*: A prospective study of the prevalence of colonic neoplasms in asymptomatic patients with an age-related risk. *Am J Gastroenterol* 1990; 85: 969-974

16. Rex DK, Lehman GA, Hawes RH, *et al*: Screening colonoscopy in asymptomatic average-risk persons with negative fecal occult blood tests. *Gastroenterology* 1991; 100: 64-67

17. Lynch HT, Rozen P, Schuelke GS: Hereditary colon cancer: polyposis and nonpolyposis variants. *CA-Cancer J Clin* 1985; 35: 95-114

18. Rozen P, Fireman Z, Figer A, *et al*: Family history of colorectal cancer as a marker of potential malignancy within a screening program. *Cancer* 1987; 60: 248-254

19. Bonelli L, Martines H, Conio M, *et al*: Family history of colorectal cancer as a risk factor for benign and malignant tumours of the large bowel. A case-control study. *Int J Cancer* 1988; 41: 513-517

20. Ponz de Leon M, Antonioli A, Ascari A, *et al*: Incidence and familial occurrence of colorectal cancer and polyps in a health-care district of northern Italy. *Cancer* 1987; 60: 2848-2859

21. Atkin WS, Morson BC, Cuzick J: Long-term risk of colorectal cancer after excision of rectosigmoid adenomas. *N Engl J Med* 1992; 326: 658-662

22. Winawer SJ, Zauber AG, O'Brien MJ, *et al*: Randomized comparison of surveillance intervals after colonoscopic removal of newly diagnosed adenomatous polyps. *N Engl J Med* 1993; 328: 901-906

23. Revision in American Cancer Society recommendations for the early detection of colorectal cancer. *CA-A* 1992; 42: 296-299

24. National Cancer Institute: *Working guidelines for early cancer detection: rationale and supporting evidence to decrease mortality.* Bethesda, Md, National Cancer Institute, 1987.

25. Solomon MJ, McLeod RS with the Canadian Task Force on the Periodic Health Examination: The Periodic Health Examination, 1994 update: 2. Screening strategies for colorectal cancer. *Can Med Assoc J* 1994; 150: 1961-1970

Screening for Colorectal Cancer

MANEUVER	EFFECTIVENESS	LEVEL OF EVIDENCE <REF>	RECOMMENDATION
Multiphase (Hemoccult)	**Asymptomatic (> 40 yrs):** Small cancer-specific mortality benefit for annual but not biennial screen after 10 yrs of screening. High false positivity (9.8%) and low sensitivity (49% for annual and 38% biennial screen) make this a poor screening method.	Randomized controlled trials<5-8> (I)	Insufficient evidence of benefit to include or exclude in the periodic health exam (PHE) of asymptomatic individuals over 40 years (C)
	Family History (1 or 2 relatives): Little evidence to confirm increased prevalence of colorectal cancer or increased associated mortality.	Case-control studies<19,20> (II-2); case series<18> (III)	Insufficient evidence to include or exclude in PHE of asymptomatic individuals over 40 yrs with a family history (1 or 2 relatives) (C)
	Cancer Family Syndrome: Risk of adenocarcinoma approaches 50%; colonoscopy has superior test characteristics.	Case series<17> (III)	Fair evidence to exclude from PHE of individuals with Cancer Family Syndrome (D)
Sigmoidoscopy	**Asymptomatic (>40 yrs) or Family History (1 or 2 relatives):** Test characteristics of sigmoidoscopy are unknown; the demonstrated survival benefit may be due to volunteer bias.	Case-control studies<13,14> (II-2)	Insufficient evidence to include or exclude in PHE of asymptomatic individuals over 40 yrs including those with a family history (1 or 2 relatives) (C)
	Cancer Family Syndrome: Risk of adenocarcinoma approaches 50%; colonoscopy superior test for detecting right-sided cancer.	Expert opinion (III)	Fair evidence to exclude from PHE of individuals with Cancer Family Syndrome (D)

(Continued on next page)

Screening for Colorectal Cancer (concl'd)

MANEUVER	EFFECTIVENESS	LEVEL OF EVIDENCE <REF>	RECOMMENDATION
Colonoscopy	**Asymptomatic (> 40 yrs) or Family History (1 or 2 relatives):** Small cancer-specific mortality benefit but poor sensitivity. Cost and compliance are potential problems.	Case series <15,16> (III)	Insufficient evidence to include or exclude in PHE of asymptomatic individuals over 40 yrs including those with a Family History (1 or 2 relatives) (C)
	Cancer Family Syndrome: Risk of adenocarcinoma approaches 50%; colonoscopy superior test for detecting right-sided cancer.	Expert opinion (III)	Fair evidence to include in PHE of individuals with Cancer Family Syndrome (B)

*   People with ulcerative colitis and familial polyposis are at higher risk of colorectal cancer. They are not "asymptomatic, otherwise healthy" individuals and have been excluded.

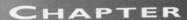

CHAPTER **67**

Screening for Prostate Cancer

By John W. Feightner

Screening for Prostate Cancer

Prepared by John W. Feightner, MD, MSc, FCFP[1]

There is poor evidence to include or exclude the digital rectal exam (DRE) from the periodic health examination for men over 50 years of age (C Recommendation). While DRE has limitations in its ability to detect early prostate cancer, there is insufficient evidence to recommend that physicians who currently include DRE in their examinations should change that behaviour.

There is insufficient evidence to include prostate specific antigen (PSA) screening in the periodic health examination of men over 50 years of age. Exclusion is recommended on the basis of low positive predictive value and the known risk of adverse affects associated with therapies of unproven effectiveness (D Recommendation).

There is also fair evidence to exclude transrectal ultrasound from the periodic health examination of asymptomatic men over 50 years of age. (D Recommendation)

Burden of Suffering

Prevalence

Prostate cancer and its early detection have received increasing attention during the early part of the 1990s. It is the second most frequent cause of death from cancer among men (an estimated 3,800 deaths in 1993), and ranks third in terms of potential years of life lost from cancer among Canadian men.<1> Excluding congenital anomalies and perinatal causes of potential years of life lost, prostate cancer ranks ninth among all causes for males. The lifetime risk of dying from prostate cancer is 3%. There is a rapid rise in incidence over the age of 60. While there has been an increase both in the overall incidence of prostate cancer and in the age-standardized incidence, there has been little change in the age-standardized mortality rate in Canada. This supports the hypothesis that the increased incidence does not reflect a true increase in the actual disease among Canadian males.

---

[1] Professor of Family Medicine, McMaster University, Hamilton, Ontario

Natural History

One of the major challenges in dealing with the early detection of prostate cancer is the lack of a clear understanding of its natural history. Autopsy studies indicate a prevalence of histologic cancer in the range of 20% of men of average age 50 and 43% of men aged 80. Hence, the often heard expression "more men die with prostate cancer than from prostate cancer". This is an indication that, particularly in older age groups, prostate cancer is often an incidental finding and can exist without creating major morbidity and mortality. Unfortunately, the natural history of this disease has not been defined. Thus, there is no way of predicting for any individual which cancer, particularly those found at an earlier stage, will progress to be clinically significant in terms of potential morbidity and/or mortality. This issue is critical to the consideration of early detection. Cancers detected at an earlier stage have a better prognosis, even if untreated, than more advanced tumours. However, if an early or small cancer is found as a result of early detection efforts, the physician cannot currently advise the patient whether he is at significant clinical risk (and thus whether therapies of unproven effectiveness are worth the risk – see discussion on *Early Detection Plus Therapy*).

Among older individuals, prostate cancer is often an incidental finding and can exist without major morbidity and mortality

Maneuver

Virtually all of the studies used to evaluate the test characteristics of the early detection maneuvers for prostate cancer have inherent methodologic study design problems.<2-4> Most significant is the reality that patients with a negative test do not undergo gold standard assessment. This is clearly not feasible when the gold standard represents prostatectomy or extensive biopsy. In the studies that have been published, however, there is no attempt to systematically monitor individuals with negative tests over time to ensure that prostate cancer does not develop subsequently. Many of the studies suffer from "filtration bias" wherein the subjects are not representative of the general population but reflect only those individuals arriving at urologists' offices or individuals with genito-urinary symptoms. More recent studies have attempted to identify the positive predictive value of screening in groups that would more closely approximate the general population.

With only a few exceptions, studies suffer from a selection bias in that some of the detection tests are only conducted on patients where there has already been a "positive" finding such as a positive digital rectal examination. This does not provide a true estimate of sensitivity and specificity.

Hence, the approximations of sensitivity and specificity are only rough estimates. While many have confidence in these estimates, slight changes in sensitivity and specificity can have a major impact on the overall accuracy of any test. This, combined with the low prevalence of clinically detectable prostate cancer leads to the concern regarding a low positive predictive value and a high rate of unnecessary biopsies.

Three strategies have been considered and used in early detection of prostate cancer.

Digital Rectal Exam

This is the oldest detection strategy and represents the simplest technology for early detection.[5-11] While easy to perform, it has serious limitations as an early detection maneuver because only the posterior and lateral aspects of the prostate can be palpated – leaving 40-50% of cancers beyond reach. The examination does appear to be skill-related and there is some evidence that the accuracy of urologists surpasses that of generalist physicians. In asymptomatic males, the estimates of sensitivity and specificity vary. Representative estimates of sensitivity and specificity range between 33-58% and 96-99%, respectively.[5,12] In one study, the sensitivity increased to 67% with repeat examinations (average 1.9 per patient) with a slightly decreased specificity of 97%.[6] A representative estimate of the positive predictive value for DRE is 28%.[12]

Transrectal Ultrasound (TRUS)

While this technique was initially promoted as a potential early detection strategy most would currently view it as a diagnostic test only. Its test characteristics have improved as the technology has improved.[13-19] The diagnostic accuracy of the image depends on the skill of the interpreter and, although it is a safe procedure, it is expensive both in terms of cost and time compared to other maneuvers. Studies have generally indicated a high sensitivity of 97% but a lower specificity at 82%.[13] While the technique can detect lesions as small as 5 mm, it has a high false positive rate which is reflected in the lower specificity.

Prostate Specific Antigen (PSA)

Between 67% and 92% of patients identified as having a positive PSA will undergo unnecessary biopsy

The prostate specific antigen represents a major development in terms of biochemical markers for the early detection of prostate cancer. Compared to DRE, the principal advantage of PSA is its ability to detect prostate cancer at an earlier stage. However, like all early detection tests, its test characteristics and ability to contribute to the net benefit of patients requires careful evaluation. As with the other tests for early detection, sensitivity and specificity can only be approximated. Because sensitivity and specificity can not be accurately estimated, most of the evaluation of PSA as a screening test has focused on its positive predictive value. A "positive" PSA level is established somewhat arbitrarily. The most common threshold is

4 µg/L although, some authors have suggested a cut point as low as 3 µg/L and others as high as 10. Most, although not all patients with an elevated PSA will move to ultrasound guided biopsy to establish whether pathological evidence of cancer can be established. Several studies have reported positive predictive values for PSA. Of concern, is that these numbers range from a low of 8% to a high of 33%.[12,20-25] This means that at best, 67% of patients identified as having a positive PSA will undergo unnecessary biopsy, and evidence indicates that this could be as high as 92%.

Because PSA is produced by the epithelial cells of the prostate rather than cancer-specific cells, its elevation can reflect benign hypertrophy of prostate tissue instead of or as well as prostate cancer. Coupled with the inherent difficulties of sampling prostate tissue using existing biopsy techniques, this creates a significant problem. In response to these concerns, investigators have begun to explore alternate approaches to using PSA. These include the use of serial PSA's looking for rapid rise, the use of PSA levels in relation to the size of the prostate on ultrasound, and the use of age-standardized levels for PSA. While these efforts may hold promise, they have been insufficiently evaluated and, hence, should not be considered for widespread use at this point in time.

To some degree the accuracy of early detection efforts begs the question of whether early detection makes a difference in terms of net benefit to the patient. For an individual patient, does early detection of prostate cancer do more good than harm?

Effectiveness of Screening and Treatment

"Is cure possible in those for whom it is necessary, and is cure necessary for those in whom it is possible?"

— Willet Whitmore

Early Detection Plus Therapy

As with all early detection efforts, the most rigorous evaluation comes in the form of a randomized controlled trial. Difficult and challenging as this may be, it is the only design which will effectively control for important biases. This situation is particularly true with a cancer whose natural history is unknown. Hence, the strongest evidence would emerge from randomized controlled trials evaluating early detection efforts that were linked to therapy. Evidence of this quality does not exist regarding the effectiveness of the early detection of prostate cancer. One case-control study (level II-2 evidence) has raised doubts about the effectiveness of early detection with the digital rectal exam.[7] In effect, there was no difference in the frequency of screening DRE's in 139 men with metastatic prostate cancer from the

Kaiser Permanente Medical Care Program compared to matched men from the program with no diagnosis of metastatic prostate cancer.

In the absence of acceptable evidence for early detection efforts, one turns to a search for sound evidence of the effectiveness of therapy for the condition once it is identified. Unfortunately, there is no adequate evidence from comparative studies to evaluate the main therapeutic options for prostate cancer, particularly for early stage lesions.

A randomized controlled trial to evaluate screening is underway and a randomized trial to evaluate therapy is in the planning stages in the U.S.. European trials evaluating various aspects of therapy are also underway but no results are as yet available.

Effectiveness of Therapy

There are essentially three approaches to dealing with prostate cancer that is detected at an early stage – no therapy but careful monitoring (sometimes referred to as "watchful waiting"), radiation therapy, and radical prostatectomy. The only data available for all three approaches come from descriptive studies which cannot rule out important biases and which often are not generalizable to the broader health care system and the population it serves.

In a Scandinavian study, Johansson and colleagues studied a population-based cohort of 223 patients with early stage prostate cancer for a mean of 123 months.[26] These individuals were selected on the basis of early stage cancer from 654 new cases of prostate cancer identified over a seven year period. The final entry of patients included some with somewhat more advanced cancers. The population was somewhat older with a mean age of 72 years. During the mean observation period of almost 10 years, only 19 patients (8.5%) died from their prostate cancer. The overall progression-free survival rate was 53.1%.

In a structured literature review focusing on articles addressing the treatment of localized prostate cancer, Wasson and coauthors concluded that they were unable to determine treatment effectiveness for localized prostate cancer as a result of the low methodologic quality of the studies.[27] They further concluded that "until better scientific evidence is available, patients and their physicians cannot make informed choices based on knowledge of the benefits of radical prostatectomy, radiation, or watchful waiting".

In the absence of evidence from properly conducted comparative studies, other approaches to weighing the available data have been attempted. Fleming and co-workers used a decision analysis strategy to evaluate alternate treatment strategies for clinically localized prostate cancer.[28] Specifically, they addressed radical prostatectomy, external beam radiation therapy and watchful waiting (with delayed hormonal therapy if and when metastatic disease developed). Their results indicated no clear net benefit for any therapy. In a selected group ages 60-65, with higher grade tumours, there was an indication that radical prostatectomy or radiation therapy might provide a small benefit. If the higher estimates of treatment efficacy were used there was a quality-adjusted survival improvement of less than one year. If the lower estimates of treatment efficacy were used, watchful waiting was always equal to or better than radical prostatectomy or radiation therapy. As with all decision analysis, the conclusions are affected by the data on which the analysis is based. Some have criticized the choice of metastatic rates and the discounting used for complications. This debate will no doubt continue until more rigorous evidence is available.

Finally, a pooled analysis of data from six non-randomized studies evaluating observation plus delayed hormone therapy for clinically localized cancer, demonstrated a 10-year disease-specific survival of 87% for men with grade one or grade two tumours.<29>

High-Risk Individuals

Men with a strong family history for prostate cancer and African-North American men carry a higher risk than the general population. However, it is not clear that an identified cancer in such individuals will behave differently biologically than cancers in normal-risk men. Hence, there is no evidence to suggest that early detection efforts will provide more benefit to such individuals than to normal-risk individuals.

Cost and Adverse Effects

While difficult to evaluate, the overall cost and adverse effects associated with a program for the early detection of prostate cancer can be substantial and can be clinically significant. Although the dollar costs of a single DRE or PSA is relatively small, subsequent biopsy costs, especially for false positive screening tests, and the cost associated with subsequent unproven therapy represent a significant cascade of costly actions.

The cost of a prostate cancer screening program can be substantial and its associated adverse effects clinically significant

Formal attempts at evaluating even this limited perspective of costs are few.

Even more challenging is the documentation of adverse effects. Case series data from the few major centres are not generalizable, and informal patient self-reports can create underestimates. Alternately, data from older populations may over-estimate adverse effect rates in younger men.

The only structured review of the available literature from 1982 to 1991 suggests the following adverse effect rates for radical prostatectomy: a surgical mortality rate of just over 1%; complete incontinence in 7% and any incontinence in 27%; impotence in 32%

with the more recent "nerve sparing" radical prostatectomy (but as high as 85% with other techniques); stricture rates of 12% and bowel injury requiring colostomy or long-term treatment of 1%.<27>

Rates for external beam radiation are lower for procedure-related mortality (0.2%), any incontinence (6.1%), complete incontinence (1.2%), and stricture (4.5%). They are higher for bowel injury (2%). The impotence rates are reported as 42%.

Risks associated with biopsy include prostatitis, epididymitis, and hematuria. It may be that the rate of 4.4% for these events reported in 1984 have improved with newer techniques.

Recommendation of Others

The U.S. Preventive Services Task Force concluded that there was insufficient evidence to recommend for or against the use of DRE in the periodic health exam;<4> PSA and TRUS were not recommended for routine screening. The National Cancer Institute in the United States concluded "there is insufficient evidence to recommend transrectal ultrasound and serum tumour markers for routine screening in asymptomatic men".

A review by the British Columbia Office of Technology Assessment recommends against the use of PSA as a routine screening test.<3> The Canadian Cancer Society does not recommend routine use of PSA.

The Canadian Urological Association and the American Urological Association recommend annual screening for men between ages 50 and 70 with both DRE and PSA. The Canadian Urological Association in its policy statement did not describe the basis on the which the evidence was reviewed nor the strength or weakness of the associated evidence. The American Cancer Society recommends annual PSA for men beginning at age 50.

Conclusions and Recommendations

There are two main philosophical views concerning early detection of cancer. One view holds that the major goal is to search aggressively for asymptomatic cancer and having found it, remove it. While the effectiveness of therapy may not be established, and its associated adverse affects may be recognized, the main mission is to detect cancer early. This view emphasizes the importance of developing tests which can detect cancer early, even if such tests may label many individuals falsely and subject them to subsequent unnecessary, invasive investigations.

The alternate view considers early detection and treatment as a single package and asks whether there is evidence that such combined efforts do more good than harm. This is the question of greatest importance, both from the individual patient's perspective as well as that of the population. Hence, while evaluating the performance of early detection tests is part of the picture, one must also evaluate the effectiveness of therapy and whether the use of available early detection tests ultimately provides overall net benefit to the patient. This is the view taken by the Canadian Task Force on the Periodic Health Examination.

Based on the absence of evidence for effectiveness of therapy and the substantial risk of adverse effects associated with such therapy; and the poor predictive value of screening tests, there is at present insufficient evidence to support wide-spread initiatives for the early detection of prostate cancer.

The Task Force does not recommend the routine use of PSA as part of a periodic health examination. While PSA can detect earlier cancer, it is associated with a substantial false positive rate. This, combined with poor evidence to support the effectiveness of subsequent therapy and clear evidence of substantial risk associated with such therapy, means that the widespread implementation of PSA would expose more men to uncertain benefit, but to definite risks. For these reasons the Task Force recommends that PSA be excluded from the periodic health examination (D Recommendation).

The Task Force debated recommending the exclusion of DRE from the periodic health examination because of its limited performance as an early detection test. However, DRE has been routine practice for many physicians for the early detection of prostate abnormalities and the available evidence was not considered sufficiently powerful to advise physicians who currently include DRE as part of a periodic health examination in men aged 50 to 70 to discontinue the practice. At the same time, the evidence is insufficient to advocate the inclusion of DRE for those physicians who do not currently include it as part of the periodic health examination for men aged 50 to 70. Hence, the decision to retain a C Recommendation for DRE – there is insufficient evidence to include DRE or exclude it from the periodic health exam.

Based on the available evidence for TRUS, the Task Force recommends against the routine use of this procedure as part of a periodic health examination (D Recommendation).

These recommendations are made on the basis of the evaluation of the best available evidence using the Canadian Task Force guidelines, and the ethical imperative that early detection efforts must be proven to result in more good than harm before being incorporated into the periodic health examination.

Patient Consent

The ethical imperative for prevention and early detection efforts is to ensure that such efforts, initiated and promoted by the physician, are proven to do more good than harm. If, in the absence of such proof, a physician decides to offer PSA to a patient, it has been argued that the patient should be fully informed of the balance of benefits and risks, and should provide informed consent for such testing. With prostate cancer screening, this should occur before ordering PSA levels, since the nature of the cascade of events which follows a positive test would make discussions occurring later in the sequence more difficult and ill-timed.

Unanswered Questions (Research Agenda)

The most important need is for randomized trials of early detection and randomized trials to evaluate the effectiveness of therapy. Such trials are underway in Europe and North America or are in the planning stages. While it will take some time before the results are available, this does not argue against the vital need for such data.

Because the natural history of prostate cancer is poorly understood, research into predicting which early cancers will become clinically significant and result in important morbidity and mortality remains a high priority.

In the absence of effectiveness of therapy and until such time as a proper trial of early detection is conducted, the importance of continued major initiatives of research into PSA may be questioned. Any efforts which do occur should focus on careful and proper evaluation of the test characteristics whether it be for serial PSA's, PSA density, or PSA age-related norms.

Evidence

The literature for this review was identified through the MEDLINE data base and from the identification of additional studies from the citations of articles from the original search.

This review was initiated in 1993 and the recommendations finalized by the Task Force in June 1994.

Selected References

1. National Cancer Institute of Canada. Canadian Cancer Statistics, 1993. Toronto, 1993

2. Canadian Task Force on the Periodic Health Examination: The periodic health examination, 1991 Update. *Can Med Assoc J* 1991; 145(5): 413-428

3. Greene CJ, Hadorn D, Bassett K, *et al*: Prostate specific antigen in the early detection of prostate cancer. British Columbia Office of Technology Assessment, Vancouver, BC, 1993

4. U.S. Preventive Services Task Force: Screening for prostate cancer: a commentary on the Canadian Task Force on the Periodic Health Examination 1991 Update on the Secondary Prevention of Prostate Cancer. *Am J Prev Med* 1994; 10(4): 187-193

5. Vihko P, Kontturi M, Likkarinen O, *et al*: Screening for carcinoma of the prostate. Rectal examination, and enzymatic and radioimmunologic measurements of serum acid phosphatase compared. *Cancer* 1985; 56: 173-177

6. Pedersen KV, Carlsson P, Varenhorst E, *et al*: Screening for carcinoma of the prostate by digital rectal examination in a randomly selected population. *BMJ* 1990; 300: 1041-1044

7. Friedman GD, Hiatt RA, Quesenberry CP, *et al*: Case-control study of screening for prostate cancer by digital rectal examination. *Lancet* 1991; 337: 1526-1529

8. Chodak GW, Shoenberg HW: Early detection of prostate cancer by routine screening. *JAMA* 1984; 252: 3261-3264

9. Guinan P, Ray P, Bhatti R, *et al*: An evaluation of five tests to diagnose prostate cancer. *Prog Clin Biol Res* 1987; 243A: 551-558

10. Thompson IM, Rounder JB, Teague JL, *et al*: Impact of routine screening for adenocarcinoma of the prostate on stage distribution. *J Urol* 1987; 137: 424-426

11. Perrin P, Maquet JH, Bringeon G, *et al*: Screening for prostate cancer. Comparison of transrectal ultrasound, prostate specific antigen and rectal examination. *Br J Urol* 1991; 68: 263-265

12. Mettlin C, Lee F, Drago J, *et al*: The American Cancer Society National Prostate Cancer Detection Project: findings of the detection of early prostate cancer in 2425 men. *Cancer* 1991; 67: 2949-2958

13. Watanabe H, Date S, Ohe H, *et al*: A survey of 3,000 examinations by transrectal ultrasonography. *Prostate* 1980; 1: 271-278

14. Rifkin MD, Friedland GW, Shortliffe L: Prostatic evaluation by transrectal endosonography: detection of carcinoma. *Radiology* 1986; 158: 85-90

15. Andriole GL, Kavoussi LR, Torrence RJ, *et al*: Transrectal ultrasonography in the diagnosis and staging of carcinoma of the prostate. *J Urol* 1988; 140: 758-760

16. Kenny GM, Hutchinson WB: Transrectal ultrasound of the prostate. *Urology* 1988; 32: 401-402

17. Brooman PJC, Peeling WB, Griffiths GJ, *et al*: A comparison between digital examination and per-rectal ultrasound in the evaluation of the prostate. *Br J Urol* 1981; 53: 617-620

18. Chodak GW, Wald V, Parmer E, *et al*: Comparison of digital examination and transrectal ultrasonography for the diagnosis of prostatic cancer. *J Urol* 1986; 135: 951-954

19. Kadow C, Gingell JC, Penry JB: Prostatic ultrasonography: a useful technique? *Br J Urol* 1985; 57: 440-443

20. Chadwick DJ, Kemple T, Astley JP, *et al*: Pilot study of screening for prostate cancer in general practice. *Lancet* 1991; 338: 613-616

21. Brawer MK, Chetner MP, Beatie J, *et al*: Screening for prostatic carcinoma with prostate specific antigen. *J Urol* 1992; 147: 841-845

22. Gustafsson O, Norming U, Almgard LE, *et al*: Diagnostic methods in the detection of prostate cancer: a study of randomly selected population of 2,400 men. *J Urol* 1992; 148: 1827-1831

23. Muschenheim F, Omarbasha B, Kardijan PM, *et al*: Screening for carcinoma of the prostate with prostate specific antigen. *Ann Clin Lab Sci* 1991; 21(6): 371-380

24. Labrie F, Dupont A, Suburu R, *et al*: Serum prostate specific antigen as a prescreening test for prostate cancer. *J Urol* 1992; 147: 846-852

25. Catalona WJ, Smith DS, Ratliff TL, *et al*: Detection of organ-confined prostate cancer is increased through prostate-specific antigen-based screening. *JAMA* 1993; 270(8): 948-954

26. Johansson JE, Adami HO, Andersson SO, *et al*: High 10-year survival rate in patients with early, untreated prostatic cancer. *JAMA* 1992; 267(16): 2191-2196

27. Wasson JH, Cushman C, Bruskewitz R, *et al*: A structured literature review of treatment for localized prostate cancer. *Arch Fam Med* 1993; 2: 487-493

28. Fleming C, Wasson JH, Albertsen PC, *et al*: A decision analysis of alternative treatment strategies for clinically localized prostate cancer. *JAMA* 1993; 269(20): 2650-2658

29. Chodak GW, Thisted RA, Gerber GS, *et al*: Results of conservative management of clinically localized prostate cancer. *N Engl J Med* 1994; 330: 242-248

Screening for Prostate Cancer

MANEUVER	EFFECTIVENESS	LEVEL OF EVIDENCE <REF>	RECOMMENDATION
Digital Rectal Examination (DRE)	Routine screening results in increased detection of early cancers but the maneuver can only detect small cancers in the posterior and lateral aspects of the prostate. The effectiveness of therapy is unproven but carries significant risks of important adverse effects.	Cohort analytic (descriptive) studies (II-3); Case control study<5-10> (II-2) Overview and decision analysis of cohort analytic (descriptive) studies<27-29> (II-3)	Poor evidence to include or exclude DRE from the periodic health examination (PHE) for men over 50 years of age (C); while DRE has limitations in its ability to detect early prostate cancer, there is insufficient evidence to recommend that physicians who currently include DRE in their examinations should change that behaviour*
Prostate specific antigen (PSA)	While PSA can identify prostate cancer at an earlier stage, the false-positive rates range from 67% to 93%. The effectiveness of therapy is unproven but carries significant risks of important adverse effects.	Cohort analytic (descriptive) studies<19-25> (II-3) Overview and decision analysis of cohort analytic (descriptive) studies<27-29> (II-3)	Exclusion is recommended on the basis of low positive predictive value and the known risk of adverse affects associated with therapies of unproven effectiveness. Fair evidence to exclude routine screening with PSA from the periodic health examination of asymptomatic men over 50 years of age (D)
Transrectal Ultrasound (TRUS)	Imaging techniques do not specifically detect malignant disease in the prostate; their routine use for screening would pose problems of feasibility and cost.	Cohort analytic (descriptive) studies<12-18> (II-3)	Fair evidence to exclude from the periodic health examination of asymptomatic men over 50 years of age (D)

*   DRE can also be done for other reasons (other than to detect prostate cancer).

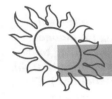

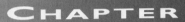

CHAPTER

68

Screening
for
Bladder
Cancer

By Sarvesh Logsetty

Screening for Bladder Cancer

Prepared by Sarvesh Logsetty, MD[1]

In 1979 the Canadian Task Force on the Periodic Health Examination addressed the question of screening for bladder cancer in the periodic health examination. The screening tool considered was urine cytology, and it was recommended that the general population not be screened (D Recommendation). The screening of high-risk groups, however, was recommended (B Recommendation) pending further information.[1] The current Task Force recommendations for urine screening for microscopic hematuria and urine cytology are a D Recommendation for the general population and a C Recommendation for the population at increased risk. The rationale for these recommendations is as follows:

1. *The screening tests, while reasonably sensitive (hematuria) and specific (cytology), have a very low positive predictive value or are prohibitively expensive.*

2. *The reason for the low positive predictive value is the rare incidence of the disease.*

3. *There is no evidence that screening identifies affected persons at an earlier stage or at a stage more amenable to treatment.*

Burden of Suffering

In 1993 the estimated incidence of bladder cancer in Canada was 4,900 cases (3,700 men and 1,200 women, a 3:1 ratio).[2] The overall age-standardized annual incidence rate in 1988, was 21.8 per 100,000 population/yr in males, 7.0 in females (see Table 1).[3] More than 95% of new cases were found in individuals over 45 years of age, especially in the 65 to 74 year age group in both sexes. Incidence rates increased with age, reaching a maximum of 313 cases per 100,000 population in males and 81 in females in those over 85 years old.

Deaths related to bladder cancer in Canada in 1993 numbered approximately 1,310.[2] The 1988 age-specific mortality rates are as high as 198 deaths per 100,000 per year in older males and 63 per 100,000 in older females.[3]

---

[1] Division of General Surgery, Department of Surgery, Hospital for Sick Children, Toronto, Ontario

Risk factors

North Americans develop predominantly transitional cell carcinoma (90%). Since 1895, when Rehn noticed an increased incidence of bladder cancer among German dye workers, a number of chemicals in the dye industry, used in developing Azo dyes, have been identified as raising the risk of bladder cancer. These compounds have been prohibited in most western countries for many years, but because of the long latent period between exposure and development of bladder cancer, people previously exposed should still be considered at risk, even decades later. Bladder cancer can develop at any time but occurs most often 20 years after exposure. Grade II-1 evidence suggests that there is a dose-dependent response, although any exposure can increase risk.[4]

Other risks consistently identified include exposure to aromatic amines (added to cutting oils and petroleum products), 4 aminobiphenyl and employment in the leather, tire and rubber industries; odds ratios range from 2.7 to 8.3.[4]

Older males, who smoke, and/or have been exposed to aromatic amines are at greatest risk of developing bladder cancer

A factor often shown to be associated with an increased incidence of bladder cancer is smoking. The rate of bladder cancer has been demonstrated to rise with increased exposure to cigarette smoking and decrease with its removal.[5] Case-control and prospective cohort studies report odds ratios and relative risks of 1.5 to 7.0.[4,5] Given the number of people who smoke relative to those working in risky occupations, and current levels of industrial control of causative chemicals, smoking is now the leading cause of bladder cancer in Canada.

Natural History

Understanding the natural history of bladder cancer is complicated by the use of two different staging systems. Comparison of data from various studies must take into account the different definitions of early disease (i.e., stage T_0, T_a, C_{is}, $T1^2$) and the grades of histopathology or the stage of disease. Authors also tend to present their data in terms of recurrence rates without giving information on length of follow-up.

Most studies show that the higher the grade or stage, the more frequent the recurrence. From 46% to 51% of stage Ta Grade I/II single tumours will recur, 71% within the first 3 months. C_{is}, a higher grade

---

[2] *American Joint Committee, Tumor staging system*
C_{is}, T_a Papillary Ca, restricted to Mucosa
T1   Lesion restricted to Lamina Propria
T2   Lesion restricted to Superficial Muscle
T3a   Lesion restricted to Deep Muscle
T3b   Lesion restricted to Perivesical fat
T4   Invading Neighboring organs

of tumour (Grade III), is associated with a higher recurrence rate (70%). Multiple tumours (up to 91%) and >10 g will also recur more frequently (80%).<6>

The propensity of the neoplasm to progress to a more advanced stage of disease is also related to the presenting stage and grade of the tumour. In a 1983 study<7> using figures provided by the National Bladder Cancer Group, 207 patients were followed with cystoscopy at regular intervals, and any recurrence was reviewed for grade and stage. Progression ranged from 2% for a TaGI lesion to 48% for a T1GIII lesion, with median follow-up of 39 months. From this and other reports, we know that C_{is} is associated with higher rates of progression and recurrence.

Maneuver

Superficial bladder cancer is asymptomatic in most patients, presenting as microscopic hematuria on routine urinalysis. Since the hematuria is usually intermittent, a single examination is not sufficient. Traditionally, the number of red blood cells per high-power field of a microscope has been the standard, reaching significance when there are more than 3 to 5 red cells per field. The advent of dipstick urinalysis has made it possible to test urine in the office quickly with relatively accurate results. Compared with microscopic hematuria testing, testing with a single dipstick is almost as sensitive (91%) as the microscope in identifying hematuria, and slightly less specific (99%). Theoretically the dipstick should be capable of detecting hemolyzed blood and thus be more sensitive generally than the microscope. The advantage of the dipstick is that it is faster and cheaper. Patients can be taught how to use the strips, sent home with a week's supply, and tested for intermittent hematuria.

In men older than 50 years with hematuria, only 14% to 24% of abnormalities will be due to bladder cancer

The reports of urine dipstick as a screening test are cohort studies.<8-11> Dipstick testing is sensitive and specific for hematuria, but hematuria is not specific to bladder cancer. Hematuria can be due to physiologic causes, such as strenuous exercise, recent sexual intercourse, first morning voiding, or to urinary tract infection. In men older than 50 years with hematuria, only 14% to 24% of abnormalities will be due to bladder cancer.<8-12> This proportion will be much lower in the younger population and in women.

The gold standard for diagnosis of bladder cancer is cystoscopy. This is routinely combined with intravenous pyelography or ultrasound to exclude more proximal pathology. Although these investigations are relatively innocuous, they do involve either significant discomfort or exposure to X-ray radiation, neither of which is warranted for a healthy person and render them inappropriate as screening tests.

Consider the following calculations regarding the utility of mass screening (dipstick for hematuria). A sensitivity of 100% and a specificity of 92%<10> will be assumed for multiple dipstick testing at home. Men aged 55 to 64 who were machine trade workers (OR = 6)<4> and have smoked heavily (OR = 7)<5> will be assessed, representative of a very high-risk group. The published odds ratios will be treated as if they are relative risks and considered independent and multiplicative. The age-specific rate in men 55 to 64 years old is about 70 per 100,000 population/yr. Thus the pretest probability in the high-risk patient is 2,940 new cases (70x6x7) per 100,000 population (3%) annually. Using these values there will be 7,765 (8%) false positives per 100,000 tested individuals who require further investigation. This is a positive predictive value of 27%. This scenario represents the best positive predictive value if bladder cancer is considered alone; the value may increase if the other causes of hematuria are taken into consideration. Therefore, even in groups at highest risk (highest possible prevalence) screening for bladder cancer using hematuria is too nonspecific to be performed on a routine basis. For each patient with bladder cancer, three healthy persons would be subjected to invasive tests.

Previously, the Canadian Task Force on the Periodic Health Examination reviewed the utility of urine cytology as a screening tool for bladder cancer.<1> It recommended that the general population not be screened (D Recommendation). The screening of high-risk groups was (B Recommendation) pending further information. This decision was based on type III evidence. Since then, we have available type II-1 evidence that characterizes the sensitivity and specificity of urine cytology in detecting bladder cancer.<13> Urine cytology may have a specificity greater than that of microscopic hematuria screening, ranging from 48% to 100%, but its sensitivity (40% to 93%) is less. Because this disease is rare, the positive predictive value is sensitive to increases in specificity: the table below demonstrates the variations in positive predictive value if the sensitivity is kept at 93% and the specificity changed from 100% to 97%.

Specificity	100%	99%	98%	97%
Positive Predictive Value	100%	74%	58%	48%

Again, because of the rare nature of the disease, there are few false negatives. Another important factor is the cost of the screening tool. Microscopic hematuria can be tested for with a dipstick in the doctor's office and costs only pennies. By contrast, urine cytology requires proper storage of the urine sample, a laboratory equipped to perform cytology, and a pathologist trained to review the specimens. The cost to Ontario Health Insurance Plan (October 1992 guide) for the hematuria testing is $3.90 per test, while urine cytology costs a total of $18.82 per test, including professional fee and pathologist's fee – almost 5 times as much. Cystoscopy would cost $120.50 per patient (surgeon's fees: $65.30; anesthetist's fees: $55.20) not including the expense of maintaining equipment and nursing support.

Effectiveness of Treatment

Intravesical immuno/chemotherapy reduces recurrence rates and BCG may also improve long-term survival

Initial therapy for superficial bladder cancer is cystoscopy and transurethral resection of the tumour. If C_{is} or multiple tumours are found, or the tumour is only partially resectable, the patient is given a course of intravesical therapy. Random biopsies of the bladder mucosa are taken beforehand. If C_{is} is found, the intravesical therapy is considered therapeutic; if not, it is considered prophylactic. Intravesical therapy can consist of either a chemotherapeutic agent (thiotepa, doxorubicin) or an immunologic agent (bacillus Calmette-Guerin (BCG)).[14-19] Several randomized trials have suggested that the use of chemotherapeutic agents intravesically after transurethral resection will delay and even reduce bladder cancer recurrence. However, many of these studies lacked controls, compared different doses of medication, or had problems with confounding factors (i.e., excluding patients with C_{is}).

There is grade I evidence both for and against the efficacy of thiotepa in reducing the recurrence rate and increasing the time to recurrence for superficial bladder cancer. The patient samples involved in the trials were similar demographically to those most likely to be identified by screening for hematuria, the over-50 white male. The associated risk factors were not presented in the studies. The grades of histopathology and tumour stage were all restricted to superficial bladder cancer, and the type of cancer was transitional cell carcinoma. The initial grade and stage of the tumour were similar among the studies, except in the few that dealt specifically with C_{is}.[15]

Comparisons of doxorubicin with both thiotepa and BCG in randomized trials have shown no significant improvement in outcome.[14,16] In fact, the outcome was worse because of the increased adverse effects of doxorubicin treatment. Almost four times as many patients suffered adverse affects from doxorubicin as from thiotepa.

In 1976, Morales et al introduced the concept of intravesical BCG as immunologic prophylaxis.[20] Since then a number of studies[14,16-18] have been published providing good evidence (grade 1) that BCG is efficacious in the treatment and prophylaxis of superficial bladder cancer.

In a randomized study comparing BCG and doxorubicin, Lamm and colleagues[14] showed that BCG reduced recurrence rates but did not improve survival. Initially, the immunotherapy consisted of bladder irrigation and subcutaneous injections, but this was subsequently refined to drop the subcutaneous injections. Thus there seems to be evidence that BCG can reduce recurrences, but no evidence that survival is affected by treatment. No information is given about the quality of life or the presence or absence of symptoms, and there is not enough information available to determine whether the treatment offers a longer symptom-free period. Herr and coauthors<17> describe results of a randomized controlled trial in which there was improved survival with BCG over the five year follow-up, but this has not been corroborated by any other trials.

Recommendations of Others

The recommendations of the U.S. Preventive Services Task Force are currently under review.

Conclusions and Recommendations

In summary, the incidence of bladder cancer increases with age, is higher in men than in women, and is strongly associated with cigarette smoking and specific chemical exposures. Removal of the chemicals or cessation of smoking have both been shown to reduce the risk of cancer. Most people with superficial bladder cancer are asymptomatic, and present with microhematuria. The current test for hematuria is the dipstick, which is very sensitive if used appropriately for intermittent hematuria. Hematuria is, however, a nonspecific sign, and many other diseases and even normal physiological states can produce a positive test. Routine screening is therefore not recommended for asymptomatic persons (D Recommendation). A high index of suspicion should be maintained in anyone with a history of smoking or exposure to any other risk factor, and at the first symptom or sign they should be investigated.

Bladder cancer is treated by local excision and intravesical therapy, either chemotherapy or immunotherapy. Chemotherapy has been shown to decrease recurrence rates and may increase long-term survival. While BCG decreases recurrence rates, there is insufficient evidence to determine its long-term effects or to assess the patient's quality of life after chemotherapy. As a result, there is insufficient evidence for or against screening of asymptomatic high-risk individuals (C Recommendation).

Unanswered Questions (Research Agenda)

Research is needed to study the usefulness of screening more rigorously and to investigate alternative forms of treatment. First, there is need for a prospective, community-based study, including subjects of all ages, to assess the usefulness of hematuria screening. One group should test urine for hematuria over a week at regular intervals, another should receive no testing beyond that performed routinely by their family physician. Once hematuria has been found, the cause should be identified and treated if possible. Patients should be followed to note any subsequent problems. Outcome assessment should include use of health resources, days of work missed, number of invasive tests "disease-free" patients undergo, and pathology found. Patients need to be followed for a long period to ensure that they do not develop any pathology heralded by the hematuria but missed on initial diagnostic tests.

More research is needed into alternate chemotherapeutic agents. Those currently used do not appear to improve long-term survival. The role of BCG instillation has to be examined in more detail. Are the early benefits from this treatment maintained over the long term? Does chemotherapy or immunotherapy improve the quality of life after treatment? Evidence is needed to support or refute the supposition that BCG will improve overall survival.

Evidence

This is a review of the incidence, associated risk factors, screening, and treatment of superficial bladder cancer. The background information, obtained from textbooks of urology, helped form an outline of pertinent issues. Information on incidence was obtained from the most recent Statistics Canada publications. A MEDLINE search was used to retrieve articles in the medical literature from 1976 to February 1993, and a review of the bibliographies identified additional articles, that appeared relevant. Information on incidence was obtained from population studies, on risk factors mainly from case-control studies, and on screening from cohort studies.

This review was initiated in January 1993, and the recommendations were finalized by the Task Force in June 1993.

Acknowledgements

The author would like to thank Task Force members, Drs. Elaine Wang and William Feldman for their special assistance.

Selected References

1. Canadian Task Force on the Periodic Health Examination: The periodic health examination. *Can Med Assoc J* 1979; 121: 1193-1254

2. National Cancer Institute of Canada: Canadian Cancer Statistics 1993. Toronto, Canada, 1993

3. Statistics Canada: Cancer in Canada. Health Reports 1992; 121(Suppl 8): 2,3,18,19,44,45,86,87,112,113,125,129

4. Anton-Culver H, Lee-Felstein A, Taylor TH: Occupation and bladder cancer risk. *Am J Epidemiol* 1992; 136(1): 89-94

5. Slattery ML, Schumacher MC, West DW, *et al*: Smoking and bladder cancer. The modifying effect of cigarettes on other factors. *Cancer* 1988; 61(2): 402-408

6. Heney NM: Natural history of superficial bladder cancer. Prognostic features and long-term disease course. *Urol Clin North Am* 1992; 19(3): 429-433

7. Heney NM: Superficial bladder cancer: progression and recurrence. *J Urol* 1983; 130: 1083-1086

8. Messing EM, Vaillancourt A: Hematuria screening for bladder cancer. *J Occup Med* 1990; 32(9): 838-845

9. Messing EM, Young TB, Hunt VB, *et al*: Home screening for hematuria: results of a multiclinic study. *J Urol* 1992; 148: 289-292

10. Britton JP, Dowell AC, Whelan P: Dipstick hematuria and bladder cancer in men over 60: results of a community study. *BMJ* 1989; 299: 1010-1012

11. Woolhandler S, Pels RJ, Bor DH, *et al*: Dipstick urinalysis screening of asymptomatic adults for urinary tract disorders: I. Hematuria and proteinuria. *JAMA* 1989; 262(9): 1214-1219

12. Mohr ND, Offord KP, Owen RA, *et al*: Asymptomatic microhematuria and urologic disease: a population-based study. *JAMA* 1986; 256(2): 224-229

13. Badalament RA, Kimmel M, Gay H, *et al*: The sensitivity of flow cytometry compared with conventional cytology in the detection of superficial bladder carcinoma. *Cancer* 1987; 59(12): 2078-2085

14. Lamm DL, Blumenstein BA, Crawford ED, *et al*: A randomized trial of intravesical doxorubicin and immunotherapy with bacille Calmette-Guerin for transitional-cell carcinoma of the bladder. *N Engl J Med* 1991; 325(17): 1205-1209

15. MRC Working Party on Urological Cancer: The effect of intravesical thiotepa on the reocurrence rate of newly diagnosed superficial bladder cancer. *Br J Urol* 1985; 57: 680-685

16. Lamm DL, DeHaven JI, Shriver J, *et al*: Prospective randomized comparison of intravesical with percutaneous bacillus Calmette-Guerin versus intravesical bacillus Calmette-Guerin in superficial bladder cancer. *J Urol* 1991; 145(5): 738-740

17. Herr HW, Laudone VP, Badalament RA, *et al*: Bacillus Calmette-Guerin therapy alters the progression of superficial bladder cancer. *J Clin Oncol* 1988; 6(9): 1450-1455

18. Herr HW, Wartinger DD, Fair WR, *et al*: Bacillus Calmette-Guerin Therapy for superficial bladder cancer: a 10-year followup. *J Urol* 1992; 147: 1020-1023

19. Zincke H, Benson RC Jr., Hilton JF, *et al*: Intravesical thiotepa and mitomycin C treatment immediately after transurethral resection and later for superficial (stages Ta and Tis) bladder cancer: a prospective, randomized, stratified study with crossover design. *J Urol* 1985; 134: 1110-1114

20. Morales A, Eidinger D, Bruce AW: Intracavitary Bacillus Calmette-Guerin in the treatment of superficial bladder tumours. *J Urol* 1976; 116: 180-183

Table 1: Incidence and Mortality Rates of Bladder Cancer in Canada

1988 Statistics Canada Data<3>	Male	Female
Number of new cases	3,406	1,206
Crude incidence rate	26.7	9.2
Age-standardized rate	21.8	7.0
Number of deaths	844	362
Crude death rate	6.6	2.8
Age-standardized death rate	5.3	1.9

Screening for Bladder Cancer

MANEUVER	EFFECTIVENESS	LEVEL OF EVIDENCE <REF>	RECOMMENDATION
Urine dipstick or microscopy for hematuria	Urine dipstick testing for hematuria is very sensitive (>98%) with poor specificity (approximately 90%).	Cohort studies<8-10> (II-2)	Fair evidence to exclude from Periodic Health Examination (PHE) for general population (D); poor evidence to include or exclude from the PHE for persons at high risk* (C)
	Cytology has low sensitivity (< 90%) and specificity (~90%) and is expensive.	Cohort and case-control studies<13> (II-2)	
	Screening yield is low and there are no studies on effectiveness of early treatment (cases identified by screening).		
	Intravesical thiotepa and Bacillus Calmette-Guerin (BCG) reduced recurrence rates but no therapeutic agent (intravesical doxorubicin, thiotepa or BCG) has improved long-term survival. Doxorubicin increased side effects.	Randomized controlled trials<14-16> (I)	

* **High-risk groups are Males > 60 years of age who smoke or have smoked, and were employed in a trade that may have exposed them to aromatic amines.**

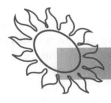

CHAPTER 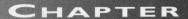 69

Prevention of Oral Cancer

By Carl Rosati

Prevention of Oral Cancer

Prepared by Carl Rosati, MD, FRCSC[1]

In 1979 the Canadian Task Force on the Periodic Health Examination identified cancers of the oral cavity as a potentially preventable cause of major morbidity and mortality. At the time, early detection was considered possible but the quality of evidence supporting the effectiveness of preventive strategies and the effectiveness of treatments for oral cancers was limited (C Recommendation). Review of the evidence from 1980 to 1993 has not changed this recommendation. However, smoking cessation counselling is highlighted as a means of preventing oral cancer and the recommendation to provide smoking cessation counselling is consistent with that made in Chapter 43 which deals more generally with the prevention of tobacco-caused disease.

Burden of Suffering

Oral cancers account for significant mortality but their prevalence is relatively low

The estimated incidence of oral cancers in Canada in 1993 was 3,120 and they accounted for 1,100 deaths, approximately 1.9% of all cancer deaths. The peak age for developing oral cancers is in the fifth to seventh decades with a male to female ratio of about 2.5:1. The lifetime probability of developing and dying from oral cancers in men is 1.71% and 0.61% and for women is 0.71% and 0.27%, respectively. The potential years of life lost (PYLL) for oral cancer was 16,000 years in Canada in 1989. Oral cancers account for significant mortality but their prevalence is relatively low. This may affect the feasibility of large scale screening with the adverse implications of the false positive and false negative diagnoses generated by such a screening program.

Over 50% of oral cancers, when diagnosed, are beyond the American Joint Committee for Cancer Staging and End Results' TNM Stage I. Consequently, there is major morbidity attributable both to the disease and to the various forms of treatment and all health status domains are affected. There is psychosocial disability in terms of appearance, self-esteem and withdrawal from familial and other social interactions. There are physical and functional disabilities in terms of personal hygiene, swallowing and maintenance of nutritional status, speaking and therapy-specific morbidities related to radical neck dissection and irradiation, thyroid and parathyroid dysfunction, mouth dryness from lack of normal secretion, osteonecrosis of facial bones and the adverse effects of chemotherapy.

---

[1] General Surgery, North York Branson Hospital, North York, Ontario

Cancer rates for both the salivary gland and nasopharynx are 10-25 times higher among the Inuit than among the general Canadian population; these cancers are associated with Epstein-Barr virus infection as well as genetic, environmental and immunologic factors. Alcohol and tobacco are major risk factors for tumours of the mouth, tongue and pharynx with a diet high in fresh fruits and vegetables acting as a protective factor. Smokeless tobacco use, including snuff and chewing tobacco is important (long-term users 50 times more likely to develop cancer of the cheek and gum than non-users) although vitamin deficiencies and occupational exposures are also implicated. Smokeless tobacco has other negative health effects[1] and in the United States use has increased over the last two decades largely due to increased consumption by young males. While smokeless tobacco use is rare in Canada (overall prevalence of use under 1% in 1986), prevalences of use of 6-30% among native children (depending on age and study population) and 1-4% among non-native adolescents have been reported.

Maneuver

There have been no randomized controlled trials to evaluate the effectiveness of oral cancer screening. In four studies, oral physical examination had a sensitivity of 59-100%, specificity of 95.9-99.7%, positive predictive value of 15-91% and negative predictive value of 99-100%;[2-5] positive predictive value is low. In addition to the psychological impact of labelling a patient with a false positive diagnosis, the added costs incurred by investigating patients so labelled would be prohibitively high. The principal reason for this problem is the low prevalence of oral cancers.

There have been no randomized controlled trials to evaluate the effectiveness of oral cancer screening

The use of tolonium chloride testing in conjunction with oral physical examination should increase the recorded prevalence of oral cancer in case-finding (average sensitivity 96.7% with 90.8 average specificity), however Rosenberg et al[6] demonstrate that the prevalence remains sufficiently low to limit its usefulness. Several other issues such as reliability of the screening test, compliance with screening (affected by the misconception that asymptomatic lesions are innocuous), follow-up, definitive therapy and cost effectiveness should be considered for large-scale programs. No cost effectiveness study has been undertaken to determine whether the reduction in morbidity or lives saved through treatment of oral cancers at an early stage is sufficient to offset the cost of an oral cancer screening program.

Effectiveness of Prevention and Treatment

Risk Factors for the Development of Oral Cancers

There is good evidence from a meta-analysis of randomized controlled trials to recommend smoking cessation counselling

There is compelling evidence from case-control and cohort analytic studies, in varied geographic locations, of a causal relationship between the use of tobacco products, the combined use of tobacco and alcohol and the development of oral cancers.[7-16] Some of these studies demonstrated a reduction in the observed oral cancer rates with cessation of tobacco and/or alcohol consumption. There is good evidence from a meta-analysis of randomized controlled trials to recommend smoking cessation counselling (see Chapter 43 on Prevention of tobacco-caused disease).[17]

School-based programs to prevent smokeless tobacco use have had mixed results.[1,18-20] Evaluation of smokeless tobacco cessation programs has been limited, generally giving inconsistent results in small case series.[1] However, one randomized trial of 518 male smokeless tobacco users found that an intervention by dental hygienists (soft-tissue exam, advice to quit, self-help materials, video, quit date) improved quit rates at three months (32% of intervention group vs. 21% of controls, p<0.01).[21]

Oral Premalignancy

A heterogeneous group of asymptomatic oral pathological entities with malignant potential includes dysplasia, erythroplasia, leukoplakia, lichen planus and submucosal fibrosis. The prevalence of oral premalignancy and its rate of malignant transformation are unknown. However, population-based studies from the U.S., Hungary, Sweden and India have estimated it to be 1.3% to over 6% and 2.2% to 6% respectively. Rates of malignant transformation of leukoplakia have been estimated at 2.2% to 6%. More recent prospective studies, with longer follow-up, and in populations with a higher proportion of dysplastic changes in their leukoplakias, suggest that the malignant transformation rates are higher than previously believed (16.2-17.5%). Although oral precancers are relatively infrequent and population screening may therefore be inappropriate, their relative importance and significant rate of malignant transformation would support case-finding strategies, particularly in high-risk populations. Arguments for adopting these strategies would be strengthened if supported by evidence of efficacious therapy for oral precancers.

Primary treatment of oral leukoplakia and therapy aimed at prevention of second primary lesions have been studied in two randomized, placebo controlled chemoprevention trials of 13-cis-retinoic acid (13cRA).[22,23] These studies demonstrated a reduction in relative risk to almost 1.0 for the complete remission of leukoplakia and a 0.83 relative risk for the occurrence of second primary oral cancers suggesting that 13cRA was highly efficacious for these purposes. However, leukoplakia relapsed within 3 to 6 months after discontinuation of therapy, the rate of mild to moderate side effects was up to 79%, dose reduction was required in 18% to 47% of patients and at least temporary cessation of therapy was required in 4.5-6.8% of patients. Furthermore, an issue not addressed by the advocates of 13cRA was the teratogenicity of retinoic acid. Results of preliminary trials of low-dose maintenance therapy using 13cRA are encouraging, though follow-up to date is limited.[24]

Trials using β-carotene demonstrated reductions (up to 71%) in the occurrence of oral leukoplakia and mucosal dysplasia to a much lesser degree than that observed with 13cRA.[24-27] Adverse effects were virtually nonexistent. Current research on low dose maintenance and alternative (β-carotene) therapies may soon resolve these issues.

Effectiveness of Treatment of Invasive Oral Cancers

The choice of therapy for early stage invasive oral cancer is controversial. Primary surgical and radiation therapy are often considered equivalent. While opinion varies considerably, particularly concerning the adverse effects of both forms of therapy and their impact on quality of life, there appears to be no difference in survival between these therapies based on the current evidence in the literature.

Multivariate analyses, in studies of both surgical and radiation therapy, have consistently identified the stage of disease as an important prognostic factor. The 1991 American Cancer Society's national five-year survival figures for oral cancer based on stage were, Local 75%, Regional 41% and Distant 18%.[23] Similar five-year survival statistics are provided in a review of the literature specifically addressing treatment of oral malignancies: Stage I 68-89%, Stage II 40-83%, Stage III 29-68%, Stage IV 6-36%.[23,28-35] These data suggest that there is a survival difference depending on the stage of the disease at the time of diagnosis but do not address lead-time or length-time bias. Two retrospective cohort studies report survival beyond five years.[23,28] Survival figures at 10 years demonstrate an increase in oral cancer-specific mortality raising concerns over lead-time bias. A single randomized controlled trial comparing elective versus therapeutic neck dissection for oral cavity carcinoma demonstrated an overall 70% survival rate for both groups at six years follow-up.[36] However the authors reported their results for all stages (I, II, III) combined. Thus, while lead-time bias may not have been an issue, it is not possible to determine the effect of treatment on early stage disease. Several large case series report similar five-year survival figures and identify second primary oral cancers as the leading cause of death in these patients after local or regional recurrence.[29-33,36]

The rates of second primary oral cancers exceeds 36% and adds further to the confusion in interpreting the effectiveness of treatment for invasive oral cancers. Definitive conclusions regarding both the most effective form of therapy and the effectiveness of treatment for early stage oral cancers await a prospective randomized trial.

Recommendations of Others

In 1989, the U.S. Preventive Services Task Force recommended counselling patients against the use of tobacco in any form, particularly with heavy alcohol consumption, based on evidence linking the adverse effects of tobacco with premalignant and malignant lesions of the oral cavity.<37> Routine screening of asymptomatic persons for oral cancer by primary care clinicians was not recommended. However, it was thought to be prudent for clinicians to perform careful examinations for cancerous lesions of the oral cavity in patients who use tobacco or excessive amounts of alcohol, as well as in those with suspicious symptoms or lesions detected through self-examination. These recommendations are currently being reviewed.

The Canadian and American Dental Associations support the concept of oral cancer screening; however, neither group has recommended specific clinical practice guidelines in this regard.<38-43>

Conclusions and Recommendations

Ample evidence establishes the causal link between use of tobacco products in any form and cancers of the aerodigestive tract, based on extensive case-control and cohort studies. In addition, there is good evidence supporting the effectiveness of counselling for smoking cessation. There is good evidence to include smoking cessation counselling in the periodic health examination to prevent oral cancer (A Recommendation).

There is insufficient evidence, however, for inclusion or exclusion of oral cancer screening in a periodic health examination (C Recommendation). Annual examination by physicians and/or dentists should be considered for men and women over 60 years of age who have known risk factors for oral pre-malignancy and invasive oral cancers, such as tobacco use in any form and regular alcohol consumption. Individual judgement should be exercised regarding the use of tolonium chloride for those identified by positive oral physical examination and referral to a specialist for further diagnostic evaluation.

Fair evidence exists supporting the efficacy of 13cRA in the treatment of oral leukoplakia; however, the high recurrence rates following cessation of therapy and the high rate of adverse effects limit its potential usefulness. Therapy with these agents remains investigational.

Unanswered Questions (Research Agenda)

Further prospective studies are required to strengthen the evidence demonstrating the effectiveness of primary prevention strategies.

Further research should be directed to determining whether current treatment modalities are in fact effective in a well designed randomized controlled trial. Once this is established then efforts to determine the reliability, validity and responsiveness of the most effective screening or case-finding maneuvers may be undertaken. Furthermore, there is evidence to suggest that screening by oral physical examination may be performed by different disciplines, using simple maneuvers. A cost effectiveness study of such a screening program is required to determine the most feasible screening strategy.

Evidence

The literature was identified with a MEDLINE search for the years 1980 to 1993, limited to studies in the English language. The following key words were used: mouth neoplasms, health status indicators, population surveillance, mass screening combined with evaluation studies, outcome and process assessment, mortality and prognosis.

This review was initiated in January 1993, and the recommendations were finalized by the Task Force in June, 1993.

Acknowledgements

Special thanks to Ms. Judy Carter and Task Force members, Elaine Wang and William Feldman, for their patience and invaluable assistance in preparing this manuscript.

Selected References

1. U.S. Department of Health and Human Services, Public Health Service, National Institute of Health: Smoking and Tobacco Control Monograph 2. Smokeless tobacco or health: An international perspective. [NIH Publication No. 93-3461], September 1992

2. Mehta FS, Gupta PC, Bhonsle RB, *et al*: Detection of oral cancer using basic health workers in an area of high oral cancer incidence in India. *Canc Detect Prev* 1986; 9: 219-225

3. Warnakulasuriya KAAS, Nanyakkara BG: Reproducibility of an oral cancer and precancer detection program using a primary health care model in Sri Lanka. *Canc Detect Prevent* 1991; 15: 331-334

4. Bouquot JE, Gorlin RJ: Leukoplakia, lichen planus and other oral keratoses in 23,616 white Americans over the age of 35 years. *Oral Surg Oral Med Oral Pathol* 1986; 61: 373-381

5. Kaugars GE, Burns JC: An education program for oral cancer detection. *J Cancer Education* 1989; 4: 175-177

6. Rosenberg D, Cretin S: Use of meta-analysis to evaluate tolonium chloride in oral cancer screening. *Oral Surg Oral Med Oral Pathol* 1989; 67: 621-627

7. Doll R, Hill AB: Lung cancer and other causes of death in relation to smoking: a second report on the mortality of British doctors. *Br Med J* 1956; 2: 1071-1081

8. Hammond EC, Horn D: Smoking and death rates: report on forty-four months of follow-up of 187,783 men. *JAMA* 1958; 166: 1159-1172

9. Rothman K, Keller A: The effect of joint exposure to alcohol and tobacco on the risk of cancer of the mouth and pharynx. *J Chron Dis* 1972; 25: 711-716

10. Wynder EL, Mushinski MH, Spivak JC: Tobacco and alcohol consumption in relation to the development of multiple primary cancers. *Cancer* 1977; 40: 1872-1878

11. Wigle DT, Mao Y, Grace M: Relative importance of smoking as a risk for selected cancers. *Can J Pub Health* 1980; 71: 269-275

12. Winn DM, Blot WJ, Shy CM, *et al*: Snuff dipping and oral cancer among women in the southern United States. *N Engl J Med* 1981; 304: 745-749

13. Zheng TZ, Boyle P, Hu HF, *et al*: Tobacco smoking, alcohol consumption and risk of oral cancer: a case-control study in Beijing, People's Republic of China. *Cancer Causes Control* 1990; 1: 173-179

14. Choi SY, Kahyo H: Effect of cigarette smoking and alcohol consumption in the etiology of cancer of the oral cavity, pharynx, and larynx. *Int J Epidemiol* 1991; 20: 878-885

15. Kato I, Nomura AM, Stemmermann GN, *et al*: Prospective study of the association of alcohol with cancer of the upper aerodigestive tract and other sites. *Cancer Causes Control* 1992; 3: 145-151

16. Winn DM: Smokeless tobacco and cancer: the epidemiologic evidence. *CA Cancer J Clin* 1988; 38: 236-243

17. Sankaranarayanan R, Nair MK, Mathew B, *et al*: Recent results of oral cancer research in Kearla, India. *Head Neck* 1992; 14: 107-112

18. Sussman S, Dent CW, Stacy AW, *et al*: Project towards no tobacco use: 1-year behavior outcomes. *Am J Public Health* 1993; 83: 1245-1250

19. Elder JP, Wildey M, de Moor C, *et al*: The long-term prevention of tobacco use among junior high school students: classroom and telephone interventions. *Am J Public Health* 1993; 1239-1244

20. Stevens MM, Freeman DH Jr, Mott LA, *et al*: Smokeless tobacco use among children: The New Hampshire study. *Am J Prev Med* 1993; 9: 160-167

21. Little SJ, Stevens VJ, Severson HH, *et al*: An effective smokeless tobacco intervention for dental hygiene patients. *J Dent Hyg* 1992; 66: 185-190

22. Hong WK, Endicott J, Itri LM, *et al*: 13-cis-retinoic acid in the treatment of oral leukoplakia. *N Engl J Med* 1986; 315: 1501-1505

23. American Cancer Society: *Cancer facts and figures 1991.* [91-500M No. 5008.91], Atlanta, GA

24. Lippman SM, Toth BB, Batsakis JG, *et al*: Low dose 13-cis-retinoic acid (13cRA) maintains remission in oral premalignancy: more effective than b-carotene in randomized trial. *Proc Am Soc Clin Oncol* 1990; 9: 59 (Abstract)

25. Malaker K, Anderson BJ, Beecroft WA, *et al*: Management of oral mucosal dysplasia with beta-carotene retinoic acid: a pilot cross-over study. *Cancer Detect Prevent* 1991; 15: 335-340

26. Garewal HS: Potential role of beta-carotene in prevention of oral cancer. *Am J Clin Nutr* 1991; 53: 294S-297S

27. Stich HF, Mathew B, Sankaranarayanan R, *et al*: Remission of precancerous lesions in the oral cavity of tobacco chewers and maintenance of the protective effect of beta-carotene or vitamin A. *Am J Clin Nutr* 1991; 53: 298S-304S

28. Ilstad ST, Tollerud DJ, Bigelow ME, *et al*: A multivariate analysis of determinants of survival for patients with squamous cell carcinoma of the head and neck. *Ann Surg* 1989; 209: 237-241

29. Vandenbrouck C, Sancho-Garnier H, Chassagne D, *et al*: Elective versus therapeutic radical neck dissection in epidermoid carcinoma of the oral cavity: results of a randomized clinical trial. *Cancer* 1980; 46: 386-390

30. Rodgers LW Jr, Stringer SP, Mendenhall WM, *et al*: Management of squamous cell carcinoma of the floor of the mouth. *Head Neck* 1993; 15: 16-19

31. Moore C, Flynn MB, Greenberg RA: Evaluation of size in prognosis of oral cancer. *Cancer* 1986; 58: 158-162

32. Khafif RA, Gelbfish GA, Attie JN, *et al*: Thirty year experience with 457 radical neck dissections in cancer of the mouth, pharynx and larynx. *Am J Surg* 1989; 158: 303-307

33. Nason RW, Sako K, Beecroft WA, *et al*: Surgical management of squamous cell carcinoma of the floor of the mouth. *Am J Surg* 1989; 158: 292-296

34. Jones JB, Lampe HB, Cheung HW: Carcinoma of the tongue in young patients. *J Otolaryngol* 1989; 18: 105-108

35. Toohill RJ, Dancavage JA, Grossman TW, *et al*: The effects of delay in standard treatment due to induction chemotherapy in two randomized prospective studies. *Laryngoscope* 1987; 97: 407-412

36. Lefebvre JL, Coche-Dequeant B, Castelain B, *et al*: Interstitial brachytherapy and early tongue squamous cell carcinoma management. *Head Neck* 1990; 12: 232-236

37. U.S. Preventive Services Task Force: *Guide to Clinical Preventive Services: an Assessment of the Effectiveness of 169 Interventions.* Williams & Wilkins, Baltimore Md, 1989: 91-94

38. Jones JA: Integrating the oral examination into clinical practice. *Hosp Pract Off Ed* 1989; 24: 23-27,30

39. Doherty SA: Basic issues in screening for oral cancer among male subpopulation. *J Tenn Dent Assoc* 1989; 69: 26-29

40. Lowry RJ: Prevention of oral carcinoma. *Dent Update* 1990; 17: 58-61

41. Melrose RJ: Regular screening leads to early diagnosis. *J Calif Dent Assoc* 1990; 18: 52

42. Fedele DJ, Jones JA, Niessen LC: Oral cancer screening in the elderly. *J Am Geriatr Soc* 1991; 39: 920-925

43. Gift HC, Newman JF: How older adults use oral health care services: results of a National Health Interview Survey. *J Am Dent Assoc* 1993; 124: 89-93

Prevention of Oral Cancer

MANEUVER	EFFECTIVENESS	LEVEL OF EVIDENCE <REF>	RECOMMENDATION
Smoking cessation counselling	Use of multiple intervention and reinforcement strategies increased 6-month and 1-year cessation rates.	Randomized controlled trials<17> (I)	Good evidence to include in periodic health exam (A)
Screening by oral physical examination	Low prevalence of oral cancers and poor positive predictive value of physical exam (even in conjunction with use of tolonium chloride testing) limit usefulness. Potential for labelling, cost of follow-up and marginal benefits demonstrated for therapy are additional considerations.	Cohort and case-control studies<2-6> (II-2)	Insufficient evidence to include or exclude from periodic health exam (C); annual examination by physician and/or dentist should be considered for men and women over age 60 years with risk factors for oral cancers and precancers; individual judgement should be exercised regarding the use of tolonium chloride for those identified as positive by oral physical exam
	Use of 13-cis-retinoic acid (13cRA) reverses or stabilizes premalignant lesions and reduces the rate of second primary malignancies. Side effects, potential teratogenicity and relapse after discontinuation limit usefulness. ß-carotene reduces occurrence of oral leukoplakia and mucosal dysplasia to a lesser degree than 13cRA, without side effects.	Randomized controlled trials<22-27> (I)	
	Survival of patients with invasive cancer appears comparable for surgical and radiation therapy; earlier stage of disease is an important prognostic factor.	Cohort studies<23,28> (II-2); case series <29-33,36> (III)	

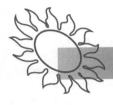

CHAPTER 70

Prevention of Skin Cancer

By John W. Feightner

Prevention of Skin Cancer

Adapted by John W. Feightner, MD, MSc, FCFP[1] from materials prepared for the U.S. Preventive Services Task Force[2]

Routine screening for skin cancer by primary care providers is not recommended for the general population (C Recommendation). For individuals with significantly increased risk (family melanoma syndrome, first degree relative with malignant melanoma) it would seem prudent to monitor regularly by physical examination and dermatologists may be the most appropriate assessors. Currently there is insufficient evidence to recommend either for or against counselling patients to perform periodic skin self-examinations. Clinicians should advise patients with increased sun exposure or at increased risk of skin cancer to protect their skin from solar rays (B Recommendation). Persons with a prior history of solar keratosis who cannot avoid sun exposure should use sunscreens that block both UV-A and UV-B radiation (B Recommendation), although there is insufficient evidence to support its use for the prevention of squamous cell carcinoma, basal cell carcinoma or malignant melanoma.

Burden of Suffering

In Canada in 1992, there were approximately 51,000 new cases of skin cancer. Of these, 47,000 were either basal cell carcinoma (BCC) and squamous cell carcinomas (SCC), commonly referred to as nonmelanomatous skin cancer (NMSC).<1> These skin cancers rarely metastasize and are generally easily treated. However, extensive lesions can cause marked tissue destruction and disfigurement as well as functional impairment if the tumours are not detected early. An increased risk for NMSC is associated with: a personal history of NMSC, older age, light eyes, skin or hair, poor ability to tan, a high density of freckles, and a marked cumulative lifetime exposure to sun.

Malignant melanoma (MM) differs considerably from these other two skin cancers. While less common, it is far more lethal. In 1993, there were an estimated 2,950 new cases of MM in Canada and in that same year, there were 560 deaths from MM. Using 1989 data, it is estimated that MM ranks 14th amongst all cancers in potential years of life lost. Over the last two decades there has been an increase in age-standardized incidence (6% in men, 4% in women) and an increase in mortality rates (3.4% in men, 1.6% in women). A number of attempts have been undertaken to identify important risk factors associated

[1] Professor of Family Medicine, McMaster University, Hamilton, Ontario
[2] by Dr. Carolyn DiGuiseppi, Science Advisor, U.S. Preventive Services Task Force, Washington, D.C.

with MM. These have included melanocytic, precursor or marker lesions (e.g. atypical moles, certain congenital moles), increased numbers of common moles, immunosuppression, and a family or personal history of skin cancer, particularly MM. A recent case-control study in Ontario identified four host risk factors associated with MM: hair colour (red haired individuals are at greater risk than those with black hair), freckled and nevus density (greater risk for those with large numbers), and a propensity to sunburn after repeated sun exposure compared to those who tan.

Some individuals are at markedly increased risk for MM. Individuals with the rare condition of "familial atypical mole and melanoma" (FAM-M) syndrome, show an increased risk of 100-fold or more. Concerns in the past have been raised around the identification of risk in individuals solely with personal or family history of extensive dysplastic nevi. However, both the clinical and pathological diagnoses of dysplastic nevi show considerable inter-observer variation, making accurate diagnosis difficult. Hence, one must be cautious to guard against inappropriate labelling.

The etiology of both NMSC and MM have been linked to ultraviolet light, particularly UV-B light. The population studies evaluating the association between NMSC and sun exposure are consistent in supporting the hypothesis that cumulative sun exposure over a lifetime is a key etiologic component. The role of ultraviolet light in the etiology of MM has received considerably more attention and debate.<2-6> Depending on the choice of confounding variables, case-control studies have shown association in conflicting directions between episodes of sunburn (particularly in early life), and the subsequent development of MM in later life. While not yet conclusive, these data plus data from migrant studies lend support to the concern that exposure to extensive sunlight in earlier years may play an etiologic role. The results, however, are not yet conclusive. Unlike NMSC, it appears as though the association with UV-B sunlight is one of "intermittent exposure" rather than cumulative exposure.

Maneuver

There are two basic approaches to skin cancer prevention, primary prevention including avoidance of sun during peak hours, use of protective clothing, and use of sunscreens; and secondary prevention, which relies on the early detection of MM or NMSC either by the patient themselves or by a physician. The primary prevention maneuvers will be discussed in the section on effectiveness.

Physical Exam by Physicians

The detection of a suspicious lesion constitutes a positive screening test which then needs to be confirmed by skin biopsy.

Studies have not been able to identify the true sensitivity and specificity of skin examination because for the most part only individuals testing "positive" have gone on to biopsy of the lesions. One study has attempted to estimate sensitivity using population incidence rates as an estimate for false negative rates and calculated sensitivities of 97% for MM, 94% for BCC and 89% for SCC.[7] The use of population incidence rates to calculate false negatives, however, is suspect in this study because over 78% of those screened had two or more risk factors for skin cancer and, hence, are not representative of the general population. In individuals with positive examinations at screening clinics, studies have indicated histologic confirmation at the rate of 40% for MM, 43% and 57% for BCC, and 14% and 75% for SCC.[7,8] The likelihood of histologic confirmation for MM in examinations by dermatologists in skin clinics ranges from 38-64% and from 72-84% for examinations by skin cancer specialists. In a randomized community study evaluating screening by expert dermatologists, histologic examination confirmed the clinical diagnosis of SCC in 38% of the cases and of BCC in 59%.[9]

Primary care physicians and other generalists who have not been trained in dermatology tend to make fewer correct diagnoses in studies using colour photographs.[10-12]

The yield in screening for skin cancer is influenced by the proportion of body surface examined. For MM, only 20% of the lesions normally occur on exposed body surfaces in contrast to 85 to 90% of NMSC. It has been estimated that the detection of MM would increase two to six times with total body skin examination (TSE). There are no data regarding the appropriate frequency of maneuvers such as TSE and as a result, those who advocate this procedure recommend annual or biennial intervals based solely on clinical judgement. This maneuver can be markedly influenced by poor patient compliance, a concern raised in one study where only 4.2% of the patients returned for a one year follow-up for TSE.[13]

There are no identified serious adverse effects associated with TSE and while theoretically complications can arise with biopsy, the actual rate of complications is small. There are, however, no controlled studies to evaluate either the detection rate or any adverse effects associated with TSE.

Patient Self-Examination

This is an option which some have advocated particularly using a seven point checklist to evaluate skin lesions. One which evaluated a seven point checklist found it had a sensitivity of 71% and a specificity of 99% with a predictive value of 7% for MM diagnosis, using a dermatologist's clinical diagnosis as the gold standard.[14] There are no data which appropriately evaluate the ability of patients to accurately detect suspicious lesions in general nor are there data regarding the accuracy of periodic skin self-examination or the efficacy of instructions in reducing self-examination errors.

Effectiveness of Prevention and Treatment

Early Detection of Lesions

Basal cell and squamous cell skin carcinomas are very common but are slow growing and rarely metastasize. While early identification and treatment of early lesions might reduce morbidity and disfigurement, no studies exist which have evaluated such early detection efforts.

Basal cell and squamous cell skin carcinomas are very common but are slow growing and rarely metastasize

The principle potential benefit of routine skin examination lies in discovering early MM. However, the sensitivity and specificity of skin examination by primary physicians and the optimal frequency of such examinations is unknown. Moreover, there are no randomized controlled trials evaluating early detection and subsequent treatment. Hence, one cannot rule out the impact of lead time and length biases on studies which employ a before/after design or use inappropriate control groups. The second challenge arises because of the relatively low lifetime risk (1%) of MM in the general population. Hence, 99% of patients from the general population would be examined with routine screening and would never be found to have MM. This raises questions, as yet unevaluated, regarding the impact of potential adverse effects as well as the cost-benefit ratio of early detection efforts for MM in the general population.

At the population level, education campaigns have been mounted to encourage MM screening by primary care providers, particularly in Scotland. One study found a trend towards a reduction in the thickness of tumours ($p<0.05$) and a trend (which was not statistically evaluated) showing a decrease in mortality in women.<15> However, there was no control group and the before/after design does not allow important confounding factors to be ruled out.

One of the difficulties in before/after studies arises when the thickness of MM is used an outcome. Studies have indicated that survival and the likelihood of recurrence after resection is correlated to the thickness of lesions. A MM <1 mm thick is associated with an eight year disease-free survival for 90% of patients compared to a rate of 74% for lesions of 1-2 mm thick. While this association exists as a prognostic variable in studies without control groups, one cannot determine whether the identification of thinner lesions is a result of early detection efforts or simply represents a natural trend in the population. Indeed, some data indicate that in certain geographic regions, there is a population trend towards thinner lesions, a phenomenon which would appear to exist quite apart from early detection efforts.

Likewise data for individuals who may be at high risk are limited. Two large case series of individuals with atypical moles, screened regularly by dermatologists indicated a tendency towards the detection of thinner lesions. Likewise before/after studies for individuals with the FAM-M syndrome and in individuals with prior MM, report that regular screening by dermatologists results in the detection of significantly thinner tumours compared to historical and other non-concurrent controls.

Primary Prevention

The approaches to the primary prevention of skin cancer include the following: limiting exposure to sunlight (by sun avoidance or by wearing protective clothing) or by applying sunscreen preparations. Such an approach has been promoted through public education campaigns including the "slip, slap, slop" program popularized in Australia (slip on protective clothing, slap on a hat and slop on sunscreen).

No randomized controlled trials or other appropriate studies evaluate avoidance of sun exposure or use of protective clothing

There are no randomized controlled trials or other appropriate comparative studies to evaluate the avoidance of sun exposure or the use of protective clothing to prevent MM and NMSC. The strongest evidence available to support what may be a prudent approach, comes from the literature which identifies an association between ultraviolet light and MM and NMSC.[2-6] Such studies, however, do not include prospective cohort studies or randomized controlled trials and do not directly address the specific prescription of avoiding sun or using protective clothing. The etiologic evidence, however, can be used to argue for the prudence of such an approach.

The effectiveness of sunscreens is unclear except for their ability to reduce recurrence or development of new solar keratoses

The evidence for the use of sunscreens is less clear cut with the exception of their ability to reduce the rate of recurrence or development of new solar keratoses. A recent randomized controlled trial evaluated the regular use of sunscreens which block UV-A and UV-B in a population of individuals over age 40 who had previous solar keratoses.[16] Over a six month period, the mean rate of solar keratoses in the control group increased by 1 per subject and decreased by 0.6 per subject in the sunscreen group. While solar keratoses are considered a precursor to squamous cell carcinoma, the risk of progression in any one year is less than 1 per 1,000 and of all squamous cell carcinomas, only 60% arise from previous solar keratoses and 40% of SCC arise from normal skin. Hence, the evidence from this study suggests sunscreen may have some impact on subsequent SCC, but the actual clinical impact is unclear. Hence, there is evidence for the prevention of solar keratoses but there is debate about the appropriateness of this as an intermediate outcome measure for squamous cell carcinoma in terms of its clinical significance. There are no randomized controlled trials of the benefits of the sunscreen in BCC or MM. However, concern has been raised by the findings from case-control and cohort studies which have indicated either no effect or a significant increased risk of BCC and MM in sunscreen users.[5,17,18] While debate continues around the potential effect of residual confounders on these results, the concerns remain unanswered. Concerns have also been raised regarding the importance of blocking UV-A as well as UV-B.

Any of the side effects of sunscreen are generally mild to moderate and occur in only 1 to 2% of users of sunscreen but these include contact and photocontact dermatitis, contact urticaria, and comedogenicity, although these are readily reversible with discontinuing the use of sunscreens.

Counselling

There are few data on the effectiveness of counselling patients to protect themselves from sunlight. One before/after study evaluating counselling at the time of skin cancer removal and on a yearly basis thereafter, reported increased use of protective clothing and sunscreen and reduced deliberate tanning in a 2-6 year follow-up.[19] The follow-up, however, involved only the two-thirds of patients who complied with follow-up visits and it was impossible to determine how much of the effect of the study was the result of surgery alone. Evidence from before/after studies indicates that public education can increase knowledge and beliefs about the health risk of sunlight, but it is not clear that individuals act on their knowledge and beliefs in this specific situation. Community and work site education interventions to reduce the risk of skin cancer, including one with a concurrent control group, have demonstrated significantly increased use of sun protection measures such as hats, shirts, and staying in the shade after the intervention. Whether the results of such education interventions can be generalized to physician counselling is not known.

Recommendations of Others

In 1989, the U.S. Preventive Services Task Force recommended routine screening for skin cancer for persons at high risk and that clinicians advise all patients with increased outdoor exposure to use sunscreen preparations and other measures to protect their skin from ultraviolet rays. There was no evidence for or against counselling patients to perform skin self-examination.[20] These recommendations are currently under review.

The (U.S.) National Institutes of Health (NIH) Consensus Panel recommended regular screening visits for skin cancer and patient education concerning periodic skin self-examinations. The NIH Consensus Panel also recommended that some family members of patients with MM be enrolled in surveillance programs. The American Cancer Society recommends monthly skin self-examination for all adults, and physician skin examination every three years in persons 20 to 39 years old and annually in persons over 40 years old. The Academy of Dermatology and the National Cancer Institute (U.S.) recommend regular screening visits for skin cancer and patient education for skin self-examination. These same agencies plus the American Cancer Society and the American Medical Association recommend patient education concerning sun avoidance and sunscreen protection.

The Canadian Dermatologists Association advocates the use of sunscreens of SPF 15 or higher for routine use by individuals who spend time outdoors exposed to the sun.

Conclusions and Recommendations

Routine screening for skin cancer by primary care providers using total-body skin examination is not recommended for the general population. Clinicians should remain alert for skin lesions with malignant features (i.e. asymmetry, border irregularity, colour variability, diameter greater than 6 mm, or rapidly changing lesions) when examining patients for other reasons, particularly in those with established risk factors. Such risk factors include clinical evidence of melanocytic precursor or marker lesions (i.e. atypical moles, certain congenital moles), large numbers of common moles, immunosuppression, a family or personal history of skin cancer, substantial cumulative lifetime sun exposure, intermittent intense sun exposure or severe sunburns in childhood, or light skin, hair, and eye colour, freckles, or poor tanning ability. Appropriate biopsy specimens should be taken of suspicious lesions (C Recommendation).

Currently, there is insufficient evidence to recommend for or against counselling patients to perform periodic self-examination of the skin. Clinicians may wish to educate patients with established risk factors for skin cancer (see above) concerning signs and symptoms suggesting cutaneous malignancy and the possible benefits of periodic self-examination (C Recommendation).

Persons with Family Melanoma Syndrome are at substantially increased risk for malignant melanoma. Clinicians examining these patients should be particularly alert to skin lesions with malignant features and should consider referral to skin cancer specialists for evaluation. For this very select subgroup there is fair evidence to offer total body skin examination (B Recommendation).

Clinicians may find it prudent to counsel persons and parents of children with established risk factors for skin cancer (including those with light skin, eyes and hair, or poor ability to tan), to avoid excessive sun exposure, especially between the hours of 10:00 a.m. and 3:00 p.m., and to use protective clothing such as shirts and hats when they are out in the sun. This recommendation is based on the etiologic evidence for UV exposure, the potential for large health benefits, low cost, and low risk of adverse effects from such counselling, even though the effectiveness of counselling is not well established (B Recommendation).

The routine use of sunscreens that block both UV-A and -B radiation is recommended for persons with prior evidence of solar keratosis who cannot avoid sun exposure (B Recommendation). There is insufficient evidence to recommend for or against counselling patients to use sunscreens to prevent malignant melanoma or basal cell carcinoma (C Recommendation).

Unanswered Questions (Research Agenda)

There is a need for continued research into the etiology of malignant melanoma. There is as well a need for further identification of individual risk factors to allow targeting of early detection and primary prevention efforts.

There is also a need for the proper evaluation of sun avoidance and the use of protective clothing as well as the effectiveness of counselling individuals to comply with these behaviours.

Finally, there is a need for further evaluation of the effectiveness of sunscreens, particularly in the prevention of malignant melanoma; and there is a need to evaluate the effect of counselling patients on the use of such agents should they be demonstrated to be effective.

Evidence

The literature was identified through a MEDLINE search for 1988 to March 1993 using the search words cancer, skin neoplasm, melanoma, dysplastic nevus, sunscreening agents, isotretinoin, and sunlight. Additional literature was identified by reviewing the citations used in articles identified in the MEDLINE search. This review was initiated in 1993 and the recommendations finalized by the Task Force in March 1994.

Selected References

1. National Cancer Institute of Canada: Canadian Cancer Statistics, 1992. NCIC, Toronto

2. Koh HK: Cutaneous melanoma. *N Engl J Med* 1991; 325: 171-182

3. International Agency for Research on Cancer: Monograph on the Evaluation of Carcinogenic Risks to Humans; Ultraviolet Radiation vol. 55, Lyon: IARC, 1992

4. Elwood JM: Melanoma and sun exposure: contrasts between intermittent and chronic exposure. *World J Surg* 1992; 16: 157-165

5. Holman CD, Armstrong BK, Heenan PJ: Relationship of cutaneous malignant melanoma to individual sunlight-exposure habits. *J Natl Cancer Inst* 1986; 76: 403-414

6. Osterlind A, Tucker MA, Stone BJ, *et al*: The Danish case-control study of cutaneous malignant melanoma. II: Importance of UV-light exposure. *Int J Cancer* 1988; 42: 319-324

7. Koh HK, Caruso A, Gage I, *et al*: Evaluation of melanoma/skin cancer screening in Massachusetts. Preliminary results. *Cancer* 1990; 65: 375-379

8. Bolognia JL, Berwick M, Fine JA: Complete follow-up and evaluation of a skin cancer screening in Connecticut. *J Am Acad Dermatol* 1990; 23: 1098-1106

9. Green A, Leslie D, Weedon D: Diagnosis of skin cancer in the general population: clinical accuracy in the Nambour survey. *Med J Aust* 1988; 148: 447-450

10. Cassileth BR, Clark WH Jr, Lusk EJ, *et al*: How well do physicians recognize melanoma and other problem lesions? *J Am Acad Dermatol* 1986; 14: 555-560

11. Ramsay DL, Fox AB: The ability of primary care physicians to recognize the common dermatoses. *Arch Dermatol* 1981; 117: 620-622

12. Wagner RF Jr, Wagner D, Tomich JM, *et al*: Diagnoses of skin disease: dermatologists vs. nondermatologists. *J Dermatol Surg Oncol* 1985; 11: 476-479

13. Lee G, Massa MC, Welykyj S, *et al*: Yield from total skin examination and effectiveness of skin cancer awareness program. Findings in 874 new dermatology patients. *Cancer* 1991; 67: 202-205

14. Keefe M, Dick DC, Wakeel RA: A study of the value of the seven-point checklist in distinguishing benign pigmented lesions from melanoma. *Clin Exp Dermatol* 1990; 15: 167-171

15. MacKie RM, Hole D: Audit of public education campaign to encourage earlier detection of malignant melanoma. *BMJ* 1992; 304: 1012-1015

16. Thompson SC, Jolley D, Marks R: Reduction of solar keratoses by regular sunscreen use. *N Engl J Med* 1993; 329: 1147-1151

17. Hunter DJ, Golditz GA, Stampfer MJ, *et al*: Risk factors for basal cell carcinoma in a prospective cohort of women. *Ann Epidemiol* 1990; 1: 13-23

18. Beitner H, Norell SE, Ringborg U, *et al*: Malignant melanoma: aetiological importance of individual pigmentation and sun exposure. *Br J Dermatol* 1990; 122: 43-51

19. Robinson JK: Compensation strategies in sun protection behaviors by a population with nonmelanoma skin cancer. *Prev Med* 1992; 21: 754-765

20. U.S. Preventive Services Task Force: *Guide to Clinical Preventive Services: an Assessment of the Effectiveness of 169 Interventions.* Williams & Wilkins, Baltimore, Md, 1989: 71-75

Prevention of Skin Cancer

MANEUVER	EFFECTIVENESS	LEVEL OF EVIDENCE <REF>	RECOMMENDATION
Total body skin examination	For normal risk individuals has not been proven as an effective early detection maneuver.	Comparison of times and places<7-9> (II-3)	There is poor evidence to include or exclude from the periodic health examination (PHE) of the general population (C); there is fair evidence for the inclusion of total body skin examination for a very select sub-group of individuals (B)
	For individuals at significantly increased risk (i.e. family melanoma syndrome (MM) first degree relative with melanoma) it is prudent to undertake regular examinations (dermatologists may be more accurate assessors).	Comparison of times and places<10-12> (II-3)	
Self-Exam	There has been no evaluation of patient ability to detect lesions or of physician ability to alter patient screening skills or behaviour except for one study with a positive predictive value of 7% for MM.	Comparison of times and places<4> (II-3)	There is poor evidence to include or exclude in the periodic health examination (C)
Avoidance of sun exposure and protective clothing	Evidence from epidemiologic studies focusing on etiology of melanoma, prudence and low cost/side-effects supports the avoidance of excessive sun exposure at mid-day, plus the use of protective clothing.	Epidemiologic and case-control studies<2-6> (II-2)	On the basis of epidemiologic data and case-control studies, and prudence, there is fair evidence to include in the periodic health examination (B)
Sunscreens (for prevention of squamous cell and basal cell carcinoma; and malignant melanoma	Studies have indicated no effect or raised concerns of increased risk among sunscreen users. At present, the evidence is inconclusive.	Cohort and case-control studies <17-19> (II-2)	There is poor evidence for the inclusion or exclusion of advice on sunscreen use in the PHE to prevent squamous cell carcinoma, basal cell carcinoma and malignant melanoma (C)*

* A randomized controlled trial<16> has demonstrated that sunscreens can reduce the rate of recurrence or development of new solar keratoses. While solar keratoses are precursor lesions for squamous cell carcinoma (SCC), they do not represent a sufficiently strong intermediate outcome measure to provide evidence of effectiveness in preventing SCC. There is fair evidence for recommending the use of sunscreens for the reduction of solar keratoses only. (B Recommendation for persons with a prior history of solar keratosis who cannot avoid sun exposure).

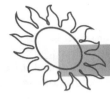

CHAPTER 71

Prevention of Pancreatic Cancer

By Brenda J. Morrison

Prevention of Pancreatic Cancer

Adapted by Brenda J. Morrison, PhD[1] from the report prepared for the U.S. Preventive Services Task Force[2]

No tests have yet been developed which are suitable for screening for pancreatic cancer in asymptomatic persons. However, counselling for smoking cessation is recommended since there is fair evidence that cessation does reduce the risk of the disease and good evidence that counselling is effective.

Burden of Suffering

Cancer of the pancreas is the fourth leading cause of cancer deaths in Canada in both men and women, accounting for 2,611 deaths in 1990 and an estimated 36,000 potential years of life lost. For 1993 it was estimated that there would be 2,750 new cases of pancreatic cancer and 2,900 deaths from the disease in Canada. In contrast with many other parts of the world, the age-specific mortality rates in Canada appear to have been dropping over the last 35 years.[1] This cancer is more common in men and older persons (the majority of cases being diagnosed between ages 60 and 80). Familial aggregations of pancreatic cancer are rare but have been described.

Since initial symptoms are usually nonspecific (e.g., abdominal pain and weight loss) and are frequently disregarded, some 80-90% of patients have regional and distant metastases by the time they are diagnosed. In Ontario only 8% of patients live more than five years after diagnosis. Pancreatic adenocarcinomas, which account for more than 90% of all pancreatic neoplasms, are only resectable in about 4-16% of cases at diagnosis and the five-year survival rate is less than 1%.

Cigarette smoking has been consistently associated with an increased risk of pancreatic cancer. The relative risk has ranged from 2 to 5 in numerous cohort and case-control studies of populations in the U.S., Canada, Europe, and Japan.[1-6] In the more recent studies, a dose-response relationship has been demonstrated.[2-4]

Several cohort studies and many population-based case-control studies have reported positive associations between pancreatic cancer and dietary factors such as meat, eggs, carbohydrates, refined sugar, cholesterol, fat and total calorie intake, as well as negative (protective) associations with intake of vegetables and fruits.[1,5,6] However, study results are inconsistent. Also, a decrease in any dietary factor

In Canada mortality rates from pancreatic cancer appear to be dropping but 5-year survival is less than 1%

---

[1] Associate Professor, Department of Health Care and Epidemiology, University of British Columbia, Vancouver, British Columbia

[2] By Carolyn DiGuiseppi, MD, MPH, Science Advisor, U.S. Preventive Services Task Force, Washington, D.C.

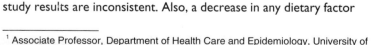

and, possibly, a substitution with another foodstuff, could cause an increase in some other disease so further research is needed. (Nutritional counselling has also been evaluated in treatment of obesity (Chapters 30 and 48) and prevention of lung cancer (Chapter 64) with more general considerations being addressed in the chapter on nutritional counselling (Chapter 49)). Studies of the relationship between increased alcohol consumption and pancreatic cancer have yielded inconsistent results;[1,6-8] few have adequately assessed level and duration of intake, or evaluated the possibility of a link between alcohol, pancreatitis and pancreatic cancer. Current epidemiologic evidence does not support an association between pancreatic cancer and coffee consumption.[1]

Many population-based epidemiologic studies have reported an association between pancreatic carcinoma and diabetes mellitus, although the excess risk for the cancer is reduced, and in some studies nullified, when cases with recent onset are excluded.[1,9] It has not been adequately determined whether diabetes is a result of the cancer, or whether it might just increase the risk for pancreatic carcinoma.

Maneuver

Adenocarcinoma is the principal form of pancreatic neoplasm for which screening has been considered; in this chapter, "pancreatic cancer" refers to adenocarcinoma unless otherwise noted. There are no reliable screening tests for detecting pancreatic cancer in asymptomatic individuals. The deep anatomic location of the pancreas makes detection of small localized tumours unlikely during routine abdominal examination. Even in patients with confirmed pancreatic cancer, an abdominal mass is palpable in only 15-25% of cases. Magnetic resonance imaging and computerized tomography (CT) are too costly to use as routine screening tests, while more accurate tests such as endoscopic retrograde cholangio-pancreatography (ERCP) and endoscopic ultrasound are inappropriate for screening asymptomatic patients due to their invasiveness. Abdominal ultrasonography is a noninvasive screening test that has a reported sensitivity of 40-98% and a specificity as high as 90-94%. However, these data are based on examinations of symptomatic patients with suspected disease. They thus provide little information on the efficacy of abdominal ultrasound as a screening test in asymptomatic persons. Conventional ultrasonography is also limited by visualization difficulties due to obesity or the presence of bowel gas and by the range of resolution, 2-3 cm. Frequently tumours ≤2 cm in diameter have produced metastatic disease,[10] thus limiting the ability of ultrasound to detect early disease.

With most cases of pancreatic malignancy there are elevated levels of certain serologic markers such as CA19-9, peanut agglutinin, pancreatic oncofetal antigen, DU-PAN-2, carcinoembryonic antigen,

No reliable screening tests exist

alpha-fetoprotein, CA-50, SPan-1, and tissue polypeptide antigen. None of these markers is, however, tumour-specific or organ-specific; elevations of various serologic markers also occur in significant proportions of persons with benign gastrointestinal diseases or malignancies other than pancreatic cancer. Most of these markers have been studied exclusively in high-risk populations, such as symptomatic patients with suspected pancreatic cancer. CA19-9 has probably achieved the widest acceptance as a serodiagnostic test for pancreatic carcinoma in symptomatic patients, with an overall sensitivity of approximately 80% (68-93%) and specificity of 90% (73-100%); sensitivity was highest in patients with more advanced disease. Among healthy subjects, CA19-9 has specificity of 94% to 99%[11-13] but nevertheless generates a large proportion of false positive results due to the low prevalence of pancreatic cancer in the general population.[14] A study of mass screening of more than 10,000 asymptomatic persons for pancreatic cancer in Japan,[8] using either ultrasonography alone or CA19-9 plus elastase-1, found the likelihood of pancreatic cancer given a positive screening test to be 0.5%; only one of the four cancers discovered could be curably resected.

The predictive value of a positive test could be improved if a population at substantially higher risk could be identified. New-onset diabetes mellitus in adult patients might be useful as a marker for a population at high risk of having pancreatic cancer[1] but not all investigations of the relationship between these diseases have shown an increased risk. If a high risk is established, studies of screening efficacy might be warranted. Screening for diabetes mellitus in the non-pregnant adult is not recommended (Chapter 50).

Effectiveness of Prevention and Treatment

Primary prevention of pancreatic cancer may be possible through clinical efforts directed at the use of tobacco products. There is good evidence from randomized trials that smoking cessation strategies are effective;[15-17] more evidence on the effectiveness of cessation strategies is presented in Chapter 43 on preventing tobacco-related illness. Former smokers have been shown to have a decreased risk of the disease compared to current smokers.[2-4]

Evidence that early detection can lower morbidity or mortality from pancreatic cancer is, however, not conclusive. The reported five-year survival for localized disease, based on 1981-1987 U.S. data, is only 7%, not substantially higher than the five-year survival with regional (4%) and distant (1%) metastases. A recent comprehensive review of published reports on surgical resection of pancreatic cancer also estimated an overall 5-year survival rate of 8% for small tumours without evidence of local or distant spread. In part, this rate may reflect the fact that a proportion of patients with localized disease cannot be operated on because of concomitant medical problems, advanced age or other reasons.<10,18> Patients who have small localized tumours that are resected for attempted cure, which account for only 4-16% of the total, may have better 5-year survival rates (as high as 37-48% in the most experienced centers<10,18>) although the designs of most studies of surgical outcome suffer from lead-time, length, and selection biases. The morbidity associated with surgical resection is high (15-53%) but perioperative mortality is now less than 7% in the hands of experienced surgeons.<9>

Reports on the effectiveness of adjuvant external beam and/or intraoperative radiotherapy in improving survival among curatively resected patients, using historical controls, have yielded inconsistent results. In one small randomized controlled trial,<19> corroborated by a subsequent case series by the same authors, an adjuvant treatment program using combined radiation and chemotherapy following curative resection was associated with a significant median survival advantage of 9 months and a 5-year survival advantage of 14.5% in treated versus control cases; however, the study was closed early due to poor subject accrual and did not control for the substantially greater frequency of clinic visits by cases. Adverse effects of combined radiation and chemotherapy include leukopenia and gastrointestinal toxicity<19> and intraoperative radiotherapy frequently causes gastrointestinal bleeding, which may be life-threatening. Additional randomized controlled trials of adjuvant therapy are needed to confirm its effectiveness in improving survival in patients with early pancreatic carcinoma. New modalities being explored include immunotherapy and hormonal therapy.

Radiation and chemotherapy have significant adverse effects

Recommendations of Others

The U.S. Preventive Services Task Force recommends against routine screening for pancreatic cancer in asymptomatic persons.<20> No organizations have published recommendations to perform routine screening for pancreatic cancer in asymptomatic persons.

Conclusions and Recommendations

Even though smoking appears to only modestly increase the risk of pancreatic cancer, smoking cessation appears to be the only intervention for which there is evidence of a reduction in risk.<15-17> Therefore physicians should counsel their patients who smoke to give up the habit (B Recommendation to prevent pancreatic cancer specifically, although an A Recommendation for preventing other tobacco-related illness, see Chapter 43). No other risk factors for pancreatic cancer have been established so no other effective primary preventive measures are known.

In terms of secondary prevention, the screening tests employing CA19-9, or CA19-9 plus elastase-1 or ultrasound have not been shown to be effective in detecting early disease in asymptomatic individuals.[8,9,12-14] Other tests have not been sufficiently evaluated to allow recommendations to be formulated. Also, since the five-year survival for localized disease is so poor, the Task Force recommends that screening not be performed (D Recommendation).

Unanswered Questions (Research Agenda)

1. The occurrence of pancreatic cancer in patients with new-onset diabetes mellitus should be investigated to determine if these patients are a high risk group.

2. Nutritional studies should be carried out to explore possible risk factors for pancreatic cancer. Primary prevention might then be possible.

Evidence

The literature was identified with a MEDLINE search in the English language for the years 1988 to October 1992 using the following key words: pancreatic neoplasms, epidemiology, United States, Europe and Canada, smoking, risk factors, primary prevention, diet therapy, monoclonal antibodies, diagnosis, sensitivity and specificity, mass screening, false positive and false negative reaction, and diabetes mellitus.

This review was initiated in October 1992 and the recommendations finalized in June 1993.

Selected References

1. Howe GR, Jain M, Burch JD, *et al*: Cigarette smoking and cancer of the pancreas: evidence from a population-based case-control study in Toronto, Canada. *Int J Cancer* 1991; 47: 323-328

2. Ghadirian P, Simard A, Baillargeon J: Tobacco, alcohol, and coffee and cancer of the pancreas. A population-based, case-control study in Quebec, Canada. *Cancer* 1991; 67: 2664-2670

3. Mack TM, Yu MC, Hanish R, *et al*: Pancreas cancer and smoking, beverage consumption, and past medical history. *J Natl Cancer Inst* 1986; 76: 49-60

4. Canadian Task Force on the Periodic Health Examination: The periodic health examination: 2. 1985 update. *Can Med Assoc J* 1986; 134: 724-727

5. Rose G, Hamilton PJ, Colwell L, *et al*: A randomized controlled trial of anti-smoking advice: 10 year results. *J Epidemiol Community Health* 1982; 36: 102-108

6. Wilson D, Wood G, Johnston N, *et al*: Randomized clinical trial of supportive follow-up for cigarette smokers in a family practice. *Can Med Assoc J* 1982; 126: 127-129

7. Boyle P, Hsieh CC, Maisonneuve P, *et al*: Epidemiology of pancreas cancer (1988). *Int J Pancreatol* 1989; 5: 327-346

8. Tsuchiya R, Tsunoda T, Ishida T, *et al*: Resection for cancer of the pancreas – the Japanese experience. *Baillieres Clin Gastroenterol* 1990; 4: 931-939

9. Kalser MH, Ellenberg SS: Pancreatic cancer. Adjuvant combined radiation and chemotherapy following curative resection. *Arch Surg* 1985; 120: 899-903

10. U.S. Department of Health and Human Services: *The Health Benefits of Smoking Cessation.* U.S. Department of Health and Human Services, Public Health Service, Centers for Disease Control, Center for Chronic Disease Prevention and Health Promotion, Office on Smoking and Health. [DHHS Publication No.(CDC) 90-8416], 1990; 155-159

11. Homma T, Tsuchiya R: The study of the mass screening of persons without symptoms and of the screening of outpatients with gastrointestinal complaints or icterus for pancreatic cancer in Japan, using CA19-9 and elastase-1 or ultrasonography. *Int J Pancreatol* 1991; 9: 119-124

12. Farrow DC, Davis S: Risk of pancreatic cancer in relation to medical history and the use of tobacco, alcohol and coffee. *Int J Cancer* 1990; 45: 816-820

13. Nix GA, Dubbelman C, Wilson JH, *et al*: Prognostic implications of tumor diameter in carcinoma of the head of the pancreas. *Cancer* 1991; 67: 529-535

14. Del Villano BC, Brennan S, Brock P, *et al*: Radioimmunometric assay for a monoclonal antibody-defined tumor marker, CA 19-9. *Clin Chem* 1983; 29: 549-552

15. Ritts RE Jr, Del Villano BC, Go VL, *et al*: Initial clinical evaluation of an immunoradiometric assay for CA 19-9 using the NCI serum bank. *Int J Cancer* 1984; 33: 339-345

16. Fabris C, Del Favero G, Basso D, *et al*: Serum markers and clinical data in diagnosing pancreatic cancer: a contrastive approach. *Am J Gastroenterol* 1988; 83: 549-553

17. Frebourg T, Bercoff E, Manchon N, *et al*: The evaluation of CA 19-9 antigen level in the early detection of pancreatic cancer. A prospective study of 866 patients. *Cancer* 1988; 62: 2287-2290

18. Hirayama T: Epidemiology of pancreatic cancer in Japan. *Jpn J Clin Oncol* 1989; 19: 208-215

19. Olsen GW, Mandel JS, Gibson RW, *et al*: A case-control study of pancreatic cancer and cigarettes, alcohol, coffee and diet. *Am J Public Health* 1989; 79: 1016-1019

20. U.S. Preventive Services Task Force: *Guide to Clinical Preventive Services: an Assessment of the Effectiveness of 169 Interventions*, Williams & Wilkins, Baltimore, Md, 1989: 87-88

Prevention of Pancreatic Cancer

MANEUVER	EFFECTIVENESS	LEVEL OF EVIDENCE <REF>	RECOMMENDATION
Screening by abdominal palpation, ultrasound or serologic tumour markers (such as CA19-9 or CA19-9 or elastase-1	Screening tests have poor yield (CA19-9, CA19-9 plus elastase-1 or ultrasound). Other tests have not been evaluated among asymptomatic individuals.	Cohort studies<8,11-14> (II-2)	There is fair evidence that routine screening should be excluded from the periodic health examination (D)
	Evidence that early detection and treatment (surgery or adjuvant therapy) can lower morbidity or mortality is not conclusive.	Randomized controlled trial<6> (I); case-control studies<5,10> (II-2)	
Smoking cessation counselling and follow-up visits	Smoking cessation strategies are effective.	Randomized controlled trials<15-17> (I)	There is fair evidence that counselling be specifically considered to prevent pancreatic cancer in a periodic health examination (B)*
	A modest increase in risk is associated with cigarette smoking.	Cohort and case-control studies <1-3,7,18> (II-2)	
	Former smokers have a decreased risk compared to current smokers.	Cohort and case-control studies<2,4,7,9,19> (II-2)	

*   There is good evidence to recommend smoking cessation counselling for other reasons (see Chapter 43).

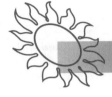

CHAPTER 72

Screening for Ovarian Cancer

By Cindy Quinton Gladstone

Screening for Ovarian Cancer

Prepared by Cindy Quinton Gladstone, MHSc, MD, FRCPC[1]

Ovarian cancer is the leading cause of gynecologic cancer mortality in North America. The disease has usually spread beyond the ovary by the time of diagnosis, and is associated with a five-year survival of 35% or less, as compared with 90% for Stage I tumours. To date, standard treatments have had little impact on mortality, and attention has focused on early detection through screening. A review of the evidence does not support such action. In fact, given the poor positive predictive value of pelvic examination, abdominal and transvaginal sonography, and/or serum CA 125 levels for ovarian cancer, as well as the potential harm of laparotomy, there is fair evidence to exclude such testing from periodic health assessments in asymptomatic pre- and post-menopausal women. The issue is less clearcut for high-risk women, with one or more first-degree relative(s) with ovarian cancer, or with one of the rare hereditary ovarian cancer syndromes. In such cases, the higher prevalence of disease may outweigh the risks of screening, although there is insufficient evidence to recommend for or against such a course of action. In all cases it would be prudent to examine the ovaries at the time of cervical cancer screening (see Chapter 73), as well as to refer women with a family history of ovarian cancer to an academic research center for follow-up.

Burden of Suffering

Ovarian cancer is the leading cause of gynecologic cancer mortality in both Canada and the U.S.

Ovarian cancer is the sixth most common female malignancy, after cancers of the breast, colon, lung, and uterus. The estimated incidence in Canada in 1993 was approximately 2100 new cases per year, about 4% of all new cancers in women.[1] Yet, because it is so lethal, it remains the leading cause of gynecologic cancer mortality in both Canada and the U.S.[2] Sparks suggests that for populations in which preventive measures have been applied for more common causes of death, the early detection of ovarian cancer "becomes the next focus of efforts to reduce premature death among women".[3]

Familial instances account for 5% to 15% of all ovarian cancers.[4,5] A recent case-control study, conducted in Alberta, Canada[6] established a relative risk of 2.61 for individuals with relatives with ovarian cancer. (The 95% confidence interval for the ratio between the observed and expected number of malignancies in cases' and controls' relatives was 1.12-1.59, significantly different

---

[1] Research Associate, Department of Preventive Medicine and Biostatistics, University of Toronto, Toronto, Ontario, 1992

from 1). Public health records in the United Kingdom showed that, if two or more close relatives were affected, the lifetime risk to a sister or mother of a patient approached 40%.[7] The rarer, hereditary cancer syndromes include: a) breast/ovary kindreds, b) Lynch II families, where both colonic and ovarian cancers occur, and c) site-specific cancers, involving only ovarian tumours. In addition to family history, other risk factors include advanced age, low parity, and nonuse of the oral contraceptive pill. At least one case-control report has shown a protective effect after as little as 3–6 months of oral contraceptive use.[8]

Ninety percent to 95% of ovarian malignancies are classified as epithelial[9] including serous, mucinous, endometrioid, clear cell, mixed epithelial, and undifferentiated histologies. Ten percent to 15% of these tumours are termed "borderline" or of "low malignant potential" because of their limited metastatic tendency and much higher 5 year survival rates. Tumour staging has been standardized by the International Federation of Gynecology and Obstetrics with Stage I tumours limited to the ovaries, Stage II including those with pelvic extension, Stage III involving those with peritoneal disease outside the pelvis and/or positive retroperitoneal or inguinal lymph nodes, and Stage IV comprising those with "distant" metastases.

At present, because of late and nonspecific symptomatology, and the relative inaccessibility of the ovaries to physical examination, only 25% of women with ovarian cancer have disease confined to the ovary at the time of diagnosis.[10] While in recent studies the five-year survival rate for this group nears 90%, the comparable rate is 35% or worse for the majority of women, who have disseminated disease when diagnosed.

Only 25% of women with ovarian cancer have disease confined to the ovary at the time of diagnosis

The natural history of ovarian cancer is not well understood. Rare case reports have suggested that malignancy may arise in benign cystadenomas. To date, however, no preinvasive lesion has been established. It may be that tumours arise *de novo* at multiple sites, as seen with primary peritoneal neoplasias. The problem of understaging due to inadequate surgery has hampered efforts to further define "typical" disease progression.

Maneuvers

Pelvic Examination

The sensitivity and specificity of the biannual examination have not been addressed. Patient size, body habitus, pelvic structure, and anxiety level would be expected to affect the accuracy of this maneuver, as would the expertise of the examiner, and the dimensions of the tumour itself. According to retrospective reports, chart reviews, and case series on this topic, pelvic examinations have missed from

10% to 100% of tumours diagnosed at laparotomy. A particularly high false positive rate would be expected in pre-menopausal women, given the increased prevalence of benign adnexal disease in this group.

One prospective comparison of preoperative ultrasound and pelvic examination in patients with pelvic masses yielded sensitivities (for detection of any pathology) of 83% and 67% respectively. Specificities were much higher at 94% and 96%.<11> The level of "blinding" of the examiners in this study, however, was questionable.

Abdominal Ultrasound

The positive predictive value of abdominal ultrasonography in asymptomatic women aged over 45 years was only 1.5%

The literature in this area is limited once again to case series.<12,13> Campbell and colleagues<14,15> performed three annual screening scans on 5,479 self-referred, asymptomatic women over 45 years of age. Of 15,977 scans, 338 were positive. Almost 4% of subsequent laparotomies were negative. Five primary ovarian malignancies, all Stage I, were diagnosed, for a prevalence of 0.09%, a specificity of 97.7%, and a sensitivity of 100%. However, even with these test characteristics, the positive predictive value in this population was only 1.5%. Furthermore, there was no independent follow-up of the women with negative scans.

Clearly, despite the impressive sensitivity and specificity reported for abdominal ultrasonography, its ability to screen for ovarian cancer is limited by the low prevalence of such tumours in the general population.

Transvaginal Sonography (TVS)

This technique is said to be superior to abdominal ultrasonography, because the transducer is closer to the area of interest, permitting the use of higher frequency ultrasound and enhancing the image quality. There have been three recent case series reported by Van Nagell's group<2,16> on screening for ovarian cancer using TVS. Specificity and sensitivity were calculated at 98.1% and 100% respectively. Other investigators have reported similar results.<17>

It has been postulated that transvaginal colour doppler may increase the specificity of TVS, because changes in tissue vascularity mediated by angiogenic tumour factors change impedance to bloodflow, even in Stage I cancers. One case series<18> supports this claim, with an abnormal colour doppler pattern seen in 0 of 30 normals, 1 of 10 benign masses, and 7 of 8 cancers.

CA 125

This tumour-associated antigen has been proposed for serologic screening for ovarian cancer. It is an antigenic determinant on a high molecular weight glycoprotein which is recognized by the monoclonal antibody OC 125.[19] Evidence concerning CA 125 screening is limited to 3 case-control studies, several case series,[19-24] and one "stochastic computer simulation".[25]

When CA 125 levels were evaluated in healthy patients, patients with benign pelvic masses, and those with malignant masses (including ovarian carcinomas), a 93.3% sensitivity and 79.7% specificity were achieved, using the usual threshold of >35 U/ml.[26] As expected, using a higher cutoff increased specificity with a concomitant reduction in sensitivity.[27] False positives were seen with leiomyomas, inflammatory masses, endometriomas, and benign epithelial neoplasms. CA 125 is less sensitive in early stage disease, as well as in borderline and mucinous tumour types.

The most interesting study[28] involved a "blind" retrospective analysis of CA 125 levels using sera obtained from the JANUS serum bank, a Norwegian repository of specimens collected since 1973 from more than 100,000 individuals. CA 125 levels were measured for women who subsequently developed ovarian cancer and from matched controls. Based on these data, the authors quote a 30-35% sensitivity (for a threshold value of 35 U/ml) for CA 125 levels drawn 2 years prior to diagnosis. Specificity was 95.4%. Specificity could be further increased when the doubling of an initially elevated CA 125 value was used as the criterion for positivity.[29]

Combination Screening

When a combination of preoperative clinical examinations, abdominal ultrasonography, and CA 125 were performed in women with ovarian masses, results in post-menopausal women suggested much lower sensitivities, but higher specificities for all maneuvers than reported elsewhere. Test characteristics were poorer in pre-menopausal women. Using this multimodal approach the authors were able to increase the positive predictive value of screening to 100% in post-menopausal women. Clearly this reflects the high prevalence of disease in this pre-selected population (24% in the pre-menopausal women and 59% in the post-menopausal group).[30]

Another multimodal screening study[31] included only post-menopausal volunteers, who underwent a routine pelvic examination and CA 125 measurement (cutoff 30 U/ml), followed by ultrasonography if indicated. Only one case of ovarian cancer was detected. As anticipated, specificities were increased to 99-100% by the combination of two or three of the maneuvers.

A recent decision analysis, designed to estimate the effectiveness of an ovarian cancer screening with CA 125 levels and transvaginal sonography in a cohort of 40-year-old women, suggested that screening increased the average life expectancy in this population by less than one day.

Costs

There are no randomized controlled trials of screening for ovarian cancer. The potential costs of screening all women over 45 years of age are prohibitive. The cost in the U.S. to screen the 43 million eligible women of this age with an ultrasound U.S. ($275 each) and a CA 125 level U.S. ($45 each) has been estimated at over U.S. $13 billion yearly, with no guarantee of a reduced death rate.[5]

Treatment Efficacy

Surgery Alone

Two recent case series have reported results of a "watch and wait" approach, without adjuvant therapy, following initial surgery. In those patients with early stage tumours who had undergone the most extensive preoperative staging, 100% 5 year disease-free survival was achieved with surgery alone.[32] Prognosis for early stage tumours with capsular rupture or positive peritoneal washings was slightly worse.[33]

Chemotherapy

The literature on chemotherapy consists mostly of trials of single-agent or combination regimens in patients with advanced ovarian cancer. Trials in early-stage disease are plagued by inconsistencies of staging and grading. In one study, patients with early stage ovarian cancer were randomized to receive melphalan or no treatment. Five-year disease-free survival for the two groups was not statistically different ($p > 0.05$) at 91% and 98% respectively.[34]

A companion study randomized women with poorly differentiated Stage I or II tumours to receive either melphalan, or a single dose of intraperitoneal Chromic Phosphate, a radioisotope. Five year disease-free survival was 80% for both groups. Overall survival for the two groups was approximately equal. The authors conclude that Chromic Phosphate is the preferred treatment, because of the risk of myelosuppression, gastrointestinal toxicity, and leukemias associated with Melphalan. Both Chromic Phospate and Melphalan toxicity have been observed by other investigators.[35]

Radiotherapy

There is a scarcity of randomized controlled trials of radiotherapy. Dembo and colleagues[36] postoperatively randomized patients with Stage I tumours to "watchful waiting" or pelvic irradiation. Relapse rates depended more on the degree of differentiation of the tumours than on treatment received.

Adverse Effects

The unfavourable effects of screening, (including patient anxiety due to false positive results, and the false sense of security occasioned by false negative results) have remained largely unquantified. In those with a family history of ovarian malignancy, the side effects of prolonged hormonal replacement therapy following prophylactic oopherectomy must also be considered.

Buchsbaum[37] reported a startling rate of adverse outcomes of surgical staging of ovarian carcinomas, including 74 complications in 154 patients and one postoperative death. Most other authors have noted far fewer adverse outcomes of diagnostic laparotomy.[38-40]

Diagnostic laparoscopy may offer a less invasive, and presumably less risky, alternative to laparotomy. However, primary endoscopic surgery is not generally accepted for routine management of suspected ovarian cancer, because of the fear of spreading malignant cells. Guidelines for the pelviscopic management of ovarian masses are currently under review.

Familial Ovarian Cancer

Routine screening has been widely advocated in this population, in which the greater prevalence of disease should markedly increase the positive predictive value of all detection measures. In a screening study in asymptomatic women with at least one first degree relative with ovarian cancer, the prevalence of ovarian cancers was 3.9 per 1,000. This is much higher than the 0.4 per 1,000 prevalence quoted for the general population. The false positive rate was also higher, however, because of the higher incidence of benign ovarian masses. The positive predictive value of ultrasonography under these circumstances was considerably higher than usual, at 7.7%.[4]

Based on such evidence, many researchers advocate combination screening in an academic centre for all women with one or more first-degree relative(s) with ovarian cancer. As tumours tend to develop at a younger age in this group, it has been suggested that such screening begin at age 30. In addition to screening, prophylactic oophorectomy is recommended, particularly where there is a history of hereditary ovarian cancer. Unfortunately, even this radical prophylaxis does not guarantee immunity from cancer, as rare case reports of postoperative disseminated intraabdominal carcinomatosis have been published.

Recommendations of Others

The U.S. Preventive Services Task Force concluded that screening of asymptomatic women for ovarian cancer is not recommended.[41] This group does indicate that it is "prudent" to examine the adnexa, if a pelvic examination is to be done for other reasons.

For pre- and post-menopausal women without a family history of ovarian cancer, the American College of Physicians (ACP) does not recommend screening (ultrasound or CA 125). For women with a family with hereditary ovarian cancer syndrome, ACP recommends referral for specialist care. ACP also recommends that for other women with a family history of ovarian cancer (in one or more relatives), decisions about screening be made based on other risk factors (age, parity and history of oral contraceptive pill use).

Conclusions and Recommendations

There is fair evidence in published clinical research to exclude screening for ovarian cancer, either by abdominal examination, pelvic or transvaginal sonography, or CA 125 levels, from the periodic health examination of asymptomatic pre- and post-menopausal women (D Recommendation). It would be reasonable to examine the adnexa if a pelvic examination were being done for another reason, such as cervical inspection or pap smear.

There is insufficient evidence to recommend for or against screening in individuals with one or more first-degree relatives with ovarian cancer (C Recommendation). However, in light of the significantly higher incidence of ovarian malignancy in such women, expert opinion currently suggests that they be referred to an academic research centre for regular combination screening with pelvic examination, ultrasonography, and determination of CA 125 levels. There is little evidence concerning the frequency of such screening.

Unanswered Questions (Research Agenda)

Well-designed clinical trials are needed to elucidate further the natural history of ovarian cancer, and to assess multimodal screening for ovarian cancer, to determine whether the combination of pelvic examination, tumour markers, and transvaginal sonography will lead to reduced mortality. Further assessment of the test characteristics for these screening maneuvers in well-defined populations, such as those with a familial risk of ovarian cancer, would also be of value. The cost-effectiveness of screening for ovarian cancer will depend on the determination of its effectiveness, if any.

Evidence

Articles assessing screening for ovarian malignancy were obtained by a computerized search (MEDLINE from 1975 onwards) using the MESH headings screening, ovarian neoplasms, and one of either ultrasonography, CA125 antigen, neoplasms-staging, surgery, chemotherapy, or radiotherapy. Only references in English were retrieved. Review articles, and those dealing with advanced stages of ovarian cancer or nonepithelial tumours (see below) were excluded. Content experts were consulted to ensure that all relevant research was analyzed. A Technical Report (1992) including a full reference list is available upon request. This review was initiated in January 1992 and recommendations finalized by the Task Force in January 1994.

Acknowledgements

The Task Force would like to acknowledge the assistance of J.L. Benedet, MD, FRCSC, Professor, Obstetrics and Gynecology, University of British Columbia, Vancouver, British Columbia, President of the Gynecologic Oncology Association of Canada and Head, Division of Gynecologic Oncology Cancer Control Agency of British Columbia; John F. Jeffrey, MD, FRCSC, Head, Division of Gynecologic Oncology, Victoria General Hospital, Halifax, Nova Scotia and Barry Rosen, MD, FRCSC, Assistant Professor, Department of Obstetrics and Gynecology/Oncology, University of Toronto, Toronto, Ontario, in the preparation of this manuscript.

Selected References

1. National Cancer Institute of Canada: *Canadian Cancer Statistics 1993*, Toronto, Canada, 1993: 14

2. Van-Nagell JR Jr, DePriest PD, Puls LE, *et al*: Ovarian cancer screening in asymptomatic post-menopausal women by transvaginal sonography. *Cancer* 1991; 68: 458-462

3. Sparks JM, Varner RE: Ovarian cancer screening. *Obstet Gynecol* 1991; 77: 787-792

4. Bourne TH, Whitehead MI, Campbell S, *et al*: Ultrasound Screening for familial ovarian cancer. *Gynecol Oncol* 1991; 43: 92-97

5. Creasman WT, DiSaia PJ: Screening in ovarian cancer. *Am J Obstet Gynecol* 1991; 165: 7-10

6. Koch M, Gaedke H, Jenkins H: Family history of ovarian cancer patients: a case-control study. *Int J Epidemiol* 1989; 18: 782-785

7. Ponder B, Easton D, Peto J: Risk of ovarian cancer associated with a family history: Preliminary report of the OPCS study. In: *Ovarian Cancer: Biological and therapeutic challenges.* London: Chapman and Hall Medical, 1990

8. The Cancer and Steroid Hormone Study of the Centers for Disease Control and the National Institute of Child Health and Human Development: The reduction in risk of ovarian cancer associated with oral contraceptive use. *N Engl J Med* 1987; 316: 650-655

9. ACOG Technical Bulletin Number 141- May 1990. Cancer of the Ovary. *Int J Gynecol Obstet* 1991; 35: 359-366

10. van Nagell JR Jr: Ovarian cancer screening. [Editorial] *Cancer* 1991; 68: 679-680

11. Andolf E, Jorgensen C: A prospective comparison of clinical ultrasound and operative examination of the female pelvis. *J Ultrasound Med* 1988; 617: 617-620

12. Goswamy RK, Campbell S, Whitehead MI: Screening for ovarian cancer. *Clin Obstet Gynaecol* 1983; 10: 621-643

13. Andolf E, Svalenius E, Astedt B: Ultrasonography for early detection of ovarian carcinoma. *Br J Obstet Gynaecol* 1986; 93: 1286-1289

14. Campbell S, Bhan V, Royston P, *et al*: Transabdominal ultrasound screening for early ovarian cancer. *BMJ* 1989; 299: 1363-1367

15. Campbell S, Royston P, Bhan V, *et al*: Novel screening strategies for early ovarian cancer by transabdominal ultrasonography. *Br J Obstet Gynaecol* 1990; 97: 304-311

16. van Nagell J, Higgins R, Donaldson E, *et al*: Transvaginal sonography as a screening method for ovarian cancer. A report of the first 1000 cases screened. *Cancer* 1990; 65: 573-577

17. Rodriguez MH, Platt LD, Medearis AL, *et al*: The use of transvaginal sonography for evaluation of post-menopausal ovarian size and morphology. *Am J Obstet Gynecol* 1988; 159: 810-814

18. Bourne T, Campbell S, Steer C, *et al*: Transvaginal colourflow imaging: a possible new screening technique for ovarian cancer. *BMJ* 1989; 299: 1367-1370

19. Tholander B, Taube A, Lindgren A, *et al*: Pretreatment serum levels of CA 125, carcinoembryonic antigen, tissue polypeptide antigen, and placental alkaline phosphatase, in patients with ovarian carcinoma, borderline tumours, or benign adnexal masses: relevance for differential diagnosis. *Gynecol Oncol* 1990; 39: 16-25

20. Kudlacek S, Schieder K, Kolbl H, *et al*: Use of CA 125 monoclonal antibody to monitor patients with ovarian cancer. *Gynecol Oncol* 1989; 35: 323-329

21. O'Connell GJ, Ryan E, Murphy KJ, *et al*: Predictive value of CA125 for ovarian carcinoma in patients presenting with pelvic masses. *Obstet Gynecol* 1987; 70: 930-932

22. Patsner B: Preoperative serum CA 125 levels in early stage ovarian cancer. *Eur J Gynaecol Oncol* 1990; 11: 319-321

23. Zurawski VR, Broderick SF, Pickens P, *et al*: Serum CA 125 levels in a group of nonhospitalized women: relevance for the early detection of ovarian cancer. *Obstet Gynecol* 1987; 69: 606-611

24. Zurawski VR, Knapp RC, Einhorn N, *et al*: An initial analysis of preoperative serum CA 125 levels in patients with early stage ovarian carcinoma. *Gynecol Oncol* 1988; 30: 7-14

25. Skates SJ, Singer DE: Quantifying the potential benefit of CA 125 screening for ovarian cancer. *J Clin Epidemiol* 1991; 44: 365-380

26. Chen DX, Schwartz PE, Li XG, *et al*: Evaluation of CA 125 levels in differentiating malignant from benign tumours in patients with pelvic masses. *Obstet Gynecol* 1988; 72: 23-27

27. Malkasian GD, Knapp RC, Lavin PT, *et al*: Preoperative evaluation of serum CA 125 levels in pre-menopausal and post-menopausal patients with pelvic masses: discrimination of benign from malignant disease. *Am J Obstet Gynecol* 1988; 159: 341-346

28. Zurawski VR, Orjaseter H, Andersen A, *et al*: Elevated serum CA 125 levels prior to diagnosis of ovarian neoplasia: relevance for early detection of ovarian cancer. *Int J Cancer* 1988; 42: 677-680

29. Zurawski VR, Sjovall K, Schoenfeld DA, *et al*: Prospective evaluation of serum CA 125 levels in a normal population, Phase I: the specificities of single and serial determinations in testing for ovarian cancer. *Gynecol Oncol* 1990; 36: 299-305

30. Finkler NJ, Benacerraf B, Lavin PT, *et al*: Comparison of serum CA 125, clinical impression, and ultrasound in the preoperative evaluation of ovarian masses. *Obstet Gynecol* 1988; 72: 659-664

31. Jacobs I, Stabile I, Bridges J, *et al*: Multimodal approach to screening for ovarian cancer. *Lancet* 1988; 1: 268-271

32. Trimbos JB, Schueler JA, van der Burg M, *et al*: Watch and wait after careful surgical treatment and staging in well-differentiated early ovarian cancer. *Cancer* 1991; 67: 597-602

33. Monga M, Carmichael JA, Shelley WE, *et al*: Surgery without adjuvant chemotherapy for early epithelial ovarian carcinoma after comprehensive surgical staging. *Gynecol Oncol* 1991; 43: 195-197

34. Young RC, Walton LA, Ellenberg SS, *et al*: Adjuvant therapy in stage I and stage II epithelial ovarian cancer. Results of two prospective randomized trials. *N Engl J Med* 1990; 322: 1021-1027

35. Klaassen D, Shelley W, Starreveld A, *et al*: Early stage ovarian cancer: a randomized clinical trial comparing whole abdominal radiotherapy, melphalan, and intraperitoneal chromic phosphate: a National Cancer Institute of Canada Clinical Trials Group report. *J Clin Oncol* 1988; 6: 1254-1263

36. Dembo A, Bush R, Beale F, *et al*: Radiotherapy in early stage ovarian cancer. *Cancer Treatment Reports* 1979; 63: 249-154

37. Buchsbaum HJ, Brady MF, Delgado G, *et al*: Surgical staging of carcinoma of the ovaries. *Surg Gynecol Obstet* 1989; 169: 226-232

38. Snider DD, Stuart GC, Nation JG: Evaluation of surgical staging in stage I low malignant potential ovarian tumours. *Gynecol Oncol* 1991; 40: 129-132

39. Lucas JA, Roberts WS, Kavanagh JJ, *et al*: Restaging laparotomy and ovarian cancer. *South Med J* 1988; 81: 584-587

40. van Lith JM, Bouma J, Aalders JG, *et al*: Role of an early second-look laparotomy in ovarian cancer. *Gynecol Oncol* 1989; 35: 255-258

41. U.S. Preventive Services Task Force: *Guide to Clinical Preventive Services: an Assessment of the Effectiveness of 169 Interventions*. Williams & Wilkins, Baltimore, Md, 1989: 81-85

Screening for Ovarian Cancer

MANEUVER	EFFECTIVENESS	LEVEL OF EVIDENCE <REF>	RECOMMENDATION
For Asymptomatic Pre- and Post-Menopausal Women			
Screening by pelvic exam, ultrasound, transvaginal sonography (TVS), serum tumour antigen (e.g CA 125) or combination	Poor positive predictive value for early detection of ovarian carcinoma. Effectiveness of screening unknown.	Case series<2,11-24,30,31> (III) and case-control studies (for CA 125 only) <26-29> (II-2)	Fair evidence to exclude screening for ovarian cancer by any means for pre- and post-menopausal women (D)
	Evidence of harm from diagnostic laparotomy.	Case series<37-40> (III)	
	Few well-controlled studies on treatment; better prognosis with early stage cancers.	Randomized controlled trials<34-36> (I) and case series<32,33> (III) for various therapies	
For High-risk Women with > 1 First-degree Relative with Ovarian Cancer			
Multimodal screening (pelvic exam, TVS, CA 125)*	Evidence of higher positive predictive value for detection because of higher prevalence in this group. Effectiveness of screening unknown.	Case series<4> (III)	Insufficient evidence to recommend for or against screening (C)

* The frequency of screening recommended by experts in this area is twice yearly. There is little evidence to support this.

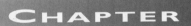

CHAPTER 73

Screening for Cervical Cancer

By Brenda J. Morrison

Screening for Cervical Cancer

Prepared by Brenda J. Morrison, PhD[1]

In 1979 the Canadian Task Force on the Periodic Health Examination found that there was fair justification for the view that the incidence and mortality of invasive cancer of the cervix could be reduced by taking cervical smears (B recommendation). The optimum age and frequency at which smears should be taken was not known but was identified as a research priority. This basic position has not changed but in 1991 the evidence was re-examined by the Task Force in response to the publication of the Report of a National Workshop on Screening for Cancer of the Cervix.<1>

Examining the ovaries at the time of cervical cancer screening should also be considered for women at high-risk of ovarian cancer (see Chapter 72).

Burden of Suffering

Cervical cancer is the eleventh most common cancer among women in Canada. In 1993, an estimated 1,300 women developed cervical cancer and about 400 died of the disease. In 1989, an estimated 10,000 potential years of life were lost due to cervical cancer. The major factors known to be associated with the occurrence of cervical cancer are age of first sexual intercourse, number of consorts, number of previous partners of consorts, smoking, low socio-economic status and possibly infections such as human papillomavirus. However, note that screening for human papilloma-virus (Chapter 63) is not recommended as part of cervical cancer screening. Rather the factors associated with the highest risk are having many sexual partners, a consort with many sexual partners and an early age of first intercourse. Most studies show that for each additional partner the risk appears to increase linearly by a factor ranging from 0.5 to 1, up to a relative risk of at least 9; for early age of first intercourse (before 17 or 18 years of age), the relative risk has been reported to range between 2 and 3.

Depending upon the stage at which the disease is detected, five-year survival rates range from 90% for stage 1 to 10-15% for stage 4, suggesting that any screening measure which permits earlier detection will improve survival.

---

[1] Associate Professor, Department of Health Care & Epidemiology, University of British Columbia, Vancouver, British Columbia

Maneuver

At present only one test is suitable for general population screening, the Papanicolaou smear test. False positive test results are not a major concern because a second smear can be taken and colposcopy done with minimal risk and relatively little expense; however some needless anxiety will be generated. False negative test results, on the other hand, allow the disease to escape detection until it reaches a less treatable stage. Even in well run laboratories estimates for false negative error rates run as high as 25%. The error can result from failure of the physician to obtain malignant cells from the cervix or failure of the laboratory process, including misinterpretation of the slide. Obtaining an adequate smear can be difficult since cytological abnormalities usually arise at the squamo-columnar junction and the site of this junction regresses up the cervical canal as a woman ages. As for laboratory error, the false negative rate appears to be lower in laboratories that process a large volume of smears.

Papanicolaou smear testing has a high false negative error rate

Effectiveness of Screening

Although the etiology of cancer of the cervix has been the subject of much debate and there are still uncertainties concerning the progression of dysplasia and carcinoma *in situ* to invasive cancer, there is evidence from both cohort and case-control studies that participation in cervical cytology screening programs reduces the incidence of invasive disease.[2-7] It has been estimated that somewhere between a quarter and one half of carcinoma *in situ* progresses; for dysplasia, the proportion is less. In the majority of cases progression appears to be slow. Models of screening frequency indicate that even a ten year smear interval would reduce the incidence of invasive cancer by about two-thirds. Because screening for this disease is so widespread, a more precise measurement of its benefit, as assessed by a randomized controlled trial, is not ethically possible.

In the majority of cases, progression of cervical cancer appears to be slow

Recommendations of Others

It is not our purpose to review the cohort and case-control evidence since this material has been presented in three major reports produced by the Canadian government during the last 15 years[2,8-9] dealing exclusively with cervical screening policy. The first, known as the Walton Report,[8] recommended that all women over the age of 18 who have had sexual intercourse should be screened and that, if the initial smear showed no atypia, a second smear be taken in a year's time to affirm that the first was not a false negative. If both these and later smears were normal, screening should be carried out every three years, until the age of 35 and every five years thereafter to age 60.

In 1982 the Walton report was revised<9> because of concerns that the sexual freedom resulting from improvements in contraceptive technology might have induced an "epidemic" of cervical cancer among younger women. The recommendation for women under thiry-five was changed to annual screening. Since that time, however, it has been concluded that for the majority of cases the progression of dysplasia and carcinoma *in situ* is slow. As a consequence the third report, *The National Workshop Report*, published in 1991, returned to the original recommendation of screening every three years and, in the interests of simplicity, suggested continuation of this frequency for women over 35. Another change was extension of the surveillance period to the age of 69, since most invasive disease occurs in post-menopausal women, many of whom have never had a smear or have had one taken infrequently. The report also dropped the recommendation for more frequent screening for high-risk women. The Workshop urged the establishment of organized cervical screening programs with a central laboratory in each province, based on the assumption that programs with centralized laboratories would be in place throughout the country.

In 1989, the U.S. Preventive Services Task Force recommended regular papanicolaou testing for all women who are or have been sexually active. Beginning with the onset of sexual activity, the test should be repeated every one to three years at the physicians discretion up to age 65 after which testing may be discontinued if previous smears have been consistently normal. This recommendation is currently under review.<10>

Frequency of Routine Screening

Since no controlled trials have been carried out, no well grounded scientific evidence exists on which to base recommendations for the optimum frequency of screening. The recommendations of the most recent National Workshop<1> are largely based on the report from the International Agency for Research on Cancer<11> which, in turn, was based on case-control studies and computer models constructed with parameters derived from cohort studies. However, Knox<12> has recently published an analysis showing that estimates of the relative protection of screening (and therapy) derived from such case-control and cohort studies are potentially invalid. The estimate depends on the true protective effect of the test and therapeutic procedures but is also determined by the ratio of the "uptake rate" of the screening procedure (or proportion being screened) in the case population and control population. If the uptake is unequal in the two groups, then the estimate may be biased. The greater the uptake of screening in the control group, relative to that for the cases, the greater the apparent protection. Many reports have documented that the women who are at highest risk of developing cervical cancer have infrequent or no smears. Therefore estimates of relative risk will be strongly confounded by the difference in uptake rates between the cases and controls.

Conclusions and Recommendations

In light of the foregoing considerations, it is difficult to formulate frequency recommendations that have solid scientific validity. On an observational basis all that can be said is that women who are presently being screened regularly have a very low rate of developing cervical cancer, whereas those who are being screened infrequently or not at all, have a much higher risk of developing the disease. In the British Columbia cohort study only 4% of cases of carcinomas *in situ* or worse were detected by smears subsequent to a third smear.[2]

There is fair evidence to include Papanicolaou smears in the periodic health examination of women who have been sexually active (B Recommendation). The Task Force concurs with the Workshop's recommendations concerning frequency of smears once central laboratories are operational. Until such time, it recommends that high-risk women be screened more frequently than every 3 years since the false negative rate may run well above 25%, and the disease progression rate is known to vary. Physicians should keep in mind, however, that these high-risk women constitute a small proportion of the population.

Because some social stigma may be attached to being labelled as being at high risk, individual physicians should consider informing a patient of the risk factors and allowing her to make the decision on the appropriate frequency of screening.

The Task Force emphasizes that the largest group of women at greatest risk of dying from cervical cancer are those who have never been screened. The majority of these are women over 50, particularly native women and women who have immigrated from poorer countries. It is more important that these women be screened, even if only once, than that average or low-risk women be screened frequently.

Unanswered Questions (Research Agenda)

Research into methodologies to reach women who have never been screened is critical. In future, most women reaching middle-age will have had many cervical smears and may therefore be at a different risk than the average middle-aged or older woman is at present. Most will have had nothing but negative smears. It is important to determine if, in well tested women, a history of numerous negative smears is associated with a substantially reduced risk.

Evidence

The evidence used in this review was taken from the collection of the author. This review was initiated in June 1989 and the recommendations were finalized by the Task Force in January, 1992. A technical report with a full reference list dated February 1992 is available upon request.

Selected References

1. Miller AB, Anderson G, Brisson J, *et al*: Report of a national workshop on screening for cancer of the cervix. *Can Med Assoc J* 1991; 145: 1301-1325

2. Boyes DA, Morrison B, Knox EG, *et al*: A cohort study of cervical cancer screening in British Columbia. *Clin Invest Med* 1982; 5: 1-29

3. Hakama M: Effect of population screening for carcinoma of the uterine cervix in Finland. *Maturitas* 1985; 7: 3-10

4. Lynge E, Poll P: Incidence of cervical cancer following negative smear. A cohort study from Maribo County, Denmark. *Am J Epidemiol* 1986; 124: 345-352

5. Clarke EA, Anderson TW: Does screening by "Pap" smears help prevent cervical cancer? *Lancet* 1979; 2(8132): 1-4

6. Stenkvist B, Bergstrom R, Eklund G, *et al*: Papanicolaou smear screening and cervical cancer. What can you expect? *JAMA* 1984; 252: 1423-1426

7. van der Graaf Y, Zielhuis GA, Peer PGM, *et al*: The effectiveness of cervical screening: a population-based case-control study. *J Clin Epidemiol* 1988; 41: 21-26

8. Task Force on Cervical Cancer Screening Programs: Cervical cancer screening programs. [The Walton Report] *Can Med Assoc J* 1976; 114: 1003-1033

9. Task Force convened by the Department of National Health and Welfare. Cervical cancer screening programs: summary of the 1982 Canadian task force report. *Can Med Assoc J* 1982; 127: 581-589

10. U.S. Preventive Services Task Force: *Guide to Clinical Preventive Services: an Assessment of the Effectiveness of 169 Interventions*. Williams & Wilkins, Baltimore, Md, 1989: 57-62

11. IARC Working Group on Evaluation of Cervical Cancer Screening Programmes: Screening for squamous cervical cancer: duration of low risk after negative results of cervical cytology and its implications for screening policies. *Br Med J* 1986; 293(6548): 659-664

12. Knox G: Case-control studies of screening procedures. *Public Health* 1991; 105: 55-61

Screening for Cervical Cancer

MANEUVER	EFFECTIVENESS	LEVEL OF EVIDENCE <REF>	RECOMMENDATION
Papanicolaou smear*	Cervical smears reduce the risk of developing invasive carcinoma of the cervix in women who have been sexually active.	Cohort and case-control studies<2-7> (II-2)	Fair evidence to include in PHE of sexually active women (B)

*   Annual screening is recommended following initiation of sexual activity or age 18; after 2 normal smears, screen every 3 years to age 69. Consider increasing frequency for women with risk factors: age of first sexual intercourse < 18 yrs, many sexual partners or consort with many partners, smoking or low socioeconomic status.

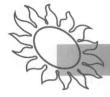

CHAPTER 74

Screening for Testicular Cancer

By R. Wayne Elford

Screening for Testicular Cancer

Adapted to the Canadian context by R. Wayne Elford, MD, CCFP, FCFP,[1] from the report prepared for the U.S. Preventive Services Task Force[2]

In 1984, the Canadian Task Force on the Periodic Health Examination recommended that screening should be performed only on patients with a history of cryptorchidism, testicular atrophy or ambiguous genitalia.<1> In our current review we find insufficient evidence to include or exclude routine screening for testicular cancer in the general population (C Recommendation).

Burden of Suffering

Testicular cancer is a relatively uncommon disease. The lifetime probability of developing the condition is 0.30% and of dying from it 0.03%. Testicular cancer represents 1.1 percent of cancers among men. Rates peaked in the age group 30 to 39 in the 1970s. By the 1980s the peak had shifted downward to the age group 25 to 34 years, where almost half the cases now occur. Testicular cancer is the most common cancer in men aged 15 to 34 years, and the incidence has been rising only in this age group. This age-specific trend has been observed in all regions of Canada, although the rates remain lowest in Quebec and the Atlantic region. Rates in the Prairies have been the most stable. Increasing rates have been observed in other countries but remain unexplained.<2> The major predisposing risk factor is cryptorchidism which increases the risk 2.5 to 40 times.<3> 80-85% of these tumors occur in the cryptorchid testicle while 15-20% occur in the contralateral testicle. Other risk factors include previous cancer in the contralateral testicle, a history of mumps orchitis, inguinal hernia or hydrocele in childhood, and high socioeconomic status.<3>

Ninety-six percent of testicular cancers are of germ cell origin of which seminoma is the most common type. Prognosis and treatment depend on the cell type and stage of disease, however recent advances in treatment have resulted in a 92% overall five-year survival.<4> Even in studies of advanced cases cure rates of 85% are now being reported.

Maneuver

Two modalities proposed as screening tests for testicular cancer are physician palpation of the testes and self-examination of the testes by the patient. Detection of a suspicious testicular mass constitutes a

---

[1] Professor and Director of Research and Faculty Development, Department of Family Medicine, University of Calgary, Calgary, Alberta
[2] By Paul S. Frame, MD, Tri-County Family Medicine, Cohocton, New York

positive test, and the diagnosis is confirmed by biopsy and histologic examination. There is no information on the sensitivity, specificity or positive predictive value of testicular examination in asymptomatic persons, whether done by physicians or by patients.

Due to the low incidence of the disease and the high cure rate, measures of sensitivity and specificity of these examinations, even if they were known, might not be very meaningful. If sensitivity is defined as the ability to detect disease at a curable stage, sensitivity is probably high since the overall cure rate is 92%. The negative predictive value is probably also quite good due to the low incidence of the disease. The positive predictive value, however, of palpation of the testes is probably very low due to the low incidence of disease and large number of other causes of scrotal masses. There is evidence, from older literature, that between 26% and 56% of patients presenting initially to their physician with testicular cancer are first diagnosed as having epididymitis, testicular trauma, hydrocele, or other benign disorders,<5> and they often receive treatment for these conditions before the cancer is diagnosed.<6>

There have been few studies of whether counselling men to perform self-examination motivates them to adopt this practice or to perform it correctly. Research to date has demonstrated only that education about testicular cancer and self-examination may enhance knowledge and self-reported claims of performing testicular examination.<7> One study found that men who reviewed an educational checklist on how to perform self-examination were able to demonstrate greater skill when self-examination was performed moments later, and they were able to recall the contents of the checklist in a telephone survey months later.<8> Few studies, however, have examined whether education or self-examination instructions actually increase the performance of self-examination. It is also unclear whether persons who detect testicular abnormalities seek medical attention promptly. Patients with testicular symptoms may wait as long as several months before contacting a physician.<9> Finally, no studies have shown that persons who perform testicular self-examination are more likely to detect early-stage tumors or have improved survival than those who do not practice self-examination.<10> Published evidence that self-examination can detect testicular cancer in asymptomatic persons is limited to a small number of anecdotal reports.

Tumor markers, including alpha-fetoprotein and human chorionic gonadotropin are useful in following non-seminomatous testicular cancers but are not useful for early detection or screening.<3>

Published evidence that self-examination can detect testicular cancer in asymptomatic persons is limited to a small number of anecdotal reports

Effectiveness of Early Detection and Treatment

Cisplatin-based chemotherapy regimes have dramatically improved the 3-5 year survival rates to greater than 90%

The prognosis for advanced stages of testicular cancer has improved dramatically in the past decade with the introduction of better chemotherapy. Current cure rates are over 80%.<10,11> However, the outcome of treatment is still better for patients with Stage I cancer than for those with more advanced disease and the treatment of early cancer has less cost and morbidity. Treatment for all types and stages of testicular cancer includes removal of the involved testicle. The current five-year survival for Stage I seminoma treated with radiotherapy is 97%.<4> Stage I nonseminomatous cancers (e.g., teratomas, embryonal carcinoma, choriocarcinoma) treated with radical retroperitoneal lymph node dissection have a reported 3- to 5-year survival approaching 90%.<12> With the advent of cisplatin-based chemotherapeutic regimens, a 3-year survival of 90-100% has been reported. Reported survival in patients with disseminated testicular cancer, however, is lower (about 67-80%), and these persons require intensive treatment with chemotherapeutic agents that produce a variety of systemic side effects.<4,11>

Although lead-time and length-time biases may account for part of the improved survival observed for persons with early-stage testicular cancer, it is likely that the prognosis is, in fact, better for persons with less advanced disease. There is, however, no evidence that screening causes more cancers to be diagnosed when Stage I, or improves outcome. Even without screening, 60-80% of seminomas are diagnosed in Stage I.<12> There is evidence that once testicular symptoms have appeared, diagnostic delays are associated with more advanced disease and lower survival.<5,9,13>

The appropriate management and follow-up of patients with a history of an undescended testicle is controversial.<14,15> It is known that orchiopexy at puberty does not prevent malignant transformation. It is uncertain whether earlier orchiopexy (prior to school age), which is now common practice, will prevent development of testicular cancer.<14> One study found carcinoma *in situ* in 1.7% of men with a history of cryptorchidism who had testicular biopsies. They projected that 50% of these lesions would progress to invasive cancer and recommended testicular biopsy be offered all men with a history of cryptorchidism.<15> Many experts recommend that intra-abdominal testes should be removed.<3> The survival for patients with a history of cryptorchidism who develop testicular cancer is excellent as it is in non-cryptorchid patients. No studies have been done to evaluate outcome benefits of formal screening of men with a history of cryptorchidism.

Discussion

There is no direct experimental evidence on which to base a recommendation for or against screening for testicular cancer by either physician examination or patient self-examination since no studies of screening have been done. One can calculate, however, that it is highly unlikely screening would significantly improve the already good outcome in this uncommon disease. If a population of 100,000 men aged between 15-35 years were screened with a 100% sensitive test, at most 10 cancers would be detected. At least 9 of these would be expected to be cured in the absence of a formal screening program. It is unknown whether the tenth patient would also be cured as a result of the cancer being detected by screening. A primary care physician with 1,500 males in his/her practice could expect to detect one testicular cancer every 15-20 years.

The vast majority of men screened by either physician or self-palpation would have normal examinations; of those with suspicious masses, most would have benign disease (false positives). Many of these cases, however, would require referral to urologists, radiographic studies, or invasive procedures (e.g., orchiectomy, inguinal exploration) before malignancy could be ruled out.[14] These interventions would incur considerable costs and possible morbidity.

Men with a history of undescended testes have a much greater incidence of testicular cancer. Although screening in this population has also not been shown to improve outcome it would be expected to have a much higher yield.

Recommendations of Others

In 1989, the U.S. Preventive Services Task Force found that there was insufficient evidence of clinical benefit or harm to recommend for or against routine screening of asymptomatic men for testicular cancer but that clinicians should advise adolescent and young adult males to seek prompt medical attention for testicular symptoms such as pain, swelling, or heaviness.[16] This recommendation is currently under review.

The American Cancer Society[17] and the National Cancer Institute[18] recommend that testicular examination be included as part of the periodic health examination of men. Recommendations differ on whether patients should be counselled to perform testicular self-examination. The American Cancer Society[19] and the National Cancer Institute[20] recommend that all postpubertal males should perform monthly testicular self-examination. Physicians have been advised to instruct male patients on how to perform this examination and some authorities believe the techniques should be reviewed at every periodic health visit beginning with puberty and continuing throughout life.[21] Others, citing the lack of evidence that self-

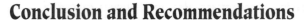

examination is effective, have advised physicians against routinely devoting time to discussing testicular self-examination.<10,22>

Conclusion and Recommendations

Selected populations (cryptorchidism, testicular atrophy, ambiguous genitalia) should be informed of their increased risk for testicular cancer

Because no studies of screening for testicular cancer by physician or patient self-examination have been reported, there is insufficient evidence to include or exclude screening for this cancer in the periodic health examination of men (C Recommendation). Based on the low incidence of disease and the current high cure rate it is unlikely formal screening would improve the already excellent prognosis. Patients with a history of cryptorchidism, orchiopexy, or testicular atrophy should be informed of their increased risk for developing testicular cancer and counselled about screening options. The optimal frequency of such examinations has not been determined and is left to clinical discretion. Clinicians should advise adolescent and young adult males to seek prompt medical attention if a testicular mass is noted.

Evidence

A MEDLINE search was conducted using the main heading of testicular cancer with subheadings of prevention, screening and epidemiology from 1986 to 1992. This review was initiated by the Task Force in November 1993 and the recommendations finalized in January 1994.

Selected References

1. Canadian Task Force on the Periodic Health Examination: The periodic health examination: 2. 1984 update. *Can Med Assoc J* 1984; 130: 1278-1285

2. Canadian Council of Cancer Registries: *The Making of the Canadian Cancer Registry: Cancer Incidence in Canada and its regions, 1969 to 1988.* Health and Welfare Canada, Statistics Canada, 1993: 55

3. Vogt HB, McHale MS: Testicular cancer. Role of primary care physicians in screening and education. *Postgrad Med* 1992; 92: 93-101

4. Boring CC, Squires TS, Tong T: Cancer statistics, 1993. *Cancer J Clin* 1993; 43: 7-26

5. Bosl GJ, Vogelzang NJ, Goldman A, *et al*: Impact of delay in diagnosis on clinical stage of testicular cancer. *Lancet* 1981; 2: 970-973

6. Prout GR, Griffin PP: Testicular tumors: delay in diagnosis and influence on survival. *Am Fam Physician* 1984; 29: 205-209

7. Marty PJ, McDermott RJ: Three strategies for encouraging testicular self-examination among college-aged males. *J Am Coll Health* 1986; 34: 253-258

8. Ostwald SK, Rothenberger J: Development of a testicular self-examination program for college men. *J Am Coll Health* 1985; 33: 234-239

9. Garnick MB: Testicular cancer. *Sem Surg Oncol* 1989; 5: 221-226

10. Westlake SJ, Frank JW: Testicular self-examination: an argument against routine teaching. *Fam Pract* 1987; 4: 143-148

11. Rowland RG: Serum markers in testicular germ-cell neoplasms. *Hematol Oncol Clin North Amer* 1988; 2: 485-489

12. Williams SD, Birch R, Einhorn LH, *et al*: Treatment of disseminated germ-cell tumors with cisplatin, bleomycin, and either vinblastine or etopside. *N Eng J Med* 1987; 316: 1435-1440

13. Fung CY, Garnick MB: Clinical stage I carcinoma of the testis: a review. *J Clin Oncol* 1988; 6: 734-750

14. Post GJ, Belis JA: Delayed presentation of testicular tumors. *South Med J* 1980; 73: 33-35

15. Giwercman A, Bruun E, Frimodt-Moller C, *et al*: Prevalence of carcinoma in situ and other histopathological abnormalities in testes of men with a history of cryptorchidism. *J Urol* 1989; 142: 998-1002

16. U.S. Preventive Services Task Force: *Guide to Clinical Prevention Services: an Assessment of the Effectiveness of 169 Interventions.* Williams & Wilkins, Baltimore, Md, 1989: 77-80

17. American Cancer Society: *Guidelines for the cancer-related checkup: recommendations and rationale.* American Cancer Society, New York, 1980

18. National Cancer Institute: *Working guidelines for early cancer detection: rationale and supporting evidence to decrease mortality.* National Cancer Institute, Bethesda, Md, 1987

19. American Cancer Society: *For men only – testicular cancer and how to do testicular self examination.* American Cancer Society, New York, 1984

20. National Cancer Institute: *Testicular self-examination.* Government Printing Office, Washington, D.C., 1986 [Publication no. DHHS (NIH) 87-2636]

21. Frame PS: A critical review of adult health maintenance. Part 3. Prevention of cancer. *J Fam Pract* 1986; 22: 511-520

22. Goldbloom RB: Self-examination by adolescents. *Pediatrics* 1985; 76: 126-128

Screening for Testicular Cancer

MANEUVER	EFFECTIVENESS	LEVEL OF EVIDENCE <REF>	RECOMMENDATION
Routine examination of testes either by physician or by patient self-examination	**General Population** No studies of screening for testicular cancer have been performed.	Expert opinion<20> (III)	Insufficient evidence to include or exclude from the periodic examination (C)
	Selected Population * Inform of increased risk and educate regarding screening options.	Expert Opinion<20> (III)	Insufficient evidence to include or exclude but it may be prudent to follow high-risk individuals with regular physician examinations (C)
Tumor markers such as alpha fetoprotein or chorionic gonadotropin	Useful in monitoring non-seminomatous cancer (infrequent type of testicular cancer).	Expert opinion <9,10> (III)	There is fair evidence to exclude from periodic health examination (D)

*   Selected populations - cryptorchidism, testicular atrophy, ambiguous genitalia

Conditions Affecting Primarily the Elderly

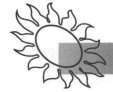

CHAPTER **75**

Screening for Cognitive Impairment in the Elderly

By Christopher Patterson

Screening for Cognitive Impairment in the Elderly

Prepared by Christopher Patterson, MD, FRCPC[1]

Cognitive impairment is a common finding in older people, as the prevalence of dementia increases with age. The most common cause of dementia is Alzheimer's disease, a slowly progressive primary dementing disorder. Intercurrent illnesses, infections, metabolic disturbances and drug intoxications may all cause or exacerbate mental confusion. Depression may worsen and occasionally mimic dementia. Identification of dementia in the early stages offers the potential to plan to deal with subsequent deterioration, organize community supports, and anticipate later incompetence, by measures such as advance directives and power of attorney. A large number of drugs have been studied for their effect on improving the cognitive and behavioural aspects of Alzheimer's disease. While beneficial effects on cognitive performance have been documented, these are rarely of sufficient magnitude to be of clinical importance. The potential harm of labelling an individual as demented must be weighed against possible benefits. There is insufficient evidence to recommend for or against measures to detect asymptomatic cognitive impairment. The prudent physician is advised to remain alert for clues that suggest deteriorating cognitive function, and then to pursue an appropriate diagnostic course of action.

Burden of Suffering

Prevalence of dementia is less than 5% below 75 years of age, but above 40% over age 80 years

Prevalence studies in Europe, the United States and Canada reveal relatively consistent findings. While methods of ascertainment vary from study to study, the prevalence of severe dementia in people aged 65 and over residing in the community is between 2.5 and 5%.<1-3> For mild degrees of dementia the prevalence is age-dependent, with rates less than 5% below 75 years, to 40% or higher above the age of 80.<4> The incidence has been estimated at 1% in persons over 65 and up to 2.5% in those over the age of 80. Projected figures for Canada are 225,000 new cases of dementia per year.<3> In addition to the cognitive deficits produced by dementia, behavioural abnormalities are common. These frequently lead to excessive caregiver stress, and may precipitate hospital or institutional admission. Behaviours such as restlessness, wandering, aggression, failure to

---

[1] Professor and Head, Division of Geriatric Medicine, McMaster University, Hamilton, Ontario

recognize relatives and locations, and inappropriate sexual behaviour are particularly troublesome. The presentation of physical disease may be altered or obscured. People with dementia have reduced survival.

Maneuver

Dementia is readily recognizable in its advanced stages. In the early stages it often goes undetected. Conventional medical histories and examinations frequently fail to identify cognitive impairment or to distinguish it from hearing impairment, depression, aphasia, bradykinesia, etc. Criteria have been established for the diagnosis of dementia.[5,6] While the "complete mental state" examination is well described in standard texts, attempts have been made to develop short mental status questionnaires to screen for cognitive impairment. The Mini Mental State examination (MMS)[7] is the most frequently used and has the most clearly defined test characteristics. Others include the Short Portable Mental Status Questionnaire (SPMSQ)[8] and the Clock Drawing test.[9] The MMS requires no special equipment and can be completed within 5-10 minutes. Little training is required, and a standardized version has been developed.[10] The sensitivity of this instrument to detect moderate dementia approaches 90% with a cut-off point of 24 out of 30. Corresponding specificity is about 80%. The test is valid and reproducible, particularly in its standardized form.[10] The SPMSQ has had similar sensitivity in published series,[11] but has been less well studied. It is a less comprehensive instrument than the MMS, as it examines principally orientation and memory, and does not cover areas of language or motor tasks. The clock drawing test, originally developed for examination of parietal lobe function, is an extremely quick test. Despite its simplicity, it offers excellent sensitivity (92%) and specificity (97%) for the detection of moderate to severe dementia.[12]

An alternative approach to the use of mental status questionnaires is screening using Instrumental Activities of Daily Living (IADL). Sixty-nine percent of a random sample of 2,792 community dwellers aged 65 years and over were subjected to a two-phase screening procedure. The first phase included a functional assessment using an IADL scale and the MMS. Subjects who fulfilled Diagnostic and Statistical Manual of Mental Disorders criteria for dementia, were evaluated by a neurologist using National Institute of Neurological Diseases and Stroke – Alzheimer Disease and Related Disease Association criteria for dementia. The prevalence of dementia in this sample was 2.4%. Subjects experiencing difficulty in telephone use, use of public transportation, responsibility for medication use and handling finances had a 12 times greater probability of being diagnosed with dementia.[13] The MMS score is correlated with the ability to perform daily activities in cognitively impaired individuals.[14]

When an older person is discovered to have cognitive impairment a search is usually made for illnesses causing cognitive impairment which may be modifiable, in the hope that the condition will be improved or reversed. Although earlier literature suggested that up to one third of cases of apparent dementia were caused by illnesses whose treatment could lead to improvement, a recent overview analysis of the subject concluded that only 11% of dementing illnesses in older people resolved during follow-up (8% partially, 3% completely). The most common underlying remediable factors were drug intoxication, depression and metabolic abnormalities.[15] Two recent large community studies have been carried out to examine the results of screening and subsequent investigations. In a three-phase study in Eastern Baltimore, Md, 78% of 3,481 subjects completed the National Institute of Mental Health Interview Survey questionnaire together with a version of the MMS. Eighty percent of a random sample of these subjects (n=1,806) were examined by psychiatrists. Thirty-six of the 44 diagnosed by a psychiatrist as having definite or probable dementia were subjected to full neurological investigations. The prevalence of dementia was 6.1% in this population and no cases of reversible dementia were found.[16] In a second large community study from East Boston, 3,624 subjects over the age of 65 were examined with a screening procedure based on detection of immediate and delayed memory. Four hundred and seventy-two who appeared to have cognitive impairment were identified. Of these, 83.5% were found to have a clinical diagnosis of probable Alzheimer's disease.[4] The vast majority of older community subjects discovered by screening to have cognitive impairment are suffering from Alzheimer's disease and do not have a correctable or even potentially correctable dementing illness. While there are theoretical reasons to identify people with dementia for early treatment, early intervention has not been shown to modify the course of the illness. Theoretically, in those who have vascular dementia, correction of risk factors (e.g. treatment of hypertension, or anticoagulation for atrial fibrillation) could delay the progress of dementia. A wide variety of agents have been tested in Alzheimer's disease. Drugs presently showing most promise increase the central levels of acetyl choline. Tacrine (tetrahydroaminoacridine), has been approved for use in the United States and is available in Canada. Modest but definite improvements in cognitive performance have been documented in some[17-19] but not all[20,21] studies. Drugs which promote enhanced cerebral metabolism have also shown some benefit, although drugs such as Hydergine have largely been abandoned in the face of recent studies which have shown no significant effect.[22] Chelation therapy with desferrioxamine has shown some promise and may delay disability in Alzheimer's disease.[23] There are no published trials examining the effects of treatment on subjects who have been discovered by community screening to suffer from cognitive impairment.

One potential benefit of early identification is the ability to plan for the anticipated further cognitive decline. For example, the assignment of a sustaining power of attorney can be made at a time before mental incompetence occurs, obviating more complex maneuvers to handle an individual's estate at a later date. The ability to discuss advance directives with an individual is another potential benefit. Planning and consideration of timely relocation to a more protected environment may also be beneficial and early involvement with caregiver support groups may assist individuals in dealing with ultimate disability. None of these theoretical advantages has been subjected to appropriate study.

Potential negative consequences of early identification of cognitive impairment clearly exist. Labelling an individual as demented may affect his or her ability to obtain life or health insurance, and may influence attitudes towards the individual by health care professionals and others. The label of Alzheimer's disease may cause prejudice and difficulty in gaining admission to some long-term facilities. The negative effects of labelling an older person as demented have not been studied systematically, although a small body of social science literature explores this important area.[24] Negative attitudes have been identified among professionals and lay people.

A label of dementia provokes negative attitudes among professionals and lay people

Recommendations of Others

The U.S. Preventive Services Task Force recommended against screening for cognitive impairment in 1989.[25]

Conclusions and Recommendations

Despite the theoretical advantages of identifying individuals with cognitive impairment, there is no evidence to indicate whether this leads to a net benefit or risk to the individual. Although pharmaceutical agents are able to produce measurable changes in cognitive performance in people with Alzheimer's disease, none has been shown to result consistently in clinically significant improvement. The high cost of investigation to exclude reversible causes of dementia, and the negative effects of labelling are examples of potential harm. Identification of asymptomatic cognitively impaired individuals by the use of short mental status tests or by any other means has not been demonstrated to produce benefit. Thus there is insufficient evidence to recommend for or against screening (C Recommendation). The prudent physician should be alert for any reports or behaviour which may indicate cognitive impairment (e.g. forgetting appointments, poor medication compliance), and then pursue appropriate strategies for further investigation and treatment.[26]

Caregivers should be alert for reports or signs of behaviour that signal the need to investigate for dementia

Unanswered Questions (Research Agenda)

1. Although two of the brief mental status instruments reviewed appear satisfactory for case finding in primary care, they are not ideal, and more sensitive and specific instruments are desirable.

2. The search for effective treatments for Alzheimer's disease should incorporate outcome measures including physical functioning, behaviour measures of caregiver burden and ability to delay or prevent institutional care.

3. Trials of screening are necessary to examine the impact of detecting cognitive impairment, its subsequent investigation and treatment.

4. Studies should be directed towards discovering any negative effects from attaching the label of Alzheimer's disease or cognitive impairment to a person.

Evidence

Subsequent to the background paper prepared in 1988, search of the recent literature (1988-Dec 1993) was carried out using the following terms: mass screening (MH), geriatric assessment (MH), cognition disorders (MH). This review was initiated in October 1993 and updates a report published in 1991.<27> Recommendations were finalized by the Task Force in January 1994.

Selected References

1. Broe GA, Akhtar AJ, Andrews GR, *et al*: Neurological disorders in the elderly at home. *J Neurol Neurosurg Psychiatry* 1976; 39: 361-366

2. Weissman MM, Myers JK, Tischler GL, *et al*: Psychiatric disorders (DSM-III) and cognitive impairment in the elderly in a U.S. urban community. *Acta Psychiatr Scand* 1985; 71: 366-379

3. Canadian Study for Health and Aging (CSHA) Unpublished results. Ottawa, 1992

4. Evans DA, Funkenstein HH, Albert MS, *et al*: Prevalence of Alzheimer's disease in a community population of older persons. *JAMA* 1989; 262: 2551-2556

5. American Psychiatric Association: *Diagnostic and statistical manual of mental disorders*. (3rd Edition) (DSM-III), Washington, D.C. 1980

6. McKhann G, Drachman D, Folstein M, *et al*: Clinical diagnosis of Alzheimer's disease: Report of the NINCDS-ADRDA Work Group under the auspices of Department of Health and Human Services Task Force on Alzheimer's Disease. *Neurology* 1984; 34: 939-944

7. Folstein MF, Folstein SE, McHugh PR: "Mini-Mental-State": A practical method for grading the cognitive state of patients for the clinician. *J Psychiatr Res* 1975; 12: 189-198

8. Pfeiffer E: A short portable mental status questionnaire for the assessment of organic brain deficits in the elderly. *J Am Geriatr Soc* 1975; 23: 433-441

9. Shulman K, Shedletsky R, Silver IL: The challenge of time: clock drawing and cognitive functioning in the elderly. *Int J Geriatr Psychiatry* 1986; 1: 135-140

10. Molloy DW, Alemayehu E, Roberts R: Reliability of a Standardized Mini-Mental State Examination compared with the traditional Mini-Mental State Examination. *Am J Psychiatry* 1991; 148: 102-105

11. Erkinjuntti T, Sulkava R, Wikstrom J, *et al*: Short portable mental status questionnaire as a screening test for dementia and delirium among the elderly. *J Amer Geriatr Soc* 1987; 35: 412-416

12. Tuokko H, Hadjistavropoulos T, Miller JA, *et al*: The Clock Test: a sensitive measure to differentiate normal elderly from those with Alzheimer Disease. *J Am Geriatr Soc* 1992; 40: 579-584

13. Barberger-Gateau P, Commenges D, Gagnon M, *et al*: Instrumental activities of daily living as a screening tool for cognitive impairment and dementia in elderly community dwellers. *J Am Geriatr Soc* 1992; 40: 1129-1134

14. Warren EJ, Grek A, Conn D, *et al*: A correlation between cognitive performance and daily functioning in elderly people. *J Geriatr Psychiatry Neurol* 1989; 2: 96-100

15. Clarfield AM: The reversible dementias, do they reverse? *Ann Intern Med* 1988; 109: 476-486

16. Folstein MF, Anthony JC, Parhad I, *et al*: The meaning of cognitive impairment in the elderly. *J Am Geriatr Soc* 1985; 33: 228-235

17. Summers WK, Majovski LV, Marsh GM, *et al*: Oral tetrahydroaminoacridine in long-term treatment of senile dementia, Alzheimer type. *N Eng J Med* 1986; 315: 1241-1245

18. Davis KL, Thal LJ, Gamzu ER, *et al*: A double-blind placebo-controlled multicentre study of tacrine for Alzheimer's disease: The Tacrine Collaborative Study Group. *N Eng J Med* 1992; 327: 1253-1259

19. Farlow M, Gracon SI, Hershey LA, *et al*: A controlled trial of tacrine in Alzheimer's disease. *JAMA* 1992; 268: 2523-2529

20. Gauthier S, Bouchar R, Lamontagne A, *et al*: Tetrahydroaminoacridine – Lethicin combination treatment in patients with intermediate stage Alzheimer's disease: results of a Canadian double-blind crossover, multicentre study. *N Eng J Med* 1990; 322: 1272-1276

21. Molloy DW, Guyatt GH, Wilson DB, *et al*: Effect of tetrahydroaminoacridine on cognition, function and behaviour in Alzheimer's disease. *Can Med Assoc J* 1991; 144: 29-34

22. Thompson TL, Filley CM, Mitchell WD, *et al*: Lack of efficacy of hydergine in patients with Alzheimer's disease. *N Eng J Med* 1990; 323: 445-448

23. Crapper McLaughlan DR, Dalton AJ, Kruck TP, *et al*: Intramuscular desferrioxamine in patients with Alzheimer's disease. *Lancet* 1991; 337: 1304-1308

24. Lasoski MC, Thelen MH: Attitudes of older and middle-aged persons towards mental health intervention. *Gerontologist* 1987; 27: 288-292

25. U.S. Preventive Services Task Force: *Guide to Clinical Preventive Services: an Assessment of the Effectiveness of 169 Interventions.* Williams & Wilkins, Baltimore, Md, 1989: 251-255

26. Clarfield AM, Bass MJ, Cohen C, *et al*: Assessing dementia: The Canadian Consensus. *Can Med Assoc J* 1991; 144: 851-853

27. Canadian Task Force on the Periodic Health Examination: The periodic health examination, 1991 update: 1. Screening for cognitive impairment in the elderly. *Can Med Assoc J* 1991; 144: 425-431

Screening for Cognitive Impairment in the Elderly

MANEUVER	EFFECTIVENESS	LEVEL OF EVIDENCE <REF>	RECOMMENDATION
Screening with short mental status instruments	The Mini Mental State examination (MMS), Short Portable Mental Status Questionnaire (SPMSQ) and clock-drawing test have high sensitivity and specificity for detection of cognitive impairment but early intervention has not been shown to modify the course of illness.	Cohort analytic studies<4,16> (II-2); case series <10-12> (III)	Insufficient evidence to recommend for or against screening (C); the prudent physician should be alert for any symptoms which suggest cognitive impairment and conduct appropriate assessment
	Potential harm of labelling individuals as demented has not been systematically studied but must be weighed against possible benefits.	Expert opinion<24> (III)	

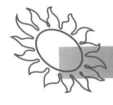

Prevention of Household and Recreational Injuries in the Elderly

By R. Wayne Elford

Prevention of Household and Recreational Injuries in the Elderly

Prepared by R. Wayne Elford, MD, CCFP, FCFP[1]

In the 1979 Canadian Task Force report, home and recreational injuries were acknowledged to constitute an important proportion of accidents.[2] The report emphasized the particular risk for the elderly.<1> At that time there was insufficient literature on the subject to justify a recommendation on scientific grounds. This lack of evidence persists for most areas of injury prevention among the elderly. New evidence has emerged, however, supporting multi-disciplinary post-fall assessment where this service is available. Accidental injury and death caused by motor vehicle accidents (46.5% of all deaths due to accidents) is covered in a separate chapter (Chapter 44).

Burden of Suffering

The seven leading causes of unintentional death in Canada are falls (21%), drowning (6.4%), burns, fire-related injuries (4.8%), suffocation (4.7%), poisonings (4.7%), bicycle and sports-related injuries (1.7%), and firearms (0.7%).<2> Injuries sustained in falls are a major cause of mortality and morbidity in the elderly population.<3> Table 1 summarizes the Canadian mortality and morbidity rates for various types of injury in the elderly. A brief description of the risk factors associated with each of the leading causes of unintentional injury in the elderly is provided.

Falls

Falls resulting in serious injury or death are among the most frequent causes of hospital admission in the elderly

In 1988 there were 2,100 deaths due to falls.<2> Falls resulting in serious injury or death were much more frequent among those aged 55 and over; 70% of fatal falls were among persons 75 years and over.<4> Ninety-five percent of injuries among the elderly living in long-term care facilities were due to falls.<5> One percent of falls by individuals aged 65 and over result in hip fracture. A descriptive study found fewer than 30% of 219 women aged 59 and over with hip fractures regained reported pre-fracture levels of physical function. Also, high post-surgery depression scores were associated with poorer recovery. A case-control study of 149 institutionalized and 68 non-institutionalized elderly persons (15% female and 87% male

---

[1] Professor and Director of Research and Faculty Development, Department of Family Medicine, University of Calgary, Calgary, Alberta
[2] "Unintentional injury" is more appropriate than "accident" in terms of terminology, however, many articles in the literature still use the term "accidental".

respectively), matched by age, sex and living location, found fallers were more physically and functionally impaired with hip weakness, poor balance and more medications predictive of falls in institutionalized patients (logistic regression $p<0.05$). Falls without fracture are among the most common causes of admission of the elderly to geriatric hospitals, residential homes and nursing homes, often due to family concerns about safety, restricted mobility and independence. Risk factors for falling include increased age, female sex, presence of more than one disease, dementia, depression, acute illness, decreased mobility, confinement to the home, postural gait instability, gait disturbance, sensory impairment, medications and possibly dietary deficiencies.[6]

Drowning

In 1987 there were 429 deaths due to drowning in Canada, including 135 boating accidents. Only 12% of drowning victims were over 65 years of age.[7]

Burns, Scalds and Fire-Related Deaths

There were 429 fire-related deaths in Canada in 1987 and 85% occurred in private dwellings.[4] Of the 402 accidental deaths among Canadians caused by fire and flames in 1988, about 21% involved persons over 65 years of age.[7] The number of fires and fire deaths (844 in 1978) has declined continually and has been attributed to better education, more widespread use of smoke detectors and fewer people smoking.[8]

Poisoning

Of the 424 fatal poisonings in Canada in 1987, 16% of the deaths were among seniors over 65 years of age.[4,7] Most were by drugs and medications (58%); 23% were by solid and liquid substances and 19% by gases and vapours. Among elderly adults, sedatives are the most commonly reported agents causing morbidity.

Suffocation

Almost two-thirds of the 415 Canadian deaths by suffocation in 1987 resulted from inhalation and/or ingestion of food; 13% were in adults over 65 years of age.[4,7]

Effectiveness of Prevention Maneuvers

During the past decade numerous descriptive studies concerning home and recreational accidents have been published. More important however, is the steady stream of experimental and quasi-experimental studies demonstrating that accidental injury and death are not random, unpredictable events, but are both predictable and preventable[9] and must be looked upon as a disease whose prevention must be approached scientifically. One model for organizing preventive measures against accidental injury and death is the Haddon Matrix,[10] named after a leading thinker in injury control. The Haddon Matrix for generating countermeasures provides a multifactorial model for developing approaches to injury prevention.[10] Three widely adopted approaches to interventions for accidental injury arising from this model are described in greater detail; namely, public health education, environmental legislation, and individual counselling.

Public Health Education

In general, modifying the environment appears more effective than trying to change behaviour among the elderly

In general, modifying the environment appears to be more effective than trying to change human behaviour among the elderly.

Legislative/Environmental

Many studies have demonstrated a far greater impact on promoting home and recreational safety by influencing legislators, who in turn can modify the environment through building codes and safety legislation (Table 2).

Individual Counselling

The elderly living alone are at particular risk for unintentional injuries due to falls, burns, and adverse reactions from medications

The "Year 2000 Injury Control Objectives for Canada" recommend that individual counselling be targeted particularly towards high risk groups; namely, the socio-economically disadvantaged, the aboriginal people, situations where alcohol and/or substance abuse is suspected, and the elderly living alone.[16] Evidence concerning the effectiveness of legislative action and individual counselling for these activities will be presented sequentially for each major type of home and recreational injury.

Falls

Systematic identification and reduction of environmental hazards prevents injuries. As with other unintentional injuries, modifying the environment (stairs, especially those with undifferentiated edges, slippery floor, surface clutter, poor lighting, unexpected obstacles and ill-fitting footwear) can be far more effective than trying to change the behaviour of people living in that environment. Several checklists for home safety evaluation[17] and for studying the epidemiology and risk of falls have been published, but none has been evaluated in clinical practice. Exercise programs have demonstrated positive effects on the muscle strength, flexibility, and cardiovascular and respiratory systems of older people. Physiotherapy improved mobility and balance in one third to one half of 100 patients over age 65 who had recently fallen; less than one half of patients fell in the 4 months following treatment. Recreational walking appeared to reduce the risk of fracture in a cohort of elderly persons.

A Falls Clinic, coordinating the expertise of a geriatrician, neurologist, cardiologist and psychiatrist, combined with resources in audiology, ophthalmology and podiatry as well as home visits by an occupational therapist eliminated falls for 1 year in 77% of patients who had fallen previously.[6,18] Another randomized controlled trial of a post-fall assessment, including a detailed physical examination and environmental assessment by a nurse practitioner, laboratory tests, electrocardiogram and 24-hour Holter monitoring reduced hospitalizations by 26% ($p<0.05$) and hospital days by 52% ($p<0.01$) for 160 elderly ambulatory residential care facility patients but did not significantly decrease falls reported on nursing incident reports (9% lower) or deaths (17% lower) with 2 years of follow-up.[19] Recommendations for rehabilitation therapies were given to 60% of intervention subjects. Recommendations for environmental alterations were made for 45% and alterations in medication for 43%. The authors concluded that though falls may not be easily prevented, they indicate the presence of important treatable conditions and some of the disability and costs associated with falls may be obviated by a thorough assessment.

An 1989 review indicated there were no controlled studies demonstrating the effectiveness of detecting disease, changing medication, promoting exercise, initiating home nursing visits to assess environmental hazards, educating patients, counselling on medication use, physical therapy or balance and gait training on reducing falls.[17]

Burns

"Granny gown" burns among elderly women are still a common problem. Cooking-related flame burns can be reduced by encouraging the independent elderly not to wear loose fitting garments in the kitchen, not to keep condiments or spices over the stove and to use the rear rather than front burner while cooking.[20] The only evidence with respect to the effectiveness of counselling on burn prevention in the elderly was at the level of expert opinion – "The physician can help reduce the incidence and the severity of fire and burn injuries by reviewing precautions with his elderly patients and their families and by stressing basic first aid procedures and the need for immediate medical attention, since even small burns can become serious if not properly treated."[21]

Recommendations of Others

In 1989, the U.S. Preventive Services Task Force recommended that it may be clinically prudent to provide counselling on measures to reduce the risk of unintentional household or environmental injuries from falls, drowning, fires or burns, poisoning, and firearms.[22]

The following recommendations from the National Institute of Aging[17] to primary care physicians concerning older patients are based on expert opinion only:

1. Assess for falls as a routine part of a physical history for those aged 65 years or older (as if falling is expected).

2. Assess for underlying disease.

3. Observe for sway or unsteady gait, using the equivalent of the "Get up and go test".

4. Weigh the benefit of each drug against its potential for contributing to falls; use those less likely to impair balance and gait.

5. Have a checklist of environmental hazards that a health educator or nurse can review with the patient. Assess home when appropriate.

6. Encourage the use of handrails and adequate lighting on stairs and in bathrooms. Advise marking the edges of steps so that they are clearly recognizable.

Conclusions and Recommendations

There is good evidence for referring elderly patients to multidisciplinary post-fall assessment teams, where such a service is available (A Recommendation).[6,18] On the other hand, there is insufficient evidence to support including assessment and counselling of elderly patients for the risk of falling in the routine health examination of the elderly (C Recommendation). It may be included, however, on other grounds. There is fair evidence that safety aids reduce the incidence and severity of injuries in the elderly[19] (B Recommendation), however, there is insufficient evidence to support counselling elderly patients and their families about acquisition of safety features, such as stair railings, bath tub railings, nonflammable fabrics. Such counselling may be included in the periodic health examination on other grounds (C Recommendation).

Unanswered Questions (Research Agenda)

The Haddon Matrix for generating countermeasures provides a model for planning research. The "human" sector presents a major challenge for behavioural medicine (e.g., medication prescribing practices in the elderly). Much remains to be learned about lifestyle patterns and behaviour change strategies. It is in this last area that individual practitioners spend most their time and energy. The "timing" of health education messages, the effectiveness of different motivational techniques, the counselling skills required by health care providers, and the atmosphere most conducive to anticipatory care, all require further elucidation.

Evidence

This review deals with household and recreational injuries without considering occupational or aviation related injuries. These limitations were incorporated in the MEDLINE search strategy: accidents as a major mesh heading under the subheadings diagnosis, economics, epidemiology, law and jurisprudence, mortality, prevention and control, standards and trends; and not aviation, occupational or traffic accidents. References were identified for the years 1981 – November 1991. Other sources included Statistics Canada, Health and Welfare Canada, the Insurance Bureau of Canada the Poison Control Centre, supporting documents of other recommending bodies and references from identified literature.

This review was initiated in January 1991 and recommendations were finalized by the Task Force in June 1993.

Selected References

1. Canadian Task Force on the Periodic Health Examination: The Periodic Health Examination. *Can Med Assoc J* 1979; 121: 1193-1254

2. Statistics Canada, Canadian Centre for Health Information: Causes of Death 1988. [Catalogue No. 82-003S]. Minister of Supply and Services Canada. *Health Reports* 1990; 2(1) Supplement 11: 146-185

3. Statistics Canada: *The Health and Activity Limitations Survey 1989.* [Catalogue No. 82-608] Ottawa, 1989

4. Canada Safety Council: *Accident Fatalities, Canada 1987.* Canada Safety Council 1988: 1-26

5. Young SW, Abedzadeh CB, White MW: A fall-prevention program for nursing homes. *Nurs Manage* 1989; 20(11): 80Y-80AA,80DD,80FF

6. Wolf-Klein GP, Silverstone FA, Basavaraju N, *et al*: Prevention of falls in the elderly population. *Arch Phys Med Rehabil* 1988; 69: 689-691

7. Laboratory Centre for Disease Control, Bureau of Chronic Disease Epidemiology, Health and Welfare Canada, Ottawa

8. McLoughlin E, Marchone M, Hanger L, *et al*: Smoke detector legislation: it's effect on owner occupied homes. *Am J Public Health* 1985; 75: 858-862

9. Francescutti LH, Saunders LD, Hamilton SM: Why are there so many injuries? Why aren't we stopping them? *Can Med Assoc J* 1991; 144(1): 57-61

10. Haddon W Jr: Advances in the epidemiology of injuries as a basis for public policy. *Public Health Rep* 1980; 95: 411-421

11. Division of Injury Control, Centre for Environmental Health and Injury Control: Childhood injuries in the United States. *Am J Dis Child* 1990; 144: 627-646

12. Nixon JW, Pearn JH, Petrie GM: Childproof safety barriers. *Aust Paediatr J* 1979; 15: 260-262

13. Webne S, Kaplan BJ, Shaw M: Pediatric burn prevention: an evaluation of the efficacy of the strategy to reduce tap water temperature in a population at risk for scalds. *J Dev Behav Paed* 1989; 10: 187-191

14. Tinetti ME, Speechley M, Ginter SF: Risk factors for falls among elderly persons living in the community. *New Eng J Med* 1988; 319(26): 1701-1707

15. Thompson RS, Rivara F, Thompson DC: A case-control study of the effectiveness of bicycle safety helmets. *N Engl J Med* 1989; 320: 1361-1367

16. Saunders LD (ed): Injury Control Objectives for Canada. Recommendations from National Working Group, May 1991 Proceedings

17. Hindmarsh JJ, Estes EH: Falls in older persons: etiology and interventions. Chapter 21 in Goldbloom RB and Lawrence RS (eds), *Preventing Disease: Beyond the Rhetoric*. Springer-Verlag, New York 1990; 186-193

18. Rubenstein L, Robbins A, Josephson R, *et al*: The value of assessing falls in an elderly population. *Ann Int Med* 1990; 113: 308-316

19. Hindmarsh JJ, Estes EH: Falls in older persons. Causes and interventions. *Arch Intern Med* 1989; 149: 2217-2222

20. Petro JA, Belger D, Salzberg CA, *et al*: Burn accidents and the elderly: what is happening and how to prevent it. *Geriatrics* 1989; 44(3): 26-48

21. Beverley EV: Reducing fire and burn hazards among the elderly. *Geriatrics* 1976; 31: 106-110

22. U.S. Preventive Services Task Force: *Guide to Clinical Preventive Services: an Assessment of the Effectiveness of 169 Interventions*. Williams & Wilkins, Baltimore, Md, 1989: 321-329

Table 1: Canadian Mortality and Morbidity Rates for Unintentional Injury in 1989[1] (per 100,000 – standardized to 1971 population)

| | Overall (0-85+ yr) | | | | Elderly (≥-65 yr) | | | |
| | Mortality | | Morbidity | | Mortality | | Morbidity | |
	M	F	M	F	M	F	M	F
Falls	6.77	4.16	425.0	384.0	59.15	45.32	1,446.5	2,161.8
Drownings	2.31	.63	2.78	1.38	2.81	.97	1.26	.57
Burns/Fire related	2.11	.91	11.52	4.23	5.39	2.33	12.82	7.02
Poisonings	1.88	.90	38.84	35.19	2.13	1.35	70.99	65.25
Suffocations	.72	.21	.39	.15	.31	.12	.17	.12
Firearms	.57	.04	4.69	.52	.17	.05	1.27	.09

[1] extracted from data Bureau of Chronic Disease Epidemiology, Laboratory Centre for Disease Control, Health and Welfare Canada

Table 2: Sample Legislative Measures to Reduce Environmental Hazards

Injury Prevention Maneuver	Quality of Evidence	Recommendation
SMOKE DETECTORS: Require that working smoke detectors be maintained in all dwellings.<8>	II-1	B
PREVENTION OF FALLS: Modify steps and stairs to decrease the likelihood that falls will occur.<6>	II-1	B
DESIGN FOR SAFER PLAYGROUNDS: Require playgrounds and play equipment to conform to Commission safety standards.<11>	II-1	B
FENCING AROUND POOLS: Reqire that all pools, private and public, be fenced on all four sides, to reduce the risk of drowning.<12>	II-2	B
WATER HEATER, THERMOSTAT CONTROL AND TAP WATER ANTI-SCALD DEVICES: Require thermostats to be set no higher than 120°F, when a new tenant occupies a dwelling or at any other specified time.<13>	II-1	B
ANTI-POISONING PACKETS: Distribute kits including ipecac, cabinet latches, emergency phone numbers, etc. to all new parents.<14>	II-2	B
BICYCLE SAFETY: Require riders to wear helmets, particularly while riding on city streets or sidewalks.<15>	II-1	B

Prevention of Household and Recreational Injuries in the Elderly

MANEUVER	EFFECTIVENESS	LEVEL OF EVIDENCE <REF>	RECOMMENDATION
Perform multidisciplinary post-fall assessment on elderly patients	Significant reduction in subsequent falls/injury in the elderly, if assessment done after first fall.	Randomized controlled trials<6,18> (I)	Good evidence to refer to multidisciplinary post-fall assessment team (where service available) (A)
Monitor elderly patients for medical impairment (balance, medication, gait abnormalities).	Association between falls in elderly and medical impairment.	Expert opinion <19> (III)	Insufficient evidence to include or exclude (C)
Use safety aides in hazardous areas such as stairs, bathtubs			
a) Legislation	Decrease rate of injury with modification of stairs.	Cohort analytic study<17> (II-2)	Fair evidence to implement (B)
b) Individual Counselling	Little information about ability of physician to influence use of safety devices.	Expert opinion <20> (III)	Insufficient evidence to include or exclude (C)
Use non-flammable fabrics and self-extinguishing cigarettes			
a) Public Health Education	Association between burns and scalds in the elderly and smoking or cooking practices.	Expert opinion <20> (III)	Insufficient evidence to implement (C)
b) Individual counselling	Little information about ability of physician to influence behaviour.	Expert opinion <14> (III)	Insufficient evidence to include or exclude (C)

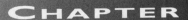

CHAPTER **77**

Secondary Prevention of Elder Abuse

By Christopher Patterson

Secondary Prevention of Elder Abuse

Prepared by Christopher Patterson, MD, FRCPC[1]

Elder abuse and mistreatment has emerged as a significant health problem, affecting all types of older individuals. While obvious cases of physical abuse are readily recognized by professionals and the lay public, subtle degrees of neglect, sexual abuse and other types of mistreatment may go unrecognized. Although it is now known to be common, affecting 4% or more of older people in Canada, the scope and definition of elder abuse lack precise boundaries, detection maneuvers are not well evaluated and there is no clear evidence that interventions are effective. For this reason, there is insufficient evidence to support inclusion or exclusion of case finding for elder abuse in the periodic health examination (C Recommendation). However, it is prudent to advise physicians to be alert for indicators of elder abuse and, if discovered, to institute measures to prevent further abuse.

Burden of Suffering

Elder abuse may be simply defined as "any act of commission or omission that results in harm to an elderly person".<1> The Department of National Health and Welfare<2> has categorized abuse and neglect as follows:

1. Physical abuse: Involves assault, rough handling, sexual abuse, or withholding of physical necessities such as food, personal care, hygiene care or medical care.

2. Psychosocial abuse: Involves verbal assault, social isolation, lack of affection, or denying the person the chance to participate in decisions in respect to his or her own life.

3. Financial abuse: Involves the misuse of money or property. This can include fraud or using the funds for purposes contrary to the needs and interests (or desires) of the older person.

4. Neglect: Can lead to any of these three types of abuse. It can be passive neglect if the caregiver does not intend to injure the dependent senior; or active when the caregiver consciously fails to meet the needs of the senior.

Other categories of abuse have been proposed;<3> the lack of consensus regarding definition of elder abuse makes the synthesis of evidence difficult.

---

[1] Professor and Head, Division of Geriatric Medicine, McMaster University, Hamilton, Ontario

There have been three studies of community prevalence of elder abuse.<4-6> Gioglio and Blakemore<4> interviewed a stratified random sample of community-dwelling people aged 65 years and older in New Jersey. Only 1% of the 342 respondents admitted to being victims of some form of abuse.<4> In a stratified random sample of all community-dwelling elderly persons in the Boston Metropolitan area, 72% of 2,813 eligible respondents were interviewed, and the prevalence of all types of elder abuse was 3.2%.<5> Podnieks and colleagues conducted a cross-Canada telephone survey of 2,000 randomly chosen elderly persons living in private houses. About 4% (95% confidence interval ± 1.5%) had experienced some form of maltreatment since their 65th birthday.<6> Two point five percent reported material abuse. Chronic verbal abuse was reported by 1.4% of the sample, 0.5% experienced family violence and 0.4% neglect. Different profiles emerged for different types of abuse. For material abuse, men and women were equally likely to be victims. They tended to live alone, and the perpetrators were often distant relatives or non-relatives. Chronic verbal abuse tended to occur between spouses, men and women being equally affected. Physical violence was most likely to occur between spouses. While men were more likely to be victims, violence perpetrated by men tended to be more severe. Prevalence estimates for elder abuse as high as 10% have been claimed.<7> While the exact prevalence of abuse and mistreatment within institutions is not clear, when a random sample of staff from 31 nursing homes in New Hampshire was interviewed, 36% reported that they had witnessed physical abuse in the preceding year.<8> Psychological abuse had been observed by 81% of staff.

Risk factors for abuse in the victim include dependency, lack of close family ties, a culture of family violence, lack of financial resources, lack of community support and factors such as low pay and poor working conditions in institutions.

The perpetrator is most often a relative, living with the victim, and may have cared for the victim for a long period of time.<9> The perpetrator often has a psychological disturbance and may be subject to external stresses such as employment loss, divorce, or illness.

Elder abuse does not usually resolve spontaneously. Abusive events tend to be repetitive, and abuse tends to continue unless a major change occurs in the milieu. In many cases victims or families have refused help. Victims are particularly afraid of reprisals, loss of autonomy or relocation.

Maneuver

Detection of elder abuse is notoriously difficult, often complicated by denial by the individual and caretaker. The victim is often reluctant to admit to abuse, for fear of abandonment, reprisal, institutionalization, or to avoid embarrassment or shame. The

Between 4 and 10% of older people experience abuse or mistreatment

Elder abuse does not resolve spontaneously and tends to escalate over time

caretaker is often reluctant to admit abuse for obvious reasons, although given appropriate circumstances (privacy and a non-judgmental listener, preferably on home territory) the caretaker is often willing to talk about difficulties and may express relief at sharing their problems with somebody else.[10] Direct questions have been suggested for incorporation in routine encounters with older people[11] in order to determine risk of abuse:

- "Has anyone at home ever hurt you?
- Has anyone ever touched you without your consent?
- Has anyone ever made you do things you didn't want to do?
- Has anyone taken anything that was yours without asking?
- Has anyone ever scolded or threatened you?
- Have you ever signed any documents that you didn't understand?
- Are you afraid of anyone at home?
- Are you alone a lot?
- Has anyone ever failed to help you take care of yourself when you needed help?"

Items in the history that should raise the possibility of abuse include: conflicting histories from patient or caregiver, denial or vague or bizarre explanation in the face of obvious injury, long delays between injury and seeking treatment, and a history of being accident prone.

While physical findings are rarely specific, unusual trauma, signs of hair pulling, human bites or unusual behaviour between client and caregiver may raise the suspicion of abuse. Social factors which may signal increased likelihood of abuse include: recent deterioration in health of patient or caregiver, evidence of increasing stress in caregiver, and unsatisfactory living arrangements.

While a number of elder abuse identification measures have been developed, an authoritative review[12] concluded that there were few items to measure categories of abuse other than physical, that the distinction of effects of disease from potential abuse was not addressed, and that assessment protocols were conceptually and operationally suboptimal, and had not been empirically tested. The Elder Assessment Instrument (EAI) has shown some promise in distinguishing individuals subsequently found to show evidence of abuse.[13]

Effectiveness of Intervention

Decisions about how and when to intervene in cases of elder abuse and neglect are among the most difficult for service providers. The causes for abuse are complex, little is really known about the causes and risk factors in the individual case. Legal and ethical issues add to this complexity. On the one hand the individual must be protected from harm, on the other, autonomy in decision making must be respected. The Criminal Code of Canada provides the legislation necessary to deal with physical, sexual and financial abuse. However, individuals are often reluctant to press charges against a close relative or caregiver.

Mandatory reporting of abuse exists in several Atlantic provinces. However, it appears that elder abuse laws have had little impact on the performance of physicians in detecting or reporting abuse in the United States. There is no evidence that mandatory reporting is effective in enhancing the treatment of elder abuse. It has been estimated that only one in 14 elder mistreatment cases is reported to a public agency.[14]

Because of the complexity of elder abuse a team approach has been advocated. The principles of intervention are to protect the victim and prevent further abuse. Principles of dealing with the abused victim include a) recognition of the problem, b) provision of information, c) assessment of decision making capacity and d) facilitating choices. After recognizing that abuse or mistreatment may be present, the physician must make an adequate assessment including determination of the safety of the victim and potential risk. Analysis of risk will include a review of the frequency and severity of abuse, and whether intent is thought to be present. The degree of stress of the perpetrator should also be assessed.

A team approach to intervention is likely to be most effective

Usually when an abusive situation is uncovered, the physician will include other health care professionals in management, most frequently a social worker and visiting nurse. In some jurisdictions multidisciplinary geriatric assessment teams may be called upon to sort out complex cases of abuse. The cognitive state must be adequately evaluated, as decision making capacity is an important factor in planning management. Evaluation of social and financial resources must also be made. Adequate documentation should occur, and where visible injuries are present, drawings or preferably colour photographs should be taken. When the victim has the capacity to make decisions about his or her actions, choices should be outlined to enable the situation to be defused. This may involve temporary relocation, involvement of community agencies, or provision of home supports. If the victim is unable by reason of temporary or permanent cognitive impairment, to make decisions about his or her future, it may be necessary to intervene and relocate the individual while appropriate arrangements for advocacy can be made. There have been no rigorous studies evaluating the outcome of interventions for elder abuse.[15] In case series where outcome has been reported,[16-19] the results have generally been disappointing. In dealing with the abuse situation the needs of the perpetrator as well as the victim should be recognized.

Recommendations of Others

The American Medical Association recommendations include incorporating routine questions related to elder abuse and neglect into daily practice.<14> The U.S. Preventive Services Task Force does not recommend routine screening interviews or examinations for evidence of violent injuries.<20> The elderly who present with multiple injuries and unplausible explanations should be evaluated with attention to possible abuse or neglect.

Conclusions and Recommendations

Elder abuse is being recognized increasingly as a health and social phenomenon. There is poor agreement on the definition and categorization of abuse. Estimated prevalence is between 1 and 10% in the community, possibly higher within institutions. There are no well-validated protocols for detection in primary care. Despite these shortcomings, the physician is uniquely equipped to recognize and address elder abuse. The primary care physician should maintain a high index of suspicion, seeking inconsistencies and anomalies in the history, and using direct questions to explore possible abuse or mistreatment. The physician should be alert to physical and psycho-social findings suggesting physical, sexual or neglectful abuse. Upon discovery of abuse, intervention may be hampered by an unwillingness on the part of the individual or the caregiver to comply with recommendations. As the causes are often complex, a team approach has been suggested, and the importance of the advocacy role of the physician is emphasized. There is insufficient evidence, however, to favour any specific protocol of treatment, and intervention should be individualized in accordance with the many factors operating in each case. A prudent recommendation is to advise physicians to be alert for indicators of elder abuse, and to institute measures to prevent further abuse. However, there is insufficient evidence to recommend for or against a search for elder abuse in the periodic health examination (C Recommendation).

Unanswered Questions (Research Agenda)

The following are research priorities:

1. To determine the causes of elder abuse in different ethnic and cultural groups in Canada.

2. To determine the prevalence of abuse in Canadian institutions.

3. To develop valid, reliable assessment tools for use in different settings (primary care, hospital emergency departments, institutions, etc.).

4. To evaluate the effectiveness of interventions for elder abuse.

Evidence

The literature was identified with a MEDLINE search using the terms elder abuse (MH) and epidemiology (SH) from 1980 to March 1993; elder abuse (MH) and clinical trials (PT) from 1980 to March 1993. Standard reference works and their bibliographies were reviewed. Consultations were held with experts in the field.

This review was initiated in June 1991 and the recommendation was finalized by the Task Force in June 1993.

Acknowledgements

The author wishes to acknowledge Elizabeth Podnieks, PhD (candidate), Professor, Ryerson School of Nursing, for her comments and critical review of the draft report. Funding for this report was provided by Health Canada under the Government of Canada's Family Violence Initiative.

Selected References

1. National Clearinghouse on Family Violence: Frail and vulnerable: Elder abuse in Canada. *Vis-à-Vis* 1983; 1(2): 1-2

2. National Clearinghouse on Family Violence: *Elder abuse.* Department of National Health and Welfare, Ottawa, 1990

3. Hudson MF: Elder mistreatment: a taxonomy with definitions by Delphi. 1990; 3: 1-20

4. Gioglio GR, Blakemore P: *Elder abuse in New Jersey: the knowledge and experience of abuse among older New Jerseyans.* Unpublished manuscript, Department of Human Services, Trenton, NJ, 1983

5. Pillemer K, Finkelhor D: The prevalence of elder abuse: a random sample survey. *Gerontologist* 1988; 28: 51-57

6. Podnieks E, Pillemer K, Nicholson J, *et al: National survey on abuse of the elderly in Canada. Preliminary findings.* Office of Research and Innovation, Ryerson Polytechnical Institute, Toronto, 1989

7. Clark CB: Geriatric abuse – out of the closet. *J Tenn Med Assoc* 1984; 77: 470-471

8. Pillemer K, Moore DW: Abuse of patients in nursing homes: findings from a survey of staff. *Gerontologist* 1989; 29: 314-320

9. Taler G, Ansello EF: Elder Abuse. *Am Fam Physician* 1985; 32: 107-114

10. Homer AC, Gilleard C: Abuse of elderly people by their carers. *BMJ* 1990; 301: 1359-1362

11. Mount Sinai Victim Services Agency Abuse Project: *Elder mistreatment guidelines for health care professional: Detection, assessment and intervention.* New York, NY, 1988

12. Sengstock MC, Hwalek M: A review and analysis of measures for the identification of elder abuse. *J Gerontological Social Work* 1987; 10: 21-36

13. Beth Israel Hospital Elder Assessment Team: An elder abuse assessment team in an acute hospital setting. *Gerontologist* 1986; 26: 115-118

14. American Medical Association: *Diagnostic and treatment guidelines on elder abuse and neglect.* AMA, Chicago, Ill, 1992

15. McDonald PL, Hornick JP, Robertson GB, *et al*: *Elder abuse and neglect in Canada.* Butterworths, Toronto, 1991: 92-95

16. Chen PN, Bell S, Dolinsky D, *et al*: Elderly abuse in domestic settings: A pilot study. *J Gerontol Social Work* 1981; 4: 3-17

17. Block MR, Sinnot JD (eds): *The battered elder syndrome: an exploratory study.* College Park Md. Centre on Aging, University of Maryland, 1979

18. O'Malley H, Segel H, Perez R, *et al*: *Elder abuse in Massachusetts: a survey of professionals and paraprofessionals.* Legal Research and Services for the Elderly, Boston, 1979

19. McLaughlin JS, Nickell JP, Gill L: An epidemiological investigation of elderly abuse in Southern Maine and New Hampshire. In: *Elder Abuse* [Publication No. 68-463], U.S. House of Representatives Select Committee on Aging, Washington, D.C., U.S. Government Printing Office, 1980: 111-147

20. U.S. Preventive Services Task Force: *Guide to Clinical Preventive Services: an Assessment of the Effectiveness of 169 Interventions.* Williams & Wilkins, Baltimore, Md, 1989: 271-275

Secondary Prevention of Elder Abuse

MANEUVER	EFFECTIVENESS	LEVEL OF EVIDENCE <REF>	RECOMMENDATION
Various questionnaires	Detection of elder abuse by questionnaire is subobtimal and/or protocols have not been adequately studied.	Descriptive studies<12> and expert opinion <14> (III)	Insufficient evidence to include or exclude in periodic health examination of elderly individuals (C)
	Intervention by professionals or teams has variable but often disappointing results.	Descriptive studies<16-19> and expert opinion <13,14> (III)	

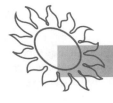

CHAPTER 78

Screening
for Visual
Impairment
in the Elderly

By Christopher Patterson

78

Screening for Visual Impairment in the Elderly

Prepared by Christopher Patterson, MD, FRCPC[1]

Visual impairment is extremely common in older people, resulting in various disabilities (e.g. inability to read, drive, watch television). Visual loss is often unreported, but may be detected readily with a sight card. Correction of refractive errors and surgery for cataracts leads to improvement in quality of life. There is fair evidence to include screening with the Snellen sight card in the periodic health examination of the elderly. Fundoscopy should be carried out regularly in diabetics. In the case of other specific diseases (i.e. age-related macular degeneration, ocular hypertension and glaucoma), there are insufficient grounds to include or exclude fundoscopy, tonometry or automated perimetry in the periodic health examination.

Burden of Suffering

Visual impairment affects at least 13% of older people; one-third of those attending geriatric clinics have severe disability

Thirteen percent of those over age 65 have some form of visual impairment. Almost 8% have severe impairment (blindness in both eyes or inability to read newsprint even with glasses).<1> About 1% of those aged over 40 years have bilateral blindness. Legal blindness (less than 20/200) occurs in up to 3% at age 60, and nearly 11% at age 80. In 1989, there were 63,576 registered blind people in Canada. The leading causes of visual impairment in older individuals are presbyopia, cataracts, age-related macular degeneration (ARMD), glaucoma and diabetic retinopathy.

In presbyopia the crystalline lens becomes thicker and less flexible, resulting in diminished accommodation, and commonly to refractive errors. This process is universal with aging, and leads to substantial visual impairment, although it does not usually result in blindness.

The presence of any opacity within the lens is defined as cataract. While cataracts may result from trauma, disease, ionizing radiation or medications (eg. corticosteroid and antineoplastic agents), in most cases they are idiopathic. The prevalence of cataracts sufficient to impair vision (less than 20/30) rises from 1.1% in the 5th decade to 100% in the 9th decade of life.

In Canada, blind registry data indicate that cataracts accounted for 15% of blindness in Canada.

---

[1] Professor and Head, Division of Geriatric Medicine, McMaster University, Hamilton, Ontario

ARMD is a leading cause of blindness in most Western countries, accounting for about 50% of new cases of blindness in Canada. It is a disease of multiple etiology, resulting in loss of central vision. The common atrophic or dry form accounts for 90% of ARMD but rarely results in vision loss greater than 20/80. Wet, exudative or disciform macular degeneration accounts for 10% of the total burden, although 90% of those with blindness (acuity less than 20/200) have this form. The prevalence of ARMD rises from less than 1% at age 55 to about 15% at age 80. If early macular changes (presence of any drusen) are included, the prevalence is 35% by age 64 and 50% by age 85. Risk factors include hyperopia, positive family history (odds ratio (OR) 2.9), smoking (OR 2.6), blue eyes (OR 1.7) and chemical exposure at work (OR 4.2). It is far more prevalent in white than in black people. It is not clear which individuals with drusen alone will develop exudative, or potentially serious changes, however, pigmentary changes, confluence of drusen and exudative changes in one eye, all increase the risk. Early symptoms include metamorphopsia or distortion of shapes, most easily recognized by viewing rectangular objects such as doors or windows.

Glaucoma is a clinical syndrome consisting of a triad of intraocular hypertension (usually greater than or equal to 20 mmHg, a characteristic peripheral visual field loss, and atrophy of the optic nerve head. The diagnosis of glaucoma requires two of these three factors in any combination. Elevation of intraocular pressure (IOP) in the absence of the other two factors is known as ocular hypertension or glaucoma suspect. Ninety percent of glaucoma is of the open angle type, and is initially asymptomatic. Prevalence estimates of glaucoma are complicated by variable diagnostic criteria in different studies. In a recent community study of over 4,000 individuals, carefully defined glaucoma was present in less than 1.5% below the age of 64 years, 2.2% (men), and 2.96% (women) between the ages of 65 and 74 years and 2.4% (men) and 6.9% (women) over the age of 75.<2> Less than 3% of people with IOP <21 mmHg will develop clinical glaucoma within 5 years. Of those with IOP >21 mmHg, 1.6% to 8.6% will develop glaucoma in 5 years. Risk factors for progression include: age, level of IOP, diabetes, myopia, black race, and vascular problems including systemic hypertension. In those with glaucoma, the visual field loss appears directly related to IOP. The fastest rate of visual loss occurs in the earlier stages of the disease.

Diabetic retinopathy (DR) occurs in both type I (ketosis-prone, insulin-dependent juvenile) and type II (non-ketosis prone, usually non-insulin requiring, adult onset) diabetes. It is recognized clinically as microaneurysms and "dot" or "blot" hemorrhages. Maculopathy is the most common cause of visual impairment in patients with diabetic retinopathy, and is more common in type II diabetics. Proliferative DR is more common in type I diabetes, and is due to new vessel formation within ischemic retinal areas. This type is particularly threatening to eyesight, which may be lost due to hemorrhage or retinal disruption. In older diabetics, DR is responsible for 33% of blindness. The prevalence of retinopathy in diabetics increases with the duration of disease and the age of the diabetic. At age 55-59 years the prevalence is about 10%, rising to 30% above age 80. By 20 years duration, virtually all type I and 60% of type II diabetes will have some degree of retinopathy. The estimated 5 year incidence of retinopathy in diabetics rises from 2.7% at age 55 to 5.4% at age 75.

Maneuver

History

Although reduced visual acuity may be noticed by individuals engaging in reading or watching television, up to one-third of older individuals have unrecognized severe visual losses. Up to 25% of older people are wearing inappropriate visual correction. Questions inquiring about visual disability have very poor sensitivity (less than 30%).

Sight Card

While the characteristics of the Snellen sight card in primary care are unknown, a portable visual acuity box used in a community survey had a sensitivity of 94% and specificity of 89% when compared to an ophthalmological clinic visit assessment.[3] Viewed through a pinhole (to minimize refractive error) sensitivity was 79% and specificity 98%.[4] Using a sight card for case finding in a geriatric clinic in Wales, 36% of 202 patients were found to have impaired vision. Thirty had refractive errors and 42 had non-refractive conditions of which 27 treatable diagnoses were discovered by an ophthalmologist. Fifteen untreatable but serious conditions (usually ARMD) were discovered. Of the 42 individuals with non-refractive errors, only 9 believed that their vision was inadequate.[5] In a case finding study from a primary care general medical clinic in Baltimore, U.S., 267 out of 458 patients were discovered to have visual problems. Of the 101 patients seen in ophthalmological consultation, 96 had serious eye diseases. Fourteen percent required immediate medical therapy and 18% required surgical intervention.[6] The vision test alone failed to identify most cases of diabetic retinopathy and glaucoma. Thus, testing with the Snellen sight card will detect visual impairment in a large percentage of older people, many of whom will benefit from refraction or referral to an ophthalmologist. In the Baltimore Eye Survey more than half the patients identified as impaired at screening subsequently showed improved vision by at least one line on the Snellen sight card, while 7.5% improved their vision by three or more lines.[7]

Fundoscopy

Fundoscopy allows the observer to detect cataracts, ARMD, diabetic retinopathy and flattening of the optic disc in glaucoma. An experienced ophthalmoscopist is able to recognize an increased optic cup to disc ratio in excess of 60%.[8] Sensitivity and specificity of this sign can exceed 90%, although it is unlikely that the same level of diagnostic accuracy could be achieved by most family physicians. In a screening study (fundoscopy followed by tonometry) of over 12,000 subjects in Australia,[9] 6.7% of individuals had suspected glaucoma. Although follow-up was far from complete, the estimated prevalence of 1.19% is close to other published studies, suggesting that most glaucoma cases would be detected by fundoscopy.

Diabetic retinopathy, age-related macular degeneration and often glaucoma can be readily diagnosed by fundoscopy

The ability to detect serious DR (proliferative retinopathy or macular edema) is dependent upon technique and experience but there was good agreement between ophthalmologists, specially trained optometrists and ophthalmic technicians (Kappa 0.75 for none, proliferative and non-proliferative DR) in a large Wisconsin case series.[10] The sensitivity of ophthalmoscopy without pupillary dilatation is 38-50% when carried out by diabetologists or experienced technicians,[11] but 0% when carried out by nurses. In these studies the gold standard was a seven field stereoscopic fundus photograph. An alternative to fundoscopy for screening diabetics to detect retinopathy is fundus photography with a single 45 degree field of the posterior pole of each eye without mydriasis.

Tonometry

While tonometry with the Schiotz tonometer has been previously recommended as a screening test for glaucoma, it has proved to have a sensitivity of only 50%[12] when used in practice. The positive predictive value has been reported to be only 5%.[13,14] This is partly due to diurnal variation in IOP, which may be as much as 5 mmHg in normal subjects, 8-10 mmHg in those with glaucoma. Only 50% of glaucomatous subjects have raised pressure in random measurement.[13] Alternative types of tonometry (aplanation, puff tonometry or a hand held Perkins model) may prove to be more sensitive. Tonometry will not detect cases of low tension glaucoma.

Perimetry will detect visual field loss, a highly sensitive but non-specific finding in glaucoma. Automated visual field screening is feasible and may be practical in the future. The Humphrey automated perimeter device has a sensitivity of 90% and specificity of 91% when compared with Goldman Perimetry. It takes about 30 minutes to perform.[15]

Effectiveness of Prevention and Treatment

Refractive errors, including those due to presbyopia are readily corrected with eye glasses or contact lenses.

For cataract, while medications to dilate the pupil may be helpful in improving vision where a small central opacity is present, the only definitive treatment is surgical removal. This procedure is highly effective in restoring vision providing the retina functions well and that adequate refraction is undertaken. When a cataract is extremely dense, it may not be possible to detect retinal disease such as macular degeneration, which may impair a successful surgical result. This supports the case for early detection of cataract. Lens removal, particularly when combined with intraocular lens implantation, results in improved vision in approximately 90% of cases.<16> In 5% of cases post-surgical visual acuity is worse, and is unimproved in another 5%. Serious complications occur in 1% or less.

Before Argon laser photocoagulation, there was no effective treatment for ARMD. Three controlled trials of this technique have demonstrated that photocoagulation of neovascular complexes preserves vision when compared with no treatment.<17-20> Older patients and those with neovascular tissue distant from the fovea were more likely to benefit. The results of these studies offer a rationale for early detection and observation of ARMD. Unfortunately, in most cases the visual deterioration continues and lesions progress beyond the point for successful treatment.

In glaucoma visual loss is not generally reversible. Measures aimed at early detection include tonometry (measuring intraocular pressure), fundoscopy to examine the optic nerve head and manual or automated perimetry to detect early peripheral field loss. Treatment is aimed at reducing intraocular pressure by topical agents (beta-adrenergic blocking drugs or pilocarpine). Some improvement in visual fields has been documented in the first six months of treatment.<21> While it is well accepted that reducing extremely high levels of IOP (>35 mmHg) prevents visual loss, such levels occur very infrequently in the general population. The benefit of treating mild to moderate intraocular hypertension is less clear. A number of randomized controlled trials of IOP reduction in intraocular hypertensives have been carried out using the development of new visual field defects as the outcome measure. Although the results of these studies are not consistently positive,<22-25> and methodological flaws are present in most studies, it has become generally accepted treatment.

In type I diabetics there is evidence that close glycemic control delays the progress of DR.<26> It remains to be seen whether retinopathy in type II diabetics can be similarly retarded. Photocoagulation by Xenon Arc or Argon laser is effective treatment for various types of DR. Several randomized studies have confirmed that photocoagulation maintains vision and reduces the risk of visual

Diabetic retinopathy, glaucoma and discoid age-related macular degeneration have been proven to benefit from early treatment

loss.[27-29] The best results occur in those whose initial vision is better than 20/30.

Recommendations of Others

The American Academy of Ophthalmology recommends that ophthalmoscopy and tonometry be performed annually in all persons over age 40. A complete ocular examination by an ophthalmologist is recommended at least once between the ages of 35 and 45 and should be repeated every 5 years after age 50. The American Optometric Association recommends a complete eye and vision examination including tonometry of people over age 35. While its recommendations are currently under review, in 1989 the U.S. Preventive Services Task Force (USPSTF) suggested it may be clinically prudent to advise persons at high risk for glaucoma such as those age 65 and older to be tested by an eye specialist; the optimal frequency was left to clinical discretion.[30] Schiotz tonometry was no longer recommended as an early-detection technique for glaucoma.[31] The USPSTF also felt that vision screening for diminished visual acuity may be appropriate in the elderly.[30]

The American College of Physicians, American Diabetes Association and the American Academy of Ophthalmology recommend regular screening of diabetics with stereoscopic fundus photography when available, or annual dilated ophthalmoscopic examination.[32]

Conclusions and Recommendations

Visual impairment and disability are common in older individuals. Snellen sight card testing detects reduced visual acuity. There is fair evidence to include this in the periodic health examination as many people with visual impairment can be readily helped (B Recommendation). In the case of diabetics, fundoscopy or retinal photography can be recommended for inclusion in the periodic health examination, to detect DR at an early stage, for monitoring and early treatment of proliferative changes by an ophthalmologist (B Recommendation).

Early identification of individuals with ARMD offers the opportunity to intervene with photocoagulation when neovascular change threatens vision. However, the ability of the primary care physician to detect such changes by fundoscopy remains uncertain, and there is insufficient evidence to guide the inclusion or exclusion of fundoscopy for this purpose (C Recommendation). It remains, however, a prudent recommendation. For early diagnosis of glaucoma, there is at present insufficient evidence to include or exclude tonometry, fundoscopy or automated perimetry in the periodic health examination (C Recommendation). For those individuals with a positive family history and for those who are black, highly myopic or diabetic, there is a greater risk of developing glaucoma. In such individuals a prudent recommendation would be to include periodic assessment by an ophthalmologist with access to automated perimetry.

Unanswered Questions (Research Agenda)

The following were identified as research priorities:

1. Evaluating fundoscopy for predicting pressure induced ocular damage.

2. Comparing the cost-effectiveness of providing currently available automated visual field screening devices to primary care practitioners and of training them to recognize reliably the fundoscopic characteristics of a glaucomatous optic disc.

3. Determine whether any simple questions have high sensitivity for detecting eye disease.

4. To determine the sensitivity and specificity of Snellen sight cards for detecting visual impairment in primary care.

5. To determine the characteristics of fundoscopy in the primary care setting for detecting age-related macular degeneration.

6. To explore the most effective method of improving the fundoscopic skills of the primary care physician.

7. Determine the most effective method of detecting glaucoma, (e.g. by puff or Perkins tonometry) in community screening.

8. To explore the role of optometrists in primary care screening for visual impairment glaucoma, diabetic retinopathy and age-related macular degeneration.

Evidence

The following search terms were used in the literature review on MEDLINE from 1986 to December 1993: glaucoma (MH), or glaucoma suspect (MH), mass screening (MH), or vision screening (MH), clinical trial (PT), glaucoma-drug therapy; intraocular pressure – drug effect; ocular hypertension – drug therapy, Timolol – administration and dosage; vision disorders; aged; diabetic retinopathy; age-related macular degeneration; cataracts; retinal diseases.

This review was initiated in March 1990 and recommendations were finalized by the Task Force in January 1994.

Acknowledgements

The Task Force thanks Drs. Vladamir Kozousek, MD, FRCSC, consultant ophthalmologist, Camp Hill Hospital, Halifax, Nova Scotia; M. Motolko, MD, FRCSC, FACS, consultant ophthalmologist, Toronto, Willowdale, Ontario; R. Pace, OD, School of Optometry, University of Waterloo, Waterloo, Ontario; Graham E. Trope, MB, DO, FRCS(Ed), PhD, FRCSC, Chairman Ophthalmology, University of Toronto, Toronto, Ontario; R. Wagg, OD, President, Nova Scotia Association of Optometrists, New Glasgow, NS, for their careful reviews and advice in the preparation of this manuscript.

Selected References

1. Nelson KA: Visual impairment among elderly Americans: statistics in transition. *J Vis Impair Blind* 1987; 81: 331-334

2. Klein BEK, Klein R, Sponsel WE, *et al*: Prevalence of Glaucoma. The Beaver Dam Eye Study. *Ophthalmology* 1992; 99: 1499-1504

3. Ederer F, Krueger DE, Mowery RL, *et al*: Lessons from the Visual Acuity Impairment Survey pilot study. *Am J Public Health* 1986; 76: 160-165

4. Loewenstein JI, Palmberg PF, Connett JE, *et al*: Effectiveness of a pinhole method for visual screening. *Arch Opththalmol* 1985; 103: 222-223

5. Long CA, Holden R, Mulkerrin E, *et al*: Opportunistic screening of visual acuity of elderly patients attending outpatient clinics. *Age Ageing* 1991; 20: 392-395

6. Strahlman E, Ford D, Whelton P, *et al*: Vision screening in a primary care setting. A missed opportunity? *Arch Intern Med* 1990; 150: 2159-2164

7. Tielsch JM, Sommer A, Witt K, *et al*: Blindness and visual impairment in an American urban population. The Baltimore Eye Survey. *Arch Ophthalmol* 1990; 108: 286-290

8. Holmin C: Optic disc evaluation versus the visual field in chronic glaucoma. *Acta Opthalmol Copenh* 1982; 60: 275-283

9. Cooper RL, Grose GC, Constable IJ: Mass screening of the optic disc for glaucoma: a follow up study. *Austr N Z J Ophthalmol* 1986; 14: 35-39

10. Moss SE, Klein R, Kessler SD, *et al*: Comparison between ophthalmoscopy and fundus photography in determining severity of diabetic retinopathy. *Ophthalmology* 1985; 92: 62-67

11. Singer DE, Nathan DM, Fogel HA, *et al*: Screening for diabetic retinopathy. *Ann Intern Med* 1992; 116: 660-671

12. Hollows FC, Graham PA: Intraocular pressure, glaucoma and glaucoma suspects in a defined population. *Br J Ophthalmol* 1966; 50: 570-586

13. Leske MC: The epidemiology of open-angle glaucoma: a review. *Am J Epidemiol* 1983; 118: 166-191

14. Ford VJ, Zimmerman TJ, Kooner A: A comparison of screening methods for the detection of glaucoma. *Invest Ophthalmol Vis Sci (Suppl)* 1982; 22: 257

15. Trope GE, Britton R: A comparison of Goldmann and Humphrey automated perimetry in patients with glaucoma. *Br J Opthalmol* 1987; 71: 489-493

16. Straatsma BR, Meyer KT, Bastek JV, *et al*: Posterior chamber intraocular lens implantation by ophthalmology residents. A prospective study of cataract surgery. *Opthalmology* 1983; 90: 327-335

17. Argon laser photocoagulation for senile macular degeneration. Results of a randomized trial. *Arch Ophthalmol* 1982; 100: 912-918

18. The Moorfields Macular Study Group: Retinal pigment epithelial detachments in the elderly: a controlled trial of argon laser photocoagulation. *Br J Ophthalmol* 1982; 66: 1-16

19. The Moorfields Macular Study Group: Treatment of senile disciform macular degeneration: a single blind randomized trial by argon laser photocoagulation. *Br J Ophthalmol* 1982; 66: 745-753

20. Coscas G, Soubrane G: Photocoagulation de néovaisseaux sou-rétiniens par le laser à argon dans la dégénérescence, maculaire sénile. *Bulletins et Mémoires de la Société Française d'Ophthalmologie* 1982; 83: 102-105

21. Messmer C, Flammer J, Stumpfig D: Influence of betaxolol and timolol on the visual fields of patients with glaucoma. *Am J Ophthalmol* 1991; 112: 678-681

22. Schulzer M, Drance SM, Douglas GR: A comparison of treated and untreated glaucoma suspects. *Ophthalmology* 1991; 98: 301-307

23. Glaucoma Laser Trial Research Group: The Glaucoma Laser Trial. *Ophthalmology* 1990; 97: 1403-1413

24. Kitazawa Y: Prophylactic therapy of ocular hypertension. A prospective study. *Trans Ophthalmol Soc NZ* 1981; 33: 30-32

25. Epstein DL, Krug JH Jr, Hertzmark E, *et al*: A long-term clinical trial of timolol therapy versus no treatment in the management of glaucoma suspects. *Ophthalmology* 1989; 96: 1460-1467

26. Reichard P, Nilsson BY, Rosenqvist U: The effect of long term intensified insulin treatment on the development of microvascular complications of diabetes millitus. *N Engl J Med* 1993; 329: 304-309

27. British Multicentre Study Group: Proliferative diabetic retinopathy: treatment with xenon-arc photocoagulation: interim report of multicentre randomized controlled trial. *BMJ* 1977; 1: 739-741

28. Early Treatment Diabetic Retinopathy Study Research Group report number 1: Photocoagulation for diabetic macular edema. *Arch Ophthalmol* 1985; 103: 1796-1806

29. British Multicentre Study Group: Photocoagulation for diabetic maculopathy. A randomized controlled trial using the xenon arc. *Diabetes* 1983; 32: 1010-1016

30. U.S. Preventive Services Task Force: *Guide to Clinical Preventive Services: an Assessment of the Effectiveness of 169 Interventions.* Williams & Wilkins, Baltimore, Md, 1989: 181-192

31. Battista RN, Huston P, Davis MW: Screening for primary open-angle glaucoma. In Goldbloom RB, Lawrence RS (eds): *Preventing Disease: Beyond the Rhetoric.* Springer-Verlag, New York, 1990

32. American College of Physicians, American Diabetes Association, American Academy of Ophthalmology: Screening guidelines for diabetic retinopathy. *Ann Intern Med* 1992; 116: 683-685

Screening for Visual Impairment in the Elderly

MANEUVER	EFFECTIVENESS	LEVEL OF EVIDENCE <REF>	RECOMMENDATION
Snellen sight card	Reliably detects reduced visual acuity in community studies.	Cohort analytic <3,4> (II-2)	Fair evidence to include screening in periodic health examination (PHE) (B)
	Population screening can lead to useful improvements in vision.	Cohort analytic <14> (II-2)	
Diabetic Retinopathy			
Fundoscopy or retinal photography in diabetics	Fundoscopy and retinal photography are sensitive for detection of diabetic retinopathy; early detection preserves vision.	Case series overview<11> and expert opinion <32> (III)	Fair evidence to include screening in PHE of diabetics (B)
	Photocoagulation in proliferative diabetic retinopathy preserves vision.	Randomized controlled trials<27-29> (I)	
Age-related macular degeneration			
Fundoscopy	(ARMD) can be detected by those trained in ophthalmoscopy.	Expert opinion <18> (III)	Insufficient evidence to include or exclude in PHE (C)
	Photocoagulation preserves vision in ARMD with neovascular changes.	Randomized controlled trials<17-20> (I)	
Glaucoma			
Fundoscopy, tonometry or automated perimetry	Examination of optic disc (fundoscopy) is sensitive for detection of glaucoma.	Cohort analytic <9> (II-2)	Insufficient evidence to include or exclude screening for glaucoma in PHE (C)
	Schiotz tonometry has poor sensitivity and specificity for early detection of glaucoma.	Case series <12-14> (III)	
	Automated perimetry (Humphrey) is sensitive for detection of glaucoma.	Case series<15> (III)	
	Topical application of beta adrenergic blockers lowers intraocular pressure and may retard vision loss.	Randomized controlled trials<22-25> (I)	

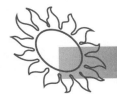

CHAPTER *79*

Hypertension in the Elderly: Case-Finding and Treatment to Prevent Vascular Disease

By Christopher Patterson
and Alexander G. Logan

79

Hypertension in the Elderly: Case-Finding and Treatment to Prevent Vascular Disease

Prepared by Christopher Patterson, MD, FRCPC[1] and Alexander G. Logan, MD, FRCPC[2]

Risks for morbid events resulting from hypertension increase with age. Results from recent large-scale randomized controlled trials have established that treatment for both isolated systolic and mixed systolic and diastolic hypertension is beneficial in terms of reduced rates of strokes, symptomatic coronary artery disease and death. While earlier recommendations have emphasized the importance of screening for hypertension in young and middle life, there is now good evidence to extend these recommendations to those aged over 65 years.

Burden of Suffering

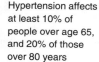

Hypertension affects at least 10% of people over age 65, and 20% of those over 80 years

Systolic hypertension is defined as an average blood pressure (BP) >160 mmHg measured on multiple readings on several occasions by sphygmomanometer cuff. Diastolic hypertension is an average diastolic BP (Korotkoff V) ≥90 mmHg. The prevalence of isolated systolic hypertension (systolic BP >160 mmHg, diastolic BP < 90 mmHg on two occasions) was about 10% of white Americans over 65 years of age, in the screening phase of the Systolic Hypertension in the Elderly Program (SHEP) study.[1] The prevalence rose to 20% in those over age 80 years. The prevalence of diastolic hypertension (diastolic BP >90 mmHg on two occasions) was found to be about 11% of white Americans and over 26% of black Americans in the screening phase of the Hypertension Detection and Follow-up Study.[2] Other estimates based upon single measurements of BP have estimated prevalence considerably higher than these figures.

Epidemiological studies, for example those arising from Framingham, Massachusetts have determined that the risks of death and morbid events relate independently to both systolic and diastolic hypertension. The risks of stroke and of cardiovascular diseases rise with age, given the same levels of BP. Thus, the rate of morbid events is age-dependent, for both men and women. In general, rates for men are higher than for women of the same age with similar levels of BP.

[1] Professor and Head, Division of Geriatric Medicine, McMaster University, Hamilton, Ontario
[2] Professor of Medicine, University of Toronto, Toronto, Ontario

Moderate degrees of hypertension are usually asymptomatic in all age groups.

Maneuver

The mercury sphygmomanometer is the instrument of choice because of its accuracy and dependability. Aneroid instruments should be calibrated twice yearly using the mercury sphygmomanometer as the standard. Guidelines for sphygmomanometry have been published<3> and include: selection of appropriate cuff size (the rubber bladder should encircle at least 2/3 of the arm); measurement should be taken after five minutes of quiet rest, with the arm bared, supported and positioned at heart level; for screening, and diagnosis the seated position should be used; if hypertension is established, subsequent readings should include a lying and standing measurement. The patient should have refrained from smoking or ingesting caffeine within 30 minutes before measurement. Two or more readings should be averaged; if the first two differ by more than 5 mmHg additional readings should be obtained. If an initial BP is elevated in a person not previously known to have hypertension, the BP should be reassessed on at least three occasions over a period of six months.

Effectiveness of Prevention and Treatment

While earlier studies have included some subjects over age 65 years, the numbers were insufficient to permit firm conclusions for this age group and decisions were based on subgroup analysis. Four large randomized controlled trials have now added persuasively to the body of knowledge about antihypertensive treatment in the elderly.

There is compelling evidence that treatment of systolic BP >160 and diastolic BP >90 reduces both morbidity and mortality

The European Working Party on High Blood Pressure in the Elderly Trial (EWPHE)<4> examined antihypertensive treatment in 840 patients over 60 years of age. These patients were recruited from hospital clinics using a sitting systolic BP of 160-239 mmHg and a sitting diastolic BP of 90-119 mmHg as entry criteria. Treatment was randomized and double-blind, using diuretics as first line treatment, subsequently adding methyldopa as necessary. After an average follow-up of nearly 5 years, there were less than 300 subjects remaining in the study (19% had died, 4% had a trial-terminating morbid cardiovascular event, 4% had a terminating non-morbid event, and 36% had left the study prematurely for other reasons). The results included a significant reduction in cardiovascular mortality (-27%, p=0.037); significant reduction in cardiac mortality, (-38%, p=0.036) and study-terminating morbid cardiovascular events were significantly reduced by 60% (p=0.064). There was a non-significant change in all cause mortality and in cerebral vascular mortality.

Criticisms of this study included the very slow recruitment rate and high dropout rate. Calculation of the number needed to treat for

5 years (NNT5) was 23 to reduce one cardiovascular death, and 37 to reduce one nonfatal cerebral vascular event (cardiovascular accident, transient ischemic attack). While no benefit was seen in subjects over age 80, only 155 completed the trial. Further analysis of the EWPHE trial indicated that the benefit of treatment occurred throughout the range of blood pressures included in the trial, whether or not the patient had cardiovascular complications at entry.<5,6>

The Systolic Hypertension in the Elderly Program (SHEP)<1,7> recruited over 4,000 subjects after a mass screening of 447,921 people over age 60. Entry criteria included systolic BP between 160 and 219 mmHg, with a diastolic BP less than 90 mmHg. Those with a history or signs of major cardiovascular diseases were excluded. The mean age of the subjects was 72 years, although 649 were over the age of 80. Treatment was randomized and double-blind, commencing with a diuretic, with beta-blockers or reserpine as second line treatment. Treatment targets were a systolic BP of less than 160 mmHg if the initial systolic BP was greater than 180 mmHg, and a reduction of 20 mmHg of mercury if initial systolic BP fell between 160 and 180. There was a significant reduction in the incidence of total stroke by 37% (p=0.0003: relative risk 0.63; 95% Confidence Internal (CI): 0.49-0.82). The incidence of myocardial infarction was reduced by one third (relative risk 0.67; 95% CI: 0.47-0.96). The incidence of left ventricular failure was reduced by one half (relative risk 0.46; 95% CI: 0.33-0.65). There was a nonsignificant reduction in all cause mortality. The NNT5 for reduction of one stroke was 40, as it was for left ventricular failure. The NNT5 to reduce a myocardial infarction was 90.

The Swedish Trial in Older Patients with Hypertension (STOP-Hypertension) was a randomized trial involving Swedish men and women between the ages of 70 and 84.<8> The entry criteria were systolic BP between 180 and 230 mmHg plus a diastolic BP of at least 90 mmHg, or a diastolic BP between 105 and 120 mmHg irrespective of systolic pressure. Treatment was randomly allocated to four drugs, one diuretic combination and three beta-blockers. This study did not exclude those with other cardiovascular diseases, except for myocardial infarction or stroke within one year, or angina requiring more treatment than glyceryl trinitrate. After an average treatment time of slightly over two years, there was a significant reduction in all cause mortality (relative risk 0.57; 95% CI: 0.37-0.87). There was a significant reduction in all strokes (relative risk 0.53; 95% CI: 0.33-0.86) and a significant reduction in fatal strokes (relative risk 0.27; 95% CI: 0.06-0.84). Treatment benefits were evident in the primary endpoints at all ages, although above age 80 the benefit was not clear. The NNT5 to prevent one stroke or death was 14.

The Medical Research Council (MRC) trial of treatment of hypertension in older adults studied the effects of antihypertensive treatment in men and women between the ages of 65 and 74 with systolic BP between 160 and 209 mmHg together with a diastolic BP of less than or equal to 114 mmHg.<9> Nearly 185,000 invitations were issued to patients in over 200 family practices. Over 20,000 were eligible for consideration, but 16,000 of these were excluded due to: prior treatment for hypertension, myocardial infarction or stroke within three months; or significant cardiovascular or other diseases. Treatment was placebo- controlled and double-blind and initiated with either diuretic or beta-blocker. The study continued for over 5 years by which time 25% of the subjects had been lost to follow-up.

The trial showed a significant reduction in all strokes of 25% (p=0.04; 95% CI: 3-42%). There was a reduction of all cardiovascular events (stroke and coronary events) of 17% (p=0.04; 95% CI: 2-29%).

These four trials confirm the beneficial effects of initiating treatment in older subjects with systolic BP >160 mmHg, and diastolic BP >90 mmHg. Treatment with diuretics is usually effective although the addition of second line drugs is often necessary.

While an exhaustive search for causes of secondary hypertension is not recommended, drugs such as alcohol and nonsteroidal anti-inflammatory drugs may contribute to blood pressure elevation.

Drugs such as alcohol and NSAIDs may contribute to elevated blood pressure

Health promotion measures such as reduction of intake of salt, cessation of tobacco use and regular exercise are usually recommended, and may influence cardiovascular disease or hypertension risk, particularly if it is borderline. Pharmacological treatment should not be delayed in those with moderate or severe hypertension.

There is evidence that conveying a diagnosis of hypertension to younger subjects may foster the development of symptoms.<10> Whether this is true in older patients is not clear.

Recommendations of Others

The U.S. Preventive Services Task Force recommends regular measurement of blood pressure for all persons above age 3.<11>

Conclusions and Recommendations

Given the high prevalence of hypertension in older people, the risks of death and morbid event resulting from untreated hypertension, and the proven effectiveness of pharmacological treatment, screening for this condition can be confidently recommended in those aged 65 to 84 years. Not withstanding problems in clinical trial methodology (e.g. slow recruitment in EWPHE, high dropout rate in MRC) efficacy of treatment has not been demonstrated in those above age 80. While definitive evidence for treatment of hypertension in those over age 85 is still lacking, it seems unlikely that judicious treatment will be detrimental. There have been no randomized trials specifically addressing this very elderly population. Caution has been advocated in the treatment of these people on the basis of two publications. The first was a small RCT (n=123) which demonstrated no benefit of treatment after 2 years. The subjects resided in residential care, the mean age was around 80 years, and no placebo was given to the control group. Given the results of recent trials, this study clearly did not have adequate power to support its conclusions of lack of effect.[12] The second was an observation from Finland that in those aged over 85, an inverse relation existed between 2 year mortality and both systolic and diastolic BP.[13]

As with management of elderly in general, close attention must be paid to the development of side effects of medications. The risks of treatment must be weighed against possible benefit in those suffering from coexistent severe diseases, such as dementia and advanced stages of other diseases.

Unanswered Questions (Research Agenda)

1. To establish efficacy of treatment for hypertensive people over age 80.
2. To determine the effects of treatment on quality of life.

Evidence

The literature was identified with a MEDLINE search using the terms hypertension (MH); aged (MH) and aged over 80 (MH); clinical trials (PT) to August 1993. Recent review articles and meta analyses were searched for additional references. Input was received from experts in the field of hypertension.

This review was initiated in April 1992 and updates a report published in 1984.[14] Recommendations were finalized by the Task Force in January 1994.

Acknowledgements

The Task Force thanks participants of the Canadian Hypertension Society Consensus Conference, April 8 and 9, 1992[15] for their assistance in reviewing the evidence.

Selected References

1. Vogt TM, Ireland CC, Black D, *et al*: Recruitment of elderly volunteers for multicenter clinical trial: the SHEP pilot study. *Controlled Clin Trials* 1986; 7: 118-133

2. Hypertension Detection Follow-up Cooperative Group: Five-year findings of the Hypertension Detection Follow-up Program. *JAMA* 1979; 242: 2562-2577

3. Logan AG: Report of the Canadian Hypertension Society's Consensus Conference on the Management of Mild Hypertension. *Can Med Assoc J* 1984; 131: 1053-1057

4. Amery A, Birkenhager W, Brixko P, *et al*: Mortality and morbidity results from the European Working Party on High Blood Pressure in the Elderly Trial. *Lancet* 1985; 1: 1349-1354

5. Amery A, Birkenhager W, Brixko R, *et al*: Efficacy of antihypertensive drug treatment according to age, sex, blood pressure, and previous cardiovascular disease in patients over the age of 60. *Lancet* 1986; 2: 589-592

6. Staessan J, Bulpitt C, Clement D, *et al*: Relation between mortality and treated blood pressure in elderly patients with hypertension: report of the European Working Party on High Blood Pressure in the Elderly. *BMJ* 1989; 298: 1552-1556

7. SHEP Cooperative Research Group: Prevention of stroke by antihypertensive drug treatment in older persons with isolated systolic hypertension. *JAMA* 1991; 265: 3255-3264

8. Dahlof B, Lindholm LH, Hansson L, *et al*: Morbidity and mortality in the Swedish Trial in Old Patients with Hypertension (STOP-Hypertension). *Lancet* 1991; 338: 1281-1285

9. MRC Working Party: Medical Research Council trial of treatment of hypertension in older adults: principal results *BMJ* 1992; 304: 405-412

10. MacDonald LA, Sackett DL, Haynes RB, *et al*: Labelling in hypertension: a review of the behavioural and psychological consequences. *J Chronic Dis* 1984; 37: 933-942

11. U.S. Preventive Services Task Force: *Guide to Clinical Preventive Services: an Assessment of the Effectiveness of 169 Interventions*. Williams & Wilkins, Baltimore, Md, 1989: 23-27

12. Sprackling ME, Mitchell JRA, Short AH, *et al*: Blood pressure reduction in elderly: a randomized controlled trial of methyldopa. *Br Med J Clin Res Ed* 1981; 283: 1151-1153

13. Rajala S, Haavisto M, Heikinheimo R, *et al*: Blood pressure and mortality in the very old. [letter] *Lancet* 1983; 2: 520-521

14. Canadian Task Force on Periodic Health Examination: The periodic health examination. 2. 1984 Update. *Can Med Assoc J* 1984; 130: 1278-1285

15. Reeves RA, Fodor JG, Gryfe CI, *et al*: Report of the Canadian Hypertension Society Consensus Conference: 4. Hypertension in the elderly. *Can Med Assoc J* 1993; 149(6): 815-820

Hypertension in the Elderly: Case-Finding and Treatment to Prevent Vascular Disease

MANEUVER	EFFECTIVENESS	LEVEL OF EVIDENCE <REF>	RECOMMENDATION
Measurement of blood pressure (BP) level used to identify hypertensive individuals	Average of at least two readings on each of at least three occasions over a period of six months. Although not evaluated for its effectiveness, case-finding should be considered in all persons aged 65 to 84 years; individual clinical judgement should be exercised in all other areas.	Expert opinion* <11> (III)	Fair evidence to include in the periodic health examination (PHE) (B)
Pharmacologic treatment of hypertension	Therapy for hypertension should be individualized, based on age, type and level of blood pressure elevation.		
	a) In persons up to 70 years with diastolic BP of 90 mmHg or over treatment lowers risk of stroke, cardiac events and death.	Randomized controlled trial<2> (I)	Good evidence to treat (A)
	b) In persons aged 70 to 84 years with diastolic BP of 90 mmHg or over and systolic BP of 160 mmHg or over treatment lowers risk of stroke and death.	Randomized controlled trials<4,5,8,9> (I)	Good evidence to treat (A)

* **High Prevalence, effective detection maneuver and efficacious treatment**

(Continued on next page)

Hypertension in the Elderly: Case-Finding and Treatment to Prevent Vascular Disease (concl'd)

MANEUVER	EFFECTIVENESS	LEVEL OF EVIDENCE <REF>	RECOMMENDATION
Pharmacologic treatment of hypertension	c) In persons aged 60 to 84 years with systolic BP of 160 mmHg or over with diastolic BP less than 90 mmHg - treatment lowers risk of stroke.	Randomized controlled trial<7> (I)	Good evidence to treat (A)
	d) In person over 84 years of age with elevated systolic or diastolic BP there is no evidence of benefit. Cautious and individualized approach is recommended.	Expert opinion <15> (III)	Insufficient evidence to include or exclude (C); cautious and individualized approach recommended
	e) In persons aged 65 to 84 years with systolic BP of 140 to 160 mmHg and diastolic BP less than 90 mmHg, there is no evidence of benefit to treatment.	Expert opinion <15> (III)	Insufficient evidence to include in or exclude from PHE (C)
	f) In persons over 70 years of age with diastolic BP 90 mmHg or over and systolic BP less than 160 mmHg, there is no evidence of benefit to treatment.	Expert opinion <15> (III)	Insufficient evidence to include in or exclude from PHE (C)

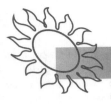

CHAPTER 80

Prevention of Hearing Impairment and Disability in the Elderly

By Christopher Patterson

Prevention of Hearing Impairment and Disability in the Elderly

Prepared by Christopher Patterson, MD, FRCPC[1]

Hearing loss is a common and potentially disabling problem in older individuals. While approximately one-quarter of older individuals complain of hearing problems, at least one-third have significant hearing impairment on audiological testing. Hearing loss may impair physical and social function, and is associated with cognitive deficits, mood disturbances and behavioral disorders. Ninety percent of hearing loss in the elderly is due to sensorineural changes, and many cases are amenable to amplification. Hearing aids improve the quality of life. On the basis of high prevalence and proven effectiveness of intervention, there is fair evidence to include screening for hearing impairment in the periodic health examination. Attempts should be made to limit environmental noise-exposure to prevent noise-induced damage to hearing.

Burden of Suffering

Age-related hearing loss (presbycusis) is a common phenomenon, due to a variety of causes. Ninety percent of presbycusis is due to sensorineural hearing loss, resulting from an interaction of age-related changes, diseases and agents that damage hearing. Changes due to aging include stiffening of the basilar membrane, hyperostosis, arteriosclerotic and rheologic changes, together with degeneration of the organ of Corti, loss of hair cells, spiral ganglion degeneration and impaired neural regulation of endolymph. Other factors include infectious diseases of the middle and inner ear, noise exposure, drugs (aminoglycoside antibiotics, salicylates, quinidine, loop diuretics) and damage to the auditory nerve.

Hearing impairment refers to limitation of function as measured by raised hearing threshold, measured as decibels of hearing loss (dB HL) relative to the hearing of a normal population, at specific frequencies, usually 250, 500, 1,000, 2,000 and 4,000 Hz. Hearing disability refers to the limitation in performing everyday tasks such as understanding speech in the presence of background noise.

Presbycusis affects primarily frequencies above 1000 Hz. While the frequency of most speech is in the 500-4000 Hz range, certain consonants (e.g. S, Th, F) have higher frequencies. The elderly hearing impaired person may have normal low frequency hearing with loss in

---

[1] Professor and Head, Division of Geriatric Medicine, McMaster University, Hamilton, Ontario

the mid and high frequencies. Thus, speech is audible but takes on a muffled character and is difficult to understand especially in the presence of background noise. As this type of hearing loss usually develops gradually over many years, the individual may be unaware of the impairment. Because of the ability to respond to low frequency sounds in speech, family and caregivers may attribute misunderstanding to confusion, forgetfulness or inattention. By preventing effective communication, hearing loss can affect physical, emotional, cognitive, behavioral and social functioning. Hearing loss is the most common chronic disability in North America.

At least 25% of individuals over the age of 65 report problems with hearing. Audiologically detectable hearing loss (HL) is present in more than one-third of all people over that age. In a large two-stage survey from the U.K. (postal questionnaire followed by clinical examination), 16% of adults (17-80 years) had a 25 dB HL or greater, 4% a 45 dB HL or greater and 1% a 65 dB HL or greater in both ears. Nine percent had a moderate (≥45 dB HL) impairment in at least one ear.[1] While the overall prevalence of 45 + dB HL in adults aged 18-80 was 4%, it rose sharply with age. Between 61 and 70 years the prevalence was 7%, between 71 and 80 years it was 18%. Eighty percent of hearing loss occurs in people over age 60 years.[2] In the U.S. hearing loss is reported by 23% of persons age 65-74, 33% of those age 75-84, and 48% of persons age 85 and over.[3] In a study of women aged 60-85 residing in two small communities in rural Idaho, 45% had a ≥25 dB HL in mid-range frequencies (1,000-4,000 Hz) and 18% had a ≥40 dB HL in the better ear.[4] In the 18th examination of the Framingham study population, 41% of 1,662 men and women between the 60th and 90th year claim to have hearing problems, and 29% had a ≥26 dB HL.[5] The prevalence of hearing loss is even greater in institutions; 45% of nursing home residents had a ≥40 dB HL at 1,000, 2,000, and 4,000 Hz.[6] The Canadian Hearing Society estimates that 10% of the population are hard of hearing or deaf, (2,535,406 Canadians) and that 84% of people tested in nursing homes have hearing impairment.

Hearing impairment is associated with diminished function in the elderly. For example, in a case series of older individuals screened in primary care practice, a 10 dB increase in hearing loss was associated with a 2.8 point increase in physical Sickness Impact Profile scores.[7] Hearing impairment is associated with more rapid decline in cognitive function in people with Alzheimer's diseases.[8] Even mild hearing loss is associated with memory failure.[9]

The rate for decline of hearing in presbycusis has been studied in a cohort of 1,475 persons over six years. The average threshold change ranged from 1-8 decibels at 250-6,000 Hz, and 10-15 decibels at 8,000 Hz.[10] In a paper drawing on data from longitudinal studies in Great Britain and Denmark, deterioration of hearing impairment

Hearing loss is the most common chronic disability in North America

appeared to be continuous and gradual for the majority (up to 97% on a two-year assessment) with a median of 5-6 decibels per decade.<11>

Maneuver

Detection maneuvers include screening questions, physical tests and pure tone audiometry. In a population of 267 women between the ages of 60 and 85 years from rural Idaho, the single question "Would you say that you have any difficulty hearing?" was found to have a 90% sensitivity for detecting a 40 dB HL at 1,000 and 2,000 kHz and an 83% sensitivity for a 40 dB HL at 1,000 and 4,000 Hz in the better ear. Corresponding specificities were 71% and 75%.<4> The whispered-voice test is administered by whispering six test words at a set distance from the patients ear (6 inches to 2 feet) out of field of vision, and asking the patient to repeat the words. Sensitivity for detecting hearing impairment is reported to be between 80% and 100%, with specificities of 82-89%.<12> The tuning fork test is performed by holding a vibrating fork one inch from the patient's ear and withdrawing it. Failure to hear a vibrating 512 Hz fork at a distance of one foot has a reported sensitivity of 80% and a specificity of 65-82%. Note that testing with a single low frequency is not suitable for screening older people who characteristically lose higher frequencies in presbycusis. The finger-rub test is carried out by rubbing thumb and forefinger together and slowly withdrawing the hand until the patient no longer hears it. Failure to hear this at a distance of 6-8 inches from the ear has a reported sensitivity of 80% and a specificity of 49%. At 3 inches, the sensitivity is reported to be 90%, and the specificity 85%.<12> Inter-observer variability data is not available for the above tests.

The audioscope (manufactured by Welch-Allyn Inc.) is an instrument which serves as both an otoscope and simplified audiometer. It delivers pure tone frequencies at thresholds of either 25 or 40 decibels at 500, 1,000, 2,000 and 4,000 Hz. This instrument has been extensively evaluated, consistently performing with a high sensitivity (87-96%) and specificity (70-90%) in four separate studies.<13-16> The advantage of this instrument is that it allows for inspection of the external auditory meatus and tympanic membrane, while providing a standardized series of pure tones giving considerable accuracy and inter-observer agreement.

Sangster and colleagues offered hearing screening to all patients aged 65 years of age or older attending a family practice over a two-month period in London, Ontario.<17> Excluding those who had ever worn a hearing aid or who had signs of active ear pathology, screening included the use of the audioscope at a setting of 40 dB together with a ten-item screening version of the hearing handicap inventory for the elderly. (HHIE-S) The inventory contains five social-situational items and five emotional response items. Individuals failed the screening if

Many hearing aid users may be unaware that they require major adjustment or replacement of their devices

there was a 40 dB HL or greater at 1,000 Hz and 2,000 Hz in one or both ears, or if they scored more than eight points on the HHIE-S. Of 115 individuals screened, 34 (30%) failed (9 failed audioscope, 14 failed HHIE-S and 11 failed both.) Twenty-five of these agreed to undergo complete audiological evaluation, and 9 declined this recommendation. Of the 25 individuals seen at the audiology clinic, 15 had severe hearing impairment. Eighteen were advised that they were candidates for a hearing aid and/or aural rehabilitation. An unexpected finding was that of 11 individuals with hearing aids, who also underwent complete audiological examination, 10 required major adjustment or replacement of their devices.[17] The sensitivity of the HHIE-10 alone is 65-75% and its specificity is 75-82%.[18,19]

Effectiveness of Prevention and Treatment

Although prevention of hearing impairment may not be possible, primary prevention of noise-induced hearing loss is achievable. Noise control programs and hearing protection are believed to be efficacious[20] based on multiple studies establishing an unequivocal relationship between noise exposure and hearing loss. It is not considered ethical to carry out a randomized trial of hearing protection. The Canadian Task Force previously recommended primary prevention of noise-induced hearing loss through noise control programs and hearing protection (A Recommendation).[21] Risk assessment for hearing loss by history was also recommended (B Recommendation).

When hearing loss is detected, the physician generally refers the patient for a complete audiological examination. Table 1 describes cases where referral is recommended. Where serious or potentially treatable pathology is detected, referral is usually made to an otolaryngologist. A common and readily reversible source of hearing loss is occlusion of the auditory meatus with cerumen.

Hearing loss due to cerumen is commonly missed through failure to examine the ear canal

Recommendations have been made on improving communication with individuals with hearing impairment (see Table 2). In those suitable for amplification, a hearing aid is often helpful. In a randomized controlled trial involving 194 elderly male veterans, subjects were randomly assigned either to receive a hearing aid or to join a waiting list. In those assigned to amplification, significant improvements occurred in social and emotional functions, depression scores, communicative and cognitive abilities by six weeks and continuing to four months.[22] For some patients, a hearing aid tuned to the individual ear with selective amplification of high frequencies, may be preferred.[23] Digital signal processing is a new technique which has shown promise for improving speech recognition by the hearing impaired. In patients with moderate sensorineural hearing loss (65 dB) amplitude processing was associated with 10-12% improvement in intelligibility, but no improvement in those with severe sensorineural loss of 95 dB. For that group, increasing consonant duration gave a modest (5%) benefit in intelligibility.<24>

Predicting who will accept amplification is a challenge because up to 50% of older individuals will not accept a hearing aid. Certain questions which explore self-perceived hearing handicap such as "Do you find it difficult to follow a conversation if there is a background noise, e.g. television, radio, children playing?" may help to distinguish those more likely to accept amplification.<25,26>

Recommendations of Others

Breslow and Somers recommend audiometry for adults every 5 years.<27> The U.S. Preventive Services Task Force previously recommended that "elderly patients should be evaluated regarding their hearing, counselled regarding the availability and use of hearing aids, and referred appropriately for any abnormalities";<28> these recommendations are presently under review. Mulrow & Lichtenstein recommend screening of elderly adults using the audioscope as the maneuver of choice.<29>

Conclusions and Recommendations

Hearing loss is a common problem in older individuals, associated with significant physical, functional and mental health consequences. The prevalence increases with age, and while many older people are aware of disability, a significant proportion are not. Screening maneuvers such as a single question and the use of an audioscope are sensitive and easily performed in the primary care setting. When hearing loss is detected, strategies to enhance communication have been suggested, but have not been critically evaluated.

On the other hand, hearing amplification has been demonstrated to improve the quality of life in a variety of domains although it is unclear whether these results can be generalized to other populations. Factors which predict acceptance of a hearing aid have not been adequately defined. Those wearing hearing aids should be reviewed periodically by an audiologist. Overall, there is fair evidence to include screening for hearing impairment in the periodic health examination in the elderly (B Recommendation) and good evidence to support noise control and hearing protection programs (A Recommendation).

Unanswered Questions (Research Agenda)

The following have been identified as research priorities:

1. Optimal methods of screening for hearing loss in primary care setting.
2. Determination of whether use of amplification changes the rate of cognitive decline in demented people.
3. Best methods of improving compliance with hearing aids.

Evidence

A literature search using MEDLINE was conducted from 1988 to March 1993, using the key words presbycusis, aged, and middle age.

This review was initiated in March 1993 and recommendations were finalized by the Task Force in March 1994.

Acknowledgements

The Task Force thanks Susan Whiteside, MClSc, Senior Audiologist, Chedoke-McMaster Hospital, Hamilton, Ontario and Sharon M. Abel, PhD, Senior Staff Scientist, Division of Clinical Epidemiology and Professor of Otolaryngology, University of Toronto, Toronto, Ontario.

Selected References

1. Davis AC: The prevalence of hearing impairment and reported hearing disability among adults in Great Britain. *Int J Epidemiol* 1989; 18: 911-917

2. Davis AC: Epidemiological profile of hearing impairments: the scale and nature of the problem with special reference to the elderly. *Acta Orolaryngol Suppl Stockh* 1991; 476: 23-31

3. Havlik RJ: Aging in the eighties: Impaired senses for sound and light in persons age 65 and over. Preliminary data from the supplement on aging to the National Health Interview Survey: United States. January-June 1984. Advance data from Vital and Health Statistics No. 125. Hyattsville, Md, National Center for Health Statistics, 1986 [Publications no DHHS (PHS) 86-1250]

4. Clark K, Sowers M, Wallace RB, *et al*: The accuracy of self-reported hearing loss in women aged 60-85 years. *Am J Epidemiol* 1991; 134: 704-708

5. Gates GA, Cooper JC, Kannel WB, *et al*: Hearing in the elderly: the Framingham cohort, 1983-1985. *Ear Hear* 1990; 11: 247-256

6.	Gutnick HN, Zillmer EA, Philput CB: Measurement and prediction of hearing loss in a nursing home. *Ear Hear* 1989; 10: 361-367

7.	Bess FH, Lichtenstein MJ, Logan SA, *et al*: Hearing impairment as a determinant of function in the elderly. *J Am Geriatr Soc* 1989; 37: 123-128

8.	Uhlmann RF, Larson EB, Koepsell TD: Hearing impairment and cognitive decline in senile dementia of the Alzheimer's type. *J Am Geriatr Soc* 1986; 34: 207-210

9.	Rabbitt P: Mild hearing loss can cause apparent memory failures which increase with age and reduce with IQ. *Acta Otolaryngol Suppl Stockh* 1991; 476: 167-175

10.	Gates GA, Cooper JC: Incidence of hearing decline in the elderly. *Acta Otolaryngol Stockh* 1991; 111: 240-248

11.	Davis AC, Ostri B, Parving A: Longitudinal study of hearing. *Acta Otolaryngol Suppl Stockh* 1990; 476: 12-22

12.	Mulrow CD: Screening for hearing impairment in the elderly. *Hosp Pract Off Ed* 1991; 26: 79-86

13.	Bienvenue GR, Michael TL, Chaffinch JO: Reference threshold sound pressure levels for the Welch-Allyn AudioScope. *J Acoust Soc Am* 1984; 75: 1887-1892

14.	Frank T, Peterson DR: Accuracy of a 40 dB HL audioscope and audiometer screening for adults. *Ear Hear* 1987; 8: 180-183

15.	Lichtenstein MJ, Bess FH, Logan SA: Validation of screening tools for identifying hearing-impaired elderly in primary care. *JAMA* 1988; 259: 2875-2878

16.	McBride WS: Screening tests for hearing loss in the elderly. *Clin Res* 1990; 38: 707A

17.	Sangster JF, Gerace TM, Seewald RC: Hearing loss in elderly patients in a family practice. *Can Med Assoc J* 1991; 144: 981-984

18.	O'Rourke CM, Britten CF, Gatschet CA, *et al*: Effectiveness of a hearing screening protocol for the elderly. *Geriatr Nurs New York* 1993; 14: 66-69

19.	Mulrow CD, Lichtenstein MJ: Screening for hearing impairment in the elderly: rationale and strategy. *J Gen Intern Med* 1991; 6: 249-258

20.	Sutor, AH: *Hearing conservation in noise and hearing conservation manual.* 4th Ed. Berger EH, Ward WD, Morrill JC, Royster LH. (Eds). American Industrial Hygiene Association. Akron, Ohio, 1986

21.	Canadian Task Force on the Periodic Health Examination: The periodic health examination. 2. 1984 Update. *Can Med Assoc J* 1984; 130: 1279-1280

22.	Mulrow CD, Aguilar C, Endicott JE, *et al*: Quality-of-life changes and hearing impairment: A randomized trial. *Ann Intern Med* 1990; 113: 188-194

23. MacKenzie K, Browning GG: Randomized, crossover study to assess patient preference for an acoustically modified hearing aid system. *J Laryngol Otol* 1991; 105: 405-408

24. Montgomery AA, Edge RA: Evaluation of two speech enhancement techniques to improve intelligibility for hearing-impaired adults. *J Speech Hear Res* 1988; 31: 386-393

25. John G, Davies E, Stephens D: Predicting who will use a hearing aid. *Practitioner* 1989; 233: 1291-1294

26. Ryding SL, Seewald RC, Corcoran DM, *et al*: Effectiveness of screening for hearing impairment in the elderly: presented at 15th Annual Conference of the Canadian Association of Speech-Language Pathologists & Audiologists, Vancouver, 1990

27. Breslow L, Somers AR: The lifetime health-monitoring program. A practical approach to preventive medicine. *N Engl J Med* 1977; 296: 601-608

28. U.S. Preventive Services Task Force: *Guide to Clinical Preventive Services: an Assessment of the Effectiveness of 169 Interventions*. Williams & Wilkins, Baltimore, Md, 1989: 193-200

29. Mulrow CD, Lichtenstein MJ: Screening for hearing impairment in the elderly: Rationale and strategy. J Gen Intern Med 1991; 6: 249-258

Table 1: Recommendations for referral to audiologist

- When an individual or family member suspects or complains of difficulty hearing or understanding.

- Tinnitus (especially if unilateral, or sudden onset).

- When a hearing aid is owned but not used, or when the device is not producing the desired compensation for hearing loss.

- Any new onset hearing loss (e.g. post traumatic).

- Pre/post exposure to ototoxic medications (e.g. aminoglycoside antibiotics).

- History of work-related noise exposure.

Table 2: Communication Strategies

- Face the person in a clear light.

- Speak clearly and slowly, don't shout.

- Rephrase a misunderstood sentence avoiding high frequency sounds ("Are you okay?" instead of "you seem to be feeling fine").

- Move away from or reduce background noise.

- Do not obscure your mouth or chew while talking.

- Ask the person what you might do to make conversation easier.

- Write down topic of conversation.

Prevention of Hearing Impairment and Disability in the Elderly

MANEUVER	EFFECTIVENESS	LEVEL OF EVIDENCE <REF>	RECOMMENDATION
Screening for hearing impairment	The audioscope has high sensitivity for detecting hearing loss.	Case series <13-16> (III)	Fair evidence to screen the elderly for hearing impairment (B)
	A single question about hearing difficulty has high sensitivity for detecting significant hearing loss.	Case series<4> (III)	
	Whispered-voice out of field of vision has high sensitivity for detecting hearing loss.	Case series<12> (III)	
	Hearing aids improve the quality of life in individuals who are hearing impaired.	Randomized controlled trial<22> (I)	
Noise control programs and hearing protection	Multiple studies demonstrate relationship between noise exposure and hearing loss.	Cohort analytic studies<20> (II-2)	Good evidence to support noise control and hearing protection programs (A)

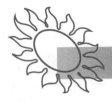

CHAPTER 81

Screening for Asymptomatic Bacteriuria in the Elderly

By Lindsay E. Nicolle

Screening for Asymptomatic Bacteriuria in the Elderly

Prepared by Lindsay E. Nicolle, MD[1]

The proportion of the Canadian population which is elderly will continue to increase over the next several decades. A high proportion of these elderly individuals will reside for at least some time in a long-term care facility. There is a marked increase in prevalence and incidence of bacteriuria in older populations. Most of this bacteriuria appears to be asymptomatic. For the institutionalized elderly with multiple co-morbidities and substantial functional impairment the prevalence of bacteriuria is extremely high. It has been argued that bacteriuria in the elderly, particularly associated with pyuria, which is evidence for a host response, should be treated. Identification and treatment of asymptomatic bacteriuria, however, would require repeated screening of elderly populations and intense antimicrobial exposure. In 1979 the Canadian Task Force on the Periodic Health Examination found that there was fair evidence that routine screening for urinary tract infection not be included among conditions sought in a periodic health examination.[1,2]

Burden of Suffering

The prevalence of asymptomatic bacteriuria increases with age for men and women, and is greater in institutionalized populations

Population studies in women report a prevalence of bacteriuria of 2-4% among sexually active young women which increases to 6-8% in women aged 60 years, and over 20% in well elderly women in the community over 80 years.[3] Bacteriuria is uncommon in younger male populations, with a prevalence of less than 1% until about age 60 years. From 1-3% of men aged 60-65 will have bacteriuria, and the prevalence increases to 10% or more for men over age 80 years.[3] The prevalence of bacteriuria is extraordinarily high for the more impaired elderly with functional deficits and co-morbid illnesses who require institutional care. Studies consistently report a prevalence of bacteriuria from 30-50% for institutionalized women and 20-30% for institutionalized men.[2] Limited studies also suggest a high incidence of bacteriuria for the institutionalized and ambulant elderly.[3,4]

Bacteriuria in the elderly is usually asymptomatic. Morbidity with asymptomatic bacteriuria may include short-term complications of acute symptomatic infection and potential long-term complications of renal failure or mortality. Measuring the burden of illness potentially related to asymptomatic bacteriuria in the elderly is, however, limited

[1] Associate Professor of Medicine/Medical Microbiology, University of Manitoba, Winnipeg, Manitoba

by several factors. First, no population-based studies in the ambulatory elderly document the occurence and impact of symptomatic urinary infection. Second, chronic genitourinary symptoms are frequent in the elderly population. Such symptoms are not ameliorated by treatment of associated asymptomatic bacteriuria and occur with equal frequency in bacteriuric and nonbacteriuric elderly populations.<5> Thus, while not due to bacteriuria, they may complicate the identification of symptomatic infection. Finally, the multiple co-morbid illnesses and functional disability of the elderly institutionalized population leads to impaired communication and identification of symptomatic infection.

Limited reports document the frequency of symptomatic infection in elderly populations. Boscia et al reported 10 of 61 elderly ambulatory women with untreated asymptomatic bacteriuria became symptomatic during 6 months of follow-up, an incidence of 0.9/1000 patient days.<6> Mims et al followed 238 elderly men from 1 to 4.5 years, 29 of whom were initially bacteriuric and 17 of 134 who were followed for one year or more who subsequently became bacteriuric.<7> Only 5 patients of the initial bacteriuric group became symptomatic and they were apparently treated with antimicrobial therapy with resolution and without further complication. In 50 elderly institutionalized women with asymptomatic bacteriuria, half of whom were treated, 4 episodes of symptomatic infection occurred in one year of follow-up, an incidence of 0.26/1000 patient days.<8> In 36 elderly institutionalized men with asymptomatic bacteriuria followed for a mean of 10.6 months, 16 of whom were treated with antimicrobials, 4 episodes of symptomatic infection or 0.34/1000 patient days developed.<9>

Urinary infection is the most common cause of bacteremia in both institutionalized and noninstitutionalized elderly populations.<3,4> Women over age 65 with acute non-obstructive pyelonephritis are more likely to be bacteremic than younger women. The case fatality rate associated with bacteremic urinary infection in the elderly has been reported to be from 10-30%. Despite these observations urinary infection is rarely a direct cause of death in elderly subjects.<3,4>

Several other clinical presentations in the elderly are frequently attributed to urinary infection because of the difficulty in ascertainment of symptoms and high prevalence of bacteriuria in this population. Where specific symptom presentations other than pyelonephritis or lower tract irritative symptoms have been critically studied, however, urinary infection has not been documented to be an important contributor to such symptoms. For instance, gross hematuria is seldom attributable to hemorrhagic cystitis in institutionalized elderly subjects despite a high prevalence of bacteriuria in residents with gross hematuria.<10> Limited studies suggest that nonspecific changes in clinical status in the absence of fever are not attributable to urinary infection.<11> The majority of febrile episodes of uncertain cause in the non-catheterized bacteriuric elderly are likely not caused by invasive urinary infection, although the contribution of urinary infection in an individual case may be impossible to ascertain.

Asymptomatic bacteriuria in the elderly is not associated with increased mortality

The contribution of asymptomatic bacteriuria to mortality in the elderly has been controversial. Initial studies from Finland[12] and Greece[13] suggested decreased survival in both women and men with asymptomatic bacteriuria. Subsequent studies in community populations from Sweden[14] and Finland[15] have not supported these initial observations. No association of bacteriuria with mortality has been reported for the institutionalized population.[16] Currently evidence does not support a direct or indirect causal association of asymptomatic bacteriuria with mortality in elderly populations. In addition, there is no evidence that asymptomatic bacteriuria, by itself, progresses to renal failure in this population.

Maneuver

Screening by culture or non-culture (e.g. leukocyte esterase/nitrate dipstick) methods of urine of asymptomatic elderly subjects to identify bacteriuria with subsequent antimicrobial treatment of bacteriuria.

Effectiveness of Prevention and Treatment

Ambulatory Elderly

Asymptomatic bacteriuria in the ambulant elderly is associated with limited morbidity

Boscia et al[5] studied 124 non-institutionalized ambulatory elderly women and reported that identification and treatment of asymptomatic bacteriuria decreased the frequency of symptomatic episodes from 16% to 8% in the subsequent 6 month period. The type of symptom presentation was not described. This difference was not statistically significant. The prevalence of bacteriuria at 6 months after treatment was 64% in the non-treated group and 35% in those who were treated. Mortality for the treated (3.2%) and untreated (4.9%) groups was not different (p=0.66). Cost analysis was not performed.

No prospective, randomized study of therapy vs. no therapy for asymptomatic bacteriuria in the non-institutionalized elderly male has been reported. One prospective cohort study provides limited data describing morbidity.[7] In this study, 234 elderly men were followed for up to 4.5 years, 134 for over one year. Twenty-nine were bacteriuric at initial screening and 20 became positive in follow-up. The majority (76%) of bacteriuric subjects spontaneously cleared bacteriuria after a mean period of 4.4 months (range 3-12 months). Only 5 (17%) bacteriuric subjects were treated for symptomatic infection and bacteriuria recurred rapidly during post-treatment in 3 of these 5. The symptom presentations were not described, and no significant detrimental outcomes with development of symptomatic infection were reported. This study suggested a high frequency of spontaneous resolution of asymptomatic bacteriuria in elderly non-institutionalized men and a low frequency of symptom development. It was concluded that screening for and treatment of asymptomatic bacteriuria was not warranted in ambulatory elderly men.

Institutionalized Elderly

Prospective, randomized studies in institutionalized women[8] and men[9] have documented no benefits of screening for and treatment of asymptomatic bacteriuria. In 36 institutionalized elderly men randomized to treatment or non-treatment and followed for 2 years, subsequent symptomatic episodes occurred with equal frequency in treated or non-treated subjects.[9] Mortality was 5 (31%) in treated and 5 (25%) in untreated subjects. In 50 institutionalized elderly women randomized to treatment or no treatment and followed for one year, morbidity from urinary infection was similar in treated and non-treated groups.[8] Antimicrobial therapy, however, was associated with significantly more adverse medication effects, increased reinfections, and a tendency to emergence of resistance. Mortality was 4 (18%) for untreated and 9 (39%) for treated subjects. Thus, these studies in the institutionalized elderly support the non-treatment of asymptomatic bacteriuria.

Trials of treatment of asymptomatic bacteriuria in institutionalized populations have not demonstrated any benefits of antimicrobial therapy

One characteristic of the institutionalized bacteriuric elderly is the rapid recurrence of bacteriuria following antimicrobial therapy.[8,9] In most individuals, treatment of asymptomatic bacteriuria is followed by an extremely short period free of bacteriuria, with over 50% recurring within 2-4 weeks of discontinuing antimicrobials. In institutionalized women with urine cultures obtained monthly, screening and antimicrobial treatment of all identified episodes decreased the overall prevalence of bacteriuria in the population by only 30% over a one year period.[8] Thus, for the institutionalized population, even intensive antimicrobial therapy for asymptomatic bacteriuria has limited impact on bacteriuria. Even if benefits of treatment of asymptomatic bacteriuria in the elderly were identified, frequent repeated screening for urinary infection would be required.

Subjects with long-term indwelling catheters are virtually always bacteriuric. Screening for bacteriuria or pyuria in these subjects will not identify those at risk for morbidity.[17] Antimicrobial therapy of asymptomatic catheter-acquired bacteriuria does not decrease morbidity from urinary infection, but will lead to emergence of organisms of increased resistance.[18]

Recommendations of Others

The recommendations of the U.S. Preventive Services Task Force on screening for asymptomatic urinary tract infection are currently under review. Other authors[19] have suggested there is no indication for screening for or treatment of asymptomatic bacteriuria in elderly populations.

Conclusions and Recommendations

There is no evidence that treatment of asymptomatic bacteriuria in elderly populations is beneficial. Treatment of asymptomatic bacteriuria will not decrease the frequency of symptomatic episodes or alter outcomes in institutionalized populations and may be associated with an increased occurence of resistant organisms. For the non-institutionalized elderly, while there may be some small decrease in the occurence of symptomatic infection, the data do not indicate sufficient impact to suggest that it would be cost effective. For men, the lack of evidence for short- or long-term adverse outcomes in those with asymptomatic bacteriuria suggests that treatment would not be indicated, although comparative randomized trials are not available for this group. Thus, there is good to fair evidence not to screen elderly populations for the presence of asymptomatic bacteriuria (D and E Recommendations depending upon subgroup). However, for ambulatory elderly women, specifically, there is insufficient evidence to recommend for or against screening (C Recommendation).

Unanswered Questions (Research Agenda)

The following have been identified as research priorities:

1. Population based studies documenting the impact of morbidity from symptomatic urinary infection in non-institutionalized elderly women and men.

2. Defining the clinical significance of a positive urine culture in ambulatory elderly men as it relates to prostatic obstruction or other genitourinary abnormalities.

3. Contribution of bacteriuria to episodes of fever in the institutionalized elderly with a positive urine culture.

Evidence

The literature was identified with a MEDLINE search to March 1993 using the following MESH headings: urinary tract infections, aged, human, case reports.

This review was initiated in June 1993 and recommendations were finalized by the Task Force in October 1993.

Selected References

1. Report of a Task Force to the Conference of Deputy Ministers of Health (cat. no. H39-3/1980E), Health Services and Promotion Branch, Department of National Health and Welfare, Ottawa, 1980

2. Canadian Task Force on the Periodic Health Examination: The periodic health examination. *Can Med Assoc J* 1979; 121: 1193-1254

3. Nicolle LE: Urinary tract infection in the elderly. *J Antimicrob Chemother* 1994; 33(Suppl A): 99-109

4. Nicolle LE: Urinary tract infections in long-term care facilities. *Infect Control Hosp Epidemiol* 1993; 14: 220-225

5. Boscia JA, Kobasa WD, Abrutyn E, *et al*: Lack of association between bacteriuria and symptoms in the elderly. *Am J Med* 1986; 81: 979-982

6. Boscia JA, Kobasa WD, Knight RA, *et al*: Therapy vs no therapy for bacteriuria in elderly ambulatory nonhospitalized women. *JAMA* 1987; 257: 1067-1071

7. Mims AD, Norman DC, Yamamura RH, *et al*: Clinically inapparent (asymptomatic) bacteriuria in ambulatory elderly men: epidemiological, clinical, and microbiological findings. *J Am Geriatr Soc* 1990; 38: 1209-1214

8. Nicolle LE, Mayhew WJ, Bryan L: Prospective, randomized comparison of therapy and no therapy for asymptomatic bacteriuria in institutionalized elderly women. *Am J Med* 1987; 83: 27-33

9. Nicolle LE, Bjornson J, Harding GKM, *et al*: Bacteriuria in elderly institutionalized men. *New Engl J Med* 1983; 309: 1420-1425

10. Nicolle LE, Orr P, Duckworth H, *et al*: Gross hematuria in residents of long-term care facilities. *Am J Med* 1993; 94: 611-618

11. Berman P, Hogan DB, Fox RA: The atypical presentation of infection in old age. *Age Ageing* 1987; 16: 201-207

12. Sourander LB, Kasanen A: A 5 year follow-up of bacteriuria in the aged. *Gerontologica Clinica* 1972; 14: 274-281

13. Dontas AS, Kasviki-Charvati P, Papanayiotou PC, *et al*: Bacteriuria and survival in old age. *New Engl J Med* 1981; 304: 939-943

14. Nordenstam GR, Brandberg CA, Oden AS, *et al*: Bacteriuria and mortality in an elderly population. *New Engl J Med* 1986; 314: 1152-1156

15. Heinamaki P, Haavisto M, Hakuline T, *et al*: Mortality in relation to urinary characteristics in the very aged. *Gerontology* 1986; 32: 167-171

16. Nicolle LE, Henderson E, Bjornson J, *et al*: The association of bacteriuria with resident characteristics and survival in elderly institutionalized men. *Ann Intern Med* 1987; 106: 682-686

17. Warren JW: Catheter-associated bacteriuria. *Clinic Ger Med* 1992; 8: 805-819

18. Warren JW, Anthony WC, Hoopes JM, *et al*: Cephalexin for susceptible bacteriuria in afebrile, long-term catheterized patients. *JAMA* 1982; 248: 454-458

19. Boscia JA, Abrutyn E, Kaye D: Asymptomatic bacteriuria in elderly persons: treat or do not treat. *Ann Intern Med* 1987; 106: 764-766

Screening for Asymptomatic Bacteriuria in the Elderly

MANEUVER	EFFECTIVENESS	LEVEL OF EVIDENCE <REF>	RECOMMENDATION
Screening urine to identify bacteriuria by culture or leukocyte esterase/nitrite dipstick in asymptomatic subjects and antimicrobial treatment of bacteriuria	Ambulatory elderly women: nonsignificant decrease in symptomatic infection in subsequent 6 months after treatment.	Randomized controlled trial<6> (I)	Insufficient evidence to recommend for or against screening and treatment (C)
	Ambulatory elderly men: no evidence for significant morbidity and mortality from untreated asymptomatic bacteriuria.	Prospective cohort study<7> (II-2)	Fair evidence to exclude screening or treatment (D)
	Institutionalized elderly women: no decrease in morbidity or mortality, increased occurrence of adverse drug effects and antimicrobial resistant organisms with antimicrobial therapy compared to no therapy.	Randomized controlled trial<8> (I)	Good evidence that screening and treatment not be included in PHE (E)
	Institutionalized elderly men: no decrease in morbidity or mortality with antimicrobial therapy compared with no therapy.	Randomized controlled trial<9> (I)	Good evidence that screening and treatment not be included (E)
	Subjects with long term indwelling catheters: morbidity similar with or without antimicrobial therapy; increased antimicrobial resistance with therapy.	Randomized controlled trials<18> (I)	Good evidence that screening and treatment not be included (E)

973

Appendix A

Previous Publications by the Canadian Task Force on the Periodic Health Examination

In English

1. *Report of a Task Force to the Conference of Deputy Ministers of Health* (cat no. H39-3/1980E), Health Services and Promotion Branch, Department of National Health and Welfare, Ottawa, 1980

2. Canadian Task Force on the Periodic Health Examination: The periodic health examination. *Can Med Assoc J* 1979; 121: 1193-1254

3. Spitzer WO: The periodic health examination: 1. Introduction. *Can Med Assoc J* 1984; 130: 1276-1278

4. Canadian Task Force on the Periodic Health Examination: The periodic health examination: 2. 1984 update. *Can Med Assoc J* 1984; 130: 1278-1285

5. Battista RN, Beaulieu MD, Feightner JW, Mann KV, Owen G: The periodic health examination: 3. An evolving concept. *Can Med Assoc J* 1984; 130(10): 1288-1292

6. Goldbloom RB, Battista RN: The periodic health examination: 1. Introduction. *Can Med Assoc J* 1986; 130: 721-723

7. Canadian Task Force on the Periodic Health Examination: The periodic health examination: 2. 1985 update. *Can Med Assoc J* 1986; 134: 724-727

8. Morrison B: The Periodic Health Examination: 3. Breast Cancer. *Can Med Assoc J* 1986 Apr 1; 134: 728-729

9. Goldbloom RB, Battista RN: The periodic health examination: 1. Introduction. *Can Med Assoc J* 1988; 138: 617-618

10. Canadian Task Force on the Periodic Health Examination: The periodic health examination: 2. 1987 update. *Can Med Assoc J* 1988; 138: 618-626

11. Battista RN, Lawrence RS (eds): Implementing preventive services. *Am J Prev Med* 1988; Suppl 4(4): i-x,1-194

12. Goldbloom RB, Battista RN, Haggerty J: The periodic health examination: 1. Introduction. *Can Med Assoc J* 1989; 141: 205-207

13. Canadian Task Force on the Periodic Health Examination: The periodic health examination: 2. 1989 update. *Can Med Assoc J* 1989; 141: 208-216

14. Idem: Periodic health examination, 1989 update: 3. Preschool examination for developmental, visual and hearing problems. *Can Med Assoc J* 1989; 141: 1136-1140

15. Idem: Periodic health examination, 1989 update: 4. Intrapartum electronic fetal monitoring and prevention of neonatal herpes simplex. *Can Med Assoc J* 1989; 141: 1233-1240

16. Idem: Periodic health examination, 1990 update: 1. Early detection of hyperthyroidism and hypothyroidism in adults and screening of newborns for congenital hypothyroidism. *Can Med Assoc J* 1990; 142(9): 955-961

17. Feightner JW, Worrall G: Early detection of depression by primary care physicians. *Can Med Assoc J* 1990; 142: 1215-1220

18. McNamee JE, Offord DR: Prevention of Suicide. *Can Med Assoc J* 1990; 142(11): 1223-1230

19. Canadian Task Force on the Periodic Health Examination: Periodic health examination, 1990 update: 2. Early detection of depression and prevention of suicide. *Can Med Assoc J* 1990; 142(11): 1233-1238

20. Goldbloom RB, Lawrence R (eds): *Preventing Disease: Beyond the Rhetoric.* Springer-Verlag, New York, 1990

21. Woolf SH, Battista RN, Anderson GM, Logan AG, Wang E and other members of the Canadian Task Force on the Periodic Health Examination. Assessing the clinical effectiveness of preventive maneuvers: Analytic principles and systematic methods in reviewing evidence and developing clinical practice recommendations. *J Clin Epidemiol* 1990; 43(9): 891-905

22. Canadian Task Force on the Periodic Health Examination: Periodic health examination, 1990 update: 3. Interventions to prevent lung cancer other than smoking cessation. *Can Med Assoc J* 1990; 143(4): 269-272

23. Idem: Periodic health examination, 1990 update: 4. Well-baby care in the first 2 years of life. *Can Med Assoc J* 1990; 143(9): 867-872

24. Idem: Periodic health examination, 1991 update: 1. Screening for cognitive impairment in the elderly. *Can Med Assoc J* 1991; 144: 425-431

25. Idem: Periodic health examination, 1991 update: 2. Administration of pneumococcal vaccine. *Can Med Assoc J* 1991; 144: 665-671

26. Idem: Periodic health examination, 1991 update: 3. Secondary prevention of prostate cancer. *Can Med Assoc J* 1991; 145: 413-428

27. Idem: Periodic health examination, 1991 update: 4. Screening for cystic fibrosis. *Can Med Assoc J* 1991; 145: 629-635

28. Idem: Periodic health examination, 1991 update: 5. Screening for abdominal aortic aneurysm. *Can Med Assoc J* 1991; 145: 783-789

29. Idem: Periodic health examination, 1991 update: 6. Acetylsalicylic acid and the primary prevention of cardiovascular disease. *Can Med Assoc J* 1991; 145: 1091-1095

30. Idem: Periodic health examination, 1992 update: 1. Screening for gestational diabetes. *Can Med Assoc J* 1992; 147: 435-443

31. Idem: Periodic health examination, 1992 update: 2. Routine prenatal ultrasound screening. *Can Med Assoc J* 1992; 147: 627-633

32. Idem: Periodic health examination, 1992 update: 3. HIV antibody screening. *Can Med Assoc J* 1992; 147: 867-876

33. Idem: Periodic health examination, 1992 update: 4. Prophylaxis for gonococcal and chlamydial ophthalmia neonatorum. *Can Med Assoc J* 1992; 147: 1449-1454

34. MacMillan HC, MacMillan JH, Offord DR with the Canadian Task Force on the Periodic Health Examination: Periodic health examination, 1993 update: 1. Primary prevention of child maltreatment. *Can Med Assoc J* 1993; 148: 151-163

35. Canadian Task Force on the Periodic Health Examination: Periodic health examination, 1993 update: 2. Lowering the blood total cholesterol level to prevent coronary heart disease. *Can Med Assoc J* 1993; 148: 521-538

36. Ismail AI, Lewis DW with the Canadian Task Force on the Periodic Health Examination: Periodic health examination, 1993 update: 3. Periodontal disease: classification, diagnosis, risk factors and prevention. *Can Med Assoc J* 1993; 149: 1409-1422

37. Canadian Task Force on the Periodic Health Examination: Periodic health examination, 1994 update: 1. Obesity in childhood. *Can Med Assoc J* 1994; 150: 871-879

38. Solomon MJ, McLeod RS with the Canadian Task Force on the Periodic Health Examination: Periodic health examination, 1994 update: 2. Screening strategies for colorectal cancer. *Can Med Assoc J* 1994; 150: 1961-1970

39. Canadian Task Force on the Periodic Health Examination: Periodic health examination, 1994 update: 3. Primary and secondary prevention of neural tube defects. *Can Med Assoc J* 1994; 151: 159-166

In French

1. L'examen médical périodique, monographie. Rapport d'un groupe d'étude à la Conférence des sous-ministres de la santé (cat. n° H39-3/1980F), Direction générale des services et de la promotion de la santé, ministère de la Santé nationale et du Bien-être social, Ottawa, 1980

2. Groupe d'étude sur l'examen médical périodique: L'examen médical périodique. *Union méd can* 1979; 108(Suppl.): 1-48

3. Spitzer WO: L'examen médical périodique: mise à jour 1984: 1. Introduction. *Union méd can* 1984; 113(9): 795-796

4. Groupe d'étude sur l'examen médical périodique: L'examen médical périodique: 2. Mise à jour 1984. *Union méd can* 1984; 113(9): 796-803

5. Battista RN, Beaulieu MD, Feightner JW, Mann KV, Owen G: L'examen médical périodique: 3. Un concept en évolution. *Union méd can* 1984; 113(9): 804-808

6. Goldbloom R, Battista RN: L'examen médical périodique: mise à jour 1985: 1. Introduction. *Union méd can* 1986; 115(4): 264-266

7. Groupe d'étude sur l'examen médical périodique: L'examen médical périodique: 2. mise à jour 1985. *Union méd can* 1986; 115(4): 266-269

8. Morrison B: 3. Le cancer du sein. *Union méd can* 1986; 115(4): 269-271

9. Goldbloom R, Battista RN: L'examen médical périodique: mise à jour 1987. *Union méd can* 1988; 117(2): 195-196

10. Groupe d'étude sur l'examen médical périodique: L'examen médical périodique (1re partie): L'ostéoporose postménopausique et les fractures en rapport avec cette maladie. *Union méd can* 1988; 118(3): 196-203

11. Groupe d'étude sur l'examen médical périodique: L'examen médical périodique (2ième partie): Les grossesses non désirées chez les adolescents. Cancer de l'endomètre. *Union méd can* 1988; 118(3): 236-237, 239-240

12. Idem: L'examen médical périodique: mise à jour 1989, Partie 1. *Union méd can* 1989; 118(6): 242, 245-248

13. Idem: L'examen médical périodique: mise à jour 1989, Partie 2. *Union méd can* 1990; 119(1): 16-17, 19-20, 23

14. Idem: L'examen médical périodique: mise à jour 1989, Partie 3. *Union méd can* 1990; 119(5): 248-250, 253

15. Idem: L'examen médical périodique: mise à jour 1989, Partie 4. *Union méd can* 1990; 119(5): 254-260

16. Idem: L'examen médical périodique, mise à jour 1990: 1. Dépistage précoce de l'hyperthyroïdie et de l'hypothyroïdie chez les adultes et dépistage de l'hypothyroïdie chez les nouveau-nés. *Union méd can* 1990; 119(6): 331-339

17. Idem: L'examen médical périodique, mise à jour 1990: 2. Dépistage précoce de la dépression et prévention du suicide. *Union méd can* 1991; 120(1): 17-22

18. Idem: L'examen médical périodique, mise à jour 1990: 3. Interventions visant à prévenir le cancer du poumon par d'autres moyens que le renoncement au tabac. *Union méd can* 1991; 120(2): 61-63

19. Idem: L'examen médical périodique, mise à jour 1990: 4. Consultations pédiatriques au cours des deux premieres années de la vie du bébé. *Union méd can* 1991; 120(5): 327-332

20. Idem: L'examen médical périodique, mise à jour 1991: 1. Dépistage des déficiences cognitives chez les personnes âgées. *Union méd can* 1991; 120(6): 425, 427, 430-432

21. Idem: L'examen médical périodique, mise à jour 1991: 2. Administration du vaccin pneumococcique. *Union méd can* 1992; 121(1): 22-28

22. Idem: L'examen médical périodique, mise à jour 1991: 3. Prévention secondaire du cancer de la prostate. *Union méd can* 1992 Jul-Août; 121(4): 243-245, 248-257

23. Idem: L'examen médical périodique, mise à jour 1991: 4. Dépistage de la fibrose kystique du pancréas (mucoviscidose). *Union méd can* 1992 Sep-Oct; 121(5): 298-306

24. Idem: L'examen médical périodique, mise à jour 1991: 5. Dépistage de l'anévrisme de l'aorte abdominale. *Union méd can* 1992 Nov-Déc; 121(6): 350-357, 388

25. Idem: L'examen médical périodique, mise à jour 1991: 6. L'acide acétylsalicylique et la prévention primaire des maladies cardiovasculaires. *Union méd can* 1993 Mars-Avr; 122(2): 109-113

26. Idem: L'examen médical périodique, mise à jour 1992: 1. Le dépistage du diabète gestationnel. *Union méd can* 1993 Mai-Juin; 122(3): 191-200

27. Idem: L'examen médical périodique, mise à jour 1992: 2. Dépistage systématique par échographie prénatale. *Union méd can* 1993 Jul-Août; 122(4): 260-265

28. Idem: L'examen médical périodique, mise à jour 1992: 3. Le dépistage des anticorps anti-VIH. *Union méd can* 1993 Sep-Oct; 122(5): 322-328, 330-332

29. Idem: L'examen médical périodique, mise à jour 1992: 4. Prophylaxie de l'ophtalmie à gonocoques et à chlamydia du nouveau-né. *Union méd can* 1993; 122(6): 406-410

30. MacMillan HC, MacMillan JH, Offord DR avec la contribution de Groupe d'étude canadien sur l'examen médical périodique: L'examen médical périodique, mise à jour 1993: 1. La prévention primaire des mauvais treatements infligés aux enfants (1re partie). *Union méd can* 1994; 123(2): 101-108

31. MacMillan HC, MacMillan JH, Offord DR avec la contribution de Groupe d'étude canadien sur l'examen médical périodique: L'examen médical périodique, mise à jour 1993: 1. La prévention primaire des mauvais traitements infligés aux enfants (2ième partie). *Union méd can* 1994; 123(3): 172-182

32. Groupe d'étude canadien sur l'examen médical périodique: L'examen médical périodique, mise à jour 1993: 2. Abaissement de la cholestérolémie dans la prévention des maladies coronariennes (1re partie). *Union méd can* 1994; 123(4): 249-258, 312-326

Appendix B

Maneuvers to be Included in Clinical Preventive Health Care

Recommendations of the Canadian Task Force on the Periodic Health Examination Not Updated Since 1979

These tables summarize maneuvers reviewed by the Canadian Task Force on the Periodic Health Examination in 1979 that were not updated in this text. However, the medical evidence at that time established that benefits outweighed potential harm. All other interventions that the Task Force has recommended in the past (A and B Recommendations) have been updated in the 1994 Guide. However, note that Duchenne muscular dystrophy, Tay-Sachs disease and Progressive incapacity with aging are currently under review.

The information is displayed with "A Recommendations" for the general population at the top (maneuvers for which there is strong evidence for inclusion in a periodic health examination). The second grouping on each page are "B Recommendations" for the general population. (Maneuvers for which there is *fair* evidence for inclusion in a periodic health examination). A subsection of each group of recommendations specifically addresses recommendations for high-risk populations.

CONDITION	MANEUVER	POPULATION
GOOD EVIDENCE TO INCLUDE (A RECOMMENDATIONS):		
Tetanus	Immunization, booster every 10 years	Adults
Immunizable conditions related to international travel	Immunization	For travellers without contraindications
Syphilis	Serologic testing	Pregnant women
High-risk populations		
Meningococcal meningitis	Immunization	Military recruits and travellers
Toxoplasmosis	Exposure history, serologic testing and hygiene counselling	Non-immune pregnant women who keep a cat at home or eat raw meat
Syphilis	Serologic testing	Individuals with a history of multiple sexual partners
FAIR EVIDENCE TO INCLUDE (B RECOMMENDATIONS):		
Hemorrhagic disease of the newborn	Vitamin K_1, 1 mg	Newborns
Hearing impairment	History and clinical examination	Adults attending for other reasons
Orthodontic conditions	Oral examination and roentgenography	Children
Progressive incapacity with aging[1]	Home visit – enquiry into physical, psychological and social competence	Elderly
High-risk populations		
Duchenne muscular dystrophy (DMD)[1]	Serum creatine phosphokinase determination	Female relatives of DMD patients
Interventricular septal defect	History and clinical examination	At birth and discharge from nursery
Tay-Sachs disease[1]	Measure resistance of serum hexosaminidase to heat inactivation	Premarital screening of high-risk including Ashkenazi Jews
Preterm labour	History; cerclage of cervix	Pregnant women

[1] Currently under review

Appendix C

List of Contributors

Author	Chapter or Contribution

Geoffrey Anderson, M.D., Ph.D.[‡]
Senior Scientist
Institute for Clinical Evaluative Sciences
Associate Professor
Department of Health Administration
University of Toronto
Toronto, Ontario
	Methodology;
	Routine prenatal ultrasound screening;
	The use of home uterine activity
	   monitoring to prevent preterm birth;
	Intrapartum electronic fetal monitoring;
	Acetylsalicylic acid and the primary
	   prevention of cardiovascular disease

John S. Andrews, M.D. Instructor Department of Pediatrics Johns Hopkins University Baltimore, Maryland, U.S	Screening for hemoglobinopathies in Canada
David Atkins, M.D., M.P.H. Clinical Assistant Professor Georgetown University Medical Center Washington, D.C., U.S.	Science Advisor U.S. Preventive Services Task Force
Robert Baldwin, M.D. Post-Doctoral Fellow Johns Hopkins University Department of Pediatrics Baltimore, Maryland, U.S.	Screening for phenylketonuria
Renaldo N. Battista, M.D., Sc.D., F.R.C.P.C.[‡] Director Division of Clinical Epidemiology Montreal General Hospital McGill University Montreal, Quebec	Methodology; Asymptomatic carotid disease

Note: [‡] = Member of the Canadian Task Force on the Periodic Health Examination
[†] = Member of the U.S. Preventive Services Task Force

Author	Chapter or Contribution
Brenda L. Beagan, M.A. Research Associate, Canadian Task Force on the Periodic Health Examination 1990-92 Dalhousie University Halifax, Nova Scotia	Primary and secondary prevention of neural tube defects; Screening for childhood obesity; Prevention of gonorrhea
Marie-Dominique Beaulieu, M.D., F.C.F.P., M.Sc.[†] Associate Professor Department of Family Medicine University of Montreal Montreal, Quebec	Screening for gestational diabetes mellitus; Primary and secondary prevention of neural tube defects; Screening for D (Rh) sensitization in pregnancy; Screening and vaccinating adolescents and adults to prevent congenital rubella syndrome; Prevention of preeclampsia; Screening for congenital hypothyroidism; Physical activity counselling; Screening for diabetes mellitus in the non-pregnant adult; Screening for thyroid disorders and thyroid cancer in asymptomatic adults
Alfred O. Berg, M.D., M.P.H.[†] Professor and Associate Chair Department of Family Medicine University of Washington Seattle, Washington, U.S.	Member, U.S. Preventive Services Task force.
Michelle Berlin, M.D., M.P.H. Assistant Professor Department of Obstetrics and Gynecology University of Pennsylvania Medical Center Philadelphia, Pennsylvania, U.S.	Prevention of Preeclampsia

Appendix C – *Cont'd*

Author	Chapter or Contribution
Donald M. Berwick, M.D., M.P.P.[†] Vice-Chair U.S. Preventive Services Task Force Associate Professor Department of Pediatrics Harvard Medical School Boston, Massachusetts, U.S.	Physical activity counselling
John Burress, M.D., M.P.H. Research Fellow Harvard School of Public Health Occupational and Environmental Medicine Boston, Massachusetts, U.S.	Physical activity counselling
Robert Côté, M.D., F.R.C.P.C. Division of Clinical Epidemiology Montreal General Hospital Associate Professor Department of Neurology and Neurosurgery McGill University Montreal, Quebec	Asymptomatic carotid disease
Deborah L. Craig, M.P.H. Health Care Consultant Halifax, Nova Scotia	Primary prevention of fetal alcohol syndrome
Orlando P. da Silva, M.D., F.R.C.P.C. Department of Pediatrics Division of Neonatology The University of Western Ontario St. Joseph's Health Centre London, Ontario	Prevention of low birth weight/preterm birth

Appendix C – *Cont'd*

Author	Chapter or Contribution
H. Dele Davies, M.D., M.Sc., F.R.C.P.C. Assistant Professor Departments of Microbiology, Infectious Disease and Pediatrics University of Calgary Calgary, Alberta	Screening for Chlamydia infection
Paul Dick, M.D.C.M., F.R.C.P.C. Assistant Professor Department of Pediatrics University of Toronto Toronto, Ontario	Prenatal screening and diagnosis for Down Syndrome prevention
Carolyn DiGuiseppi, M.D., M.P.H. Science Advisor U.S. Preventive Services Task Force Office of Disease Prevention and Health Promotion Washington, D.C., U.S.	Screening for D (Rh) sensitization in pregnancy; Screening and vaccinating adolescents and adults to prevent congenital rubella syndrome; Screening children for lead exposure in Canada; Hepatitis B immunization in childhood; Screening for thyroid disorders and thyroid cancer in asymptomatic adults; Prevention of skin cancer; Prevention of pancreatic cancer
Jennifer L. Dingle, M.B.A. Coordinator, Canadian Task Force on the Periodic Health Examination Department of Pediatrics Dalhousie University Halifax, Nova Scotia	Methodology; Prevention of periodontal disease; Prevention of tobacco-caused illness; Prevention of unintended pregnancy and sexually transmitted diseases in adolescents
James Douketis, M.D. Clinical Research Fellow in Thromboembolism Department of Medicine McMaster University Hamilton, Ontario	Prevention of obesity in adults

Appendix C – *Cont'd*

Author	Chapter or Contribution
R. Wayne Elford, M.D., C.C.F.P., F.C.F.P.[‡] Professor and Director of Research and Faculty Development Department of Family Medicine University of Calgary Calgary, Alberta	Overview tables Prevention of household and recreational injuries in children (<15 years of age); Prevention of motor vehicle accidents; Prevention of household and recreational injuries in adults; Prevention of influenza; Screening for testicular cancer; Prevention of household and recreational injuries in the elderly
Denice S. Feig, M.D., F.R.C.P.C. Assistant Professor Department of Medicine University of Toronto Toronto, Ontario	Prevention of osteoporotic fractures in women by estrogen replacement therapy
John W. Feightner, M.D., M.Sc., F.C.F.P.[‡] Professor Department of Family Medicine McMaster University Hamilton, Ontario	Routine iron supplementation during pregnancy; Prevention of iron deficiency anemia in infants; Preschool screening for developmental problems; Routine preschool screening for visual and hearing problems; Early detection of depression; Screening for prostate cancer; Prevention of skin cancer

Author	Chapter or Contribution
William Feldman, M.D., F.R.C.P.C.[‡] Professor of Pediatrics and of Preventive Medicine and Biostatistics University of Toronto Head, Division of General Pediatrics Hospital for Sick Children Toronto, Ontario	Screening for phenylketonuria; Screening for cystic fibrosis; Well-baby care in the first 2 years of life; Screening children for lead exposure in Canada; Screening for childhood obesity; Dipstick proteinuria screening of asymptomatic adults to prevent progressive renal disease; Prevention of unintended pregnancy and sexually transmitted diseases in adolescents; Prevention of obesity in adults
Paul S. Frame, M.D.[†] Clinical Associate Professor Department of Family Medicine and Department of Community and Preventive Medicine University of Rochester School of Medicine and Dentistry Rochester, New York, U.S.	Nutritional counselling for undesirable dietary patterns and screening for protein/calorie malnutrition disorders in adults; Screening for testicular cancer
Dennis G. Fryback, Ph.D.[†] Department of Preventive Medicine University of Wisconsin-Madison Madison, Wisconsin, U.S.	Member, U.S. Preventive Services Task Force.
Ronald Gold, M.D., M.P.H. Professor of Pediatrics and Microbiology University of Toronto Toronto, Ontario	Childhood immunizations
Richard B. Goldbloom, O.C., M.D., F.R.C.P.C.[‡] **Editor** Professor Department of Pediatrics Dalhousie University Halifax, Nova Scotia	Introduction; Prophylaxis for gonococcal and chlamydial ophthalmia neonatorum; Screening for hemoglobinopathies in Canada; Screening for idiopathic adolescent scoliosis

Appendix C – *Cont'd*

Author	Chapter or Contribution
David A. Grimes, M.D.[†] Professor and Vice-Chairman Department of Obstetrics, Gynecology and Reproductive Sciences University of California at San Francisco (UCSF) San Francisco, California, U.S	Member, U.S. Preventive Services Task Force
Jean L. Haggerty, M.Sc. Coordinator Canadian Task Force on the Periodic Health Examination, 1987-89 Faculty Lecturer McGill University Montreal, Quebec	Early detection and counselling of problem drinking
Amid I. Ismail, B.D.S., M.P.H., Dr.P.H. Associate Professor and Chair Department of Pediatric and Community Dentistry Dalhousie University Halifax, Nova Scotia	Prevention of dental caries; Prevention of periodontal disease
J. Kenneth Johnson, M.D. At time of writing: Research Associate Department of Preventive Medicine and Biostatistics University of Toronto Toronto, Ontario	Screening for human papillomavirus
Douglas B. Kamerow, M.D., M.P.H. Director, Clinical Preventive Services Staff Office of Disease Prevention and Health Promotion Clinical Associate Professor Department of Community and Family Medicine Georgetown University Washington, D.C., U.S.	Staff Director, U.S. Preventive Services Task Force and, Managing Editor, *Guide to Clinical Preventive Services*

Author	Chapter or Contribution
Murray Krahn, M.D., M.Sc. Assistant Professor Departments of Medicine and Clinical Biochemistry University of Toronto Toronto, Ontario	Hepatitis B immunization
Robert S. Lawrence, M.D.[†] Director, Health Sciences The Rockefeller Foundation New York, New York, U.S.	Nutritional counselling for undesirable dietary patterns and screening for protein/calorie malnutrition disorders in adults
Donald W. Lewis, D.D.S., D.D.P.H., M.Sc.D., F.R.C.D.C. Professor of Community Dentistry Faculty of Dentistry University of Toronto Toronto, Ontario	Prevention of dental caries; Prevention of periodontal disease
Ellen L. Lipman, M.D., F.R.C.P.C. Assistant Professor Department of Psychiatry McMaster University Hamilton, Ontario	Disadvantaged children
Alexander G. Logan, M.D., F.R.C.P.C.[‡] Professor of Medicine Department of Medicine University of Toronto Toronto, Ontario	Methodology; Screening for hypertension in young and middle-aged adults; Lowering the blood total cholesterol level to prevent coronary heart disease; Hypertension in the elderly: case-finding and treatment to prevent vascular disease
Sarvesh Logsetty, M.D. Division of General Surgery Department of Surgery Hospital for Sick Children Toronto, Ontario	Screening for bladder cancer

Author	Chapter or Contribution
Ariane Mackey, M.D., F.R.C.P.C. Fellow (Cerebro-Vascular) Division of Neurology Department of Medicine Montreal General Hospital Montreal, Quebec	Asymptomatic carotid disease
Harriet L. MacMillan, M.D., F.R.C.P.C. Assistant Professor Departments of Pediatrics and of Psychiatry McMaster University Hamilton, Ontario	Primary prevention of child maltreatment
James H. MacMillan, M.Sc. Biostatistician Glaxo Canada Inc. Mississauga, Ontario	Primary prevention of child maltreatment

Anne Martell, M.A., C.M.C.
Martell Consulting Services Ltd.
Halifax, Nova Scotia
	Childhood immunizations;
	Prevention of unintended pregnancy and
	  sexually transmitted diseases in
	  adolescents

Robin S. McLeod, M.D., F.R.C.S.C., F.A.C.S. Associate Professor Department of Surgery University of Toronto Toronto, Ontario	Screening for colorectal cancer

Jane E. McNamee, M.A.
Research Associate
Department of Psychiatry
Chedoke-McMaster Hospitals and
  Centre for Studies of Children at Risk
Chedoke-McMaster Hospitals and
  McMaster University
Hamilton, Ontario
	Prevention of suicide;
	Children of alcoholics

Author	Chapter or Contribution
Susan E. Moner, M.D. At time of writing: Research Associate Department of Preventive Medicine and Biostatistics University of Toronto Toronto, Ontario	Smoking and pregnancy

Brenda J. Morrison, Ph.D.[‡]
Professor
Department of Health Care and
  Epidemiology
University of British Columbia
Vancouver, British Columbia
	Interventions other than smoking
	  cessation to prevent lung cancer;
	Screening for breast cancer;
	Prevention of pancreatic cancer;
	Screening for cervical cancer

Ryuta Nagai, M.D., F.R.C.P.C.
At time of writing:
Research Associate
Department of Preventive Medicine and
  Biostatistics
University of Toronto
Toronto, Ontario
	Dipstick proteinuria screening of
	  asymptomatic adults to prevent
	  progressive renal disease

Lindsay E. Nicolle, M.D.
Associate Professor
Departments of Medicine and of
  Medical Microbiology
University of Manitoba
Winnipeg, Manitoba
	Screening for asymptomatic bacteriuria
	  in pregnancy;
	Screening for asymptomatic bacteriuria
	  in the elderly

David R. (Dan) Offord, M.D.[‡]
Professor
Department of Psychiatry
McMaster University
Hamilton, Ontario
	Primary prevention of fetal alcohol
	  syndrome;
	Primary prevention of child
	  maltreatment;
	Disadvantaged children;
	Prevention of suicide;
	Children of alcoholics

Appendix C – *Cont'd*

Author	Chapter or Contribution
Christopher Patterson, M.D., F.R.C.P.C.[‡] Professor and Head Division of Geriatric Medicine Department of Medicine McMaster University Hamilton, Ontario	Nutritional counselling for undesirable dietary patterns and screening for protein/calorie malnutrition disorders in adults; Screening for abdominal aortic aneurysm; Screening for cognitive impairment in the elderly; Secondary prevention of elder abuse; Screening for visual impairment in the elderly; Hypertension in the elderly: case-finding and treatment to prevent vascular disease; Prevention of hearing impairment and disability in the elderly
Cindy Quinton Gladstone, M.H.Sc., M.D., F.R.C.P.C. At time of writing: Research Associate Department of Preventive Medicine and Biostatistics University of Toronto Toronto, Ontario	Screening for ovarian cancer
Patricia Randel, M.Sc. Research Associate, Canadian Task Force on the Periodic Health Examination Department of Pediatrics Dalhousie University Halifax, Nova Scotia	Screening children for lead exposure in Canada
M. Carrington Reid, M.D. Fellow Robert Wood Johnson Clinical Scholar Yale School of Medicine New Haven, Connecticut, U.S.	Screening for diabetes mellitus in the non-pregnant adult

Author	Chapter or Contribution
Carl Rosati, M.D., F.R.C.S.C. General Surgery North York Branson Hospital North York, Ontario	Prevention of oral cancer
Michael B.H. Smith, M.B., B.Ch., C.C.F.P., F.R.C.P.C. Lecturer in Pediatrics Dalhousie University Halifax, Nova Scotia	Screening for urinary infection in asymptomatic infants and children
Michael J. Solomon, M.B., B.C.H., B.A.O.(Hons), F.R.A.C.S. Director of Research University of Sydney Department of Colorectal Surgery Royal Prince Alfred Hospital Newtown, NSW, Australia	Screening for colorectal cancer
Harold C. Sox, Jr., M.D.[†] Chairman U.S. Preventive Services Task Force Joseph M. Huber Professor and Chairman Department of Medicine Dartmouth-Hitchcock Medical Center Lebanon, New Hampshire, U.S.	Screening for diabetes mellitus in the non-pregnant adult
Sylvie Stachenko, M.D., M.Sc., F.C.F.P. Director Preventive Health Services Division Health Programs and Services Branch Health Canada Ottawa, Ontario	Preventive guidelines: their role in clinical prevention and health promotion
Michael Tarrant, M.D., C.C.F.P., F.C.F.P. Associate Professor Department of Family Medicine University of Calgary Calgary, Alberta	Prevention of influenza

Appendix C – *Cont'd*

Author	Chapter or Contribution
Mark C. Taylor, M.D., F.R.C.S.C. Clinical Fellow The Toronto Hospital Toronto, Ontario	Prevention of tobacco-caused disease

Robert B. Wallace, M.D.[†]
Professor and Head
Department of Preventive Medicine and
    Environmental Health
University of Iowa College of Medicine
Iowa City, Iowa, U.S.
	Member, U.S. Preventive Services Task
	    Force

**Sharon L. Walmsley, M.D.,
F.R.C.P.C.**
Assistant Professor
Department of Medicine and
    Microbiology
University of Toronto
Toronto, Ontario
	Screening and isoniazid prophylactic
	    therapy for tuberculosis

**Elaine E. L. Wang, M.D., C.M.,
F.R.C.P.C.**[‡]
Associate Professor
Department of Pediatrics and of
    Preventive Medicine and Biostatistics
Faculty of Medicine
University of Toronto
Toronto, Ontario
	Methodology;
	Prevention of neonatal herpes simplex;
	Breast feeding;
	Administration of pneumococcal vaccine;
	Dipstick proteinuria screening of
	    asymptomatic adults in the prevention
	    of progressive renal disease;
	Screening for HIV antibody;
	Prevention of spread of gonorrhea

A. Eugene Washington, M.D., M.Sc.[†] Director Medical Effectiveness Research Center University of California School of Medicine San Francisco, California, U.S.	Prevention of preeclampsia

Appendix C – *Concl'd*

Author	Chapter or Contribution
Modena E.H. Wilson, M.D., M.P.H.[†] Associate Professor Department of Pediatrics Johns Hopkins University Baltimore, Maryland, U.S.	Screening for phenylketonuria; Screening for hemoglobinopathies in Canada
Steven H. Woolf, M.D., M.P.H. Science Advisor U.S. Preventive Services Task Force Washington, D.C., U.S.A. Assistant Clinical Professor Department of Family Practice Medical College of Virginia Richmond, Virginia, U.S.	Methodology; Routine iron supplementation during pregnancy; The use of home uterine activity monitoring to prevent preterm birth; Screening for idiopathic adolescent scoliosis; Nutritional counselling for undesirable dietary patterns and screening for protein/calorie malnutrition disorders in adults

Index

Intrauterine device (IUD)   543-544,
    552-553
Intrauterine growth retardation (IUGR)   4,
    7, 86, 136
IOP   933, 935-936
IPV   375-376
IQ, maternal   361
IQ   182, 190-191, 274, 279, 291, 361-362,
    472-473
Iron deficiency (IDA)   64-66, 68-70,
    217-218, 235, 244-247, 249-251, 254,
    262, 359, 368, 543, 586, 588
Iron deficiency anemia in infants   244-255
Iron-fortified formula or cereal   248-249,
    251, 254
Iron supplementation, in pregnancy   64-66,
    68-70, 72
IRT   197-198, 201
Ischemic attacks, transient (TIAs)   692,
    697, 703
Isoniazid chemoprophylactic therapy
    (INH)   754, 757-763, 765
IUAT   759-760
IUD   543-544, 552-553
IUGR   4, 7, 86, 136

Jansky Screening Index (JSI)   291, 295
JSI   291, 295

Labelling   19, 213, 218, 223, 292-293, 322,
    326, 478-479, 591, 606, 652, 661, 712,
    717, 756, 771, 776, 839, 847, 851,
    902, 905, 909
Laboratory Center for Disease Control
    (LCDC)   130, 725
Lateral Electrical Surface Stimulation
    (LESS)   348-349, 354
LDL cholesterol   335, 650-654, 658-661,
    666, 669
Lead exposure (BPb)   268-281, 287-288,
    360, 368
Lead exposure, children in Canada,
    screening for   268-288
Lead mobilization tests (LMT)   277
LESS   348-349, 354
Leukocyte esterase/nitrite dipstick
    (LE)   101, 222, 791, 968, 973
Lipid-lowering drugs   653, 659-660, 669
Liver disease   398-399
Low birth weight (LBW)   26-27, 29-30, 32,
    36, 38-46, 50, 66-67, 69, 101, 103,
    160, 245, 255, 358-359, 364, 541, 586,
    735
Low-calorie diets (LCD)   576
Low-density lipoprotein (LDL)   650

Lung cancer   501, 503, 586, 592, 780-783,
    786, 863, 870

Macrosomia   16-19, 21, 23
McCarthy Screening Test   291
Macular degeneration, age-related
    (ARMD)   932-933, 935-936, 938, 942
Malignant melanoma (MM)   420, 590, 637,
    755-756, 761, 803, 814, 850-857, 859
Malnutrition, protein/calorie (PCM)   586,
    588, 590, 599
Malnutrition   197, 280, 359, 364, 400, 586,
    588-590, 595, 599, 765
MAMC   590
Mammography   788-791, 795
Mantoux tuberculin test   755, 765
MAST   54, 474, 489-491, 494
Maternal serum alpha-fetoprotein (MSAFP)
    screening   74-75, 77-79, 81
MCV   208-209, 218
Mean arterial pressure (MAP)   138
Mean corpuscular volume (MCV)   208-209
Measles-mumps-rubella (MMR)
    vaccine   128, 130, 372, 376-379,
    381-384
Measles   130, 258, 372, 376-379, 381, 384
Medical impairment, elderly   920
Medical impairment, motor vehicle accident
    injuries   515, 517-518, 524
Melanoma, malignant (MM)   850-855
Mental development   57, 74, 183, 194,
    246, 250, 263, 266, 357, 362, 459, 473
Mental retardation   52, 57, 84, 180,
    182-183, 190, 260, 263, 266, 359, 362,
    471
Mental status instruments   903, 906, 909
Mental Status Questionnaire, Short
    Portable (SPMSQ)   903, 909
Michigan Alcoholism Screening Test
    (MAST)   54, 489-491, 494
Micopurulent cervicitis (MPC)   732, 737
Microcytosis   208, 214, 217-218
Microscopy   222-223, 836
Midarm muscle circumference
    (MAMC)   590
Milk, whole cow's (WCM)   245
Mini Mental State examination
    (MMS)   903, 909
Minneapolis Preschool Screening
    Instrument   291
MM   420, 590, 637, 755-756, 761, 803,
    814, 850-857, 859
MMR (vaccine)   128, 130, 372, 377-379,
    381-384
MMS   903, 909